Human Disease and Pathology

Neighbors | Tannehill-Jones

CENGAGE Learning®

Australia • Brazil • Japan • Korea • Mexico • Singapore • Spain • United Kingdom • United States

CENGAGE Learning

Human Disease and Pathology

Senior Project Development Manager:
Linda deStefano

Market Development Manager:
Heather Kramer

Senior Production/Manufacturing Manager:
Donna M. Brown

Production Editorial Manager:
Kim Fry

Sr. Rights Acquisition Account Manager:
Todd Osborne

Human Diseases, 3rd Edition
Neighbors | Tannehill-Jones

For product information and technology assistance, contact us at
Cengage Learning Customer & Sales Support, 1-800-354-9706
For permission to use material from this text or product,
submit all requests online at **cengage.com/permissions**
Further permissions questions can be emailed to
permissionrequest@cengage.com

This book contains select works from existing Cengage Learning resources and was produced by Cengage Learning Custom Solutions for collegiate use. As such, those adopting and/or contributing to this work are responsible for editorial content accuracy, continuity and completeness.

ISBN-13: 978-1-285-55487-7

ISBN-10: 1-285-55487-6

Cengage Learning
5191 Natorp Boulevard
Mason, Ohio 45040
USA

Cengage Learning is a leading provider of customized learning solutions with office locations around the globe, including Singapore, the United Kingdom, Australia, Mexico, Brazil, and Japan. Locate your local office at:
international.cengage.com/region.

Cengage Learning products are represented in Canada by Nelson Education, Ltd.
For your lifelong learning solutions, visit **www.cengage.com/custom.**
Visit our corporate website at **www.cengage.com.**

Printed in the United States of America

CHAPTER 4

Contents

CHAPTER 18

Integumentary System Diseases and Disorders 395

List of Tables

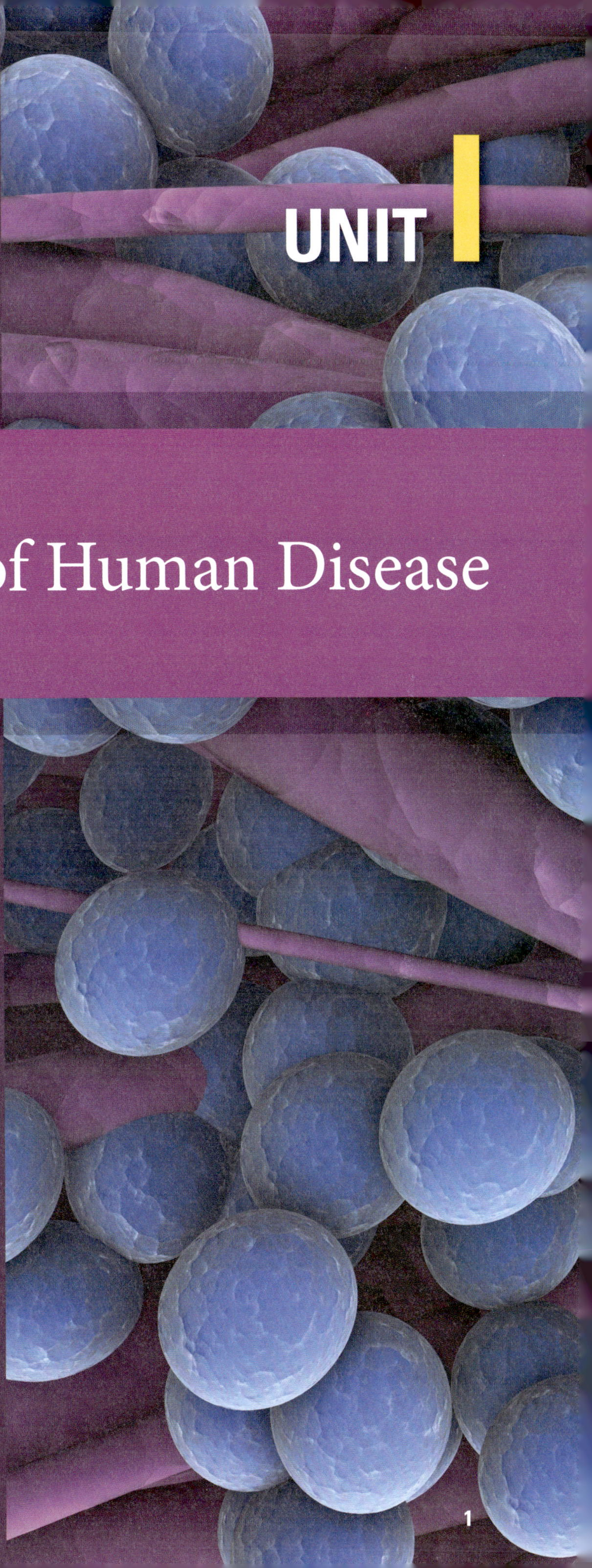

UNIT I

Concepts of Human Disease

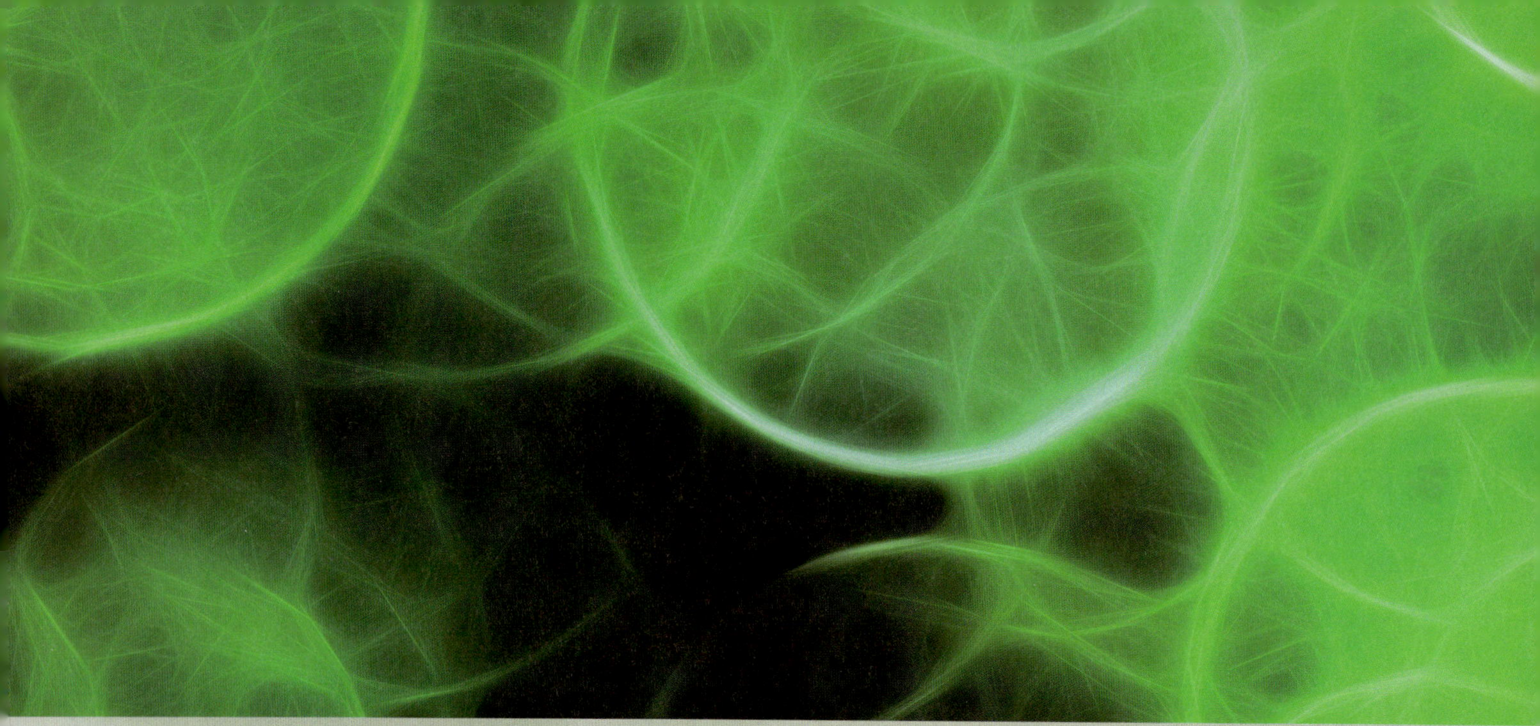

OUTLINE

- Disease, Disorder, and Syndrome
  - *Disease*
  - *Disorder*
  - *Syndrome*
- Pathology
- Pathogenesis
- Etiology
- Predisposing Factors
  - *Age*
  - *Sex*
  - *Environment*
  - *Lifestyle*
  - *Heredity*
- Diagnosis
- Prognosis
  - *Acute Disease*
  - *Chronic Disease*
  - *Complication*
  - *Mortality Rate*
  - *Survival Rate*
- Treatment
- Medical Ethics
- Summary
- Review Questions
- Case Studies
- Bibliography

KEY TERMS

Acute (p. 5)
Auscultation (p. 8)
Chronic (p. 5)
Complication (p. 9)
Diagnosis (p. 7)
Disease (p. 4)
Disorder (p. 4)
Etiology (p. 6)
Exacerbation (p. 9)
Fatal (p. 9)
Holistic medicine (p. 9)
Homeostasis (p. 4)
Iatrogenic (p. 6)
Idiopathic (p. 6)
Lethal (p. 9)
Mortality (p. 9)
Nosocomial (p. 6)
Palliative (p. 10)
Palpation (p. 8)
Pathogenesis (p. 5)
Pathogens (p. 4)
Pathologic (p. 4)
Pathologist (p. 4)
Pathology (p. 4)
Percussion (p. 8)
Predisposing factors (p. 7)
Prevalent (p. 7)
Preventive (p. 10)
Prognosis (p. 8)
Remission (p. 9)
Signs (p. 8)
Symptoms (p. 8)
Syndrome (p. 4)

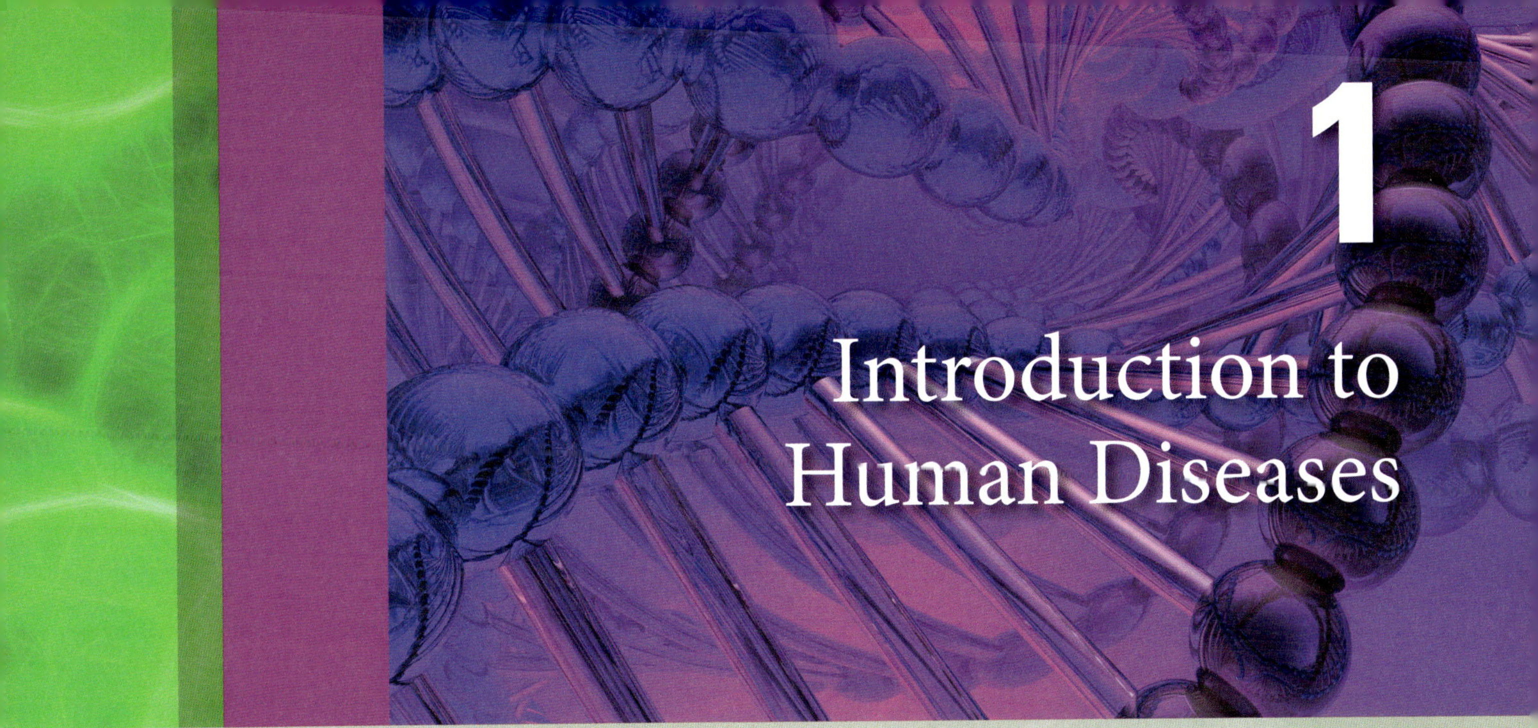

1 Introduction to Human Diseases

LEARNING OBJECTIVES

Upon completion of the chapter, the learner should be able to:

1. Define basic terminology used in the study of human diseases.
2. Discuss the pathogenesis of disease.
3. Describe the Standard Precaution guidelines for disease prevention.
4. Identify the predisposing factors to human diseases.
5. Explain the difference between diagnosis and prognosis of a disease.
6. Describe some common tests used to diagnose disease states.

OVERVIEW

The study of human diseases is important for understanding a variety of other topics in the health care field. Diseases that affect humans can range from mild to severe and can be acute (short term) or chronic (long term). Some diseases affect only one part of the body or a particular body system, whereas others affect several parts of the body or body systems at the same time. Many factors influence the body's ability to stay healthy or predispose the body to a disease process. Some of these factors are controllable, but some are strictly related to heredity. Diseases can be diagnosed by professional health care providers using a variety of techniques and tests. ■

DISEASE, DISORDER, AND SYNDROME

In the study of human disease, several terms used are similar and often used interchangeably but might not have identical definitions.

Disease

Disease may be defined in several ways. It may be called a change in structure or function that is considered to be abnormal within the body, or it may be defined as any change from normal. It usually refers to a condition in which symptoms occur and a pathological state is present such as in pneumonia or leukemia. Both of these definitions have one underlying concept: the alteration of **homeostasis** (HOME-ee-oh-STAY-sis).

Homeostasis is the state of sameness or normalcy the body strives to maintain. The body is remarkable in its ability to maintain homeostasis, but when this homeostasis is no longer maintained, the body is diseased or "not at ease."

Disorder

Disorder is defined as a derangement or abnormality of function. The term *disorder* can also refer to a pathological condition of the body or mind but more commonly is used to refer to a problem such as a vitamin deficiency (nutritional disorder). It is also used to refer to structural problems such as a malformation of a joint (bone disorder) or a condition in which the term *disease* does not seem to apply, such as dysphagia (swallowing disorder). Because *disease* and *disorder* are so closely related, they are often used synonymously.

Syndrome

Syndrome (SIN-drome) refers to a group of symptoms, which might be caused by a specific disease but might also be caused by several interrelated problems. Examples include Tourette's syndrome, Down syndrome, and acquired immunodeficiency syndrome (AIDS), which are discussed later in the text.

PATHOLOGY

Pathology (pah-THOL-oh-jee) can be broadly defined as the study of disease (patho = disease; ology = study). A **pathologist** (pah-THOL-oh-jist) is one who studies disease. Even a student studying diseases might be considered a pathologist, using the strict definition of the word.

There are many types of pathologists because there are numerous ways to study disease. One of the more commonly known pathologists is the surgical pathologist, who inspects surgical tissue or biopsies for evidence of disease (Figure 1–1). The medical examiner or coroner can be a pathologist who studies human tissue to determine the cause of death and provide evidence of criminal involvement in a death. Other types of pathologists are outlined in Table 1–1.

The prefix *patho-* can be used in a variety of ways to describe disease processes or the disease itself. Microorganisms or agents that cause disease are called **pathogens** (PATH-oh-jens). These include bacteria, viruses, fungi, protozoans, and helminths (worms). All are pathogens that cause a pathogenic reaction. Fractures that are caused by a disease process that weakens the bone, such as osteoporosis, would be called **pathologic** (path-oh-LODGE-ick) fractures.

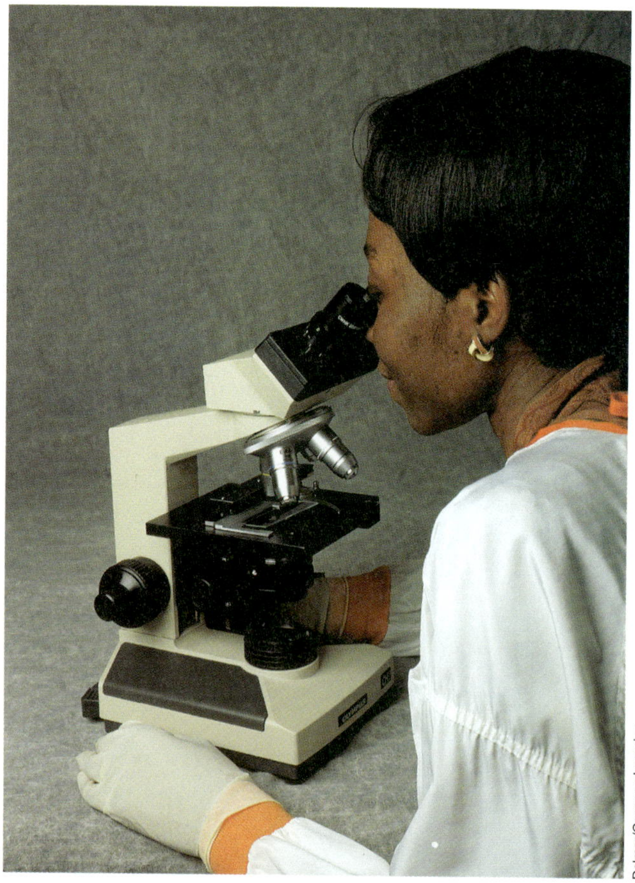

FIGURE 1–1 Pathologist looking through a microscope.

TABLE 1–1 Types of Pathologists

Pathologist	Role or Subject
Experimental	Research
Academic	Teaching
Anatomic	Clinical examinations
Autopsy	Postmortem
Surgical	Biopsies
Clinical	Laboratory examinations
Hematology	Blood
Immunology	Antigen/antibodies
Microbiology	Microorganisms

PATHOGENESIS

The **pathogenesis** (PATH-oh-JEN-ah-sis; patho = disease; genesis = arising) is a description of how a particular disease progresses. Many of us are familiar with the pathogenesis of the common cold.

A cold begins with an inoculation of the cold virus. This can occur following a simple handshake with someone who has a cold. Afterward, the target person might rub his or her eyes or nose, allowing entry of the virus into the body. After the inoculation period comes incubation time. During this period, the virus multiplies, and the target person begins to have symptoms such as a runny nose and itchy eyes. The pathogenesis of the cold then moves into full-blown illness, usually followed by recovery and return to the previous state of health.

The pathogenesis of a disease can be explained in terms of time. An **acute** (a-CUTE) disease is short term and usually has a sudden onset. If the disease lasts for an extended period of time or the healing process is progressing slowly, it is classified as a **chronic** (KRON-ick) condition. See Table 1–2 for examples of acute and chronic diseases.

TABLE 1–2 Examples of Acute and Chronic Diseases

Acute	Chronic
Upper respiratory infections	Arthritis
Lacerations	Hypertension
Middle ear infections	Diabetes mellitus
Gastroenteritis	Low back pain
Pneumonia	Heart disease
Fractures	Asthma

HEALTHY HIGHLIGHT

Hand-Washing Technique

To prevent the spread of disease between oneself and others, good and frequent hand washing is the best prevention. Follow these good hand-washing steps.

- Use an antimicrobial soap when possible. Have paper towels available to dry hands and to turn off the water.
- Adjust water temperature and force. Wet hands and wrists and use a fingernail cleaner (if available) to clean under the nails gently on both hands while holding hands under the running water.
- Apply a small amount of liquid soap. Work into a lather on wrists and hands. Briskly rub hands together for 15 seconds being sure to wash areas between fingers and around each wrist.
- Rinse well from wrists to fingertips. Be careful not to touch the sides of the basin or let the water run down the arm off the elbow.
- Dry each hand from fingertips to wrist using a paper towel. When finished, turn off the water, using a paper towel as a barrier between the hands and the faucet.
- Discard soiled towels in the trash basket.

Source: Centers for Disease Control and Prevention (CDC) (2002).

ETIOLOGY

The **etiology** (EE-tee-OL-oh-jee) of a disease means the study of cause. The term *etiology* is commonly used to mean simply "the cause." One might say that the cause is unknown or "of unknown etiology." The cause or etiology of pneumonia can be a virus or a bacterium. The etiology of athlete's foot is a fungus named tinea pedis.

Another term used to mean "the cause is unknown" is **idiopathic** (ID-ee-oh-PATH-ick). If an individual is diagnosed as having idiopathic gastric pain, it means the cause of the pain in the stomach is unknown.

Other terms related to cause of disease are **iatrogenic** (eye-AT-roh-JEN-ick) and **nosocomial** (NOS-oh-KOH-me-al). Iatrogenic (iatro = medicine, physician; genic = arising from) means that the problem arose from a prescribed treatment. An example of an iatrogenic problem is the development of anemia in a patient undergoing chemotherapy treatments for cancer.

Nosocomial is a closely related term; it implies that the disease was acquired from a hospital environment. An example would be a postoperative patient developing an incisional staphylococcal infection. The best way to prevent nosocomial infections is through the practice of good hand washing. A good hand-washing technique is described in the preceding Healthy Highlight.

HEALTHY HIGHLIGHT

Standard Precautions

Using standard precautions is recommended by the Centers for Disease Control and Prevention for the care of all patients or when administering first aid to anyone. These standards also include respiratory hygiene and cough etiquette, safe injection techniques, and wearing masks for spinal insertions.

- **Hand washing** Wash hands after touching blood, body fluids, or both, even if gloves are worn; use an antimicrobial soap.
- **Respiratory etiquette** Cover mouth, nose, or both with a tissue when coughing and dispose of used tissue immediately. Wear mask if possible. Maintain distance from others, ideally greater than three feet. Wash hands after contact with secretions.
- **Gloves** Wear gloves when touching blood, body fluids, and contaminated items; change gloves after patient contact or contact with contaminated items; wash hands before and after.
- **Eye wear, mask, and face shield** Wear protection for the eyes, mouth, and face when performing procedures when a risk of splashing or spraying of blood or body secretions exists. This includes insertion of catheters or injection of material into spinal or epidural spaces. A mask should also be worn if the caregiver has a respiratory infection but cannot avoid direct patient contact.
- **Gown** Wear a waterproof gown to protect the clothing from splashing or spraying blood or body fluids.
- **Equipment** Wear gloves when handling equipment contaminated with blood or body fluids; clean equipment appropriately after use; discard disposable equipment in proper containers.
- **Environment control** Follow proper procedures for cleaning and disinfecting the patient's environment after completion of a procedure.
- **Linen** Use proper procedure for disposing of linen contaminated with blood or body fluids.
- **Blood-borne pathogens** Do not recap needles; dispose of used needles and other sharp instruments in proper containers; use a mouthpiece for resuscitation; keep a mouthpiece available in areas where there is likelihood of need.

PREDISPOSING FACTORS

Predisposing factors, also known as risk factors, make a person more susceptible to disease. Predisposing factors are not the cause of the disease, and people with predisposing factors do not always develop the disease. These factors include age, sex, environment, lifestyle, and heredity. Some risk factors are controllable, such as lifestyle behaviors, whereas others, such as age, are not.

Age

From the beginning of life until death, our risk of disease follows our age. Newborns are at risk of disease because their immune systems are not fully developed. On the other hand, older persons are at risk because their immune systems are degenerating or wearing out. Girls in their early teens and women over the age of thirty are at high risk for a difficult or problem pregnancy. The older we become, the higher the risk for diseases such as cancer, heart disease, stroke, senile dementia, and Alzheimer's.

Sex

Some diseases are more **prevalent** (occurring more often) in one gender or the other. Men are more at risk for diseases such as lung cancer, gout, and parkinsonism. Other disorders or diseases occur more often in women including osteoporosis, rheumatoid arthritis, and breast cancer.

Environment

Air and water pollution can lead to respiratory and gastrointestinal disease. Poor sanitation, excessive noise, and stress are also environmental risk factors. Occupational diseases such as lung disease are high among miners and persons working in areas where there are increased amounts of dust or other particles in the air.

Farmers are considered to be at higher risk for diseases because of their increased exposure to dust, pesticides, and other pollutants. Farmers are also at higher risk for trauma injuries due to safety problems around farm machinery. People living in remote, rural areas do not have health care availability comparable to those living in urban areas. This increases their risk for chronic illnesses.

Lifestyle

Lifestyle factors fall into a category over which the individual has some control. Choosing to improve health behaviors in these areas could lead to a reduction in risk and thus a possibility of avoiding the occurrence of the disease. Such factors include smoking, drinking alcohol, poor nutrition (excessive fat, salt, and sugar and not enough fruits, vegetables, and fiber), lack of exercise, and stress.

Practicing health behaviors to prevent contamination, and thus disease, is also an important lifestyle behavior. The Centers for Disease Control and Prevention recommend the use of standard precautions when caring for any individual when there is a chance of being contaminated with blood or body fluids (see Healthy Highlight on page 6). This is an important measure to prevent transmission of any disease that can be passed between humans in blood or body fluids, such as hepatitis, E. coli infections, and AIDS.

Heredity

Although one cannot change genetic makeup, being aware of hereditary risk factors might encourage the individual to change lifestyle behaviors to reduce the risk of disease. For example, coronary heart disease has been shown to have a high familial tendency. Persons with this family inheritance are compounding their chances if they smoke, have poor nutritional intake, and do not exercise routinely.

Breast cancer and cervical cancer also have familial tendencies. Women with family members who have been diagnosed with breast cancer or cervical cancer are at a higher risk for developing these diseases. These women should be screened routinely for evidence of cancer and should complete monthly breast self-exams. With this knowledge about hereditary factors, individuals can choose to decrease their overall risk by improving their lifestyle health behaviors.

DIAGNOSIS

Diagnosis (DIE-ag-KNOW-sis) is the identification or naming of a disease. When an individual seeks medical attention, it is the duty of the physician to determine a diagnosis of the problem. A diagnosis is made after a methodical study by the physician,

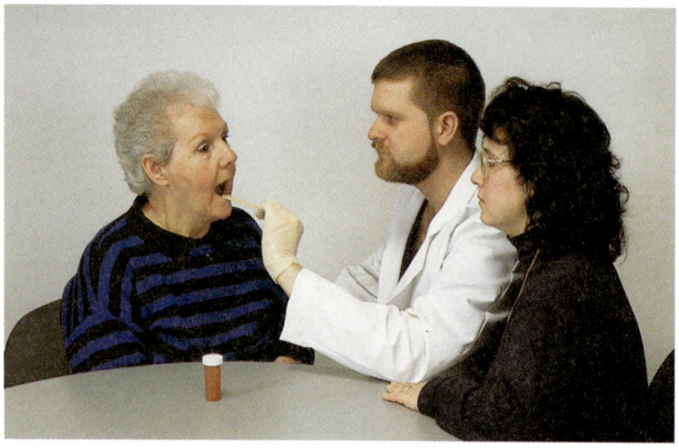

FIGURE 1–2 Physician checking a patient.

using data collected from a medical history, physical examination, and diagnostic tests (Figure 1–2).

A medical history is a systems review that might include such information as previous illnesses, family illness, predisposing factors, medication allergies, current illnesses, and current **symptoms** (SIMP-tums, what patients report as their problem or problems). Examples of symptoms might include stomach pain, headache, and nausea.

The physician proceeds with a head-to-toe physical examination of the patient, looking for signs of the disease. **Signs** differ from symptoms in that signs are observable or measurable. Signs are what the physician sees or measures. Examples of signs could include vomiting, elevated blood pressure, and elevated temperature.

In some cases, a patient's concern might be considered as both a symptom and a sign. Some references call this an objective or observable symptom, whereas others state that it is also a sign. An example would be a patient complaining of a runny nose. The runny nose is the patient's symptom and, because it is observable to the physician, it is also a sign.

During the physical examination, the physician might use other skills such as **auscultation** (AWS-kul-TAY-shun, using a stethoscope to listen to body cavities), **palpation** (pal-PAY-shun, feeling lightly or pressing firmly on internal organs or structures), and **percussion** (per-KUSH-un; tapping over various body areas to produce a vibrating sound). All the results are compared to a normal standard to identify problems.

Diagnostic tests and procedures to assist in determining a diagnosis are numerous. The routine or most common include urinalysis, complete blood count (CBC), chest x-ray (CXR), and electrocardiography (EKG or ECG). See Table 1–3 for examples of common diagnostic tests and procedures.

PROGNOSIS

Prognosis (prawg-KNOW-sis) is the predicted or expected outcome of the disease. For example, the prognosis of the common cold would be that the individual should feel better in 7 to 10 days.

Acute Disease

The duration of the disease can be described as acute in nature. An acute disease is one that usually has a sudden onset and lasts a short amount of time (days

TABLE 1–3 Examples of Common Diagnostic Tests and Procedures

Test	Description
Complete blood count (CBC)	An examination of blood for cell counts and abnormalities
Urinalysis (UA)	An examination of urine for abnormalities
Chest x-ray (CXR)	X-ray examination of the chest cavity
Electrocardiography (ECG or EKG)	A procedure for recording the electrical activity of the heart
Blood glucose	A test of the blood to determine its glucose or sugar levels
Computerized axial tomography (CT or CAT)	A special X-ray examination showing detailed images of body structures and organs
Serum electrolytes	An examination of blood serum to determine the levels of the common electrolytes (sodium, potassium, and chloride)

or weeks). Most acute diseases are related to the respiratory system. Again, the common cold would be a good example.

Chronic Disease

If the disease persists for a long time, it is considered to be chronic. Chronic diseases might begin insidiously (slowly and without symptoms) and last for the entire life of the individual. As one ages, the occurrence of chronic disease increases. One of the most common chronic diseases is hypertension, or high blood pressure.

Chronic diseases often go through periods of **remission** and **exacerbation** (ex-AS-er-BAY-shun). Remission refers to a time when symptoms are diminished or temporarily resolved. Exacerbation refers to a time when symptoms flare up or become worse. Leukemia is a disease that progresses through periods of remission and exacerbation. Both acute and chronic diseases can range from mild to life threatening.

Complication

The prognosis might be altered or changed at times if the individual develops a **complication**. A complication is the onset of a second disease or disorder in an individual who is already affected with a disease. An individual with a fractured arm might have a prognosis of the arm healing in 6 to 8 weeks. If the individual suffers the complication of bone infection, the prognosis maight change drastically.

Mortality Rate

Diseases commonly leading to the death of an individual have a high **mortality** rate. Mortality is defined as the quality of being mortal, that is, destined to die. The mortality rate of a disease is related to the number of people who die with the disease in a certain amount of time. Other terms the medical community uses to refer to a deadly disease include **fatal** and **lethal**.

Survival Rate

A physician's prognosis can also consider survival rate. Survival rate is the percentage of people with a particular disease who live for a set period of time. For example, the 2-year survival rate of individuals with lung cancer would be the percentage of people alive 2 years after diagnosis.

TREATMENT

After the diagnosis is established, the physician will work with the individual to explain or outline a plan of care. The physician might offer treatment options to the individual with expected outcomes or prognoses. The individual's entire being should be taken into consideration. The concept of considering the whole person rather than just the physical being is called **holistic medicine**.

From a holistic viewpoint, there is interaction between the spiritual, cognitive, social, physical, and emotional being. These areas do not work independently, but have a dynamic interaction (Figure 1–3).

Treatment interventions might include (1) medications, (2) surgery, (3) exercise, (4) nutritional modifications, (5) physical therapy, and (6) education. Individuals and family members should be educated and involved in the treatment plan. Failure to involve the individual and family can decrease compliance and lead to failure of the plan.

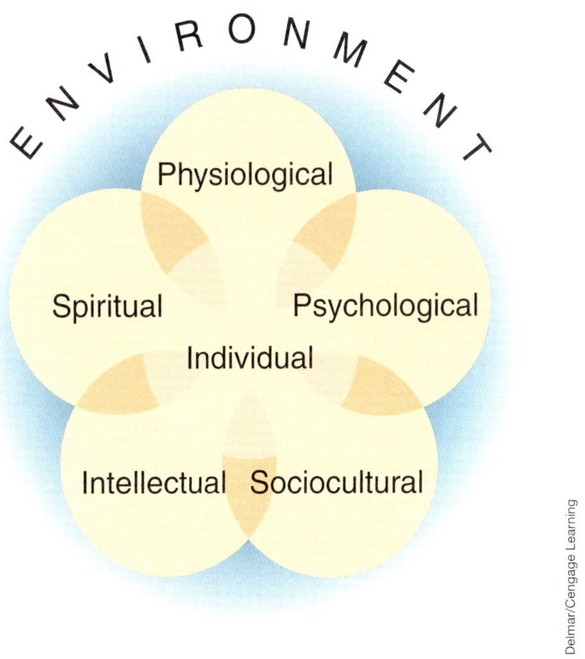

FIGURE 1–3 Holistic medicine.

After the treatment plan is implemented, the physician will follow up with the individual to determine effectiveness. The individual and physician should work together to modify the plan if it is found to be ineffective. Implementation of the plan usually requires an entire health care team. The team can include nurses, a physical therapist, a social worker, clergy, and other health care professionals as needed.

The best treatment option is a **preventive** plan. In preventive treatment, care is given to prevent disease. Examples of preventive care are breast mammograms to screen for breast cancer, blood pressure screening for hypertension, routine dental care to prevent dental caries, and Hemoccult stool test to screen for colon cancer.

Other treatment plans might include **palliative** (PAL-ee-uh-tiv) treatment. Palliative treatment is aimed at preventing pain and discomfort but does not seek to cure the disease. Treatment for end-term cancer and other serious chronic conditions can be palliative.

Decisions concerning treatment plans can be very difficult for the patient, the patient's family, and the health care team. This is especially true when those decisions involve palliative treatment and end-of-life issues. During these times, professionals often seek assistance in decision making by using their knowledge of medical ethics.

MEDICAL ETHICS

Webster's dictionary defines ethics as "the study of standards of conduct and moral judgment." More simply put, ethics deals with the "rightness and wrongness" or "goodness and badness" of human actions. Ethics covers many areas of conduct and judgment in our society.

Bioethics is a branch of ethics concerned with what is right or wrong in bio (life) decisions. Because bioethics is a study of life ethics, it covers or becomes entwined with medical ethics. Medical ethics includes the values and decisions in medical practice, including relationships to patients, patients' families, peer physicians, and society.

Part of the ethical challenge in this age of rapidly advancing technologies is actually determining what is right, wrong, good, or bad. New scientific discoveries are challenging familiar or usual human behaviors, leading to reconsideration of actions, thoughts, and emotions. Ethical dilemmas, once rare, are now common and often happen so quickly that society is unable to understand completely the impact these decisions will have on the future.

Bioethical decisions are often very difficult because they touch the core of humanity in dealing with issues of birth, death, sickness, health, and dignity. This generation and generations to come will be faced with ethical decisions formerly unknown to man. Many of these decisions will have great impact on medical ethics and will actually shape the future of mankind.

When challenges concerning medical ethics arise in a health care facility, an ethics committee might be called on to make a decision. This committee might involve one or more persons at each of these levels: physician, nurse, ethicist, social worker, case manager, chaplain, legal representative, and administrator, or director.

Groups or committees involved in decision making might need to consider previous works of philosophy, history, law, and religion to assist them in reaching a conclusion. Participation in ethical decision making requires members to follow some basic rules, which can include:

- Keeping the discussion focused and civil.
- Listening with an open mind to all opinions.
- Entertaining diverse ideas.
- Weighing the pros and cons of each idea.
- Considering the impact of the decision on all persons involved.

Every individual at some time or another will encounter or be called on to make a decision that is bioethical in nature. Examples of these can include one's willingness to:

- Use a surrogate mother or father to have a biological child.
- Control the sex of children through chromosome selection.
- Use fetal stem cells to grow new organs and tissues.
- Use prescription stimulants in children.
- Legalize abortion.

- Use mood-altering drugs for older persons.
- Clone humans.
- Treat disease by replacing damaged or abnormal genes with normal genes.
- Use animal organs or tissues (xenotransplants) in humans.
- Support euthanasia.
- Allow physician-assisted suicide.

Each of the preceding issues can be overwhelming. Even so, yet another concern must be addressed, involving the economics of these choices.

Consider, for example, the economics of human cloning. How will research, technology, and intervention be funded? If costs are funded by individuals, only wealthy individuals would be able to afford clones. Is that fair or right? If costs are funded by the government, what criteria will be used for selection? Will selection be based on intelligence, physical ability, or artistic skills? Who decides?

Medical ethics includes some very complicated life issues. Bioethical decision making, or determining the rightness or wrongness of such issues, will continue to be a challenge for society well into the future.

SUMMARY

The study of human diseases is important to any health care or allied health professional. Disease can affect any body system or organ and can range from mild to severe, depending on many factors. Several risk factors for disease can be controlled to some extent by one's lifestyle. Other diseases might not be preventable or controlled but need medical intervention for treatment or cure. Diagnosis and treatment of a disease is usually accomplished by a team of health care professionals led by the physician. Ethical decision making has become a challenge in health care today and, as technology continues to grow and develop, medical ethics will become more challenging than ever.

REVIEW QUESTIONS

Short Answer

1. Identify why it is important to study human diseases.

2. Describe the types of pathologists and their roles in the study of disease.

3. List the five predisposing factors for disease and one disease related to each factor.

Matching

4. Match the terms in the left column with the correct definition in the right column.

_____ Pathogenesis	a. the cause of a disease
_____ Etiology	b. interventions to cure or control a disease
_____ Diagnosis	c. the development of a disease
_____ Prognosis	d. the identification or naming of a disease
_____ Treatment	e. the predicted or expected outcome of a disease

CASE STUDIES

■ Stan Cotton was accidentally tripped by another player while running down the field at a soccer game you were coaching. He is able to walk to the sideline with assistance but has obvious bleeding on his legs and one arm. You grab the first-aid box and go to his side. What do you do next? What equipment might you use to give aid to Stan? What standard precautions should apply to this case?

■ Jane Swenson has been suffering from a cold for about a week and has missed 3 days of work. She decides to return to work at the local senior citizen center. She is still coughing at intervals and has a runny nose but has improved since last week. Should she still use some precautions to prevent spreading her illness? If so, what should she do?

*Study*WARE™ Connection

To help you learn the content in this chapter, take a practice quiz or play an interactive game on your StudyWARE™ CD-ROM.

Workbook Practice

Go to your Workbook and complete the practice questions.

BIBLIOGRAPHY

Centers for Disease Control and Prevention (CDC). (2002). Guideline for hand hygiene in health care setting. *Morbidity and Mortality Weekly Report*. Atlanta, GA: Centers for Disease Control (CDC), 51 (RR 16), 20–25

Hussar, D. A. (2007). New drugs. *Nursing 37*(2), 51–60.

Landsdown, A. B. G. (2007). The role of the pathologist in wound management. *British Journal of Nursing 16*(20), S24–S33.

O'Fallon, L. I. (2006). Fostering the relationship between public health and nursing. *Public Health Nursing 23*(5), 377–380.

Schapira, A. (July 7, 2006). Mitochondrial disease. *Lancet 368*(9529), 70–82.

Scully, L. R., & Bidochka, M. J. (2006). Developing insect models for the study of current and emerging human pathogens. *FEMS Microbiology Letters 263*(1), 1–9.

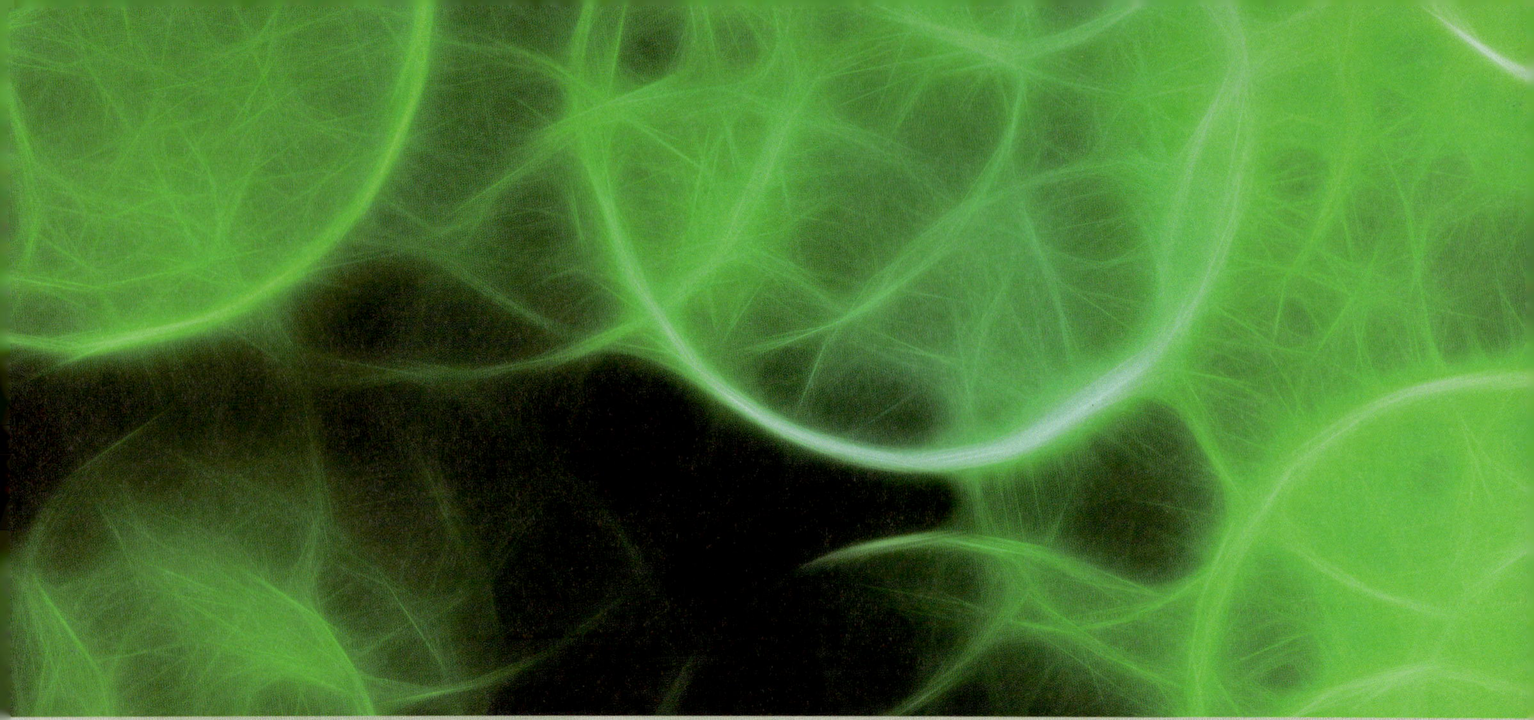

OUTLINE

- Causes of Disease
  - *Heredity*
  - *Trauma*
  - *Inflammation and Infection*
  - *Hyperplasias and Neoplasms*
  - *Nutritional Imbalance*
  - *Impaired Immunity*
- Aging
- Death
  - *Cellular Injury*
  - *Cellular Adaptation*
  - *Cell and Tissue Death*
  - *Organism Death*
- Summary
- Review Questions
- Case Studies
- Bibliography

KEY TERMS

AIDS (p. 20)
Allergen (p. 20)
Allergy (p. 20)
Anoxia (p. 22)
Antibodies (p. 20)
Antigens (p. 20)
Atrophy (p. 22)
Autoimmunity (p. 20)
Benign (p. 18)
Cachexia (p. 19)
Cancer (p. 18)
Congenital (p. 16)
Degenerative (p. 21)
Dysplasia (p. 22)
Encapsulated (p. 18)
Enteral (p. 19)
Gangrene (p. 24)
Hyperplasias (p. 17)
Hypertrophy (p. 22)
Hypoxia (p. 22)
Immunodeficiency (p. 20)
Infarct (p. 24)
Infection (p. 17)
Inflammation (p. 17)
Ischemia (p. 23)
Malignant (p. 18)
Metaplasia (p. 22)
Metastasize (p. 18)
Metastatic (p. 18)
Morbidity (p. 24)
MVA (p. 16)
Necrosis (p. 24)
Neoplasia (p. 22)
Neoplasms (p. 17)
Oncology (p. 17)
Organ rejection (p. 21)
Parenteral (p. 19)
TPN (p. 19)
Trauma (p. 16)
Triage (p. 17)
Tumors (p. 17)

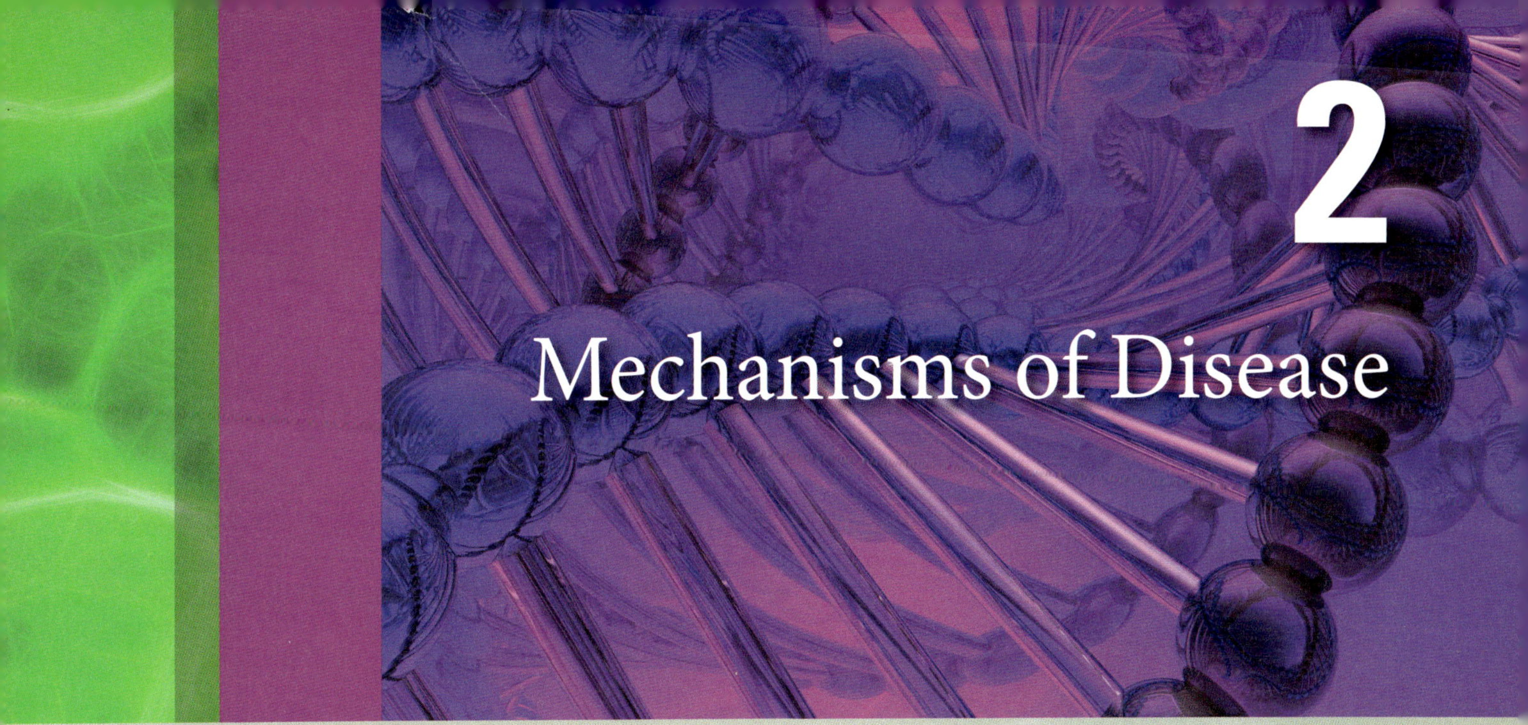

2 Mechanisms of Disease

LEARNING OBJECTIVES

Upon completion of the chapter, the learner should be able to:

1. Identify important terminology related to the mechanisms of human disease.
2. Describe the causes of disease.
3. Identify disorders in each category of the causes of disease.
4. Describe behaviors important to a healthy lifestyle.
5. Compare the various types of impaired immunity.
6. Identify the basic changes in the body occurring in the aging process.
7. Describe the process of cell and tissue injury, adaptation, and death.

OVERVIEW

The human body is a complex machine that normally runs in an efficient, balanced manner, but when changes occur in the body due to lifestyle behaviors, abnormal growths, nutritional problems, bacterial invasion, or any other factor that upsets the balance, the result might be a disease process. Human disease can be very minor or life threatening. Diseases are caused by a variety of factors; some are controllable and some are not. Even normal changes such as aging can put the individual at higher risk for developing disease. Many changes or alterations in cell and tissue structure can occur. Some of these changes are reversible, but some might cause cellular, tissue, organ, or system death. ■

CAUSES OF DISEASE

To gain a better understanding of the different causes of diseases, it is usually helpful to classify or divide them into smaller groups. This classification can be approached in several different yet logical ways. One commonly used approach is to divide the causes of disease into the following six categories:

1. Heredity
2. Trauma
3. Inflammation and infection
4. Hyperplasias and neoplasms
5. Nutritional imbalance
6. Immunity

Heredity

Hereditary diseases are caused by an abnormality in the individual's genetic or chromosomal makeup. These diseases might or might not be apparent at birth. Hereditary diseases that are present at birth, even if not apparent, are called **congenital** (kon-JEN-ih-tahl) disorders. However, not all congenital disorders are inherited. Some other causes of congenital disorders include disease during pregnancy (fetal alcohol syndrome) or difficulty with delivery (cerebral palsy), to name only a couple.

Hereditary diseases are classified in three basic ways, as (1) a single gene abnormality, (2) an abnormality of several genes (polygenic), or (3) an abnormality of a chromosome (either entire absence of a chromosome or the presence of an additional chromosome). See Table 2–1 for the classification of hereditary diseases and examples.

Chromosomal and genetic abnormalities might or might not be compatible with life. Some abnormalities might be present but cause no effect on the individual, whereas others might lead to the death and spontaneous abortion of the unborn child.

More information related to hereditary diseases can be found in Chapter 19, "Genetic and Developmental Diseases and Disorders."

Trauma

Traumatic diseases are caused by a physical injury from an external force. Trauma is the leading cause of death in children and young adults. The type of **trauma** (TRAW-mah) or traumatic disease most commonly affecting individuals varies with age, race, and residence. For example, accidents, especially falls, are a common cause of traumatic disorders in older adults, whereas gunshot wounds are the most common cause of traumatic disease and even death in young adult black males living in urban areas. However, **motor vehicle accidents (MVAs)** are the most frequent cause of serious injury overall.

The Centers for Disease Control and Prevention (CDC) lists deaths caused by trauma, in order of prevalence (or occurrence), as follows:

- Motor vehicle accidents
- Firearms
- Poison
- Falls
- Suffocation
- Suicide
- Homicide

Emergency management of trauma is often necessary to prevent the complications of shock, hemorrhage, and infection. On arrival at an emergency department, patients are assessed according to signs and symptoms, age, and medical history. Needs are then prioritized and care is given in order of severity

TABLE 2–1 Classification of Hereditary Disease with Examples

Single Gene	Polygenic	Chromosomal
Cystic fibrosis Phenylketonuria Sickle cell anemia	Gout Hypertension Congenital heart anomalies	Klinefelter's syndrome Turner's syndrome Down syndrome

of injury. This prioritizing of care is called **triage** (tree-AUZH) and incorporates an ABC prioritizing method with A for Airway, B for Breathing, and C for Cardiac function. After these areas are assessed, other areas of trauma such as bleeding and fractures are addressed. An example of triage, in general, would be giving priority care to a patient who is not breathing before assisting a patient who has a bleeding leg wound.

Types of trauma commonly occurring in each body system are discussed in the specific system chapters.

Inflammation and Infection

Inflammation (IN-flah-MAY-shun) is a protective immune response that is triggered by any type of injury or irritant. Even the slightest trauma can initiate the inflammatory response. Signs of inflammation are redness, heat, swelling, pain, and loss of motion. An example of inflammation is sunburn. The tissue is red, warm to the touch, swollen, painful, and uncomfortable when moving. Although this area is inflamed, it is usually not infected.

Infection (in-FECT-shun) refers to the invasion of microorganisms into tissue that causes cell or tissue injury. Inflammation and infection are often used synonymously even though they are quite different. A tissue can be inflamed but not infected, as in sunburn, but usually, tissue that is infected will also be inflamed.

For tissue to be infected or for infection to occur, there has to be an invasion of microorganisms. Usually, inflammation and infection go hand in hand. For example, when the skin is cut, the tissue around the cut will undergo a mild inflammation. As skin bacteria invade the cut tissue, the area becomes infected and usually becomes even more inflamed due to the irritation to the tissue caused by the bacteria (Figure 2–1).

Diseases that are related to inflammation are identified with the suffix "itis." Examples include appendicitis (inflammation of the appendix), gastritis (inflammation of the stomach), colitis (inflammation of the colon), and encephalitis (inflammation of the brain). In many cases, the inflammation will progress to an infection due to the presence of bacteria in the region. For example, appendicitis can be caused by an obstruction of the appendix. Because the bacteria *Escherichia coli* (E. coli) are commonly found in the colon, the appendix becomes infected.

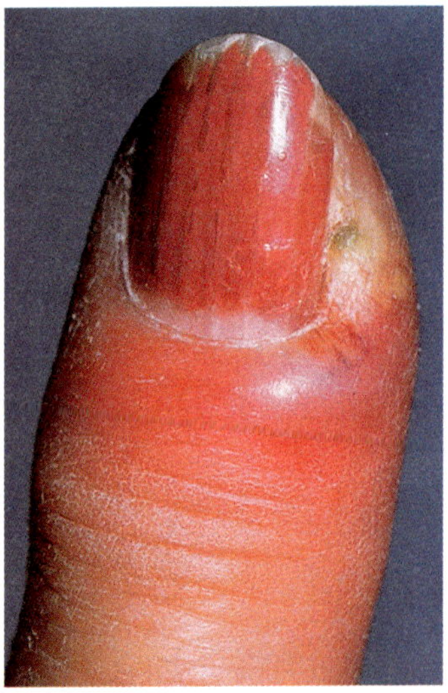

FIGURE 2–1 Inflammation of a finger.

Hyperplasias and Neoplasms

Hyperplasias (HIGH-per-PLAY-zee-ahs; hyper = excessive, plasia = growth) and **neoplasms** (NEE-oh-plazms; neo = new, plasm = growth) are similar because, in both, an increase in cell number leads to an increase in tissue size.

Hyperplasias

Hyperplasias differ from neoplasms in terms of cause and growth limits. Hyperplasias are an overgrowth in response to some type of stimulus. An example of a hyperplasia would be enlargement of the thyroid gland (goiter) in response to a hormone deficiency.

Neoplasms

Neoplasms (new growths) are commonly called **tumors**. The Latin word *tumor* means "swelling" and originally was used in the description of the swelling related to inflammation. The Greek term for swelling is *onkos*, which has been used to construct the word **oncology** (ong-KOL-oh-jee; onco = tumor, logy = study of, or the study of cancer). Although all tumors are not neoplasms, as described in more detail in Chapter 3, "Neoplasms," the words are often used synonymously.

Diseases with tumor involvement usually end with the suffix *oma*. Examples include lipoma, carcinoma, melanoma, and sarcoma (Table 2–2). An exception to

TABLE 2–2 **Examples of Neoplasms or Tumors**

Neoplasm/Tumor	Description
Adenoma	Usually benign tumor arising from glandular epithelial tissue
Carcinoma	Malignant tumor of epithelial tissue
Fibroma	Benign encapsulated tumor of connective tissue
Glioma	Malignant tumor of neurological cells
Lipoma	Benign fatty tumor
Melanoma	Malignant tumor of the skin
Sarcoma	Malignant tumor arising from connective tissue such as muscle or bone

this is the word *hematoma*, which is a clot of blood in an area. A hematoma on the head due to a blunt blow would be an example.

Neoplasms or tumors (omas) may be classified as **benign** (beh-NINE) or **malignant** (mah-LIG-nant). Generally speaking, benign tumors have a limited growth, are **encapsulated** (enclosed in a capsule) and thus easily removed, and are not deadly. Malignant tumors are just the opposite. These tumors grow uncontrollably; have finger-like projections into surrounding tissue, making removal very difficult; and are usually deadly. *Malignant* means deadly or progressing to death. With these definitions, it is understandable why the terms *tumor*, *malignancy*, and *cancer* bring fear to an individual. Some -omas, or tumor diseases, are commonly called cancer. **Cancer** is defined as any malignant tumor.

The finger-like or crab-like projections that characterize malignant tumors give cancer its name, from the Greek *karkinos*, meaning "crab." This characteristic makes surgical removal of cancer quite difficult (Figure 2–2). Another characteristic of malignant neoplasms is that they **metastasize** (meh-TAS-tah-sighz), or move. **Metastatic** (MET-ah-STAT-ic) cancers move from a site of origin to a secondary site in the body. For example, lung cancer commonly metastasizes to the bone. Chapter 3 discusses more detailed information about hyperplasias and neoplasms.

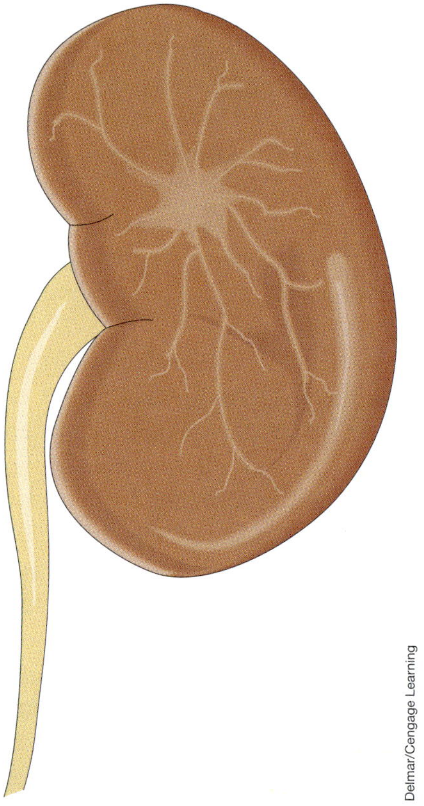

FIGURE 2–2 Crab-like appearance of cancer in a kidney.

Nutritional Imbalance

Good nutrition is important in maintaining good health and reducing the chance of disease. Nutritional disorders can cause problems with physical growth, mental and intellectual retardation, and even death in extreme cases. Most nutritional diseases are related to overconsumption or underconsumption of nutrients. Specific problems are malnutrition, obesity, and excessive or deficient vitamins, minerals, or both.

Malnutrition

Malnutrition can be due to inadequate nutrient intake or to intake of an adequate amount with poor nutritive value. Diseases that cause a problem with absorption of nutrients can also lead to malnutrition. Children and older persons are the age groups most affected

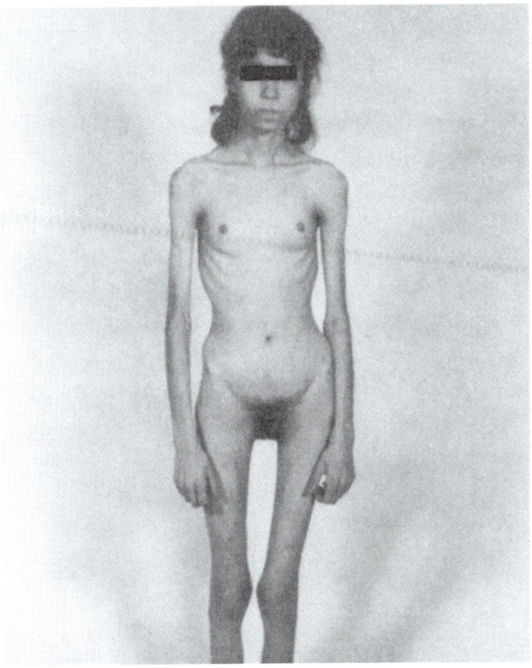

FIGURE 2–3 Cachexia.

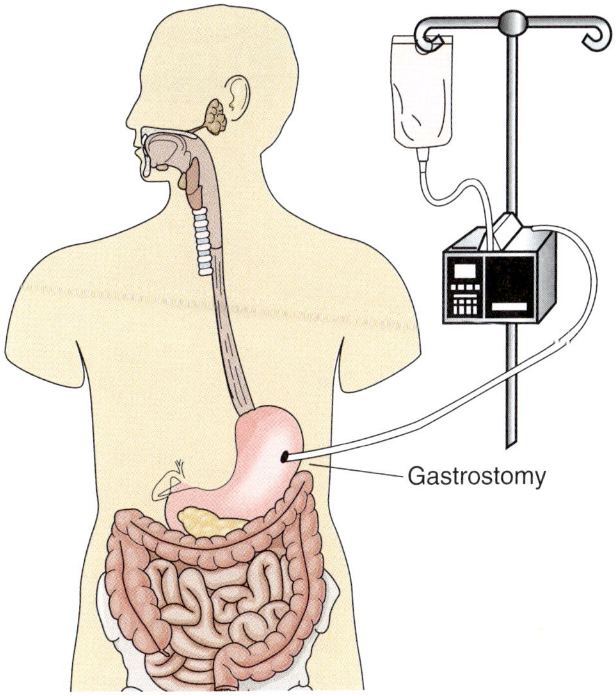

FIGURE 2–4 Gastrostomy feeding.

by malnutrition. Persons suffering with cancer often experience problems with malnutrition and develop cachexia. **Cachexia** (ca-KECK-see-ah) is a term that describes any individual who has an ill, thin, wasted appearance (Figure 2–3).

Persons who are unable to eat enough to maintain their body weight can receive nutritional supplements in a liquid drink. Another way to supplement or provide for total nutritional intake is not through the alimentary canal or digestive system but through a **parenteral** (pah-REN-ter-al; to administer by injection) route. Parenteral routes can include subcutaneous (sub = under, cutaneous = skin), intramuscular (intra = within, muscular = muscle), or intravenous (intra = within, venous = vein) administration. The intravenous route is the most commonly used parenteral route. Providing the total nutrition needed by giving nutritive liquid through a venous (vein) route is called **total parenteral nutrition (TPN)**.

Nutrition can also be provided through an **enteral** (small intestine) route. A nasogastric (naso = nose, gastric = stomach) tube or a tube running through the nose and into the stomach can be used for feedings if the supplement is planned short term. For longer term enteral feeding, a gastrostomy (gastro = stomach, ostomy = opening; opening into the stomach) procedure is performed to place a tube through the abdominal and stomach wall. Enteral feeding, commonly called "tube feeding," is accomplished by this method (Figure 2–4).

Obesity

Although many individuals in the United States have a nutritional deficiency, the most common problem is obesity, which is primarily due to overconsumption of nutrients and lack of exercise. Although obesity is difficult to define specifically for each individual, it is obviously a major nutritional problem. Obesity shortens the life span of the individual by increasing the chance for arteriosclerosis, leading to cardiovascular diseases. It also affects the individual's risk for developing bone or joint problems due to the increased pressure on the skeletal system.

Vitamin or Mineral Excess or Deficiency

Vitamin and mineral excesses and deficiencies are usually related to diet, metabolic disorders, and some medications. Hypervitaminosis can occur in individuals who consume large amounts of vitamins for an extended period of time.

HEALTHY HIGHLIGHT

General Guidelines for a Healthy Lifestyle

General guidelines for a healthy lifestyle include the following tips:

- Maintain proper body weight.
- Eat a variety of foods.
- Avoid excessive fat, salt, and sugar.
- Eat adequate amounts of fiber.
- Consume alcohol in moderation, no more than two drinks per day for men and one for women.
- Get enough rest and sleep, at least 7 or more hours per day.
- Always eat breakfast.
- Maintain a moderate exercise schedule.

Nutritional guidelines for a healthy lifestyle are difficult to determine because they must cover a variety of ages and nutritional needs. Children, teens, and pregnant women have very specific nutritional needs. The Healthy Highlight on this following page lists general guidelines for a healthy lifestyle.

Impaired Immunity

The immune system of the body is a specialized group of cells, tissues, and organs that are designed to defend the body against pathogenic attacks. The body's first line of defense against pathogens is its normal structure and function, including an intact skin; mucous membranes; tears; and secretions. The immune system protects the body in two additional ways, through:

1. The inflammatory response in which leukocytes play a vital part in killing foreign invaders.
2. The specific antigen–antibody reaction in which the body responds to antigens (AN-tih-jens) by producing antibodies. **Antigens** are substances that cause the body some type of harm, thus setting off this specific reaction. **Antibodies**, also called immune bodies, are proteins that the body produces to react to the antigen and render it harmless.

Impaired immunity occurs when some part of this system malfunctions. Following are some common ways the system malfunctions.

Allergy

The immune response is too intense or hypersensitive to an environmental substance. The **allergen** (environmental substance that causes a reaction) in an **allergy** might be such things as house dust, grass, pets, perfumes, or insect bites, to name a few. These allergens do not usually cause this type of reaction in most persons but do cause an allergic reaction in persons sensitive to them.

Autoimmunity

The immune response attacks itself. In **autoimmunity** (auto = self), the body's lymphocytes (a white blood cell that produces antibodies) cannot identify the body's own self-antigens, which are harmless. In response, the lymphocytes form antibodies that then attack the body's own cells. Examples of autoimmune diseases include rheumatoid arthritis and rheumatic fever.

Immunodeficiency

The immune response is unable to defend the body due to a decrease or absence of leukocytes, primarily lymphocytes. Persons with **immunodeficiency** are usually asymptomatic (without symptoms) except for recurrent infections. It is these recurrent infections that often lead to death. An example of an immunodeficiency disease is **AIDS (acquired immunodeficiency syndrome)**. Immunodeficiency also can be caused by medications, chemotherapy, or radiation. Organ recipients are intentionally immunosuppressed or immunodeficient to save their transplanted organ. Without immunosuppressant medications, the body's immune system would recognize the organ as foreign and attack it, leading to organ death. This process is called **organ rejection**. Cancer patients often undergo chemotherapy and radiation treatments that can cause immunodeficiency. Some medications also affect the system by depressing its ability to function properly. Chapter 5, "Immune System Diseases and Disorders," discusses the immune system and related diseases in more detail.

AGING

There is no definite age in years when an individual becomes aged. However, some statisticians consider the retirement age of 65 as aged. An individual's body actually begins to age at physical maturity, around age 18, in a complicated process that is not completely understood but is progressive and irreversible. Diseases related to aging are often called **degenerative** diseases. Tissue degeneration is a change in functional activity to a lower or lesser level. Examples of degenerative diseases are degenerative joint disease and degenerative disk disease.

The mechanisms of aging are complex and thought to include such factors as heredity, lifestyle, stress, diet, and environment. One might slow the process of aging to some degree by living a healthy lifestyle and controlling stress and environmental factors.

Hereditary factors can include increased life span related to an inherited ability to resist disease. Just as families have a history of disease patterns, they also appear to have a pattern of longevity. Thus, individuals who have relatives who live to be in their nineties might themselves live to that age. Individuals with a family history of members who have died of heart disease in their early years might also suffer the same problem. Although hereditary patterns cannot be controlled, longevity can be increased and disease decreased by controlling lifestyle behaviors that increase risk of chronic disease.

The body replaces and repairs itself throughout its lifetime, but with aging, this process slows. As early as age 40, there are changes in skin, endocrine function, vision, and muscle strength. Other changes in the aging process might include bone loss leading to osteoporosis, decreased melanin pigment production leading to graying of the hair, decreased immunity leading to an increase in infections and possible development of cancer, loss of brain and nerve cells that might lead to senile dementia, and decrease in intestinal motility leading to constipation and possible diverticulosis.

HEALTHY HIGHLIGHT

The Use of Herbal Therapies Is Increasing

The use of herbal remedies has been well known to be increasing among older persons, but it is not also increasing among all age groups. A reliable risk–benefit profile of the most commonly used herbal preparations is needed so both medical practitioners and lay consumers can understand the best use of these products. Millions are spent each year on herbal remedies. The most common include *Ginkgo biloba*, St. John's wort, ginseng, garlic, echinacea, saw palmetto, and kava. The literature reports there is evidence that *Ginko biloba* might affect memory loss and that St. John's wort might affect depression, but both of these also might interact with other drugs the person consumes. There is little support for any positive effects of ginseng. Saw palmetto has been shown to decrease the symptoms of prostate problems and kava might be helpful in treating anxiety. However, because the research is still incomplete on the benefits of these products, consumers should be cautious in using them, especially when combining them with other prescription medications.

Ernst (2002).

DEATH

Humans are mortal, so eventually, everyone will die. Even though we are unable to understand the aging process fully, cellular, tissue, and organ death can be reviewed in an effort to understand the death of the organism as a whole.

Cellular Injury

Cellular injury and death can be due to some type of trauma, **hypoxia** (HIGH-POCK-see-ah; not enough oxygen), **anoxia** (ah-NOCK-see-ah; no oxygen), drug or bacterial toxins, or viruses. Cells can undergo near-dcath experiences and actually recuperate in what is considered to be reversible cell injury.

The ability of the cell to survive depends on several factors, including the amount of time the cell suffers and the type of cell injury that occurred. If the cause of the injury is short term, the cell has a greater chance of survival.

The type of cell also plays a part in its ability to recuperate. The heart, brain, and nerve cells are easily injured and often suffer death. This is particularly important because these cells do not replace themselves. Even short-term injury might readily lead to death in these cells. Other cells are not as easily damaged. Connective and epithelial cells often recuperate and even readily replace themselves by mitosis (cell division).

Cellular Adaptation

Cells that are exposed to adverse conditions often go through a process of adaptation. When the condition is changed, these cells might be able to change back to their normal structure and function. However, some adaptations are permanent, so even if the condition improves, the cells are not able to return to normal. Types of adaptation include **atrophy** (AT-tro-fee), **hypertrophy** (HIGH-PER-tro-fee), **hyperplasia**, **dysplasia** (dis-PLAY-zee-ah), **metaplasia** (MET-ah-PLAY-zee-ah), and **neoplasia** (nee-oh-PLAY-zee-ah).

Atrophy

Atrophy (a = without, trophy = growth) is a decrease in cell size, which leads to a decrease in the size of the tissue and organ (Figure 2–5). Atrophy is often due to the aging process itself or to disease. An example of atrophy related to aging would be the smaller size of

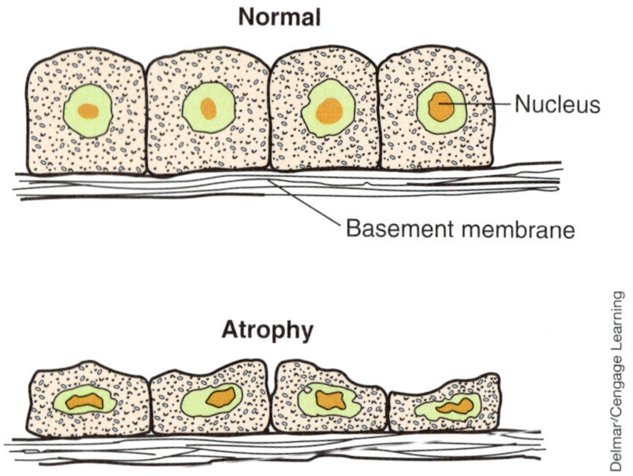

FIGURE 2–5 Normal cell versus atrophied cell.

the muscles and bones of older people. As the female ages, the breasts and female reproductive organs atrophy, especially after menopause. Examples of disease or pathologic atrophy are usually related to decreased use of the organ, especially muscles. Spinal cord injuries lead to an inability to move muscles. Without use, muscle cells decrease in size and the muscle atrophies.

Hypertrophy

Hypertrophy (hyper = excessive, trophy = growth) is an increase in the size of the cell leading to an increase in tissue and organ size (Figure 2–6). Skeletal muscle and heart muscle cells do not increase in number by mitosis. Literally, what an individual has at birth is what the individual has throughout life. This helps explain why some athletes bulk up with exercise while others do not. The inherited number of muscle cells does not change with exercise; only the size of each cell changes. To adapt to an increased workload,

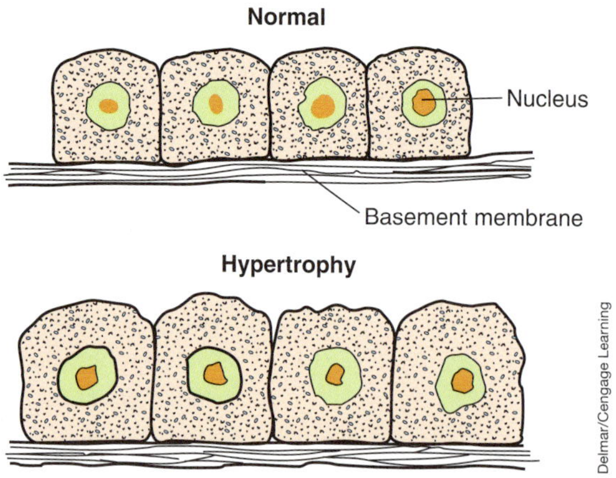

FIGURE 2–6 Normal cell versus hypertrophied cell.

muscle cells increase in size. Increased workload on the skeletal muscles causes cellular hypertrophy and an increase in muscle size. Heart muscle hypertrophy is usually seen in the left ventricle of the heart (left ventricular hypertrophy) when the left ventricle must work harder to pump blood through diseased valves and arteries. To adapt to this need, the cells increase in size and the left side of the heart enlarges.

Hyperplasia

Hyperplasia (hyper = increased, plasia = growth) is an increase in cell number that is commonly due to hormonal stimulation (Figure 2–7). Hyperplasia is discussed in more detail in Chapter 3.

Dysplasia

Dysplasia (dys = bad or difficult, plasia = growth) usually follows hyperplasia. It is an alteration in size, shape, and organization of cells (Figure 2–8). Dysplastic cells might change back to the normal cell structure if the irritant or stimulus is removed, but usually, these cells progress to neoplasia.

Metaplasia

Metaplasia (meta = changed, plasia = growth) is a cellular adaptation in which the cell changes to another type of cell (Figure 2–9). An example is the columnar epithelial cells of the respiratory tree, which often change to stratified squamous epithelial cells when exposed to the irritants of cigarette smoking. This protective adaptation might be reversible if the individual quits smoking.

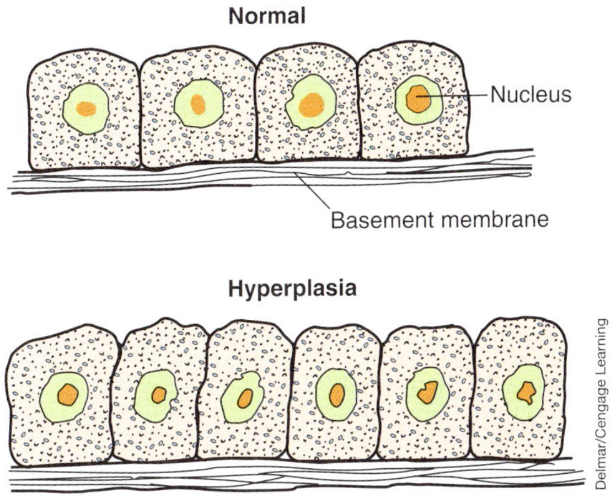

FIGURE 2–7 Normal tissue versus hyperplasia.

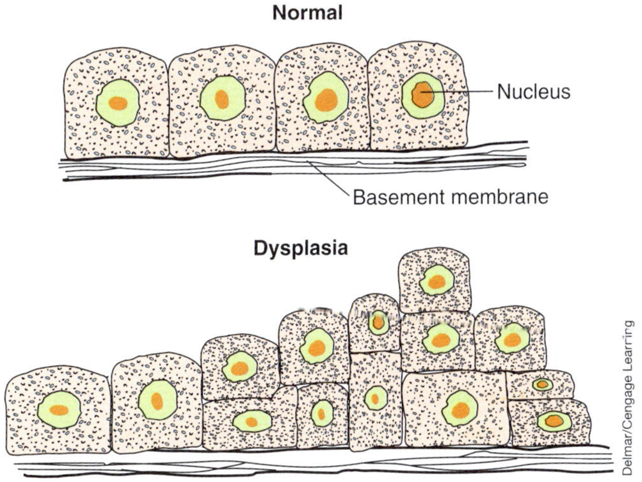

FIGURE 2–8 Normal tissue versus dysplasia.

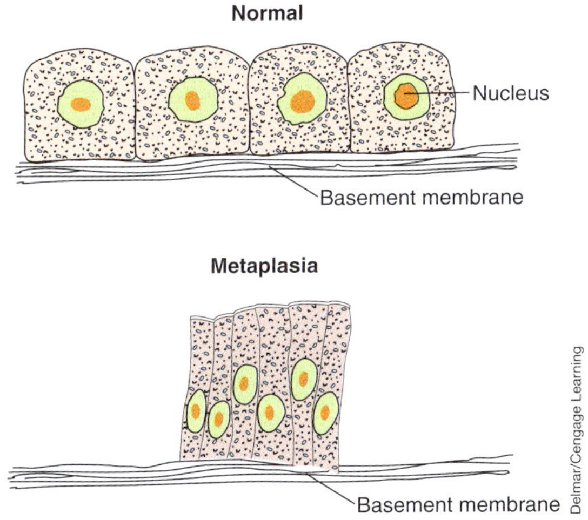

FIGURE 2–9 Normal tissue versus metaplasia.

Neoplasia

Neoplasia (neo = new, plasia = growth) is the development of a new type of cell with an uncontrolled growth pattern (Figure 2–10). Neoplasia is discussed in more detail in Chapter 3.

Cell and Tissue Death

Cell death, as previously mentioned, can be caused by trauma, hypoxia, anoxia, drug or bacterial toxins, or viruses. The most common causes of cell death are hypoxia and anoxia.

Cell hypoxia caused by decreased blood flow is called **ischemia** (iss-KEE-me-ah; isch = hold back,

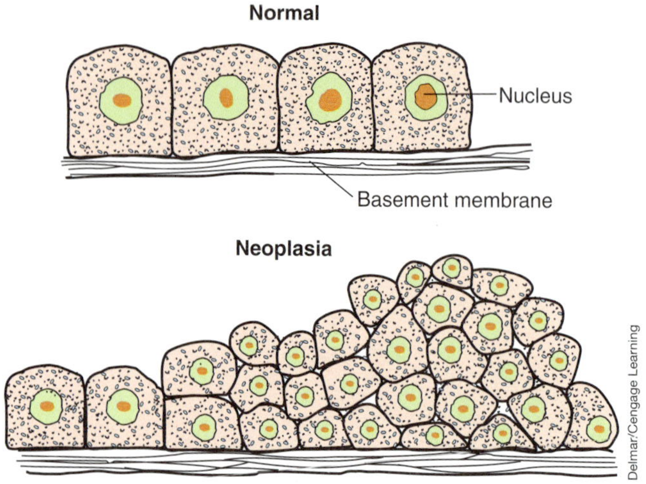

FIGURE 2–10 Normal tissue versus neoplasia.

emia = blood). A cell without oxygen cannot produce needed energy and eventually dies.

Cellular death, called **necrosis** (neh-CROW-sis), can involve a group of cells and, thus, tissue. When referring to dead cells or tissue, one would describe the area as necrotic. When necrosis occurs due to ischemia, the area of dead cells (ischemic necrosis) is called an **infarct** (IN-farkt). Infarcts are commonly due to obstruction of arteries. The most common infarct affects tissues of the heart, leading to a myocardial infarction, or heart attack.

Cells that are injured and not able to recover eventually die. The cause of cell death can be determined by a pathologist because the gross (visible with the eye) and microscopic appearance of the tissue differs with the type of death. There are several types of necrosis, primarily named by the microscopic appearance of the dead cells.

The most common type of necrosis is called coagulation necrosis and is due to cellular anoxia. Coagulation necrosis is the type of cell death experienced with myocardial infarction.

A common alteration in necrosis occurs when saprophytic (dead tissue–loving) bacteria become involved in the necrotic tissue. With this occurrence, the necrotic tissue is now described as gangrenous or having **gangrene** (GANG-green). The type of gangrene can be wet, dry, or gas, depending on the appearance of the necrotic tissue.

Wet gangrene usually occurs when the necrosis was caused by the sudden stoppage of blood flow, as in the trauma of burning, freezing, or embolism.

Dry gangrene occurs when blood flow has been slowed for a long period of time before necrosis occurred, as in the case of arteriosclerosis and advanced diabetes. In dry gangrene, the tissue is black, shriveled, or mummified. This type of gangrene occurs on the extremities only, primarily on the feet and toes.

Gas gangrene occurs with dirty, infected wounds. The tissue becomes infected with anaerobic (growing without oxygen) bacteria that produce a toxic gas. This is an acute, painful, and often fatal type of gangrene.

Organism Death

Human death can be related to any of the aforementioned causes of disease. The aging process leads to death due to a change in the normal structure of the individual's organs or a decrease in the ability to fight disease. Diseases that would not be lethal in our younger years, such as respiratory infections, can be the cause of death in an older individual.

According to Centers for Disease Control (CDC), the most common cause of death in the United States is heart disease, followed by cancer and strokes (cerebrovascular accident). Although heart disease is the leading cause of death, stroke is the leading cause of serious, long-term disability in the United States. See Chapter 8, "Cardiovascular System Diseases and Disorders," for more information.)

Many times, the human organism—like the cell—does not die but becomes disabled. Disability is called **morbidity** (state of being diseased). Oftentimes, morbidity is so extreme that the individual's quality of life is severely limited. This is often seen in cases of severe brain injury or even in some congenital disorders.

Prior to death, major organs such as the heart, lungs, and brain stop functioning. When the brain ceases to function, the individual is considered brain dead. Although death is difficult to define and difficult to determine in some cases, one guideline used is that of brain death. The criteria for determining brain death include:

- Lack of response to stimuli.
- Loss of all reflexes.
- Absence of respirations or breathing effort.
- Lack of brain activity as shown by an electroencephalogram (EEG).

This issue of defining death and when an individual is actually dead is still controversial in the medical profession.

SUMMARY

Human diseases are caused by heredity; trauma; inflammation, infection, or both; hyperplasias, neoplasms, or both; nutritional imbalances; impaired immunity; or some or all of these. Lifestyle behaviors can also be contributing factors to disease development, as can the aging process. Eventually, all organisms die, and the process of death can occur at the cellular, tissue, or whole organism level.

REVIEW QUESTIONS

Matching

1. Match the cause of diseases in the left column with the example of a disease for that category in the right column.

_____ Heredity	a. pneumonia
_____ Trauma	b. motor vehicle accident
_____ Inflammation/infection	c. cancer
_____ Hyperplasias/neoplasms	d. obesity
_____ Nutritional imbalance	e. allergies
_____ Impaired immunity	f. cystic fibrosis

True or False

2. T F In autoimmunity, the body's immune system attacks itself.

3. T F Some medications used to prevent or cure some diseases can cause immunodeficiency.

4. T F Diseases related to the aging process are called regenerative disorders.

5. T F All congenital disorders are easily recognized at birth.

6. T F Heart and brain cells are easily injured by hypoxia.

7. T F Heredity does not affect the aging process.

8. T F Cellular death occurs only in the event of hypoxia (lack of oxygen).

Short Answer

9. List the factors that affect a cell's ability to survive after injury.

10. How do cells adapt when exposed to adverse conditions?

CASE STUDIES

- Cann Ragland, age 29, was seriously injured in a motorcycle accident. He is comatose and on life support equipment to maintain his breathing. He has not improved in 2 weeks with aggressive medical treatment. The family is questioning whether he is alive or dead at this time. What criteria can be used to determine this? What are the issues surrounding this determination? How could you help the family through this difficult time? What resources are available to help people make decisions about end-of-life care?

- Jessie Leher, age 69, is concerned about her aging status and loss of short-term memory at times. Her sister told her to take *Ginko biloba* and Co-Q10, over-the-counter herbal products. Jessie has high blood pressure and some circulatory problems. She takes several prescription medications for these disorders and for a couple of other problems, such as arthritis. Should she be cautioned about also taking the herbal remedies? How effective are these products? What would you tell Ms. Leher if she asked you whether she should take the herbal remedies? What sources of more detailed information about these products could you review?

*Study***WARE**™ Connection

To help you learn the content in this chapter, take a practice quiz or play an interactive game on your StudyWARE™ CD-ROM.

Workbook Practice

Go to your Workbook and complete the practice questions.

BIBLIOGRAPHY

American Heart Association. (2008). Heart disease and stroke statistics: 2008 update. *www.americanheart.org*

Centers for Disease Control and Prevention. (2006). Deaths, injuries. *National Vital Statistics Report, 2002.* Atlanta, GA: Centers for Disease Control and Prevention.

Dowd, J. B., Haan, M. N., Blythe, L., Moore, K., & Atello, A. E. (2008). Socioeconomic gradients in immune response to latent infection. *American Journal of epidemiology 167*(1), 112.

Ernst, E. (January 1, 2002). The risk–benefit profile of commonly used herbal therapies: Ginko, St. John's wort, ginseng, Echinacea, saw palmetto, and kava. *Annals of Internal Medicine 136*(1), 42–53.

Daviri, C., Demakakos, P., Charizani, F., Tigani, X., Tsiou, C., Chalamandaris, A., et al. (2008). Assessment of the health status of Greek centenarians. *Archives of Gerontology and Geriatrics 46*(1), 67–78.

Noonan, K. (2007). Introduction to B-cell disorders. *Clinical Journal of Oncology Nursing 11*(Supplement), 3–12.

Pan, P., Ozao, J., Zhou, Z., & Chen, S. (2008). Advancements in immune tolerance. *Advanced Drug Delivery Reviews 60*(2), 91–105.

Prinz, P. N. (2004). Age impairments in sleep, metabolic and immune functions. *Experimental Gerontology 39*(11/12), 1739–1743.

Sehgal, V. N., & Srivastava, G. (2006). Vitiligo: Autoimmunity and immune responses. *International Journal of Dermatology 45*(5), 583–590.

Simmons, F. E. R., Frew, A. J., Ansotegui, I. J., Bochner, B. S., Golden, D. B. K., Finkelman, F. D., et al. (2008). Practical allergy (PRACTALL) report: Risk assessment in anaphylaxis. *Allergy 63*(1), 35–37.

Shi, Y., Sun, G., Zhao, C., & Stewart, R. (2008). Neural stem cell self-renewal. *Critical Reviews in Oncology/Hematology 65*(1), 43–53.

Short, R. (2006). Boosting the immune system. *Nursing Older People 18*(8), 18–21.

Ting, A. E., Mays, R. W., Frey, M. R., Hof, W. V., Medicetty, S., & Deans, R. (2008) Therapeutic pathways of adult stem cell repair. *Critical Reviews in Oncology/Hematology 65*(1), 81–93.

Zhang, S., Li, X., Johnson, M. A., & Pankratx, M. T. (2008). Human embryonic stem cells for brain repair? *Biological Sciences 363*(1489), 87–99.

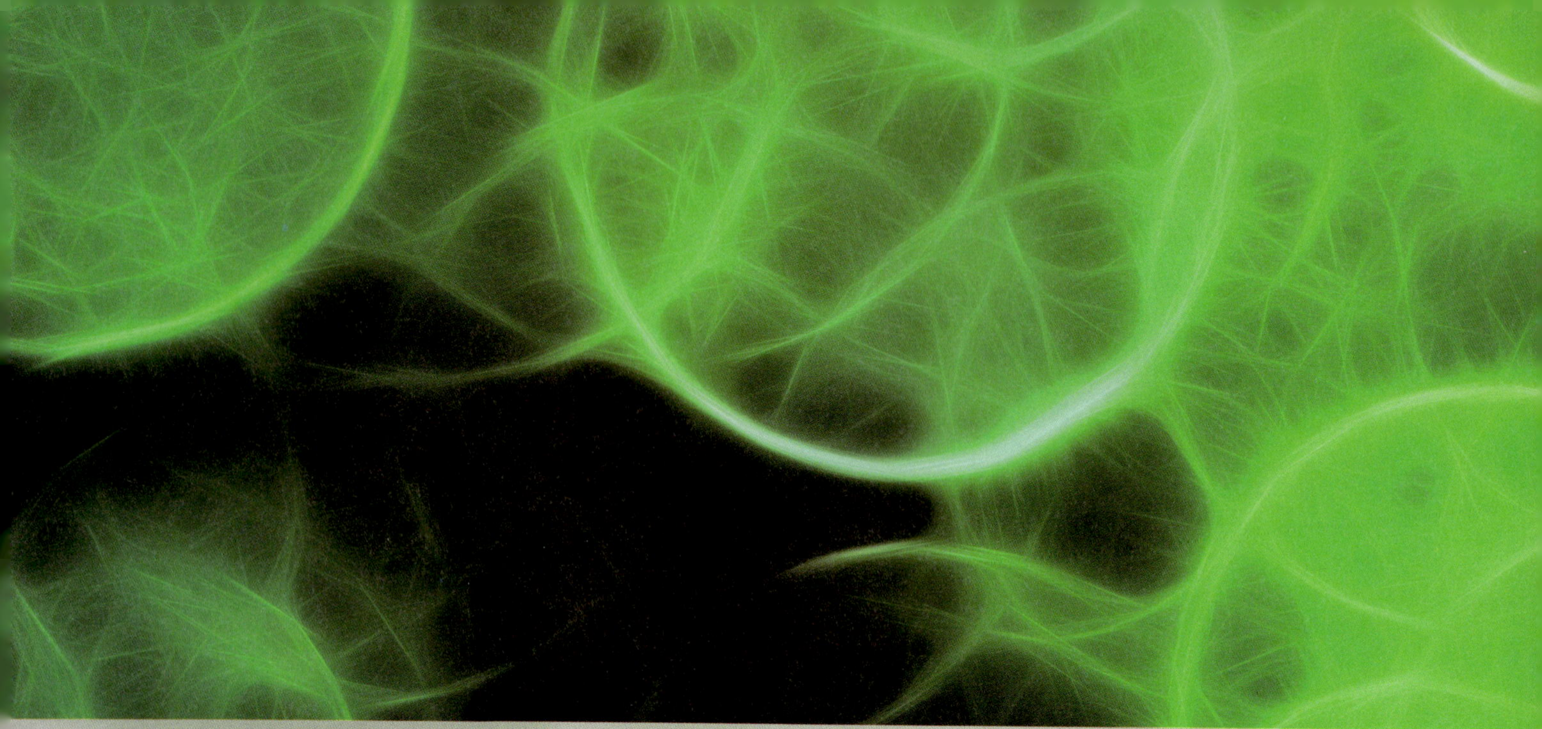

OUTLINE

- Terminology Related to Neoplasms and Tumors
- Classification of Neoplasms
  - *Appearance and Growth Pattern*
  - *Tissue of Origin*
- Growth of Benign and Malignant Neoplasms
  - *Benign Neoplasm Growth*
  - *Malignant Neoplasm Growth*
- Hyperplasias and Neoplasms
  - *Hyperplasias*
  - *Neoplasms*
- Development of Malignant Neoplasms (Cancer)
- Invasion by and Metastasis of Cancer
  - *Lymphatic System Metastasis*
  - *Bloodstream Metastasis*
  - *Cavity Metastasis*
- Grading and Staging of Cancer
  - *Grading*
  - *Staging*
- Causes of Cancer
  - *Chemical Carcinogens*
  - *Hormones*
  - *Radiation*
  - *Viruses*
  - *Genetic Predisposition*
  - *Personal Risk Behaviors*
- Cancer Prevention
- Frequency of Cancer
- Diagnosis of Cancer
- Signs and Symptoms of Cancer
  - *Pain*
  - *Obstruction*
  - *Hemorrhage*
  - *Anemia*
  - *Fractures*
  - *Infection*
  - *Cachexia*
- Cancer Treatment
  - *Surgery*
  - *Chemotherapy*
  - *Radiation*
  - *Hormone Therapy*
- Summary
- Review Questions
- Case Studies
- Bibliography

KEY TERMS

Anaplastic (p. 36)
Angiogenesis (p. 33)
Benign (p. 30)
Biopsy (p. 36)
Cachexia (p. 33)
Carcinogen (p. 34)
Carcinogenesis (p. 36)
Carcinoma (p. 30)
Carcinoma in situ (p. 34)
Chemotherapy (p. 45)
Curative (p. 45)
Cytology (p. 44)
Differentiation (p. 32)
Dysplasia (p. 34)
Frozen section (p. 45)
Grading (p. 36)
Hematoma (p. 30)
Hyperplasia(s) (p. 33)
Invasion (p. 30)
Leukemia (p. 30)
Lymphomas (p. 31)
Malignant (p. 30)
Metaplasia (p. 36)
Metastasis (p. 30)
Neoplasm(s) (p. 30)
Palliative (p. 45)
Pap test (p. 40)
Preventive (p. 39)
Radiation (p. 34)
Sarcoma (p. 30)
Staging (p. 36)
Tumor (p. 30)

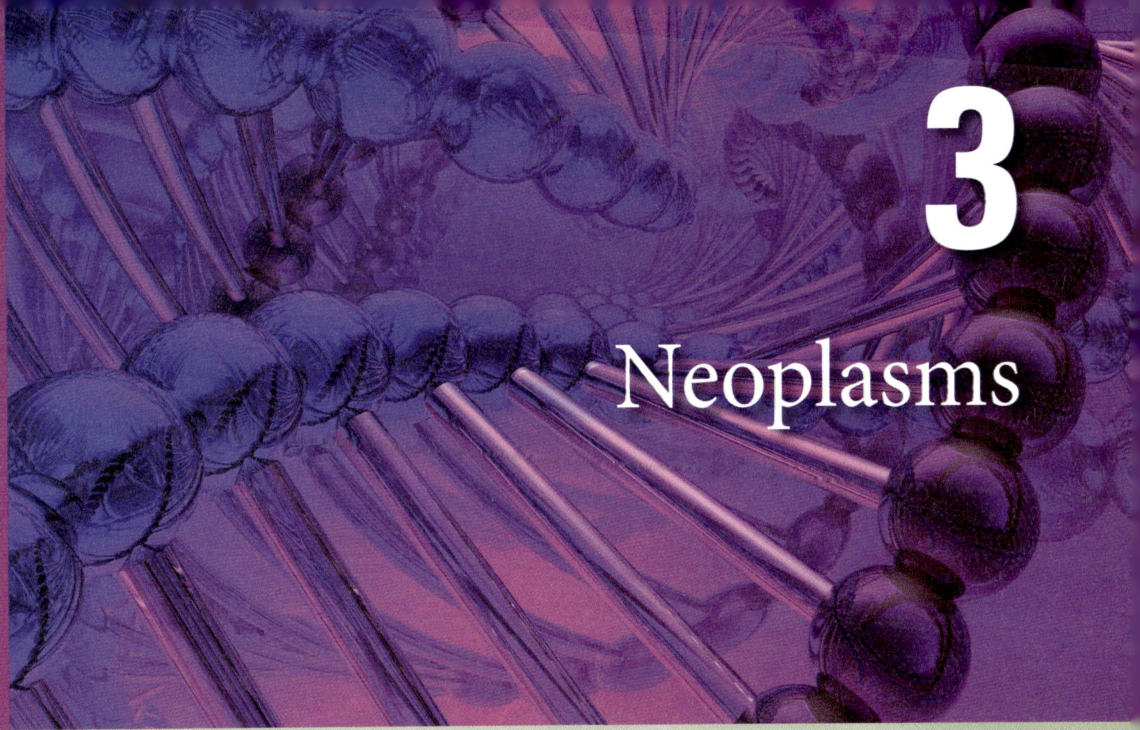

3 Neoplasms

LEARNING OBJECTIVES

Upon completion of the chapter, the learner should be able to:

1. Define basic terminology used in the study of neoplasms.
2. Explain the system used to classify neoplasms.
3. Compare hyperplasias to neoplasms.
4. Identify the progression of cancer development.
5. State the signs and symptoms of cancer.
6. Identify some common carcinogenic substances.
7. Identify high-risk behaviors for cancer development.
8. State the frequency of cancer development in the population.
9. Describe the curative, palliative, and preventive methods used in cancer treatment.

OVERVIEW

Thousands of individuals are diagnosed with neoplasms each year. The diagnostic statement, "You have a tumor," often causes instant fear, dread, and tears for the individuals and families involved; few statements in our society carry the emotional impact this one does. To most people, this diagnosis is equivalent to a pronouncement of death. But not all tumors are malignant, and not all are deadly. However, more than 1.3 million individuals are diagnosed with malignant neoplasms each year. This includes all types of cancers. Prostate cancer is the most commonly diagnosed cancer among men, whereas breast cancer is the most commonly diagnosed type in women (American Cancer Society, 2007). Cancer can be diagnosed using a variety of diagnostic tests, and treatment of cancer is most successful when the cancer has been diagnosed early. Individuals can reduce their risk of developing some types of cancer by following preventive measures recommended by the American Cancer Society. ■

TERMINOLOGY RELATED TO NEOPLASMS AND TUMORS

The term **neoplasm** (NEE-oh-plazm; neo = new, plasm = growth) means a new growth. The term **tumor** may be defined simply as a swelling or as a neoplasm. Tumor is used as a sign of inflammation and, in this instance, describes swelling. The term *tumor* as related to neoplasm means a new growth. Even though the terms *tumor* and *neoplasm* are used synonymously, not all neoplasms form tumors (Table 3–1). For instance, **leukemia** (loo-KEE-me-ah; leuk = white, emia = blood) is a malignant disease of the bone marrow that causes an increase in white blood cell production and might not form distinctive tumors. Likewise, not all tumors are neoplasms—a **hematoma** (HEM-ah-TOH-mah; hemat = blood, oma = tumor) is a large tumor or swelling filled with blood, commonly called a bruise or contusion (Figure 3–1).

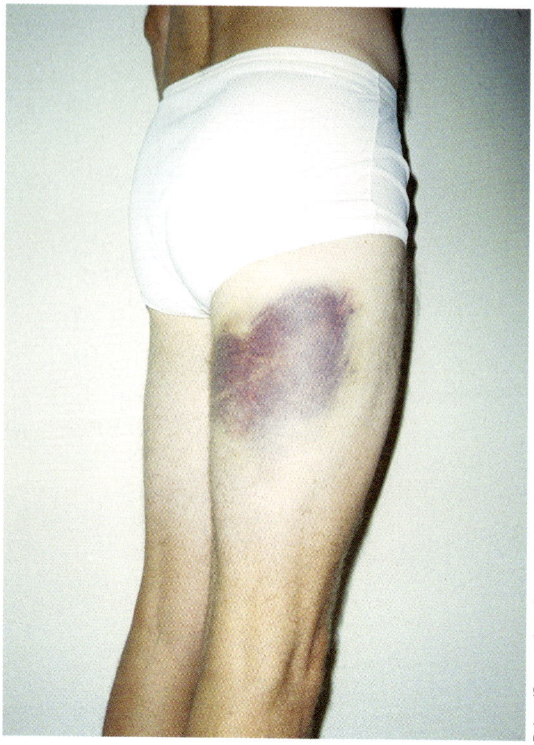

FIGURE 3–1 Hematoma.

CLASSIFICATION OF NEOPLASMS

Neoplasms may be classified in a variety of ways. Two of the most common ways are according to the (1) appearance and growth pattern and (2) tissue of origin, or type of body tissue from which they grow.

Appearance and Growth Pattern

Classification by appearance and growth pattern identifies neoplasms (tumors) as **benign** (beh-NINE) or **malignant** (mah-LIG-nant).

Benign Neoplasm

Neoplasms that are confined to a local area and do not spread are called benign. Benign neoplasms are more commonly called tumors. They are generally harmless unless they are growing in a confined space such as the brain.

TABLE 3–1 **Neoplasm vs Non-neoplasm**

Neoplasm-new growth	Swelling: Can be called tumor No Swelling: No tumor, but is a neoplasm—e.g., leukemia
Non-neoplasm	Swelling: Hematoma, inflammation

Malignant Neoplasm

Malignant (deadly) neoplasms are so named because they exhibit characteristics of invasion and metastasis. **Invasion** refers to the spreading of the neoplasm into local or surrounding tissue. **Metastasis** (meh-TAS-tah-sis) is the spread of the neoplasm to distant sites. The general term for any malignant neoplasm is *cancer*.

Tissue of Origin

Neoplasms are classified or named according to the tissue from which they grow along with the suffix "oma" for tumor. A benign tumor will have the suffix "oma" added after the name of the tissue. An example would be lipoma, a benign tumor of fatty tissue. A malignant neoplasm will have the term **carcinoma** (KAR-sih-NO-mah) or **sarcoma** (sar-KOH-mah) added to the name of the tissue type.

Epithelial Tissue (Skin or Gland)

A benign tumor of epithelial tissue such as a gland would be adenoma; if it is a malignant neoplasm, the name becomes adenocarcinoma. *Carcinoma* denotes the largest group of malignant neoplasms and indicates

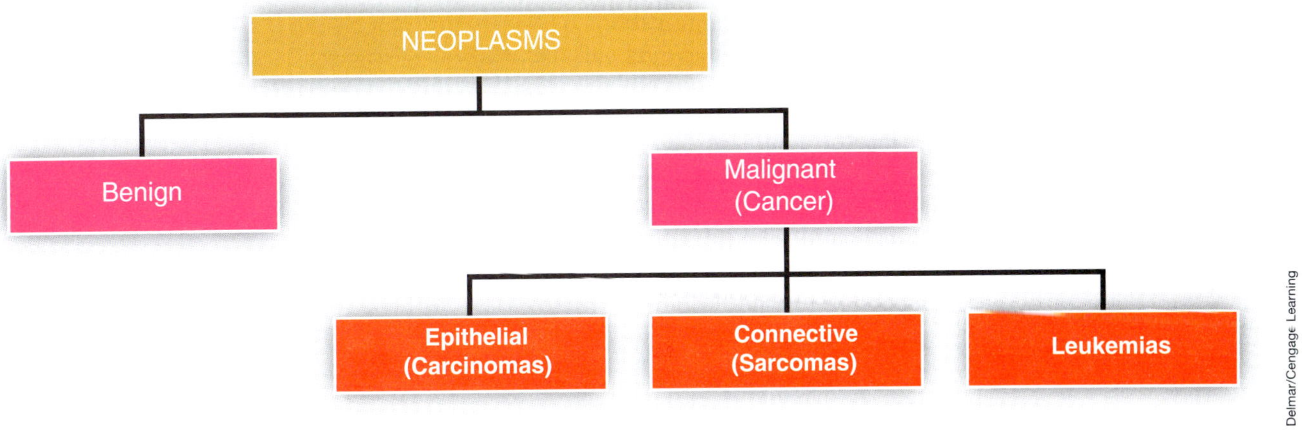

FIGURE 3–2 Classification of neoplasms.

a tumor of epithelial tissue found on external or internal body surfaces.

Connective Tissue (Bone, Muscle, or Fat)

A benign tumor of connective tissue such as bone would be an osteoma; if it is a malignant neoplasm, the name is osteosarcoma—*sarcoma* is the term used if the neoplasm is from connective tissue such as muscle, fat, and bone. Sarcomas are less common than carcinomas but spread more rapidly and are highly malignant.

Lymphatic or Blood-Forming Tissue

Lymphomas (lim-FOH-mas) and leukemias are malignant neoplasms of lymphatic and blood-forming organs and lymphatic tissues, respectively. These malignant neoplasms do not have benign counterparts. All leukemias and lymphomas are malignant, although their prognoses can vary considerably (Figure 3–2).

Other Tissues

Some tumors, of course, do not follow this pattern. For example, malignant melanoma, a malignant neoplasm of melanocytes (skin cells), is not a benign tumor, as its name would suggest. *Glioma* refers to all tumors of the glial cells of the brain, but gliomas do not fit truly the terms of this classification system. They are benign in appearance and do not metastasize, but they are malignant (deadly) because most are fatal. Examples of benign and malignant neoplasms are listed in Table 3–2.

GROWTH OF BENIGN AND MALIGNANT NEOPLASMS

Normal cells grow and function for a purpose and are regulated by several factors. First, the built-in genetic program of each cell regulates its growth pattern. Second, normal cellular growth is limited by contact with other cells. When two normal cells come in

TABLE 3–2 Origins and Names for Benign and Malignant Neoplasms

Cell or Tissue of Origin	Name of Benign Neoplasm	Name of Malignant Neoplasm
Glandular epithelium	Adenoma	Adenocarcinoma
Squamous epithelium	Epithelioma	Squamous cell carcinoma
Adipose (fat)	Lipoma	Liposarcoma
Cartilage	Chondroma	Chondrosarcoma
Bone	Osteoma	Osteosarcoma
Glial		Glioma
Blood		Leukemia

contact with one another, they tend to stick together and transmit a signal called contact inhibition to each other to stop growing (Figure 3–3).

Finally, normal cellular growth is regulated by growth-promoting or growth-inhibiting substances. When the normal cells stop growing, they begin performing their specialized function. For example, epithelial cells begin functioning to cover and protect the organism, whereas bone cells function to provide structure and support. This process of individual specialization is called **differentiation** (Figure 3–4).

Benign Neoplasm Growth

Benign neoplasm or tumors might retain some normal structure and function. These cells often resemble cells of their origin, and even though they have an abnormal appearance, their appearance is uniform. Benign neoplasms also can function to some degree like normal cells. They are encapsulated, or covered with a capsule-like material, that makes removal or excision easier. These tumor cells have a limited growth potential and are slower growing than metastatic neoplasms.

Benign neoplasms are expansive (grow and enlarge in the area) but are not invasive or metastatic. This does not mean that benign tumors are harmless. The presence and growth of any tumor can obstruct passageways such as those in the digestive and respiratory systems, leading to difficulty with eating or breathing.

Tumors also can exert pressure on nerves, causing pain and loss of sensation or movement.

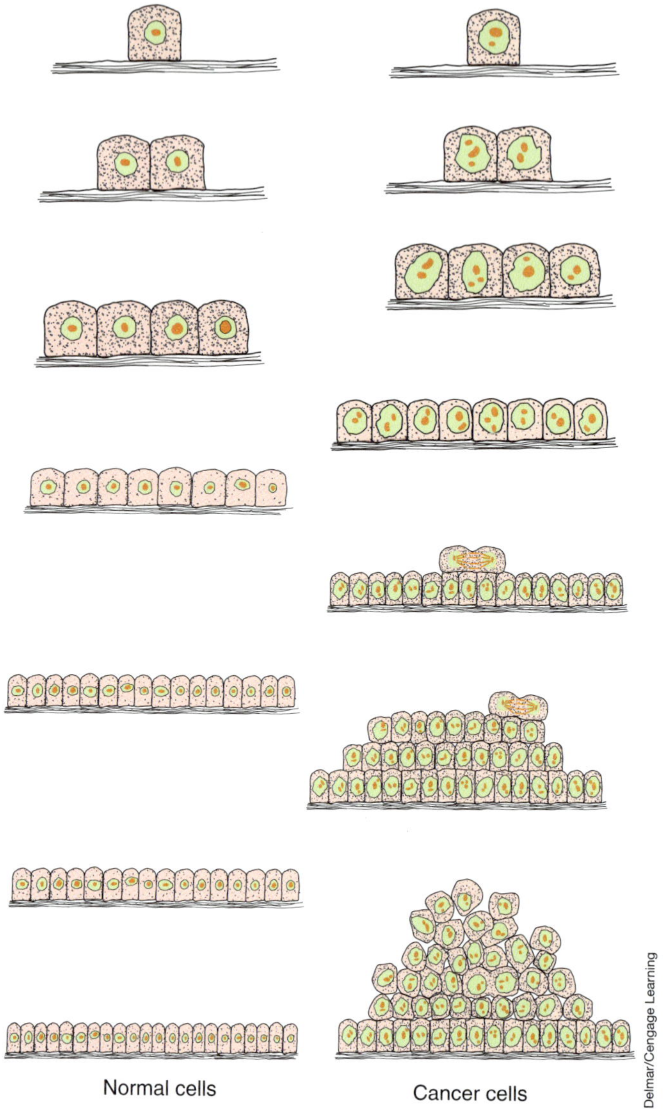

FIGURE 3–3 Cellular growth patterns.

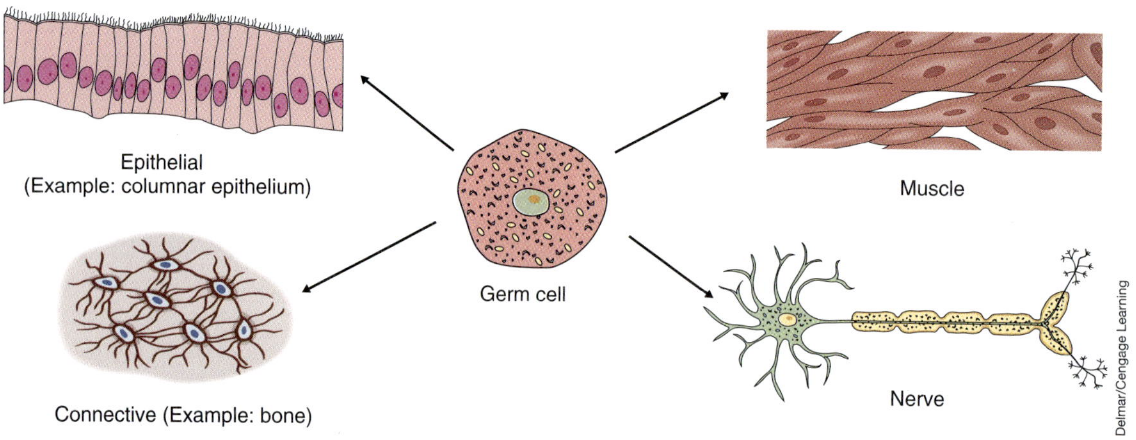

FIGURE 3–4 The process of cell differentiation.

Benign tumors affecting a gland might cause over- or under-secretion of hormones, with resulting disorders. A benign tumor growing in an enclosed area such as the brain can place pressure on normal tissue, leading to death of the tissue and, potentially, death of the individual.

Malignant Neoplasm Growth

Malignant neoplasms are cells whose growth pattern has no purpose and is uncontrollable. Neoplastic cells grow autonomously or independent of growth factors. These cells grow excessively, without regard to normal regulatory factors such as contact inhibition.

Malignant neoplastic cells do not have the structure or function of the cells of their origin. Unlike benign tumor cells, neoplastic cells do not look alike. Their structure is not uniform but rather is haphazard and inconsistent. They are not differentiated and do not perform specialized functions. The surface area of the malignant neoplasm is not encapsulated. Rather, it is more crab-like in appearance, with multiple claw-like extensions that invade surrounding tissue. A malignant neoplasm (cancer) also metastasizes to distant areas or organs. A comparison of benign and malignant neoplasms is listed in Table 3–3.

Cancer (malignant neoplasm) cells are fast growing. The entire metabolism of the cancerous cell is aimed at rapid reproduction and growth, far outpacing the growth of the normal cell, and leads to an increase in the need for nutrients and oxygen. To meet this need, **angiogenesis** (AN-jee-oh-JEN-eh-sis; angio = vessel, genesis = growth or new growth of blood vessels) occurs to increase blood flow, providing increased nutrients to the neoplasm and allowing it to continue this rapid, uncontrolled growth. During this time, normal cells are deprived of needed nutrients, and the individual begins to lose weight and appear thin, frail, and weak, a condition called **cachexia**.

HYPERPLASIAS AND NEOPLASMS

It is important to note that there is another type of cellular growth that closely resembles a neoplasm. **Hyperplasia** (HIGH-per-PLAY-zee-ah; hyper = too much, plasia = growth) and neoplasia (neo = new, plasia = growth) are both overgrowths of cells that cause an increase in the size of the tissue.

Both commonly produce masses that, once discovered, must be identified as either hyperplasia or neoplasm because the treatment of each is drastically different. Hyperplasias and neoplasms differ in the cause and extent of their growth.

Hyperplasias

Hyperplasia usually occurs in response to a stimulus, and the growth stops when the stimulus stops. Hyperplasias can be caused by a variety of stimuli. An example of a hyperplasia caused by tissue irritation is a skin callus on the foot; the stimulus is the irritation or rubbing of a shoe on that particular area. When the shoe size is corrected, the stimulus ends, the hyperplasia stops, and the callus eventually disappears.

Hyperplasias can develop due to hormone excess or deficiency such as the hormone deficiency hyperplasia causing enlargement of the thyroid gland, called goiter. Chronic inflammation can also lead to hyperplasia, as in lymph node hyperplasia or adenoid hyperplasia. Finally, hyperplasia can be caused by an unknown stimulus, as in the case of prostatic hyperplasia in older men.

TABLE 3–3 Comparison of Benign and Malignant Neoplasms

Feature	Benign	Malignant
Growth	Slow, expansive	Fast, invasive, metastatic
Appearance	Symmetrical	Crab-like
Capsule	Yes	No
Tissue type	Resembles tissue of origin	Does not resemble tissue of origin
Cells	Differentiated	Undifferentiated
Surface	Smooth	Irregular, may ulcerate and hemorrhage

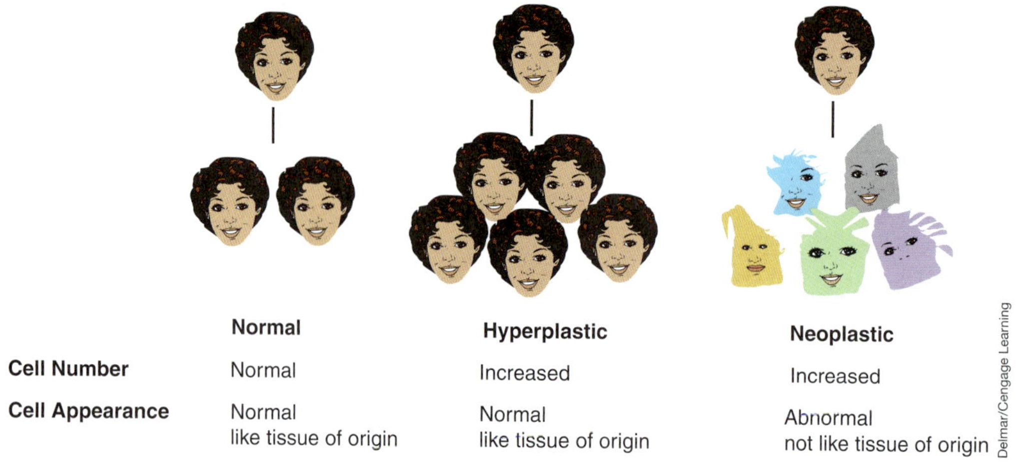

FIGURE 3–5 Comparison of hyperplasia and neoplasm.

Hyperplasias are an increase of cells that look like cells of their origin. To simplify this concept, one might consider the cells as daughter cells that still look like their mother (Figure 3–5).

Neoplasms

Hyperplasias and neoplasms both represent an increase in cell number, but neoplasms grow independently, excessively, and usually unceasingly.

Neoplasms are not only an increase in cell number but new (neo = new) or different in their appearance from their cell of origin, or mother, unlike hyperplasia. This difference in appearance is important to the clinical pathologist who determines or diagnoses the mass as hyperplasia or neoplasm.

DEVELOPMENT OF MALIGNANT NEOPLASMS (CANCER)

Genetic alteration is the basis for the development of malignant neoplasm, or cancer. Cells throughout the body can undergo genetic alteration or mutation, but amazingly, few develop into cancer. A cell must undergo a change or series of changes in its DNA structure to acquire the altered growth pattern of cancer. Genetic mutation or change is brought about by a virus, chemicals, **radiation** (the process of using light, short waves such as ultraviolet or X-ray), or other biologic agent called a **carcinogen** (kar-SIN-oh-jen; carcino = cancer, gen = arising), or cancer-causing agent or substance.

Continued exposure to a carcinogen or to several carcinogens can increase or promote the abnormality of the cell. Abnormal cells might revert to normal cells, appear as benign tumors, or digress to a malignant neoplasm. The body's immune system might prevent or reverse the development of cancer. Just removing or stopping the carcinogen can also reverse cancer development.

If development is not halted, abnormal cells begin to establish themselves in an effort to become cancerous and must now grow rapidly enough to establish a site. They must fight for space and nutrition, so the body and the abnormal cells are at odds with each other at this point. If the body wins, the abnormal cells might die out and disappear. If the abnormal cells attain the upper hand, they can become established and thrive.

As long as the abnormal cells are not firmly established, they are considered preneoplastic or precancerous. If these cells are discovered at this point, surgical removal can occur before cancer actually develops. Unfortunately, very few potential cancers are discovered at this stage. Squamous epithelial tissue often progresses through a slow series of changes, including hyperplasia, abnormal hyperplasia called **dysplasia** (DIS-PLAY-zee-ah), and, finally, a stage called **carcinoma in situ**.

In carcinoma in situ, the atypical cells are "just sitting" in the epithelial layer of the tissue and have not broken through the basement membrane and invaded the surrounding tissue. Carcinoma in situ commonly occurs in the uterine cervix, larynx, and mouth. Cancer can be avoided at this stage by surgical removal of the dysplasia, or in situ tumor.

The final stage in cancer development is the invasion by the precancerous cells into the surrounding tissue, signifying a change from precancerous to malignant neoplasm. In epithelial tissue, this is the point at which neoplastic cells (carcinomas) break

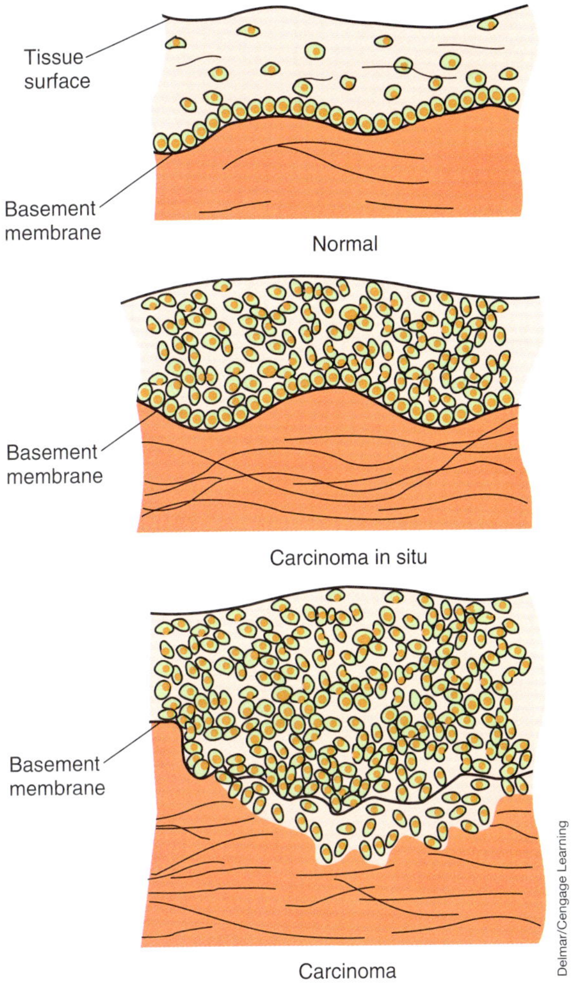

FIGURE 3–6 Normal, carcinoma in situ, and carcinoma tissue.

through the basement membrane that separates the epithelium from the connective tissue below (Figure 3–6). When this break occurs, the neoplastic cells can spread quickly, not only with local tissue invasion but via the lymphatic system (lymph fluid) and circulatory system (blood).

INVASION BY AND METASTASIS OF CANCER

Local invasion by cancer is similar to the way plants sink their roots into the soil. The finger-like projections of the neoplasms force themselves along the lines of least resistance. Pressure from the growing tumor occludes blood supply, leading to local tissue necrosis, weakening the tissue, which eases further spread of the neoplasm.

Spread of cancer from this primary location or site to secondary sites in the body is called metastasis. Cancer cells are carried, or metastasize, through the lymphatic system or through the blood. In some cases, metastasis occurs by seeding or spreading within a cavity.

Lymphatic System Metastasis

Carcinomas—epithelial tissue neoplasms—commonly spread through the lymphatics or lymphatic system. Because lymph nodes can catch or filter cancer cells, lymph nodes are commonly removed surgically and examined for the presence of cancerous cells. Lymph nodes near the tumor are generally the first to filter cancerous cells. As more and more neoplastic cells spread into the lymphatic system, the filters fill with neoplastic cells and, eventually, the nodes become full and unable to filter more cells. When this occurs, the neoplastic cells can spill over into the bloodstream.

Absence of lymph node involvement with cancer is a favorable sign and can mean that surgical cure is possible. Usually, the higher the number of lymph nodes involved, the poorer the chance of survival.

Bloodstream Metastasis

Sarcomas do not use the lymphatic system as readily as carcinomas (Table 3–4). These tumors shed neoplastic cells directly into the blood, by which they can be widely distributed throughout the body. Common sites of bloodstream metastasis are the liver, lungs, and brain. Frequently, and unfortunately, it is the secondary cancer site that is discovered first.

Cavity Metastasis

Metastasis can also occur by invasion and implantation within a serous (watery or fluid-filled) cavity. When neoplastic cells reach a serous cavity such as the pleural or peritoneal cavity, they can seed and implant freely within that cavity.

TABLE 3–4 Comparison of Carcinomas and Sarcomas

Feature	Carcinoma	Sarcoma
Tissue	Epithelial	Connective
Occurrence	Very common	Less common
Growth	Slow	Rapid
Metastasis	Primarily through lymph	Primarily through blood

StudyWARE™ Connection

View an animation about the metastasis of cancer on your StudyWARE™ CD-ROM.

GRADING AND STAGING OF CANCER

Grading and **staging** of malignant tumors are used to plan treatment and predict possibility of a cure. Grading determines the degree of abnormality of the neoplasm, and staging considers the degree of spread.

Grading

Grading is the microscopic examination of the tumor to determine the degree of differentiation. The more differentiated the tumor, the more it looks like the tissue of its origin. The more abnormal the tissue appears in comparison to its normal tissue, the more undifferentiated or **anaplastic** (AN-ah-PLAST-ic) it is. The higher the degree of differentiation, the better the prognosis.

Tumors that are undifferentiated or anaplastic do not resemble the tissue of origin, are highly malignant, and offer a poor prognosis. Tumors are typically placed into grades from I to IV. Grade I tumors are the less aggressive and serious, whereas grade IV tumors are the most aggressive and serious in nature.

Staging

Staging determines the extent of spread of the neoplasm. Clinical examination, X-rays, **biopsy** (BYE-op-see; removing a small piece of tissue for microscopic examination), and surgical exploration can be used to evaluate the degree of spread. Tumors can be placed in stages according to a numerical system (I to IV), much like the system described for grading.

A second, more detailed staging is the TNM system. In this system, tumors are staged according to the size and extent of the primary tumor, number of lymph nodes involved, and metastasis to other sites.

Grading and staging are two predictors of prognosis. Of the two predictors, staging is the better indicator.

CAUSES OF CANCER

Unfortunately, the actual cause of most cancer is unknown. Cancer appears to occur due to a variety of circumstances, which suggests that more than one factor is involved in its development. One thing remains constant in the development of cancer: the genetic alteration that allows the cell to grow independently and uncontrollably. It is thought that cellular mutations actually occur frequently in humans. It is further theorized that the human immune system catches and destroys these abnormal cells as soon as they occur. So, in some respects, cancer might represent some failure of the immune system in the individual. Prevention and cure of cancer will depend on finding the initiating agents that cause the genetic alteration in the cell or the event that causes an altered cell to become malignant. Currently, hundreds of carcinogenic compounds have been identified.

The process of **carcinogenesis** (KAR-sin-oh-JEN-eh-sis; cancer development) in an individual might take many years to develop, might stop and start, or might even be reversed, but usually there will be a continual progression of cellular changes from hyperplasia to dysplasia to **metaplasia** (MET-ah-PLAY-zee-ah) to neoplasia (Figure 3–7).

Chemical Carcinogens

Chemical carcinogenesis is quite complex. The frequency of exposure and the strength or potency of the chemical are important factors in the development of cancer. Chemicals that do not cause a problem by themselves might enhance cancer development when used in combination with other chemicals.

Chemical carcinogens abound in our environment, and exposure to certain chemicals used in industry can lead to cancer among workers. For instance, naphthylamine, found in certain types of dye, has been found to cause bladder cancer; asbestos, previously used in roofing and insulating materials, has been identified as a carcinogen leading to lung cancer. Miners of nickel ore have a high rate of nasal cancer, and farmers using arsenic as an insecticide often suffer from skin and lung cancers.

Currently, chemicals used as food additives, cosmetics, and certain plastics are the focus of intensive research investigating the possible relationship of these chemicals to cancer.

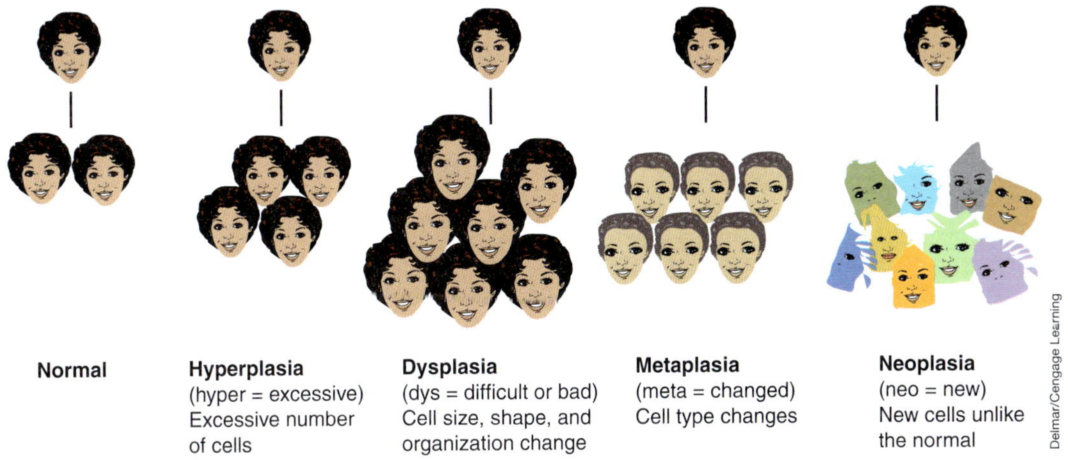

FIGURE 3–7 Cellular changes progressing to neoplasm.

Hormones

Hormones can increase the incidence of cancer, yet, at times, hormones can be used as a form of cancer treatment. The action of hormones as related to cancer is not clearly understood. For example, a benign mole normally does not become malignant until sex hormones increase at puberty, but administration of diethylstilbestrol, a synthetic estrogen compound, to pregnant women during the 1940s and 1950s led to an increase in a rare vaginal adenocarcinoma in their female children and to testicular abnormalities in their male children.

Excessive production of estrogen in the female can lead to cancer of the breast and uterus. Estrogen medication used to treat menopausal symptoms in women has been shown to lead to an increase in endometrial cancer. The ovaries are sometimes removed after a female has breast cancer in an effort to decrease stimulation of other possible tumors.

Although much research had been done to correlate cancer with birth control pills, the findings are inconclusive. The most widely used combination pill, combining estrogen and progestin, a synthetic form of progesterone, might actually decrease the risk of ovarian and endometrial cancer.

Cancer of the prostate is stimulated by the male hormone testosterone but is slowed or inhibited by estrogen treatment. Males who suffer with prostatic cancer can undergo treatment with estrogen medication to counteract the effects of testosterone. Treatment to decrease testosterone production might also include an orchiectomy—removal of the testes—in an effort to decrease or slow the growth of the prostatic tumor or decrease stimulation of other possible tumors.

Radiation

Ultraviolet (UV) radiation, X-radiation, and radioactive materials are all known carcinogens. More than 1 million cases of skin cancer are diagnosed each year (American Cancer Society, 2008). Sunbathers, farmers, fishermen, construction workers, mariners, and anyone else with an extended exposure to the UV rays of the sun or tanning lights have an increased risk of developing basal or squamous cell carcinomas. Although basal and squamous cell carcinomas tend to occur from cumulative exposure to the sun, melanoma occurs more frequently due to extreme, blistering burns at a young age. Fair-skinned people are at greatest risk for skin cancer because they lack the protective effects of melanin. UV-related skin cancer is uncommon among the black population.

X-rays have been used extensively as a diagnostic tool since discovery by Wilhelm Roentgen in 1895. Radiologists commonly developed cancers before the correlation of radiation and cancer—Roentgen himself developed skin cancer. In the late 1800s, radiation dosage was determined by taking repeated X-rays of the operator's hand, and soon after X-ray discovery, the development of the first hand cancer was reported. Presently, radiation is considered a professional risk for radiologists and those working in the field of radiology, but with proper use of protective clothing and equipment, the risk is minimal.

High doses of radiation might actually be used as treatment for some cancers, but this treatment does carry a risk of developing secondary tumors. These tumors usually develop after a lengthy period of time (20 to 25 years), which makes the benefits of radiation therapy far outweigh its risk.

Radioactive materials that emit alpha, beta, and gamma rays are potential carcinogens. Most of these materials are used in medicine and research and are under strict regulation. With the use of protective clothing, the risk to workers in these areas is minimal. The most devastating and dramatic link between radiation and cancer was the increase shown in leukemia and thyroid cancers in the survivors of the atomic bombs dropped on Hiroshima and Nagasaki in 1945.

Viruses

Viruses have been proven to cause cancer in laboratory animals, but the proof is not as clear-cut in humans. Some examples worth noting include the Epstein-Barr virus, which causes infectious mononucleosis and has been associated with Burkitt's lymphoma, a malignant neoplasm seen primarily in Africa. Hepatitis B virus has been closely connected to liver cancer. Individuals with cervical cancer also tend to have the herpes simplex virus.

Genetic Predisposition

There is some evidence of genetic predisposition for cancer, as demonstrated by the increased occurrence of certain types of cancers in the same family. This knowledge has led to intensive research. Discovery of certain cancer suppressor genes, and most recently a breast cancer gene, has aided research efforts, but complete understanding of the correlation of genetics and cancer has not yet been reached.

It is known that colon and breast cancer have a higher incidence in certain families. A woman whose mother or sisters have or have had breast cancer runs a fivefold greater chance of developing breast cancer than women who do not have this family history. Genetic testing is now available for the breast cancer gene.

Personal Risk Behaviors

Several personal behaviors common in our society—smoking cigarettes and other tobacco product use, some dietary practices, alcohol use, and certain sexual behavior—put an individual at increased risk for developing cancer.

Smoking and Tobacco Product Use

Cigarette smoking is carcinogenic. Approximately 440,000 deaths occur yearly from tobacco use (Centers for Disease Control [CDC], 2005). According to the CDC, smoking kills more people in the United States each year than car accidents, alcohol, AIDS, murders, illegal drugs, and suicides combined. It is the major cause of lung cancer. Cancer of the lung is 15 times greater in smokers than in nonsmokers.

Smoking also doubles the incidence of cancer of the bladder and pancreas. Chemicals in cigarette smoke affect all organs of the body because the chemicals are absorbed from the lungs into the blood and circulated to all organs. These chemicals are found in increased concentrations in the urine of smokers. Secondhand smoke has now also been proven to be detrimental, leading to approximately 3,000 deaths per year in nonsmokers.

The chemicals in smokeless tobacco are absorbed into the blood and, again, circulate to the entire body with detrimental effects. Oral cancer occurs more frequently in users of smokeless tobacco than in nontobacco users.

Diet

Identifying the carcinogenic nature of dietary practices is difficult because many factors are involved. Diet seems to function over a period of time to place an individual at risk for cancer. There is a consistent relationship between increased weight in women and the risk of cancer, although there is not a relationship between the two for men. Obesity and a high consumption of dietary fat in women is a consistent risk factor for endometrial, breast, and colon cancer.

Much controversy exists concerning food additives, especially saccharin and nitrates. Saccharin has been shown to cause bladder cancer in rats, but this correlation has not been clear in humans. Nitrates are used as preservatives in meat and fish and have been shown to produce stomach cancer in animals. Countries with high nitrate consumption, Japan for example, have high rates of gastric cancer.

Colon cancer rates are lower in countries that have a lower consumption of dietary fat and a higher consumption of dietary fiber than the United States. The western plains area of the United States is high in selenium and has the lowest colon cancer rates, thus supporting the concept of some correlation between selenium levels and colon cancer.

Alcohol Use

Cancer of the mouth, throat, and esophagus occurs more often in people who smoke and consume large quantities of alcohol. Alcohol has not been proven as a carcinogen per se, but recent studies have also shown a higher incidence of breast cancer in women who drink even moderate amounts (three drinks per week).

Sexual Behavior

The risk of developing cervical cancer is related to the age of first sexual intercourse and the number of sexual partners. The younger the female and the larger the number of sex partners, the greater the risk, and females who have only one sexual partner are at risk if that partner has had multiple partners. Recent medical studies have confirmed that human papilloma virus (HPV) is associated with most cervical cancers and that it is easily transmitted between partners (American Cancer Society, 2008).

The incidence of cervical cancer is two times greater in black women than in white and is found more commonly in women from lower socioeconomic groups. Women marrying men whose previous sexual partners had developed cervical cancer also are at greater risk of developing cervical cancer.

Pregnancy and childbirth appear to be protective mechanisms from cancer of the ovary, endometrium, and breast for women. Females who start menstrual cycles at a later age, have early menopause, bear the first child at an early age, or experience some or all these behaviors are at decreased risk for breast cancer.

CANCER PREVENTION

Cancer of the lung, breast, and colon are responsible for the majority of cancer deaths. Many of these cancers can be prevented by lifestyle changes. Smoking and tobacco use lead to approximately 30% of all cancers. Cigarette smoking is considered the single most preventable cause of lung cancer, other diseases of the lung, and heart disease.

Diet and nutrition play a significant role in the prevention of cancer. **Preventive** measures include reduction of fat intake and an increase in consumption more high-fiber food such as bran, whole grains, and fibrous vegetables and fruits. Monitor caloric intake and exercise properly.

Americans' passion for a suntan encourages people to lie in the sun and use tanning lights. The most widespread cancer—skin cancer—can be prevented by avoiding unnecessary exposure to the sun and tanning lights. If exposure to the sun is necessary, the use of a sunblock agent with 15 or higher sun protection factor (SPF) is recommended.

The American Cancer Society recommends the following preventive measures.

- Do not smoke. Smoking damages nearly every organ in the body, is associated with at least 15 cancers, and accounts for about one third of all cancer deaths. This lifestyle behavior choice is the most preventable cause of early death in our society.
- Limit alcohol intake. Women should not drink more than one drink per day and men no more than two per day. Heavy drinking increases the risk of cancer of the esophagus, mouth, throat, larynx, and liver.
- Protect skin from excessive sun exposure. Use SPF 15 or greater when outdoors. Approximately 1 million cases of nonmelanoma skin cancer diagnosed yearly in the United States is thought to be sun-related.
- Refuse needless X-rays. Take special precautions to protect the unborn child if X-rays are necessary.
- Avoid heavily polluted air and long exposure to household solvent cleaners, paint thinners, and the like.
- Follow label instructions carefully when using pesticides, fungicides, and other home garden and lawn chemicals.
- Maintain a healthy body weight. Eat fewer fatty foods and more high-fiber food such as bran, whole grains, and fibrous vegetables and fruits.
- Women should perform breast self-examinations regularly.
- Exercise regularly. The recommendation is 30 minutes of moderate to vigorous activity at least 5 days a week. Those who engage in regular moderate exercise might lower their chance of developing cancer by 30%.
- Routine HPV vaccination is recommended for girls 11–12 years old to prevent HPV infection. Gardasil is the only FDA-approved vaccine. It will not treat an existing infection.

GLIMPSE OF THE FUTURE

Dendritic Cell Vaccines for Cancer

Researchers are testing the effectiveness of dendritic cell vaccines for preventing tumor growth and extending life in patients with cancer. Dendritic cells are immune-stimulating cells in the human body. These cells occur naturally in tissues such as the skin and the lining of nose, lungs, stomach, and intestines. Because they stimulate antigen-specific immunity after injection, they may be used for cancer treatment in the future.

Source: Ballestrero, et al. (2008).

- Have regular checkups by physicians. For women over 50, a mammogram is recommended as part of the routine examination. Also, the **Pap test** (a test to screen for cervical cancer) should be performed at regular intervals.
- The American Cancer Society no longer recommends monthly testicular self-exams for men because it has not been shown to affect early diagnosis. However, the Society does recommend that men report to their health care provider changes in how the testicle feels or looks (American Cancer Society, 2007).
- A rectal examination should be part of every medical checkup for men and women, and stool samples should be examined for blood, which might be an indication of colon cancer.

HEALTHY HIGHLIGHT

Breast Awareness and Self-Examination

Beginning in their 20s, women should be told about the benefits and limitations of breast self-exam (BSE). Women should be aware of how their breasts normally look and feel and report any new breast changes to a health professional as soon as they are found. Finding a breast change does not mean there is cancer.

Women can notice changes by being aware of how their breasts normally look and feel and by feeling their breasts for changes (breast awareness) or by choosing to use a step-by-step approach and using a specific schedule to examine their breasts.

Again, women with breast implants can do BSE. It may be helpful to have the surgeon help identify the edges of the implant so that you know what you are feeling. There is some thought that the implants push out the breast tissue and actually make it easier to examine.

If you choose to do BSE, the following information provides a step-by-step approach for the exam. The best time for a woman to examine her breasts is when the breasts are not tender or swollen. Women who are pregnant, breast-feeding, or have breast implants can also choose to examine their breasts regularly. Women who examine their breasts should have their technique reviewed during their periodic health exams by their health care professional. It is acceptable for women to choose not to do BSE or to do BSE occasionally.

Women who choose not to do BSE should still be aware of their breasts and report any changes without delay to their doctor.

HEALTHY HIGHLIGHT

How to Examine Your Breasts

1. Lie down and place your right arm behind your head. The exam is done while lying down and not standing up. This is because when lying down, the breast tissue spreads evenly over the chest wall and it is as thin as possible, making it much easier to feel all the breast tissue.
2. Use the finger pads of the three middle fingers on your left hand to feel for lumps in the right breast. Use overlapping, dime-sized circular motions of the finger pads to feel the breast tissue.

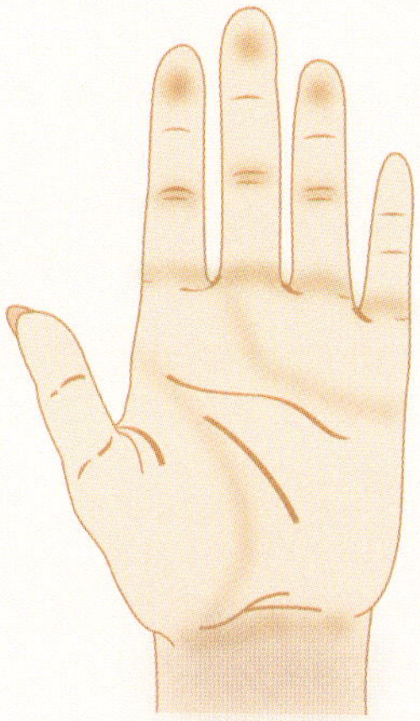

American Cancer Society, Inc.

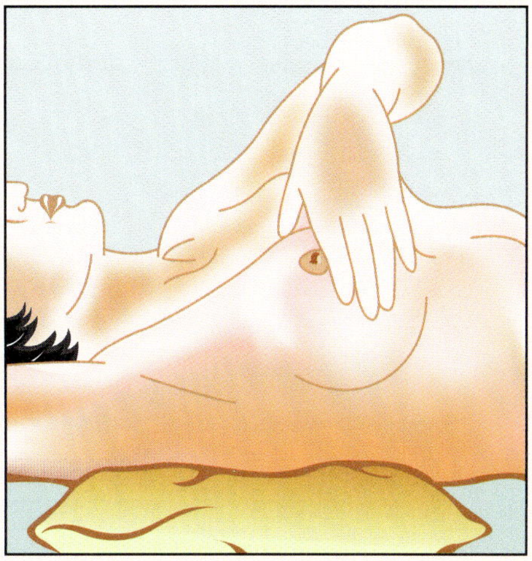

American Cancer Society, Inc.

3. Use three levels of pressure to feel all the breast tissue. Light pressure is needed to feel the tissue closest to the skin, medium pressure to feel a little deeper, and firm pressure to feel the tissue closest to the chest and ribs. A firm ridge in the lower curve of each breast is normal. If you are not sure how hard to press, talk to your doctor or nurse. Use each pressure level to feel the breast tissue before moving on to the next spot.
4. Move around the breast in an up-and-down pattern, starting at an imaginary line drawn straight down your side from the underarm and moving across the breast to the middle of the chest bone (sternum or breastbone). Be sure to check the entire breast area, going down until you feel only ribs and up to the neck or collar bone (clavicle).
5. There is some evidence to suggest that the up-and-down pattern (sometimes called the vertical pattern) is the most effective pattern for covering the entire breast without missing any breast tissue.
6. Repeat the exam on your left breast, using the finger pads of the right hand.
7. While standing in front of a mirror with your hands pressing firmly down on your hips, look at your breasts for any changes of size, shape, contour, dimpling, or redness or scaliness of the nipple or breast skin. (The pressing down on the hips position contracts the chest wall muscles and enhances any breast changes.)
8. Examine each underarm while sitting up or standing and with your arm only slightly raised so you can easily feel in this area. Raising your arm straight up tightens the tissue in this area and makes it difficult to examine.

(*continued*)

HEALTHY HIGHLIGHT (continued)

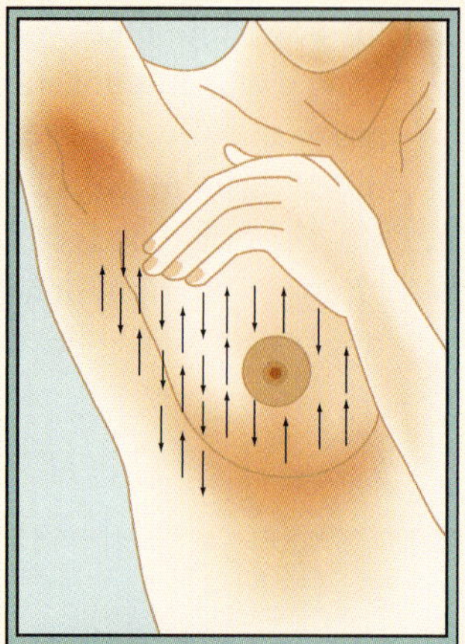

Breast Self Examination
Examine up to the collarbone, out to armpit, in to middle of chest, and down to bottom of rib cage

This procedure for doing breast self-exam is different than previous procedure recommendations. These changes represent an extensive review of the medical literature and input from an expert advisory group. There is evidence that the woman's position (lying down), area felt, pattern of coverage of the breast, and use of different amounts of pressure increase the sensitivity of BSE as measured with silicone models. Lying down also made it easier to feel lumps while doing CBE using patient models with known small noncancerous lumps in their breasts.

Source: American Cancer Society Web site, www.cancer.org. Reprinted by the permission of the American Cancer Society, Inc.

FREQUENCY OF CANCER

Cancer is a focus of major concern for our society because it strikes more than a million individuals per year. Cancer, along with heart disease, causes more than half of all deaths in the United States. One in two men and one in three women will be diagnosed with cancer during their lifespan. Since 1990, over 11 million cases of cancer have been diagnosed, with 5 million deaths occurring. One out of four deaths (1,500 per day) is due to cancer. It affects many lives, causing extreme grief, suffering, and financial loss. However, over 7.5 million Americans who have or have had cancer are still alive.

The term *cancer* covers a large number of specific types of malignant neoplasms. Each of these types might vary considerably from each other in behavior and treatment, and the prognosis for these individual types will depend on the individual cancer's metastatic rate, the extent of spread when discovered, and the effectiveness of current treatments.

In general, the survival rate of cancer is approximately 50%. Even though all malignant neoplasms might fit into a classification of carcinomas, sarcomas, leukemias, or lymphomas, there is a great difference in the way they behave. Some types, such as pancreatic carcinoma, are usually deadly, whereas skin carcinoma seldom is.

Cancer affects people of all ages and both male and female. The most common type of cancer is basal and squamous cell skin cancer. These neoplasms are seldom fatal because they are very visible, slow growing, and can be completely excised. Because these tumors are generally treated in a physician's office, they are difficult to track statistically and are usually excluded in statistical data. Malignant melanoma, however, is a deadly form of skin cancer that comprises approximately only 1% of all skin malignancies but is statistically recorded as skin cancer.

The most common types of cancer, excluding skin cancers, are cancers of the lung, colon, breast, uterus, and prostate. The common sites for cancer in the male and female are presented in Figures 3–8 and 3–9.

Lifetime Probability of Developing Cancer, Men, US, 2002–2004*

Site	Risk
All sites†	1 in 2
Prostate	1 in 6
Lung & bronchus	1 in 13
Colon & rectum	1 in 18
Urinary bladder‡	1 in 27
Melanoma	1 in 41
Non-Hodgkin lymphoma	1 in 46
Kidney	1 in 59
Leukemia	1 in 67
Oral cavity	1 in 71
Stomach	1 in 88

*For those free of cancer at beginning of age interval.
† All Sites exclude basal and squamous cell skin cancers and in situ cancers except urinary bladder.
‡ Includes invasive and in situ cancer cases
Source: DevCan: Probability of Developing or Dying of Cancer Software, Version 6.2.1 Statistical Research and Applications Branch, NCI, 2007. http://srab.cancer.gov/devcan

Lifetime Probability of Developing Cancer, Women, US, 2002–2004*

Site	Risk
All sites†	1 in 3
Breast	1 in 8
Lung & bronchus	1 in 16
Colon & rectum	1 in 19
Uterine corpus	1 in 41
Non-Hodgkin lymphoma	1 in 53
Melanoma	1 in 61
Ovary	1 in 71
Pancreas	1 in 76
Urinary bladder‡	1 in 85
Uterine cervix	1 in 142

*For those free of cancer at beginning of age interval.
† All Sites exclude basal and squamous cell skin cancers and in situ cancers except urinary bladder.
‡ Includes invasive and in situ cancer cases
Source: DevCan: Probability of Developing or Dying of Cancer Software, Version 6.2.1 Statistical Research and Applications Branch, NCI, 2007. http://srab.cancer.gov/devcan

FIGURE 3–8 Lifetime probability of developing cancer by site and sex.

2009 Estimated US Cancer Cases*

Men 766,130		Women 713,220	
Prostate	25%	27%	Breast
Lung & bronchus	15%	14%	Lung & bronchus
Colon & rectum	10%	10%	Colon & rectum
Urinary bladder	7%	6%	Uterine corpus
Melanoma of skin	5%	4%	Non-Hodgkin lymphoma
Non-Hodgkin lymphoma	5%	4%	Melanoma of skin
Kidney & renal pelvis	5%	4%	Thyroid
Leukemia	3%	3%	Kidney & renal pelvis
Oral cavity	3%	3%	Ovary
Pancreas	3%	3%	Pancreas
All other sites	19%	22%	All other sites

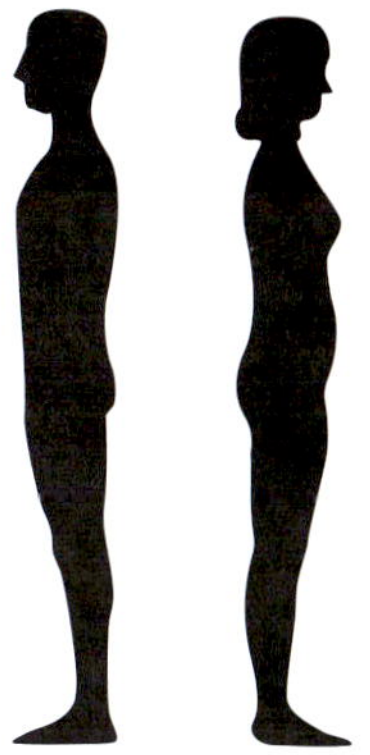

*Excludes basal and squamous cell skin cancers and in situ carcinomas except urinary bladder.
Source: American Cancer Society, 2009.
Source: American Cancer Society, 2004.

2009 Estimated US Cancer Deaths*

Men 292,540		Women 269,800	
Lung & bronchus	30%	26%	Lung & bronchus
Prostate	9%	15%	Breast
Colon & rectum	9%	9%	Colon & rectum
Pancreas	6%	6%	Pancreas
Leukemia	4%	5%	Ovary
Liver & intrahepatic bile duct	4%	4%	Non-Hodgkin lymphoma
Esophagus	4%	3%	Leukemia
Urinary bladder	3%	3%	Uterine corpus
Non-Hodgkin lymphoma	3%	2%	Liver & intrahepatic bile duct
Kidney & renal pelvis	3%	2%	Brain/ONS
All other sites	25%	25%	All other sites

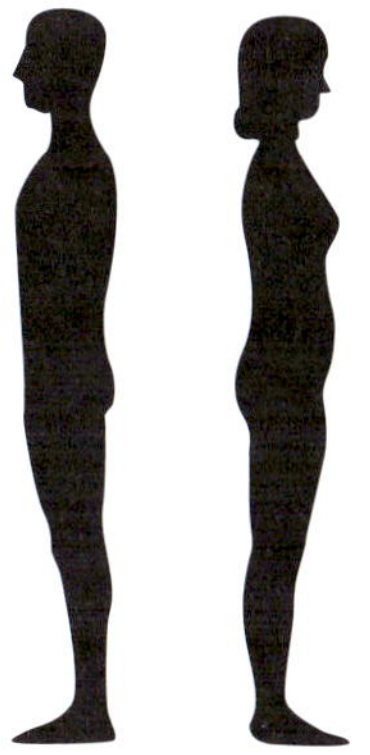

ONS=other nervous system.
Source: American Cancer Society, 2009.

FIGURE 3–9 Leading sites of new cancers and deaths.

DIAGNOSIS OF CANCER

The prognosis for the individual with a malignant neoplasm is best if the cancer is located and treated early. Routine screening can be very effective in discovery and early diagnosis of cancer. Screening measures include monthly breast self-examinations, regular Pap tests, and mammograms for females. Screening for males no longer includes a routine testicular self-examination, but any change in how the testicle feels or looks should be noticed and reported to the individual's physician. Occult stool examinations after age 40 to screen for colon cancer is important for both sexes.

Discovery of tumors can occur through routine screening or accidentally during other diagnostic procedures. For instance, X-ray examinations of the chest prior to surgery might reveal a mass, or annual physical examinations can lead to the discovery.

Recognition of cancer warning signs by an individual is important. The American Cancer Society lists several of these signs, with the initial letters forming the acronym CAUTION. They might be indicative of cancer development, so the individual with one or more of these signs should be evaluated immediately by a physician.

- Change in bowel or bladder habits
- A sore that does not heal
- Unusual bleeding or discharge
- Thickening or lump in breast or elsewhere
- Indigestion or difficulty swallowing
- Obvious change in a wart or mole
- Nagging cough or hoarseness

When discovered, more detailed radiologic exams such as computerized tomography (CT), magnetic resonance imaging (MRI), and positron emission tomography (PET) can be used to gain more information on size and location of tumor(s). (More detailed information on these exams can be found in Chapter 6, "Musculoskeletal System Diseases and Disorders," and Chapter 8, "Cardiovascular System Diseases and Disorders.")

Diagnosis of a tumor is made by microscopic examination of the cells and tissue. Examination of cells is called **cytology** (sigh-TOL-oh-jee; cyto = cell, ology = study) or a cytologic examination. Live tissue examination is a biopsy, which is the most definitive (clear-cut or without question) test used to diagnose a tumor.

A Papanicolaou, or Pap test, named after its developer, Dr. George Papanicolaou, can be used to examine the cells. Although most people think of a Pap test as a test only for cervical cytology, in reality, this simple staining test can be used to examine other body fluids such as urine, feces, sputum, prostatic fluid, or vaginal fluids. After the sample is stained, it is placed under a microscope and examined for abnormal cells.

To microscopically examine live tissue, a biopsy must be done. A biopsy can be obtained by aspiration, needle biopsy, endoscopy, or surgery. Aspiration biopsy uses a needle attached to a suction device to remove a small piece of tissue from the tumor. Needle biopsy is obtained by punching a needle through the tumor and using the tissue caught in the lumen of the needle for examination. If the size of the needle is quite small, the biopsy is called a fine needle biopsy. During endoscopy, the tissue is removed by use of the appropriate scope, for example, bronchoscope, colonoscope, or gastroscope. For surgical biopsy, the tissue is removed by cutting or incising the tissue (Figure 3–10).

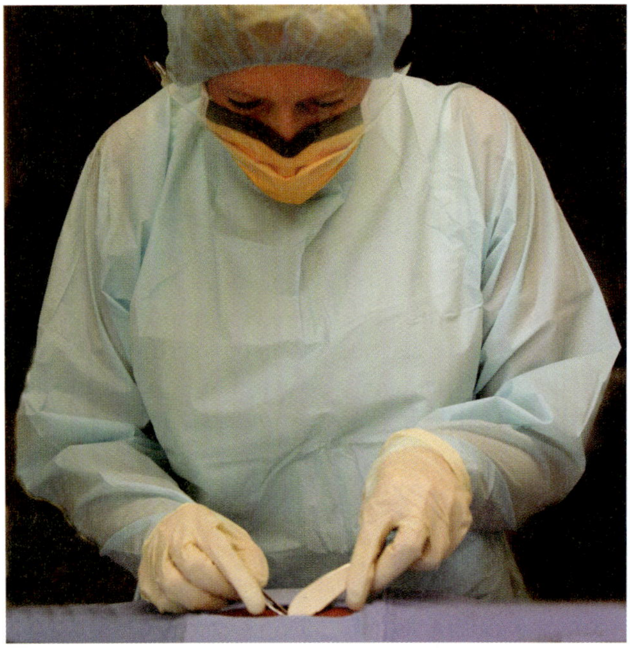

Courtesy of Mark L. Kuss

FIGURE 3–10A Tissue biopsy. A small piece of tissue is surgically removed.

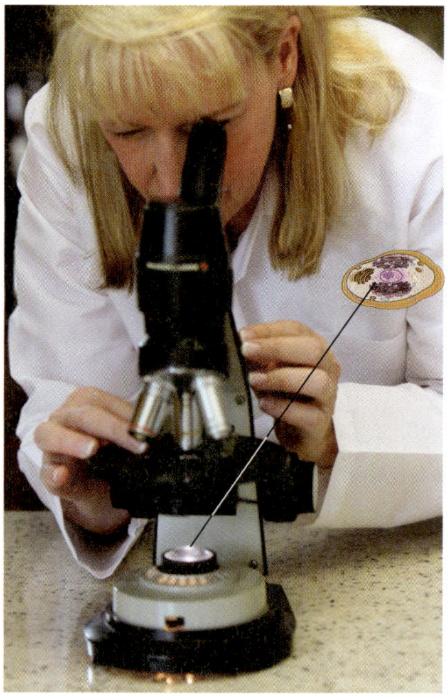

Courtesy of Mark L. Kuss

FIGURE 3–10B Pathologist views tissue under microscope looking for presence of disease.

Surgical biopsy can be performed with the patient's consent to excise the tumor if it is found to be cancerous. After the biopsy is obtained, it is sent immediately to the pathologist for diagnosis. The patient often remains in the surgical suite under anesthesia while the surgeon awaits these results. A technique called a **frozen section** enables the pathologist to make a rapid determination of the tumor condition: benign or malignant.

SIGNS AND SYMPTOMS OF CANCER

Signs and symptoms of cancer are highly variable according to the site and type of malignancy. Pain, obstruction, hemorrhage, anemia, fracture, infection, and cachexia might be manifestations of cancer. Any one of these or a combination can be present, but often, cancer is asymptomatic until late in its developmental stage, including metastasis.

Pain

Pain from cancer is usually not an early symptom. Cancer causes pain by growing to the point of causing destruction of normal tissue, obstructing the lumen of hollow organs like the intestine, placing pressure on nerve endings, causing inflammation leading to discomfort, or any of these.

Obstruction

Obstruction of a hollow organ can occur from a tumor growing inside the organ or from tumor growth outside the organ that compresses or pushes into the organ. Examples of obstruction could include the bronchus of the lung and any area of the intestine.

Hemorrhage

Hemorrhage can be caused by the cancerous tissue ulcerating and bleeding. This might lead to acute or chronic blood loss and often results in anemia. Hidden blood in the feces can be detected by a Hemoccult® stool test.

Anemia

Anemia is very common in individuals with malignant neoplasm and might be the result of tumor hemorrhage or a decrease in red blood cell production as a result of cancer treatments.

Fractures

Pathologic fractures might occur if a tumor has invaded the bone and caused weakness at that site. A fracture occurring from a minimal injury might be indicative of a cancer but, in an older person, might also be due to osteoporosis. The bone tumor might be primary or secondary with cancer of the lung, breast, or prostate readily metastasizing to the bone.

Infection

Infection is common and can lead to the demise of the individual. Tumor ulceration can allow entry of microorganisms that cause infection, or the individual might have impaired immunity due to **chemotherapy** (chemo = chemical, therapy = treatment) and radiation treatments, affecting the bone marrow and causing a decrease in production of white blood cells.

Individuals with cancer often have a loss of appetite, leading to a poor nutritional state and an increase in the chance of infection. Immune deficiency often leads to infection of the individual by a host of organisms such as fungi, viruses, protozoa, and bacteria that are not usually pathogenic.

Cachexia

Cachexia is a condition of general ill health and malnutrition often seen in the terminally ill patient. (Refer to Figure 2–3 in Chapter 2, "Mechanisms of Disease.") This condition is evidence of the demands on the body by the rapidly growing tumor and treatment modalities, coupled with poor nutritional intake.

CANCER TREATMENT

New technological advances lead to ever-changing treatment of malignant neoplasms. Treatment might be aimed at cure (**curative**), at relief of symptoms (**palliative**; PAL-ee-AY-tiv), or at prevention (preventive). Major types of treatment include surgery, chemotherapy, and radiation, and hormone treatment might be the treatment of choice in some instances. The oncologist might recommend one of these treatments or a combination of them, depending on the type of cancer and treatment plan.

Surgery

Surgery for cancer can be curative, palliative, or preventive.

Curative surgery is aimed at complete removal of the tumor. Cancer of the lung, stomach, skin, breast, intestine, and female reproductive organs respond well to this type of surgery.

Palliative surgery is usually indicated when cure is not possible but when surgery will alleviate pain and discomfort. The intestine is an area commonly undergoing this type of surgery for obstruction, bleeding, or perforation. Surgery also might be performed to sever nerves in an effort to reduce pain.

Preventive surgery might be performed to prevent development of cancer. Polyps in the colon can be removed if they are thought to be precancerous, and a woman might choose to undergo prophylactic mastectomy if she has been identified as one at high risk for breast cancer.

Chemotherapy

Chemotherapy can be the medication of choice or used in combination with surgery and radiation therapy. Generally, chemotherapy is effective to treat rapidly growing metastatic neoplasms. It is aimed at rapidly growing neoplastic cells with the idea that it will kill or inhibit the growth of these cells while having minimal effect on normal cells.

In some instances, the growth rate of normal cells and neoplastic cells is not varied enough, and normal body cells suffer from the effects of the treatment. Rapidly growing normal cells such as those found in the epithelium, hair, and bone marrow suffer the most, leading to nausea, vomiting, loss of appetite, hair loss, anemia, and impaired immunity.

Radiation

Radiation is generally used in treatment of residual neoplasm postoperatively and to treat tumors that are not surgically accessible or operable. Palliative radiation treatments can shrink the tumor and relieve discomfort. Radiation treatment can be external with direct radiation or internal, using radioisotope beads, seeds, or ribbons that are implanted inside the body. Both methods are aimed at disrupting DNA and interfering with cell growth and replication.

The goal is to destroy as much of the tumor as possible without affecting the normal tissue surrounding it. Adverse effects generally occur in the skin, mucous membranes, and bone marrow, leading to nausea, vomiting, loss of appetite, hair loss, and impaired immunity.

Hormone Therapy

Hormone therapy can cause regression in tumors of the breast and prostate. Administration of antagonistic hormones or excision of hormone-producing organs such as the ovaries and testes can be effective in prolonging life. Hormone therapy is generally used as a palliative treatment for metastatic tumors.

COMPLEMENTARY AND ALTERNATIVE THERAPY

Alternative Therapies for Breast Cancer: A Good Idea or Not?

Alternative therapies are frequently used by breast cancer patients. Many women choose alternative treatments in lieu of the standard treatments. There are some significant outcome issues that women who choose to use these therapies need to consider. This research study showed that alternative therapies used as the main treatment for breast cancer may result in increased recurrence of the disease and even death. Most women in the study who delayed or opted out of surgical intervention, chemotherapy, or radiation had greater progression of the disease. This information might assist women to make a knowledgeable decision about treatment for breast cancer.

Source: Chang, et al., (2006).

SUMMARY

Neoplasms are new growths, either benign or malignant, that can arise from cells almost anywhere in the body. *Tumor* is the term commonly used to describe a neoplasm, but not all neoplasms form tumors. Hyperplasias are similar to neoplasms because they are an overgrowth of cells, but they resemble their cell of origin, whereas neoplasms do not. Neoplasms that are malignant are usually called cancers and are usually named for the type of tissue from which they developed. Metastatic cancers are those that spread to other parts of the body.

The cause of most cancer is unknown, but research has identified high-risk behaviors as well as some carcinogens in the environment that might contribute to cancer development. The American Cancer Society has recommended preventive measures and lists seven warning signs of cancer. Although the mortality rate for cancer in general is still very high in the United States, early diagnosis and treatment can yield a good prognosis for many types of cancer.

REVIEW QUESTIONS

Short Answer

1. What is the difference between a neoplasm and a tumor?

2. How are neoplasms classified?

3. What is the largest group of malignant neoplasms?

4. When a malignant neoplasm moves to various parts or organs of the body, it is said to be a _____ tumor.

5. What is the difference between hyperplasia and neoplasms?

True or False

6. T F Grading is the microscopic examination of the tumor to determine the degree of differentiation.

7. T F Tumors that are undifferentiated or anaplastic do not resemble the tissue of origin, are highly malignant, and have a poor prognosis.

8. T F Radioactive materials that emit alpha, beta, and gamma rays are not considered to be potential carcinogens.

9. T F There is no known genetic predisposition for cancer.

10. T F There are several personal risk behaviors common in our society that put an individual at increased risk for developing cancer.

Matching

11. Match the term in the left column with the phrase that best describes it from the column on the right.

_____ Metastatic neoplasm	a. known carcinogens
_____ Cancer of the lung, breast, and colon	b. an acronym for the seven warning signs of cancer
_____ CAUTION	c. microscopic examination of live tissue
_____ Basal and squamous cell skin cancer	d. responsible for the majority of cancer deaths
_____ Biopsy	e. cells whose growth pattern has no purpose and is uncontrollable
_____ Liver, lungs, and brain	f. common sites of bloodstream metastasis
_____ Ultraviolet (UV) radiation, x-radiation, and radioactive materials	g. the most common type of cancer
_____ Routine screening	h. major types of cancer treatment
_____ Surgery, chemotherapy, and radiation	i. treatment aimed at relieving symptoms
_____ Palliative	j. very effective in the discovery and early diagnosis of cancer

CASE STUDIES

■ Mr. Holloway is a 65-year-old man who has made an appointment for a routine checkup. He has not complained of any unusual symptoms but feels he should have a yearly examination because of his age. What are some routine screening tests that should be performed on Mr. Holloway because of his age and gender? What important cancer prevention strategies should you discuss with Mr. Holloway during his visit?

■ Mrs. Holloway, age 55, is also visiting her physician for routine screening. She is concerned because her sister who is age 47, was recently diagnosed with breast cancer. What types of cancer are most commonly diagnosed in patients like Mrs. Holloway, based on her age and gender? Should she be concerned about developing breast cancer? If she has never performed breast self-exams, what would you tell her about this screening procedure? How could you help her understand the correct procedure for completing a breast self-exam?

*Study***WARE**™ Connection

To help you learn the content in this chapter, take a practice quiz or play an interactive game on your StudyWARE™ CD-ROM.

Workbook Practice

Go to your Workbook and complete the practice questions.

BIBLIOGRAPHY

American Cancer Society. (2007). Cancer statistics 2006. *www.cancer.org* (accessed January 2008).

American Cancer Society. (2007). Detailed guide: Testicular cancer. *www.cancer.org* (accessed January 2008).

American Cancer Society. (2007). How to perform a breast self-exam. *www.cancer.org* (accessed January 2008).

American Cancer Society. (2007). Resources for healthy living, prevention, and early detection. *www.cancer.org* (accessed May 2008).

Ballestrero, A., Boy, D., Moran, E., Cirmena, G., Brossart, P., & Nencioni, A. (2008). Immunotherapy with dendritic cells for cancer. *Advanced Drug Delivery Reviews 60*(2), 173–183.

Centers for Disease Control and Prevention (CDC). (2005). Smoking deaths cost nation 92 billion in lost productivity annually. Atlanta, GA: Centers for Disease Control and Prevention (CDC).

Centers for Disease Control and Prevention. (2007). United States cancer statistics. *www.cdc.gov/uscs/* (accessed January 2008).

Chang, E. Y., Glissmeyer, M., Tonnes, S., Hudson, T., & Johnson, N. (2006). Outcomes of breast cancer in patients who use alternative therapies as primary treatment. *American Journal of Surgery 192*(4), 471–473.

Esper, P., Gale, D., & Muehlbauer, P. (2007). What kind of rash is it? *Clinical Journal of Oncology Nursing 11*(5), 659–666.

Jain, R. K. (2008). Taming vessels to treat cancer. *Scientific American 298*(1), 56–63.

Kandsberger, D. (2007). Factors influencing the successful utilization of home health care in the treatment of children and adolescents with cancer. *Home Health Care Management & Practice 19*(6), 450–455.

Mayo Clinic. (2007). Women's health, birth control pill FAQ: Benefits, risks and choices. Rochester, MN: Mayo Clinic.com Health Library.

McCaughan, E., & McKenna, H. (2007). Never-ending making sense: Towards a substantive theory of the information-seeking behavior of newly diagnosed cancer patients. *Journal of Clinical Nursing 16*(11), 2096–2104.

Molnar, S., Guglielmone, H., Lavarda, M., Rizzi, M. L., & Jarchum, G. (2007). Procoagulant factors in patients with cancer. *Hematology 12*(6), 555–559.

Motzer, R. J., & Basch, E. L. (December 22, 2007). Targeted drugs for metastatic renal cell carcinoma. *Lancet 370*(9605), 2071–2073.

Ortholan, C., Gerald, J. P., Benezery, K., & Francois, E. (2007). State of the art and recent advance in the treatment of resectable nonmetastatic rectal cancer. *Surgical Oncology 16*(Supplement), 125–128.

Radiologic Society of North America. (2008). Positron emission tomography (PET) scanning. *RadiologicInfo* (April 14, 2008), p. 1.

Reis-Fiho, J. S., & Tutt, A. N. (2008). Triple negative tumors: A critical review. *Histopathology 52*(1), 108–118.

Sara, C., Werner, P., & Ziedenberg, H. (2007). Physicians' and nurses' preferences in using life-sustaining treatments. *Nursing Ethics 14*(5), 665–674.

Schwabe, M., & Luppert, M. (2007). Epigenetic lesions in malignant melanoma. *Pharmaceutical Biotechnology 8*(6), 382–387.

Verhoef, M., Weeks, L., Brazier, A., & Leis, A. (2007). Evaluating supportive cancer care: Are we missing an opportunity? *Supportive Care in Cancer 15*(8), 905–907.

Voltz, E., & Gronemeyer, H. (2008). A new era of cancer therapy: Cancer cell targeted therapies are coming of age. *International Journal of Biochemistry & Cell Biology 40*(1), 1–8.

Ward, W. (2007). Tumors masquerading as hematomas. *Clinical Orthopaedics & Related Research 465*(1), 232–240.

Wood, L. S., & Machen, B. (2007). Sorafenib: A promising new targeted therapy for renal cell carcinoma. *Clinical Journal of Oncology Nursing 11*(5), 649–656.

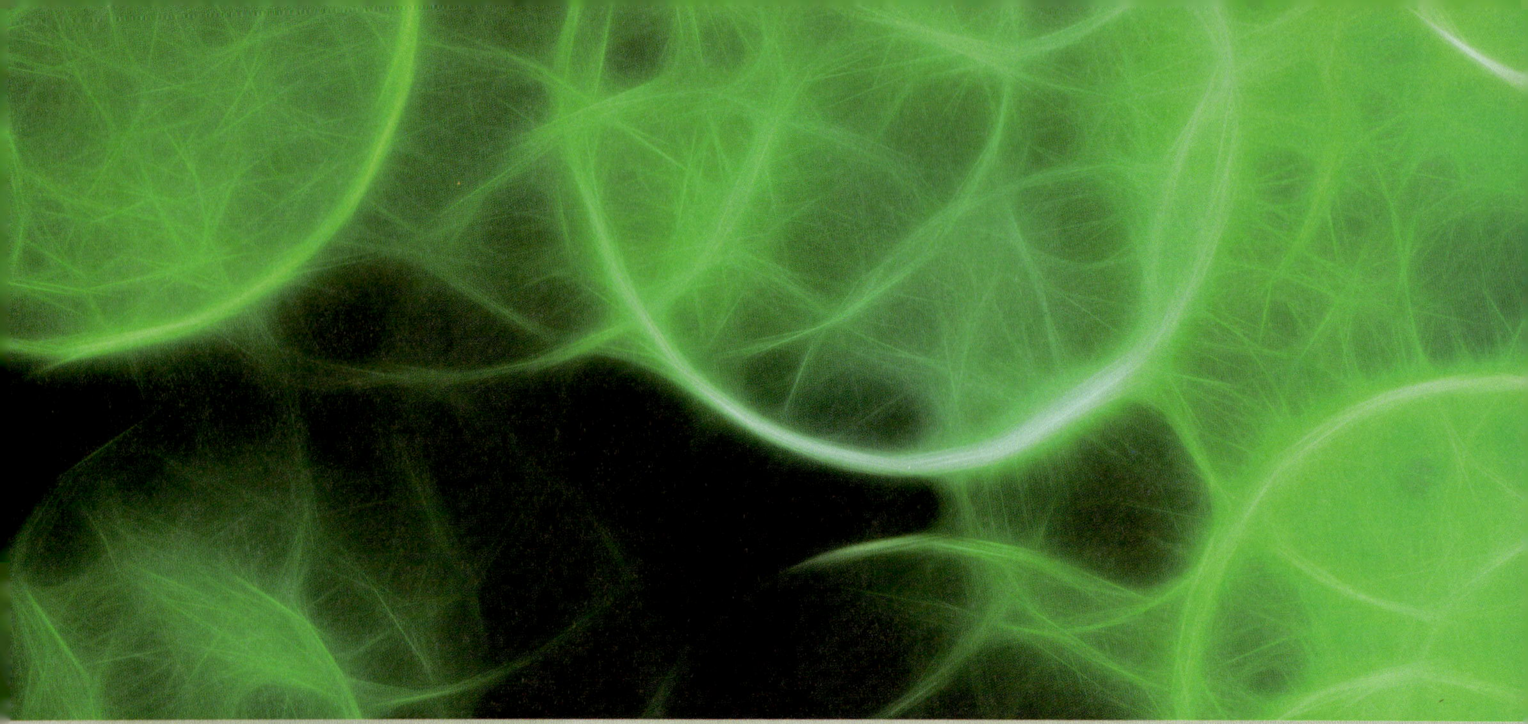

OUTLINE

- Defense Mechanisms
  - *Physical or Surface Barriers (Nonspecific)*
  - *Inflammation (Nonspecific)*
  - *Immune Response (Specific)*
- Inflammation
  - *The Inflammatory Process*
  - *Chronic Inflammation*
  - *Inflammatory Exudates*
  - *Inflammatory Lesions*
- Tissue Repair and Healing
  - *Tissue Repair*
  - *Tissue Healing*
  - *Delayed Wound Healing*
  - *Complications of Wound Healing*
- Infection
  - *Frequency and Types of Infection*
  - *Testing for Infection*
- Summary
- Review Questions
- Case Studies
- Bibliography

KEY TERMS

Abscess (p. 55)
Adhesion (p. 60)
Antibody (p. 55)
Antigen (p. 53)
Bacteria (p. 52)
Cellulitis (p. 55)
Chemotaxis (p. 53)
Culture and sensitivity (p. 64)
Débridement (p. 59)
Dehiscence (p. 59)
Diapedesis (p. 53)
Empyema (p. 55)
Exudate (p. 53)
Fistula (p. 56)
Fungi (p. 60)
Helminths (p. 60)
Histamine (p. 53)
Hyperemia (p. 53)
Induration (p. 65)
Infection (p. 60)
Inflammation (p. 54)
Keloid (p. 59)
Lesion (p. 55)
Leukocytosis (p. 64)
Macrophage (p. 54)
Malaise (p. 64)
Mast cells (p. 53)
Opportunistic (p. 60)
Primary union (p. 57)
Protozoa (p. 60)
Purulent (p. 55)
Pus (p. 54)
Pyogenic (p. 55)
Rickettsiae (p. 60)
Scar (p. 57)
Secondary union (p. 58)
Septicemia (p. 64)
Sinus (p. 56)
Tachycardia (p. 64)
Trauma (p. 53)
Ulcer (p. 56)
Virulent (p. 59)
Virus(es) (p. 60)

4

Inflammation and Infection

LEARNING OBJECTIVES

Upon completion of the chapter, the learner should be able to:

1. Identify important terminology related to the defense mechanisms.
2. Describe the basic defense mechanisms in the body.
3. Explain the steps in the inflammatory process.
4. Describe the process of tissue repair and healing.
5. Identify complications of wound healing.
6. Describe the process of infection development.
7. Identify the common infectious microorganisms and the resulting diseases.
8. Identify the common laboratory test conducted to identify pathogenic organisms.

OVERVIEW

The human body is in a constant state of activity, part of which is to prevent trauma and maintain homeostasis against foreign invaders and pathogens. It maintains defense mechanisms—inflammation is a natural one—for this protection, but when these protective mechanisms fail, the usual result is an infection. Infections are diagnosed and treated in a variety of ways. ■

DEFENSE MECHANISMS

The immune system has the difficult job of protecting the body against foreign invasion. Defense can be nonspecific, protecting the body against any and all invaders; or it can be specific, identifying the invader prior to killing it. This system uses three basic lines of defense to accomplish its protective goals.

Physical or Surface Barriers (Nonspecific)

An intact skin is the body's first line of defense. The skin is a physical barrier and an acidic, antimicrobial surface that is an effective barrier against infection most of the time. The skin has more than 650,000 microorganisms per square inch on its surface, adding up to more than 100 trillion microorganisms per person. The normal bacterial flora of the skin acts as a placeholder, preventing habitation by other **bacteria** (microscopic, one-celled organisms). Sebaceous (oil secreting) and odoriferous (perspiration secreting) glands secrete antibacterial acids and enzymes. Mucous membranes serve to trap invaders.

Inflammation (Nonspecific)

If physical barriers are broken and the foreign invader penetrates the cells and tissues, it triggers the inflammatory response. This response begins a stereotypic vascular response within seconds of an unwanted invasion. In other words, the process unfolds or follows the same pattern regardless of the type of invader. The primary goals of the inflammatory response are to isolate the invader, destroy it, and clean up the debris, thereby promoting healing.

Immune Response (Specific)

The third and last line of defense reacts to invasion much slower than inflammation but with specific killing ability. All cells, even human body cells, have

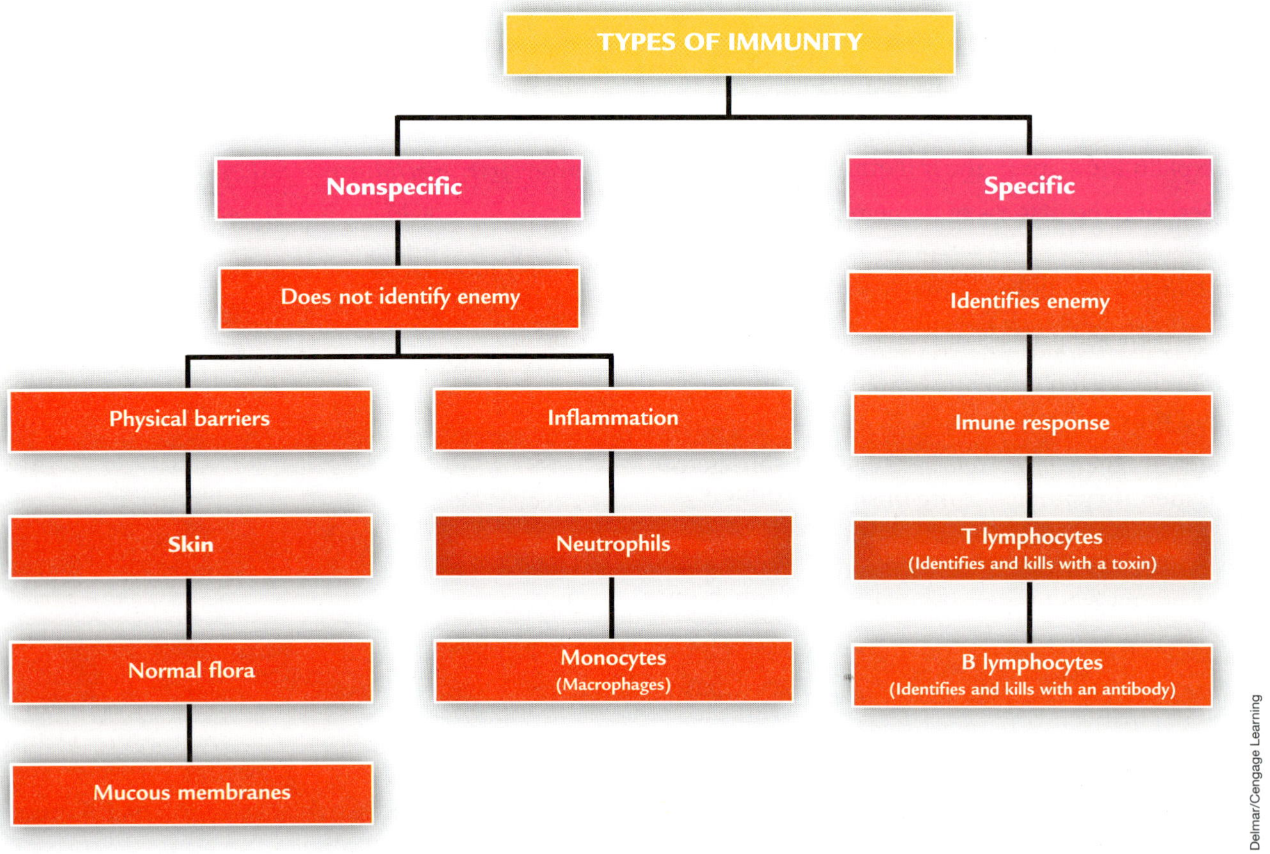

FIGURE 4–1 Immunity—lines of defense.

protein or saccharide markers called **antigens** (AN-tih-jenz) on their surfaces that identify the cell. During the immune response, the body actually identifies the invader by the antigen. Once the antigen is identified, lymphocytes produce **antibodies**. These antibodies link with the cell antigen, thus killing the cell or disabling it. This immunologic defense has the unique ability to remember the invader and produce more antibodies if the invader returns (Figure 4–1).

INFLAMMATION

Inflammation is a nonspecific cellular and vascular reaction to any tissue **trauma** (TRAW-mah; injury). One limiting factor of inflammation, however, is that it cannot occur in tissue that does not have a blood supply.

If tissue is destroyed by injury, the inflammatory process will occur only along borders of the injury where blood supply is maintained. In gangrenous tissue, for example, inflammation cannot occur in the dead or necrotic tissue, but there is an observable reaction along its borders.

The fact that inflammation occurs only in vascularized (supplied with blood) tissue is important in forensic medicine. Evidence of inflammation in tissue confirms that an injury occurred while the individual was alive. If no evidence of inflammation exists, the pathologist can be assured that the person was dead when the injury was inflicted.

Inflammation is designed to be a beneficial, protective defense mechanism. In some instances, the reaction can become so intense that it becomes harmful to tissues. Such an acute hypersensitive reaction can lead not only to local tissue damage but also to anaphylactic shock and death of the individual. If the process goes awry, producing an autoimmune reaction, the body basically begins to destroy itself, and anti-inflammatory medications might be needed to stop the reaction if it becomes injurious.

The Inflammatory Process

When any tissue undergoes trauma, regardless of the cause—physical injury, invasion of microorganisms, ischemia (decreased oxygen in cells), freezing, burning, electrocution, radiation, or chemical irritation, for instance—inflammation will occur.

Mast cells, also called tissue histocytes, exist in all tissues of the body and play a major role in the inflammatory process. When injured or irritated, these cells release **histamine**. Histamine causes local arterioles, venules, and capillaries to dilate, resulting in an increase in blood flow to the area. This increase in blood flow, called **hyperemia** (HIGH-per-EE-me-ah; hyper = increased, emia = blood), causes increased redness and heat in the area.

Hyperemia also brings increased numbers of leukocytes (white blood cells) to the area. The white cells that move into this area first and in the greatest numbers are neutrophils, also called polymorphonuclear cells (PMNs) (poly = many, morphic = shaped nucleus). These white cells line the endothelium of the vessels, awaiting the opportunity to move into the tissue.

As the capillaries dilate under the influence of histamine, vascular permeability occurs. In other words, the capillary becomes permeable, or leaky, as the endothelial cells are stretched apart. This permeability allows blood fluid called **exudate** (ECKS-you-dayt) to leak into the tissue. This leakage of fluid is the cause of the swelling or edema observed with inflammation.

As edema increases, more pressure is exerted on nerve endings, leading to increased pain. With increased pain and tenderness, the individual tends to guard the area and experience loss of function. These vascular and cellular responses produce the five cardinal signs of inflammation: heat, redness, swelling, pain, and loss of function (Figure 4–2).

Vascular permeability also allows the waiting neutrophils to escape into the tissue. The neutrophils extend part of their bodies between the epithelial cells and squeeze through the capillary wall by a process called **diapedesis** (DYE-ah-pe-DEE-sis) (see Figure 4–2). The process of diapedesis is very effective, delivering millions of neutrophils to the area within a few hours.

Neutrophils can be considered the foot soldiers of the inflammatory process. They arrive first, they arrive in great numbers, and they readily move into action in the tissue, drawn or directed to the injured area by a process called **chemotaxis**. One might think of this process as a chemical taxi cab. Chemicals, detected through chemoreceptors on the neutrophil's outer membrane, are released by a variety of elements such as bacteria, injured tissue, and plasma proteins. These chemoreceptors also draw the neutrophil in the direction of the highest chemical concentration (see Figure 4–2).

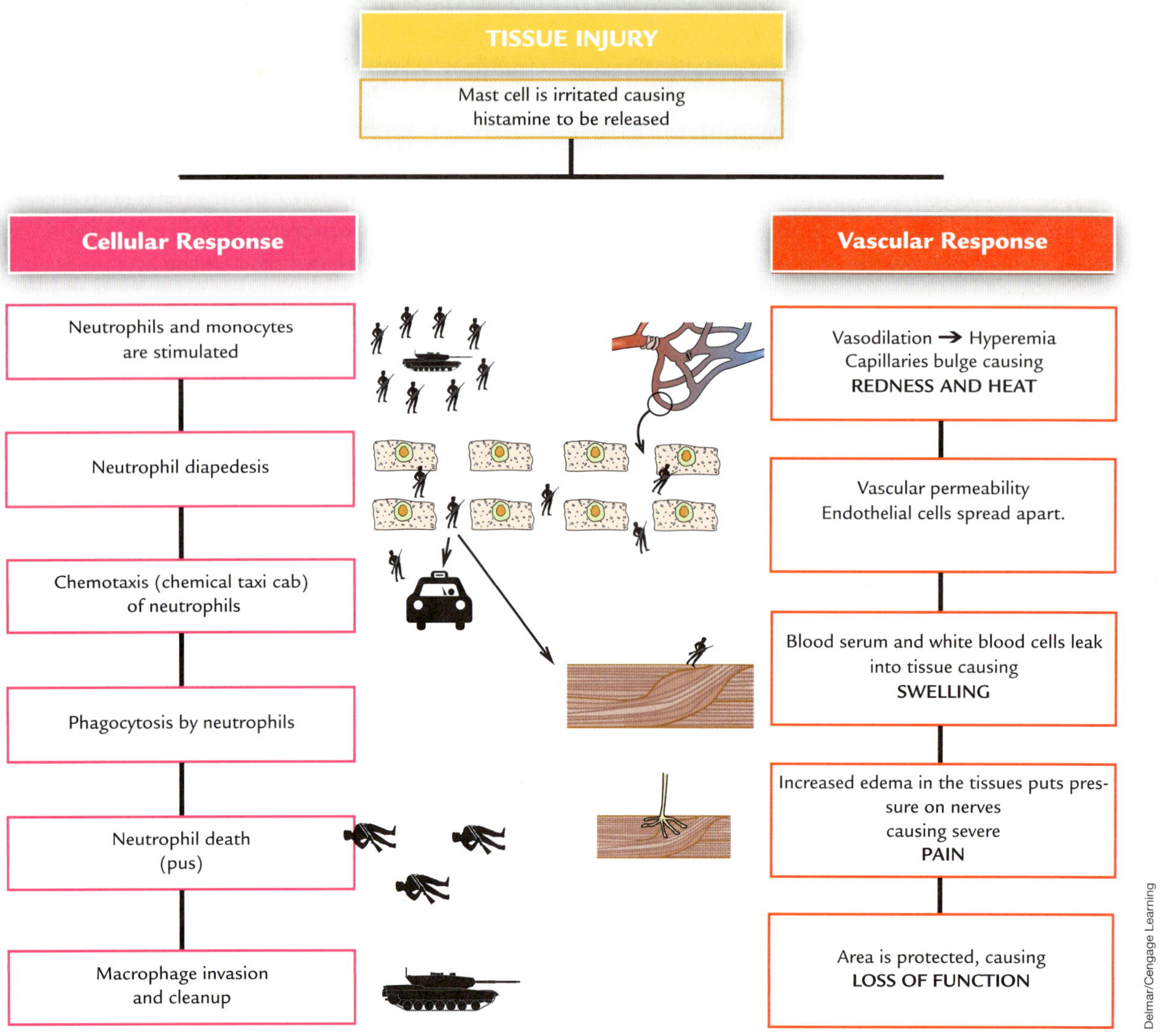

FIGURE 4–2 Acute inflammation—cellular and vascular response.

When the neutrophil arrives at the scene of the trauma, it begins the job of phagocytosis, or cell eating. The neutrophil eats and destroys microorganisms, foreign materials, and dead cells. However, the life of the neutrophil is short. The death of numerous neutrophils mixed with exudate or blood fluid make up, in part, the white fluid identified as **pus**.

Approximately 3 to 4 days after the inflammatory process begins, large numbers of another type of white cell, the large, slow-moving monocyte, begins to arrive at the scene. As the monocyte leaves the bloodstream and moves into the tissue, it too becomes phagocytic and is called a **macrophage** (macro = large, phage = eat). As the name suggests, a macrophage is a large eater of microorganisms, foreign material, and dead cells. This cell might be considered the tank of the war because it is slower moving but has more killing power than the neutrophil. Another job of the macrophage is to act as the clean-up crew, removing the dead neutrophils and tissue debris in the inflamed area.

Until this point, the **inflammation** is considered an acute (short-lived) situation. If the inflammation persists for a longer period of time, it is considered a chronic problem. This time period is difficult to establish because some chronic inflammations will exhibit periods of exacerbation (flare up), eliciting a new outpouring of neutrophils. Likewise, some acute inflammations will trigger the response of an unusually high number of macrophages.

After approximately 7 to 10 days, if the inflammatory process has not overcome the invader, the nuclear warheads of the defense system—the lymphocytes—are called on to respond. Lymphocytes are slow but powerful, specific killers, part of the body's third line of defense: the immune response. They identify the enemy, make an antibody to kill it, and then remember the enemy and the killing process (see Figure 4–1). Refer to Chapter 5, "Immune System Diseases and Disorders," for more detailed information on the immune system.

Chronic Inflammation

Generally speaking, a chronic inflammation can be considered one that lasts 2 weeks or longer. If the acute attack by neutrophils and macrophages is unsuccessful, the battle can become chronic. Microscopic examination of chronic inflammation will reveal a large number of macrophages and fewer neutrophils.

If macrophages are unable to overcome the invader and protect the host, the body might try to isolate the area by forming a granuloma. A granuloma is formed by macrophages and fibrous deposits of collagen and may be hardened by calcium deposits. This granuloma protects the surrounding tissue and allows healing to begin. A classic cause of granuloma formation is tuberculosis. These granulomas may become quite large, form a fibrous rim, and eventually calcify. Another cause of granuloma is foreign body involvement such as a wood splinter, gravel, suture, glass sliver, or metal fragments embedded in the tissue. The body walls off the material to protect the adjacent tissue. This granuloma may become hardened with fibrous tissue and remain for the life of the individual.

Inflammatory Exudates

The duration and extent of an inflammatory **lesion** (LEE-zhun; any discontinuity of tissue) may be determined by direct visualization of the site. External inflammatory lesions are observed easily, whereas internal inflammatory lesions in organs and cavities might require surgical or endoscopic examination. The appearance and amount of exudate or blood fluid can assist in identifying an acute or chronic condition.

Serous Exudate

Serous exudate is a clear, serum-like fluid containing small amounts of protein. It implies a lesser degree of damage and occurs in the acute stage of inflammation. Examples of serous exudate include the fluid in skin blisters, cold sores, and injured joints, for example. Serous exudate is easily reabsorbed after the inflammatory response is halted and healing begins.

Fibrinous Exudate

Fibrinous exudate is composed of fluid and large amounts of fibrinogen. In comparison to serous exudate, the leakage of fibrinogen indicates a larger injury with more severe inflammation. Fibrinous exudate can be observed in strep throat or bacterial pneumonia, forming a mesh-like lesion. A superficial skin wound might be covered with dried fibrinous exudate commonly called a scab.

Purulent Exudate

Purulent (PURR-you-lent) exudate is loaded with dead and dying PMNs or neutrophils, tissue debris, and **pyogenic** (PYE-oh-JEN-ick; pyo = pus, genic = arising), or pus-forming, bacteria. Purulent exudate is commonly called pus. A localized collection of pus is called an **abscess**; an accumulation of pus in a body cavity is called **empyema** (EM-pye-EE-mah). For example, pus accumulated in the chest or thoracic cavity would be called thoracic empyema.

Inflammatory Lesions

Any discontinuity or abnormality of tissue is called a lesion, a broad term that includes wounds, ulcers, wheals, blisters, vesicles, pustules, or tumors, to name a few. Lesions are due to physical or pathologic injury. Inflammatory lesions include abscesses, ulcers, and **cellulitis** (SELL-you-LYE-tis; inflammation of connective tissue).

Abscesses

Abscesses are typically caused by streptococcal and staphylococcal (pyogenic) bacteria. During the inflammatory response, the body attempts to contain or stop the spread of the bacteria into adjacent tissue by forming a wall around the area. When this wall forms around a purulent exudate, an abscess is formed. Boils, furuncles, and pimples are examples of abscesses.

Typically, a small abscess shows signs of acute inflammation: redness, heat, swelling, and pain. When the central portion of the abscess softens or develops a head, puncturing the head will cause an outpouring of pus, relief of pain, and onset of healing. Puncturing the abscess before the area is walled off and the head is soft, however, can lead to a spread of the infecting organism.

A small abscess might rupture and heal spontaneously, but a large abscess might need to be surgically incised and drained. Draining an abscess speeds healing; without drainage, the body must continue to battle the invading organisms. If the body is successful, it will eventually win the battle, reabsorb the exudate, and replace the area with fibrous tissue. A large abscess, such as in appendicitis, can spread and become fatal if not contained. If a large abscess ruptures, it tends to form a tract, or opening to the surface of the skin called a **sinus**. If this tract connects two organs or cavities to each other or to the surface of the skin, it is called a **fistula** (FIST-you-lah) (Figure 4–3).

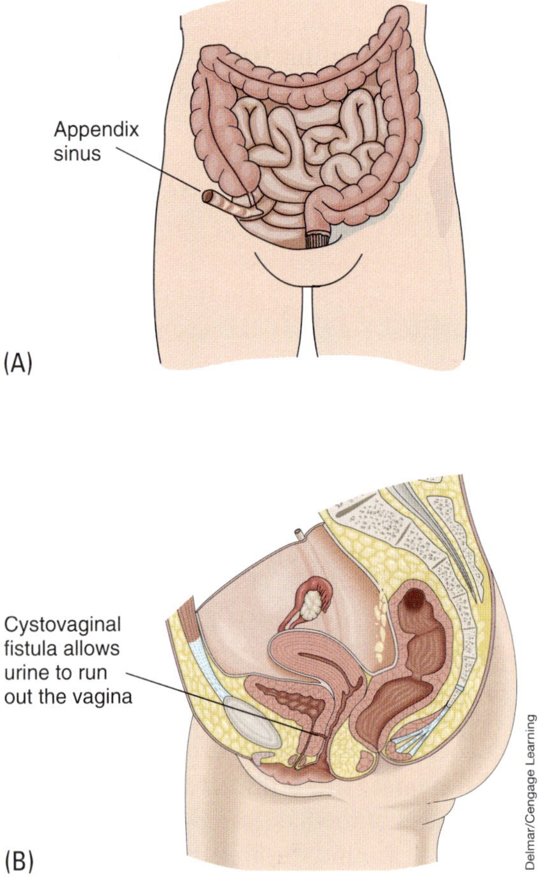

FIGURE 4–3 (A) sinus and (B) fistula.

Ulcer

An **ulcer** is a crater-like lesion in the skin or mucous membrane. It is the result of an injury and the subsequent inflammatory response. The tissue in this area becomes necrotic (dead) and sloughs off, leaving a crater or excavated area. Ulcers are commonly seen in the stomach and duodenum as a result of injury by bacteria and stomach acid. Pressure ulcers, commonly called bedsores or decubitus ulcers, are caused by excessive pressure on tissue. Pressure ulcers primarily appear over bony prominences of the body, especially those affected in the reclining position, such as the heel, sacrum, hip, elbow, and scapula (Figure 4–4).

Cellulitis

Cellulitis is a diffuse, or widespread, acute inflammatory process. It is commonly seen in the skin and subcutaneous tissues. Cellulitis is characterized by general edema and redness. Cellulitis of the face primarily involves the cheeks and periorbital (peri = around, orbital = eye) areas. This type of cellulitis must receive special attention because it can spread to the sinuses of the brain. Cellulitis is often caused by streptococcus or staphylococcus bacteria and is due to the body's inability to confine or wall off the causative organism. Cellulitis is potentially dangerous but usually can be treated effectively with antibiotics.

TISSUE REPAIR AND HEALING

Proper tissue repair and healing is an ongoing process much like any other body process and occurs in most instances, but this process can be influenced by many

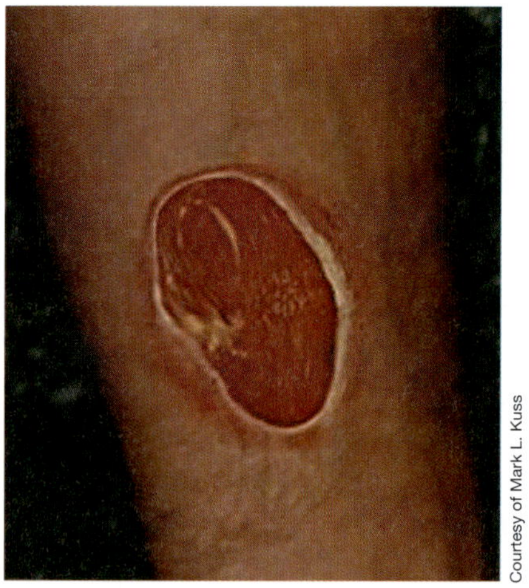

FIGURE 4–4 Pressure ulcer.

other factors. Healing can be impaired or slowed when secondary diseases are present, the body is malnourished, or the immune system is compromised.

Tissue Repair

During the final phase of the inflammatory process, macrophages are responsible for cleaning up the area and producing growth factors that aid the repair process. Repair of tissue also depends on cellular regeneration and the type of cells that make up the tissue. Some cells divide quite readily, but others do not. Cellular proliferation, or division, can be grouped into three general categories.

1. **Mitotic cells** continuously divide throughout life. They exist in the skin and mucosa of internal organs and readily replace damaged tissue.
2. **Facultative mitotic** cells do not divide regularly but can be stimulated to divide when necessary. They exist in such organs as the liver and kidney. Some part of these organs must remain intact for these cells to be available to divide and replace the lost tissue.
3. **Nondividing cells** do not divide under any condition. Cells of this type include central nerves, brain cells, and heart muscle cells. Repair of these tissues is by fibrous scarring.

The body's two basic methods of repair involve healing by regeneration and by fibrous connective tissue repair, or **scar** formation. Regeneration is the best type of repair because it usually leads to restoration of normal function, whereas fibrous connective tissue repair does not.

Regeneration

Regeneration involves mitotic cell division. During regeneration, the damaged tissue is replaced by cellular division of healthy tissue. For example, skin tissue is replaced by epithelial cell division, and bone tissue is replaced by osteocyte division. Regeneration can usually occur in internal organs if the major framework of the organ has not been destroyed. Complex structures such as lung tissue and glomeruli (in the kidney), however, do not regenerate. Regeneration is particularly important when there is damage to a large amount of tissue; for instance, epithelial regeneration is very beneficial with massive burns. Bone cells, osteocytes, and blood-forming bone cells have a remarkable ability to regenerate from a few remaining cells and can be transplanted from another individual by bone marrow transplant.

Fibrous Connective Tissue Repair (Scar Formation)

Fibrous connective tissue repair, or scar formation, can occur in any tissue and produces the same result, no matter the location—a tough, fibrous tissue called a scar. A scar provides a bridge between the normal tissue and the wound, but it does not restore function. Wound repair of nerves, brain tissue, and heart muscle is by fibrous connective tissue repair (Figure 4–5).

Tissue Healing

Tissue healing can be separated into categories of healing by primary union or secondary union. Categorization is determined by whether the wound edges are approximated (pulled together) or left separated during the healing process.

Primary Union (First Intention)

Primary union, also called healing by first intention, involves approximating the edges of the wound. A classic example of healing by primary union is the healing process following a clean surgical incision. The wound edges are clean, there is minimal tissue damage, and the edges are approximated with sutures, staples, or tape.

Primary healing occurs in an orderly fashion. The steps of primary healing include the following:

1. The incisional line quickly fills with serum, forming a scab.
2. Within 1 to 2 days, new capillaries begin to bridge the gap between the wound edges.
3. In the next few days, fibroblasts grow across the deeper wound layers and begin to deposit collagen in this fibrous network. This tissue is called granulation tissue.
4. The collagen begins to contract, pulling the wound edges together and forming a scar.

After a few weeks, the incision might appear healed, but the deeper layers of tissue might not be healed for a month or more. Usually, an incisional scar will pale in color and shrink in size over a period of months or years.

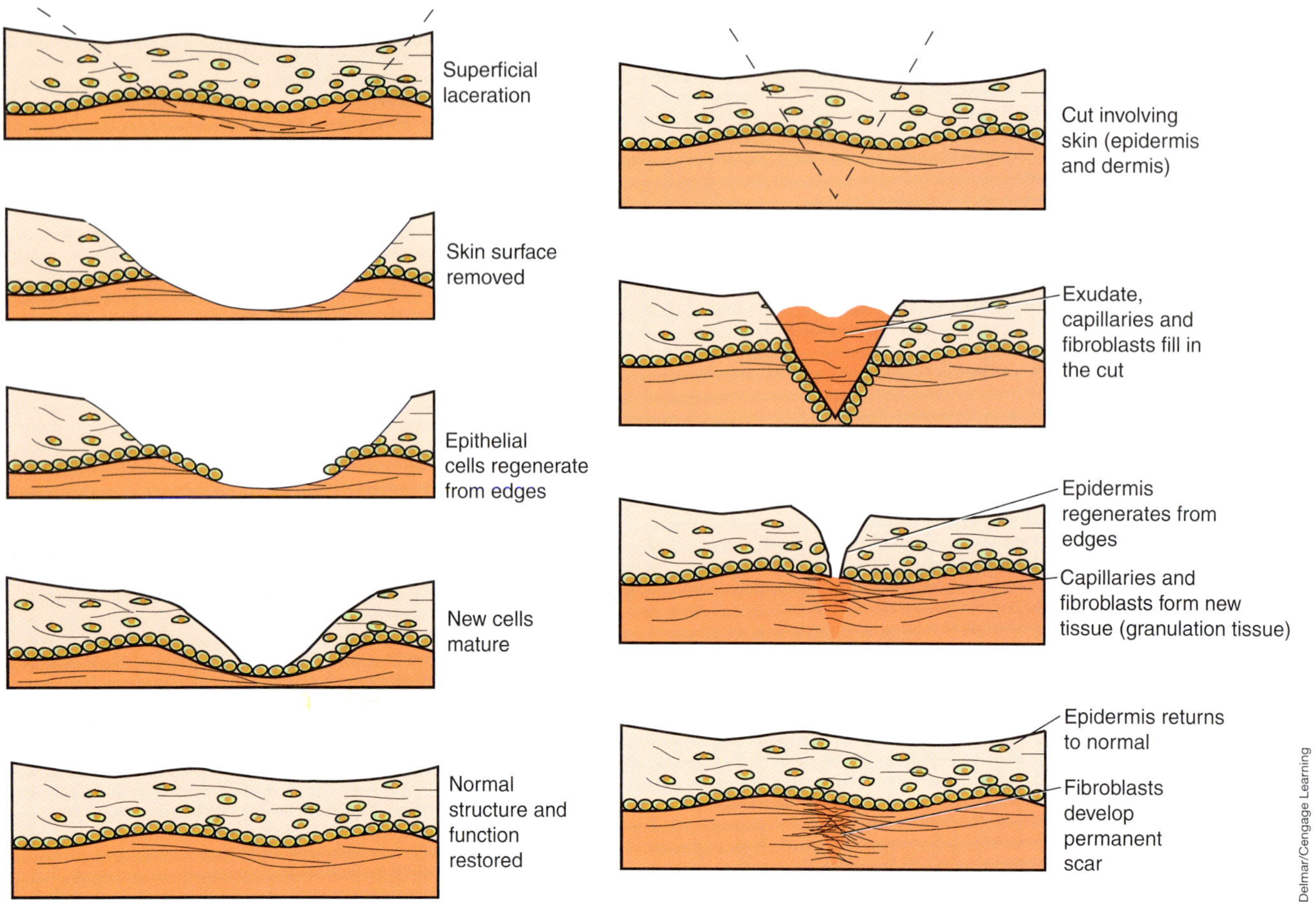

FIGURE 4–5 Tissue repair—complete regeneration and fibrous connective tissue repair.

Secondary Union (Secondary Intention)

Large wounds and those infected by dirt, debris, and bacteria cannot be pulled together to heal by primary intention. The process of healing by **secondary union** is the same process as that of primary union but involves a larger degree of tissue damage and more inflammation to resolve (Figure 4–6). To fill the wound, large numbers of capillaries, fibroblasts, and collagen must be produced. After a week or so, the new, soft, red tissue is called granulation tissue, which is eventually replaced as more collagen is deposited in the area. The collagen contracts, pulling the

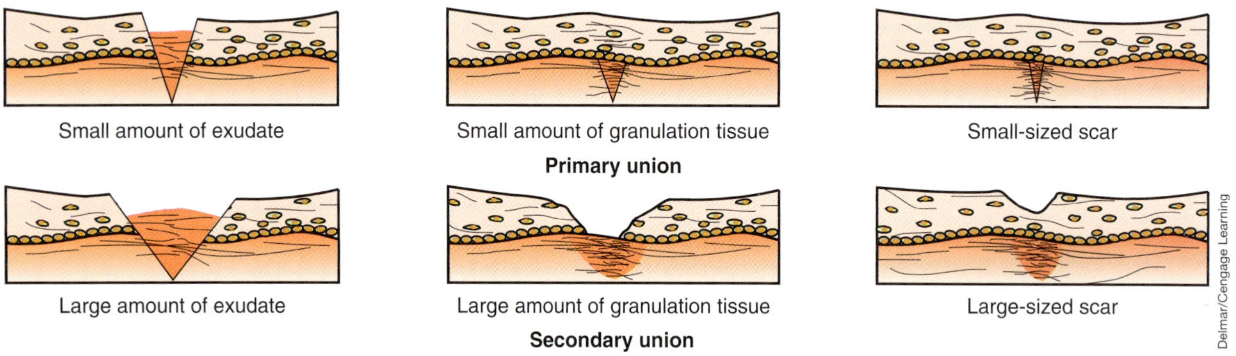

FIGURE 4–6 Tissue healing—primary and secondary union.

wound edges together and beginning the formation of a scar. Healing time varies depending on the size of the wound; large wounds can take a long time to heal by secondary union because additional time will be needed for the scar to develop the strength of the surrounding tissue. If the wound is too large, the epithelium might not be able to bridge the gap, and a skin graft might be needed.

*Study***WARE**™ Connection

View an animation on tissue repair and healing on your StudyWARE™ CD-ROM.

Delayed Wound Healing

One of the greatest impediments to wound healing is the amount of dead tissue and debris—dirt, bacteria, dead leukocytes, or a variety of other contaminates—in the wound. It might take the body's leukocytes weeks or months to phagocytize (eat up) all the debris. In the meantime, bacteria might be producing dead cells and necrotic tissue as fast as the cleanup effort can advance. To speed healing, dirty wounds must be cleaned and débrided. **Débridement** (day-breed-MON), commonly pronounced (day-breed-MENT), is a process of washing or cutting away necrotic tissue and foreign material.

Other factors affecting healing time include the following:

1. **Age** Younger people heal more rapidly than older people.
2. **Size** Smaller wounds heal faster than larger ones.
3. **Location** Epithelial tissue heals rapidly, compared to other tissue types.
4. **Nutrition** Good nutritional status promotes wound healing. Protein and vitamin C are essential to healing.
5. **Immobility** Wound tissue heals more rapidly if it is kept immobile.
6. **Circulation** Tissue with good blood supply heals more rapidly. Epithelial tissue heals more readily than cartilage. Individuals with diabetes have small-blood-vessel disease (diabetic microangiopathy), leading to ischemia of the tissue and poor wound healing.
7. **Organism virulence** Wounds infected with **virulent** (VIR-you-lent; poisonous) microorganisms are slower to heal than those that are not infected.
8. **Steroids** Steroid therapy inhibits the inflammatory response, giving the invading offender the upper hand.

Complications of Wound Healing

Prolonged wound healing can occur as a result of any one or a combination of the factors previously discussed. Other complications of wound healing involve poor or excessive scar formation. A scar that does not have adequate strength can lead to wound **dehiscence** (dee-HISS-ens), or separation of tissue margins. Excessive collagen formation often results in a hard, raised scar called a **keloid** (KEE-loid) (Figure 4–7). Keloid scars are often unsightly but harmless and occur more often in the African-American population. Surgical removal can result in the formation of another keloid.

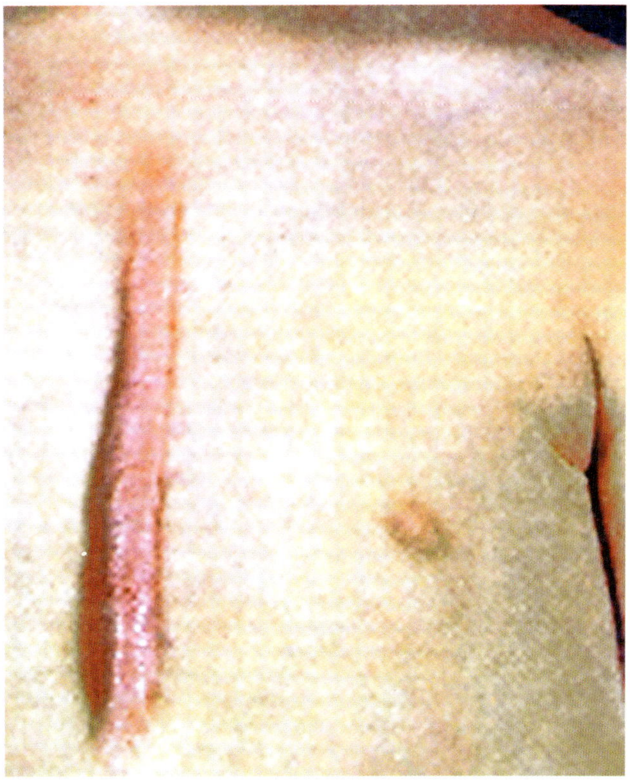

Courtesy of Mark L. Kuss

FIGURE 4–7 Keloid.

Adhesions (ad-HE-zhuns) from scar tissue can be a complication of surgery, especially abdominal surgery. As normal fibrous scar tissue develops in the operative organ, part of this tissue can cling to the surface of the adjoining organs, forming a fibrous band called an **adhesion**. Adhesions are often asymptomatic and cause no difficulties, but in some cases, they can become painful and lead to obstruction of the adjacent organ. The intestine frequently is obstructed by adhesions following abdominal surgery. Further surgery to release painful or obstructive adhesions may be needed.

INFECTION

In Chapter 2, "Mechanisms of Disease," the fact that inflammation and infection are different responses or reactions was introduced. Inflammation is a protective immune response and can occur without bacterial invasion. **Infection**, however, refers to the invasion of microorganisms in the tissue, causing cell or tissue injury and leading to the inflammatory response.

Humans live with disease-causing microorganisms all around them. Some bacteria even live on the skin surface, in the respiratory tract, and in the intestine without causing illness, and some are actually beneficial. These bacteria are called *normal flora*.

Microorganisms that produce disease are called pathogenic. Normal flora can become pathogenic under certain conditions. When this occurs, the normal flora bacteria become **opportunistic** because they take the opportunity to cause infection in the host.

Certain conditions must be present for a microorganism to cause an infection in the host. Pathogens must have an area to enter, be resistant enough and enter in great enough numbers to survive, and overcome the defenses of the individual.

First, the microorganism must successfully gain access into the body through a portal of entry; any break in the skin offers this. Common openings such as the nose, mouth, eyes, and ears are also portals of entry. The most common port of entry is the respiratory system. Other portals include the digestive system, urinary tract, and reproductive tract.

Second, the pathogen must be resistant to the defenses of the host. The ability of a microorganism to overcome the defense of the host is its virulence. A virulent microorganism has an aggressive or invasive nature and can produce a toxin, or poison, that injures tissues. The degree of virulence of a microorganism varies. Generally speaking, organisms that come from an infected host are more virulent than those grown in laboratory conditions.

Third, the number of invading pathogens can determine the risk for infection—even weak pathogenic organisms can cause infection if they invade in large enough numbers to overcome the body's defense system. Generally speaking, the higher the number of invading pathogens, the greater the risk of infection.

Finally, the condition of the individual or the host is a determinant of infection risk. An individual who is in good physical and emotional health, has good nutrition, practices risk-reducing habits, and is relatively young has a good chance of avoiding infection.

Frequency and Types of Infection

Infectious diseases are the leading cause of death in the world, so a country's ability to track and identify infectious diseases is an important weapon in the control of disease. In the United States, the Centers for Disease Control and Prevention (CDC), based in Atlanta, provide these services.

Respiratory infections, including upper respiratory infections, influenza-like infections, pneumonia, and bronchitis account for more than 80% of all infections. Childhood infections, wound infections, viral infections, and other types of infection account for the remaining number of infections diagnosed.

Microorganisms that produce infection in humans include bacteria, **viruses, fungi, rickettsiae** (ric-KET-see-ah), **protozoa**, and **helminths** (Table 4–1). These organisms can produce infections in the host that range from very mild to life threatening.

Bacteria

Bacterial infections can occur as a primary or secondary disease. Primary bacterial infections occur when a person is exposed to a pathogen. Secondary infection occurs after the onset of another disease process or condition. Secondary infections are very common. The most common cause for them is obstruction of a body passageway. For example, nasal obstruction can lead to sinusitis, and obstruction of the eustachian tubes can lead to otitis media, or middle-ear infection.

Normal flora bacteria live on or in the skin, mouth, nose, genital tract, and intestines of humans. These bacteria often become pathogenic when they

TABLE 4–1 Some Common Infections Caused by Microorganisms in Humans

Bacteria	Virus	Fungus
Staphylococcus Streptococcus *Escherichia coli* *Klebsiella* *Pseudomonas* *Shigella* *Salmonella*	Common Cold Herpes Simplex Mononucleosis HIV Measles Mumps Rubella Influenza (flu)	Ringworm (Tinea) Athlete's Foot Candidiasis Thrush Vaginitis Histoplasmosis Coccidioidomycosis
Rickettsial	**Protozoan**	**Helminths**
Rocky Mountain Spotted Fever	Malaria Giardiasis	Roundworms Flatworms Pinworms Tapeworms

gain access into the body or when the body's resistance is less robust than normal. *Staphylococcus* is a bacterium of the skin that often enters the body and can infect any organ. *Staph aureus* is an important member of the staphylococcus family because it can develop strains, such as methicillin-resistant staphylococcus aureus (MRSA), that are resistant to penicillin and other antibiotics. These antibiotic-resistant strains are particularly dangerous because they are difficult to control and eliminate. For instance, a form of MRSA called community-acquired MRSA (CA-MRSA) is the most dangerous form of MRSA. It has become epidemic in the United States in the past few years with an estimated 2.3 million people carrying the infection without symptoms. It is second only to HIV as the major public health threat. CA-MRSA starts out as a skin infection but soon becomes a serious systemic infection. It can rapidly cause severe respiratory distress leading to respiratory failure.

Streptococcus bacteria normally live on the skin and in the throat. Common infections caused by streptococcus bacteria include strep throat, scarlet fever, pneumonia, and meningitis. In a select group of individuals, strep throat can lead to rheumatic fever and glomerulonephritis.

Enteric bacteria are those living in the intestinal tract, and common forms include *Escherichia coli* (*E. coli*), *Klebsiella*, *Pseudomonas*, *Shigella*, and *Salmonella*. *E. coli* causes enteritis in infants and adults and can be the cause of travelers' diarrhea. *E. coli* and *Klebsiella* are common causes of urinary tract infections. *Pseudomonas* commonly infects wounds and is associated with a foul odor and green pus production. *Shigella* and *Salmonella* infections cause diarrhea; *Salmonella* is the causative organism of food poisoning.

Viruses

Viruses are the smallest infective organisms and must be visualized by an electron microscope. They cannot reproduce or live outside the cell and must invade the cell and use it to reproduce their genetic information. Lymphocytes of the immune system are the body's primary defense against viruses. Some viruses can mutate or change, so the body must develop more than one kind of antibody to kill that type of virus.

Viral infections cannot be treated easily. Some antiviral agents can be given to individuals who have reduced resistance to infections to try to prevent such infection. Antibiotic therapy does not kill a virus. Usually, supportive care is given by treating the symptoms the virus causes, such as fever, sore throat, runny nose, headache, and chest congestion. Antibiotics will

COMPLEMENTARY AND ALTERNATIVE THERAPY

Aromatherapy

Aromatherapy has been used in a variety of ways for treating ailments such as skin wounds, headaches, depression, anxiety, nausea, and complications of burns. Its effects have not been well understood by either medical providers or the patients, but there is some evidence that it is effective for isolated problems. Several hospitals have developed policies and protocols for using aromatherapy. There is also ongoing research on using this therapy for patients with radiation burns, nausea from chemotherapy, and slow-healing wounds. It is also being studied for its effects on infection in burn patients. It has often been combined with massage to increase patient satisfaction and relaxation.

Source: Bukel (2007).

help in treatment of a secondary bacterial infection occurring with the viral infection.

Viral infections of the upper respiratory system, including the common cold, far outnumber other viral diseases. Cold sores, also known as herpes simplex, are very common and affect many individuals. Infectious mononucleosis frequently affects adolescents and young adults. Human immunodeficiency virus (HIV) causes acquired immune deficiency syndrome (AIDS) and has become the most noted virus due to its fatal outcome.

Immunizations are effective in preventing many viral diseases such as measles, mumps, rubella, and small pox. Influenza virus (flu) mutates and requires new vaccines with each mutation. Some viruses are latent types, meaning they live inside the cell, causing no harm until the body becomes stressed or impaired. Latent viruses, such as those in the herpes family, replicate and cause symptoms during stressful periods.

Fungi

Fungi are microscopic plant-like organisms that cause diseases referred to as mycoses. Fungi are larger than bacteria, and only a few types are pathogenic. Single-celled forms of fungi are called yeast.

Fungal infections of the skin such as those of the tinea family (ringworm and athlete's foot) are common. Candida, commonly called candidiasis or yeast infection, often occurs in individuals with suppressed immune systems, anyone on long-term antibiotic

HEALTHY HIGHLIGHT

Medication Precautions

WARNING! Anyone taking a prescribed antibiotic medication should always take ALL of the medication even if the symptoms stop. Antibiotics should not be saved for the next illness. Failure to complete antibiotic therapy can lead to the development of antibiotic-resistant strains of bacteria because the first doses of medication might kill weaker bacteria and stun the stronger ones, but if therapy is halted prematurely, the stronger bacteria might survive and reproduce strains that can resist the antibiotic. When this occurs, stronger and usually more expensive medications must be used to treat the same infection at a later date. Mismanagement of antibiotic therapy has led to development of strains of bacteria that now must be treated with stronger oral antibiotics or intravenous (IV) antibiotics.

HEALTHY HIGHLIGHT

Prevention for the Common Cold

The common cold virus has more than 100 strains, which the body must identify and kill each as the body becomes infected. An individual will not suffer with the same cold virus twice, which explains why young children have more colds than adults. As we age, we have become ill with many cold viruses and have developed immunity to this greater number. Cold viruses are very contagious, entering the body primarily through the respiratory tract. Good hand washing is the best preventive measure for the common cold, and using antibacterial hand gels and sanitizers is also recommended.

therapy, and in individuals with diabetes. Candida is a superficial infection of the skin and mucous membranes, appearing commonly in the moist folds of the skin, the mouth (thrush), vaginal cavity (vaginitis), and genital area.

Other fungal infections include histoplasmosis and coccidioidomycosis (cok-sid-e-oyd-o-my-CO-sis). These infections are common to certain geographical locations but are not common in the general population. Fungal infections can be treated with antifungal and antibiotic medications but often are difficult to cure and might require long-term therapy.

Rickettsiae

Rickettsiae are microscopic organisms that are intermediate between bacteria and viruses. They must live in the host cell like a virus. Rickettsiae are spread by fleas, ticks, mites, and lice and can cause fatal infections in humans, the most common of which is Rocky Mountain Spotted Fever.

Protozoa

Protozoa are single-celled microscopic members of the animal kingdom. They are found in the soil and live on dead or decaying material. Infection is by ingestion of spores or by infected insect bites.

Malaria, which is spread by mosquitoes, is the most prevalent protozoan infection worldwide but is uncommon in the United States. The protozoa causing malaria live in and destroy the red blood cell of the host. Giardiasis (gee-ar-DIE-a-sis) is an intestinal infection caused by drinking water infected with the *Giardia lamblia* protozoan; it is treated with antibiotic therapy.

Helminths

Helminths are any of the roundworms or flatworms. Helminth infestation is common worldwide but not as common in the United States. Pinworms and tapeworms are the most common helminths. Pinworms cause anal itching but do not cause serious illness. Tapeworms, acquired by eating uncooked or inadequately cooked meat, can cause intestinal disease in humans.

GLIMPSE OF THE FUTURE

Myrrh: The Age Old Perfume May Have New Uses

Myrrh comes from the dried sap of the tree *Commiphora myrrha* and other species of plants. It has been used in incense and perfume since biblical times. Chinese medicine used myrrh for liniments and painful disorders such as arthritis or gum infections. It is used in Western medicine as antiseptic in mouthwashes and toothpastes. Myrrh has also been used to lower blood glucose and to treat circulatory problems in many cultures and by herbalists in the United States. New research is looking at products containing myrrh as an anticancer and antiparasitic treatment. It is also being tested for its benefits in wound healing.

Source: Nomicos (2007).

Testing for Infection

Symptoms of infection in an individual can include fever, **tachycardia** (TACH-ee-KAR-dee-ah; tachy = rapid, cardia = heart rate), and **malaise** (general ill feeling). Often, blood studies will reveal **leukocytosis** (leuko = white, cyto = cell, osis = condition), or an increase in the white cell count, and blood from an individual with **septicemia** (SEP-tih-SEE-me-ah) will reveal the presence of the pathogen in the blood. Infection in the meninges, or meningitis, can show presence of pathogens in the individual's spinal fluid.

A culture is the process of growing pathogenic cells on or in a gelatin-like substance called media that pathogenic organisms use for food (Figure 4–8). Media can be made of different nutrient agars of which a common one is sheep's blood agar. Laboratory studies of how the microorganism uses this food assist in the determination of the type of pathogen.

A culture is the most definitive test for organisms in a lesion or wound Cultures are most commonly used for bacteria identification, but can also identify fungal infections. Most bacterial specimens are obtained from the throat, urine, sputum, purulent wound lesions, feces, blood, and spinal fluid.

After identification of the pathogen, a sensitivity test is used to identify the type of treatment needed. The combined test for these is called a **culture and sensitivity** test. During a sensitivity test, the microorganisms are smeared on the nutrient agar, and small antibiotic-permeated disks are placed on the agar (Figure 4–9). After incubation, the agar plate is observed for killing zones around the disk; disks that display a large kill zone are the most effective in treatment.

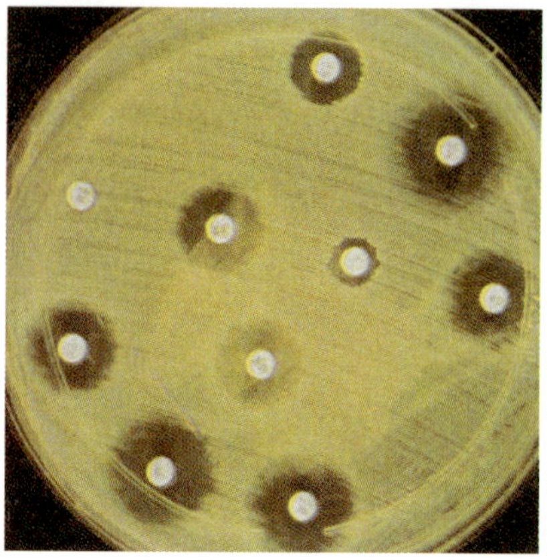
Delmar/Cengage Learning

FIGURE 4–9 Bacterial sensitivity.

Specific antigen–antibody reactive tests can be used to determine the presence of pathogens. For example, a rapid diagnosis of strep throat can be made by testing for the presence of an antigen in a throat specimen. The streptococcus antigen will clot or clump when mixed with laboratory streptococcus antibody.

Bacterial, rickettsial, and some other pathogenic infections can be determined by serologic testing, which uses the individual's blood serum to test for antibodies against the pathogen.

Skin testing also uses antibody presence to determine exposure to pathogens. Tuberculosis (TB) skin testing (also called the Mantoux test) is one of the most common skin tests and involves the intradermal (under the skin) injection of tuberculin bacteria particles (antigen) (Figure 4–10). If an individual has been exposed to TB and has developed the TB antibody, this antibody will attack the

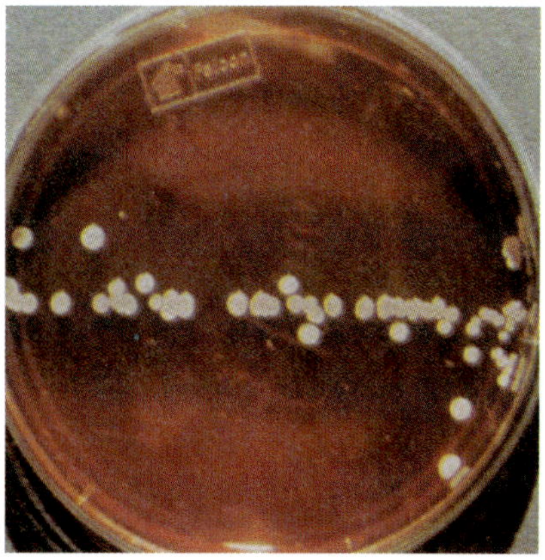
Delmar/Cengage Learning

FIGURE 4–8 Bacterial culture.

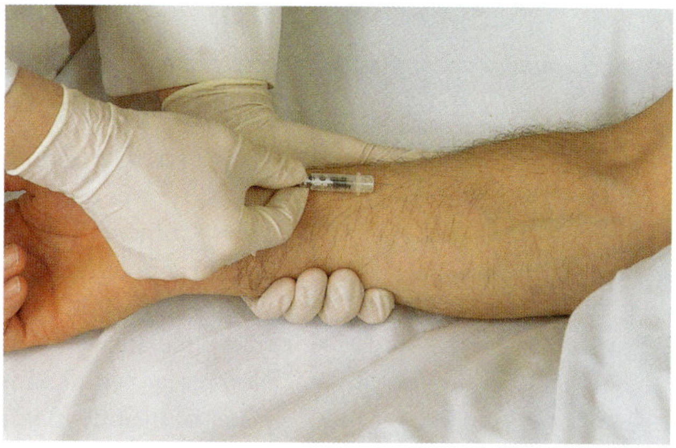
Delmar/Cengage Learning

FIGURE 4–10 Tuberculosis (TB) skin test.

antigen and cause an **induration** (IN-dur-RAY-shun; hardened tissue), displaying a positive skin test (Figure 4–11).

In 2007, the FDA approved the Xpert MRSA test, which uses DNA-type technology to test for the drug-resistant strain. Tissue sampling testing should be available soon.

A positive skin test and serology testing might not indicate current infection or the degree of infection. These tests are only a few of the many laboratory tests used in diagnosing pathogenic infections and indicate only that the individual has been exposed to the pathogen and has developed antibodies.

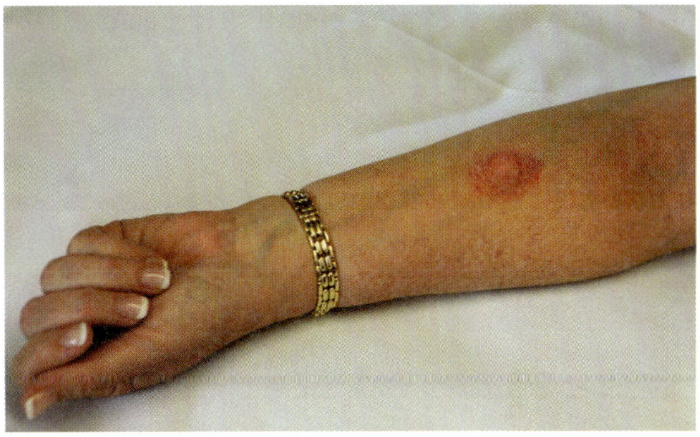

Courtesy of Mark L. Kuss

FIGURE 4–11 Positive skin test.

SUMMARY

The body responds to the invasions of pathogens by using its defense mechanisms. Inflammation is a natural protective mechanism that occurs when physical barriers are broken and the invader penetrates the tissues. The inflammatory process consists of a series of events that eventually, if functioning properly, destroy the invading pathogen. When this system of protection fails, infection can occur. Infections are caused by a variety of organisms, most commonly by bacteria and viruses. They are diagnosed and treated in a variety of ways. Several kinds of laboratory tests can be used to identify the organism and determine the appropriate therapy.

REVIEW QUESTIONS

Short Answer

1. What are the three defense mechanisms of the body? (Describe them.)

2. What are the steps in the inflammatory process?

3. How do inflammatory exudates and inflammatory lesions differ?

4. What are the five cardinal signs of inflammation?

5. What is the difference between a keloid and an adhesion?

6. Compare and contrast some microorganisms that produce infection in humans.

7. What type of testing is used to identify the organism causing an infection?

Fill in the Blanks

8. Cellular proliferation can be grouped into the three categories of ___________, ___________, and ___________.

9. The body's two main methods of repair involve ___________ and ___________.

10. Primary union is also called ___________.

11. The process of secondary union involves a larger degree of ___________ and more ___________ to resolve it than primary union requires.

12. The greatest impediments to wound healing are ___________ and ___________.

CASE STUDIES

- Ms. Jannicet is an 85-year-old resident in a local long-term care facility. She is very thin and frail and, except for meals, stays in bed most of the day. This puts her at risk for developing pressure ulcers. On what ares of her body would she most likely develop pressure ulcers? How can they be prevented? How would you describe a pressure ulcer? Describe the healing process of a pressure ulcer.

- Mr. Jordan has a sore throat and frequent cough, so he made an appointment with his physician for an evaluation. He was diagnosed with an upper respiratory infection. The physician prescribed an antibiotic to be taken four times a day for 10 days. What are some important points about taking the medication that Mr. Jordan should know? Although he already has an infection, is good hand washing still important? If so, why?

*Study*WARE™ Connection

To help you learn the content in this chapter, take a practice quiz or play an interactive game on your StudyWARE™ CD-ROM.

Workbook Practice

Go to your Workbook and complete the practice questions.

BIBLIOGRAPHY

Buckel, J. (2007). Literature review: Should nurisng take aromatherapy more seriously? *British Journal of Nursing 16*(2), 116–120.

Duimel-Peeters, I. (2005). Preventing pressure ulcer with massage? *American Journal of Nursing 105*(8), 31–33.

Gauldie, J. (2007). Inflammation and the aging process: Devil or angel? *Nutrition Reviews Supplement 65* (supplement), S167–S169.

Langkamp-Henken, B., Hudgens, J., Stechmiller, J. K., & Herrlinger-Garcia, K. A. (2005). Mini-nutritional assessment and screening scores are associated with nutritional indicators in elderly people with pressure ulcers. *Journal of the American Dietetic Association 105*(10), 1590–1596.

Mennick, F., Chu, J. J., & Walters-Fischer, P. (2005). Acute infection and vaccination. *American Journal of Nursing 105*(7), 72C.

New MRSA test: Pathologist invents easy way to diagnose MRSA. (2007). Science Daily. Institute of Physics. *www.sciencedaily.com*

Nomicos, E. Y. (2007). Myrrh: Medical marvel or myth of the magi? *Holistic Nursing Practice 21*(6), 308–323.

Parkes, G. C. (2007). An overview of probiotics and prebiotics. *Nursing Standard 21*(20), 43–47.

Schwartz, R. A., & Nervi, S. (March 1, 2007). Erythema nodosum: A sign of systemic disease. *American Family Physician 75*(5), 695–700.

Stuber, F., Klaschik, S., Lehmann, Le. E., Schewe, J., Weber, S., & Book, M. (November 15, 2005). Cytokine promoter polymorphisms in severe sepsis. *Clinical Infectious Diseases 41*(supplement), S416–S420.

Wound management. (2006). *Paediatric Nursing 18*(8), 30.

UNIT II

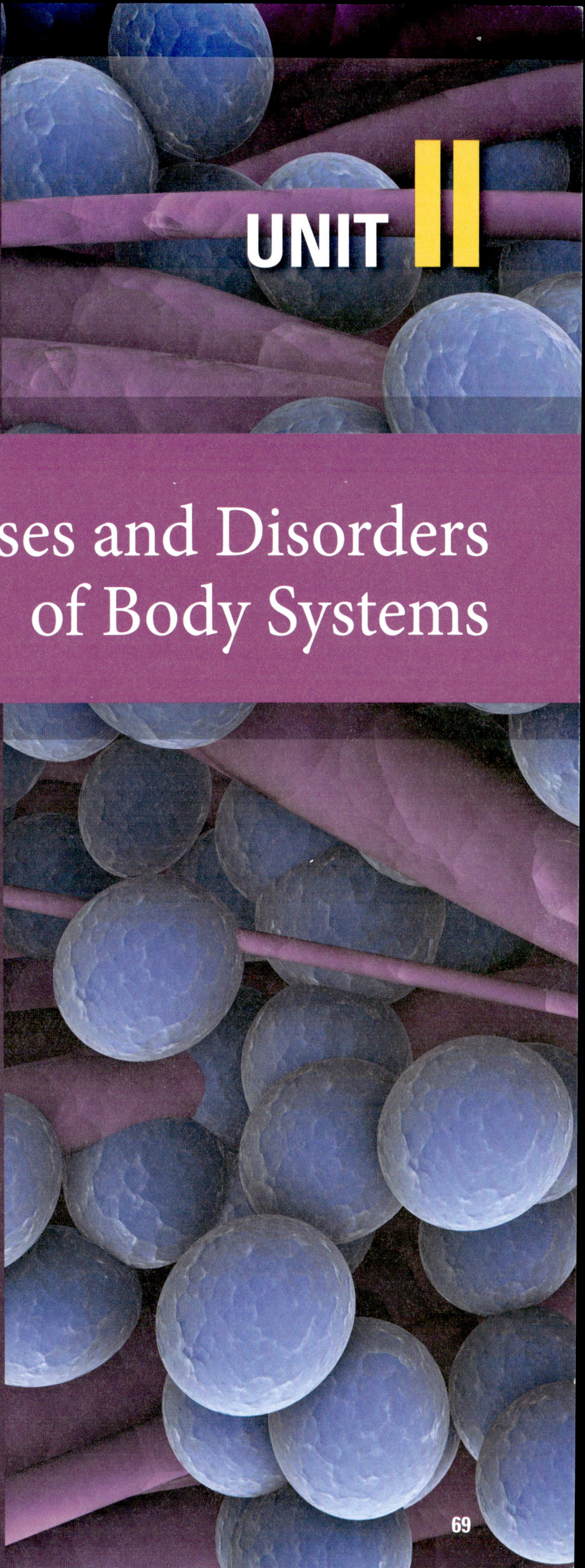

Common Diseases and Disorders of Body Systems

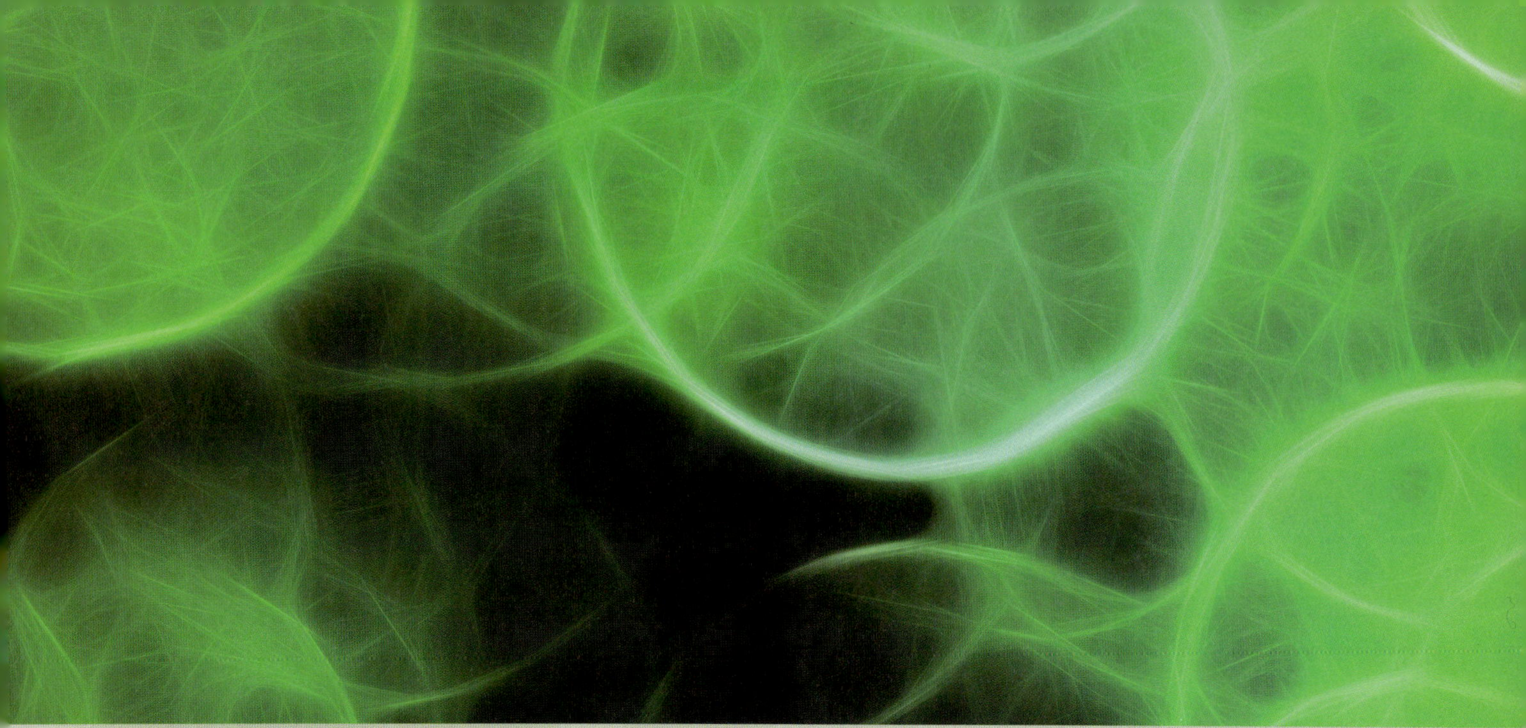

OUTLINE

- Anatomy and Physiology
- Common Signs and Symptoms
- Diagnostic Tests
- Common Diseases of the Immune System
  - *Hypersensitivity Disorders*
  - *Immune Deficiency Disorders*
- Trauma
- Rare Diseases
  - *Severe Combined Immunodeficiency Disease (SCID)*
- Effects of Aging on the Immune System
- Summary
- Review Questions
- Case Studies
- Bibliography

KEY TERMS

Allergen(s) (p. 73)
Allergy (p. 74)
Anaphylaxis (p. 78)
Antigen(s) (p. 73)
Autoimmune (p. 73)
Bronchospasm (p. 76)
Corticosteroid(s) (p. 78)
Cytotoxic (p. 87)
Hemolytic (p. 74)
Hypersensitivity (p. 74)
Immunodeficiency (p. 73)
Isoimmune (p. 73)
Kaposi's sarcoma (p. 88)
Pneumocystis carinii (p. 88)
Prophylactic (p. 79)
Self-antigen (p. 79)
Status asthmaticus (p. 77)
Streptococcal (p. 79)
Urticaria (p. 75)

5

Immune System Diseases and Disorders

LEARNING OBJECTIVES

Upon completion of the chapter, the learner should be able to:

1. Define the terminology common to the immune system and the disorders of the system.
2. Discuss the basic anatomy and physiology of the immune system.
3. Identify the important signs and symptoms associated with common immune system disorders.
4. Describe the common diagnostics used to determine type, cause, or both of an immune system disorder.
5. Identify disorders of the immune system.
6. Describe the typical course and management of common immune system disorders.
7. Describe the effects of aging on the immune system and the common disorders of the system associated with aging.

OVERVIEW

The immune system protects the body through the processes of defense, attack, and removal of pathogens. The immune system also helps the body by removing aged or dead cells and other debris. Diseases or disorders of the immune system can range from mild to severe and can affect individuals of any age, race, or gender. Many of the disorders of the system are extremely debilitating and require long-term therapy. If the immune system is not functioning properly due to disease or other influencing factors, the result may be a secondary disease of the body resulting from the compromised immune system. ■

ANATOMY AND PHYSIOLOGY

The immune system is made up of a complex group of cells and organs found throughout the body. The system includes primary organs, such as the thymus gland and the bone marrow, and secondary organs such as the lymph nodes, spleen, liver, and tonsils (Figure 5–1). Lymphocytes, the major cells of the immune system, arise and develop in the primary organs. The secondary organs are responsible for filtering foreign substances and providing the space for antigen reactions.

The cells of the immune system include four types of leukocytes: polymorphonuclear leukocytes, monocytes, macrophages, and lymphocytes. The polymorphonuclear leukocytes (PMNs), also known as granulocytes, are active in the inflammatory process. Some leukocytes react when infection threatens the body; others respond to prevent damage to cells and tissues from an allergic reaction. The monocytes and macrophages become phagocytic in the presence of pathogens and foreign substances. The lymphocytes are the major players in the immune response (Table 5–1).

Lymphocytes are formed in the bone marrow. Those remaining and maturing in the bone marrow become B lymphocytes. Others migrate and mature in the thymus and become T lymphocytes. When mature, both B and T lymphocytes enter the blood and circulate and colonize the lymphatic organs, predominately the spleen and lymph nodes.

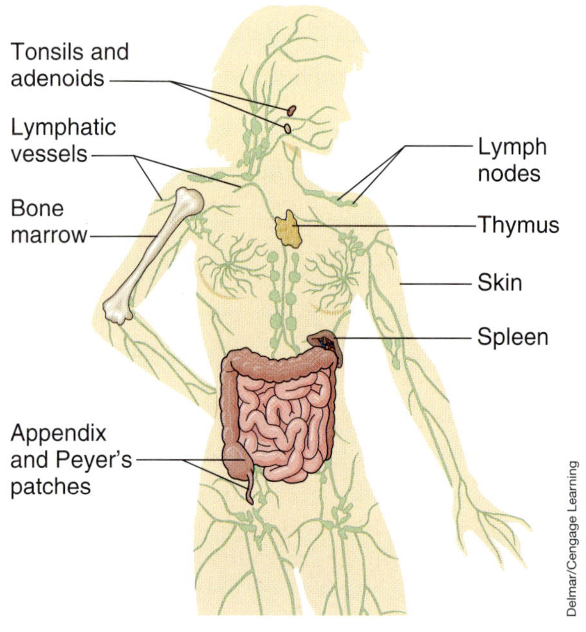

FIGURE 5–1 Organs of the immune system.

TABLE 5–1 Types and Functions of Leukocytes

Type	Function
Polymorphonuclear leukocytes	
Neutrophils	Phagocytosis
Eosinophils	Allergic response
Basophils	Histamine release
Monocytes	Become macrophages (phagocytosis)
Macrophages	Phagocytosis
Lymphocytes	
T lymphocytes	Cell-mediated immunity
B lymphocytes	Humoral immunity
Plasma cells	Antibody production

T lymphocytes, or T cells, are responsible for the cell-mediated response. These cells destroy microorganisms that invade the body. These reactions do not require antibodies produced by the B lymphocytes or B cells because the T cells have been previously sensitized by circulating antigens. Several types of T cells function to stimulate B cells to produce antibodies, destroy foreign cells in the body, stop the immune response, and remember previous exposure to antigens.

B lymphocytes are responsible for humoral immunity. Humoral immunity is associated with circulating antibodies in contrast to cell-mediated immunity. The B lymphocytes enlarge and divide to become mature plasma cells. The plasma cells secrete antibodies into the blood and lymph to protect the body against infections and toxins produced by microorganisms.

There are two types of immune responses in the body: specific and nonspecific. Specific immune response is associated with antigens and the antibody reaction. It is the body's watch-guard system for foreign invaders. The antibody response occurs after exposure to an antigen. Antibodies may neutralize, kill, or cause clumping of the foreign microorganism. Antibodies may be assisted by the complement system. This system is a group of proteins that are formed in the liver and circulate in the serum. The complement system works with and enhances the work of the antibodies to destroy the invader.

The nonspecific immune response includes inflammation, phagocytosis, physical barriers (the skin and mucous membranes), and chemical barriers

TABLE 5–2 Types of Immunity

Type of Immunity	Example
Active natural immunity	Having the disease (such as mumps)
Active artificial immunity	Receiving a vaccination (such as MMR)
Passive natural immunity	Antibodies produced by the body itself or received from maternal–fetus transmission
Passive artificial immunity	Injection of antibodies

(acids and other secretions). These immune response defenses are the body's first line of protection against foreign invaders.

There are several ways to classify types of immunity, but the most common method is to divide immunity into passive and active and natural and artificial. Table 5–2 outlines the types of immunity and gives examples of each. In addition, some classification systems use the term *natural resistance* when describing immunity. Natural resistance is the inherited immunity the individual may possess due to race, species, or ethnic background. Some races, species, or particular groups of populations are naturally resistant to certain diseases, just as some are more susceptible to certain diseases.

COMMON SIGNS AND SYMPTOMS

In some cases, a patient's concern can be considered as both a symptom and a sign. Some references call this an objective or observable symptom, whereas others state that it is also a sign. An example would be a patient complaining of a runny nose. The runny nose is the patient's symptom and, because it is observable to the physician, it is also a sign.

The common signs and symptoms related to the various immune system diseases are quite varied, depending on the organ or organ system affected. Symptoms common to allergic reactions include local or systemic inflammatory responses (redness, heat, swelling, and itching) and respiratory symptoms (runny nose, coughing, sneezing, and nasal congestion).

The classic clinical problem with immune deficiency disorders is the development of unusual and severe infections such as pneumonia, meningitis, or septicemia, to name just a few. Also, the development of infections by microorganisms that are not usually pathogenic (opportunistic infections) might be indicative of an **immunodeficiency** (lack of immunity) disorder. The common signs and symptoms related to the various **autoimmune** (immunity against self) and **isoimmune** (immunity against other humans) disorders are also varied, depending on the organ or organ system affected and the invading pathogen. For this reason, signs and symptoms of these diseases are identified in the discussion of the specific disease.

DIAGNOSTIC TESTS

Determining the cause of an allergic reaction might be quite difficult. There are hundreds of possible **antigens** (**allergens**) that cause allergic reactions. Some of the more common allergens are house dust, pet hair, chocolate, ragweed, cigarette smoke, pollen, seafood, nickel, plants, paints, dyes, and chemical cleaners.

The most important test for diagnosing allergies is the skin test. A skin test may be performed by intradermal injection involving injection of a small amount of the suspected antigen under the skin. A skin patch

GLIMPSE OF THE FUTURE

Altering the Immune Response to Prevent Tumor Growth

Research is now being conducted to determine if altering adaptive immunity can reduce tumor growth and cancer spread. The immune system is important in preserving the body's immunity by eliminating tumors that produce antigens. These antigens have to be identified and then targeted. It is a very complex process that involves the T cells. In the future, vaccines may be developed through this research that will help the immune system reduce tumor growth and prevent cancer metastasis.

Source: Franco, (2008).

test utilizes placement of a small antigen-soaked patch placed against the individual's skin. Another skin test is a scratch test in which a small amount of suspected antigen is placed in a small scratch. All three types of tests are used to identify an allergen.

Allergy to the antigen is positive if an inflammatory response or wheal occurs at the injection site. The size of the wheal is usually indicative of the individual's sensitivity to the allergen. There are hundreds of allergic antigens that may be used in skin testing.

After an antigen has been identified, a desensitization treatment may be attempted. Desensitization requires the injection of an increasing amount of allergen over a long period of time with the goal of desensitizing the body to the allergen. Other treatments include antihistamine medications and avoiding exposure to the allergen.

Hypersensitivity reactions to transfused blood cells are usually identified by a blood count indicating low levels of red cells, white cells, and platelets. Antibodies can form against all these blood elements, leading to anemia, leukopenia, and thrombocytopenia, respectively.

A Coombs test will indicate the formation of antibodies on the red blood cell. This test can be used to determine blood type and diagnose certain **hemolytic** (HE-moh-LIT-ick; hemo = blood, lytic = destroying) anemias. A coombs test can also indicate the presence of maternal antibodies against the fetal blood type, as occurs in erythroblastosis fetalis.

Autoimmune disorders can be diagnosed using blood tests that measure for specific diseases. For example, individuals with systemic lupus erythematosus will have a positive antinuclear antibody (ANA) test. Rheumatoid factor (RF) in the blood is often indicative of rheumatoid arthritis.

Immunodeficiency disorders are usually diagnosed by blood testing that reveals low white cell counts, specifically B and T lymphocytes. Presence of an antibody in the blood against a causative pathogen can also be used. Finding an antibody against the human immunodeficiency virus (HIV) is indicative of exposure to AIDS.

COMMON DISEASES OF THE IMMUNE SYSTEM

Diseases of the immune system can be divided into two main groups: hypersensitivity disorders and immune deficiency disorders. Several specific diseases are within each grouping. Each of these has some unique

COMPLEMENTARY AND ALTERNATIVE THERAPY

Echinacea, Vitamin C, and Zinc for Colds

Echinacea (purple cornflower), vitamin C, and zinc have all been promoted as cold remedies. Some sources state they prevent colds or reduce the effects of colds by boosting the immune system. Many studies have been conducted on these products, attempting to decide if they have any effectiveness in reducing the length of time a person suffers from the common cold. They have also tried to determine if echinacea, vitamin C or zinc lozenges can prevent a cold when the individual has been exposed to the viruses that cause colds. The consensus of the various research studies is that echinacea seems to help fight the common cold but that vitamin C and zinc have very little effect if any. However, some researchers found that people who engage in heavy exercise might benefit from taking vitamin C to prevent colds. Another study saw some positive results from zinc nasal gel rather than lozenges. Part of the problem in reaching a consensus about the effects of the products is that they each come in many different strengths and preparations and all studies did not use the same dosages and preparations. That could have altered the results and conclusions. Further study is needed to really determine the effectiveness of these treatments.

Source: Tufts University Health & Nutrition Letter, (October 2007).

COMPLEMENTARY AND ALTERNATIVE THERAPY

Use of Herbal Therapy by Food-Allergic Patients

Research is being done on food-allergic patients who use complementary and alternative therapies. One study looked at the frequency that these patients used alternative therapies and their effectiveness. The results showed that, although most patients liked using herbal preparations more than traditional drugs, they did not receive the beneficial effects they needed from the alternative therapies.

Source. Goldsobel, (2007).

problems associated with the disease, but some of the signs and symptoms may be quite similar.

Hypersensitivity Disorders

Hypersensitivity disorders are the result of an overreaction of the immune system to an antigen or allergen. Hypersensitivity disorders can be further classified as those related to allergy, autoimmunity, and isoimmunity (Figure 5–2).

ALLERGIES

DESCRIPTION. Allergies are among the most prevalent types of hypersensitivity problems. Millions of people suffer from some type of allergy. Hay fever, asthma (AZ-ma), **urticaria** (UR-tih-KAR-ree-ah; a

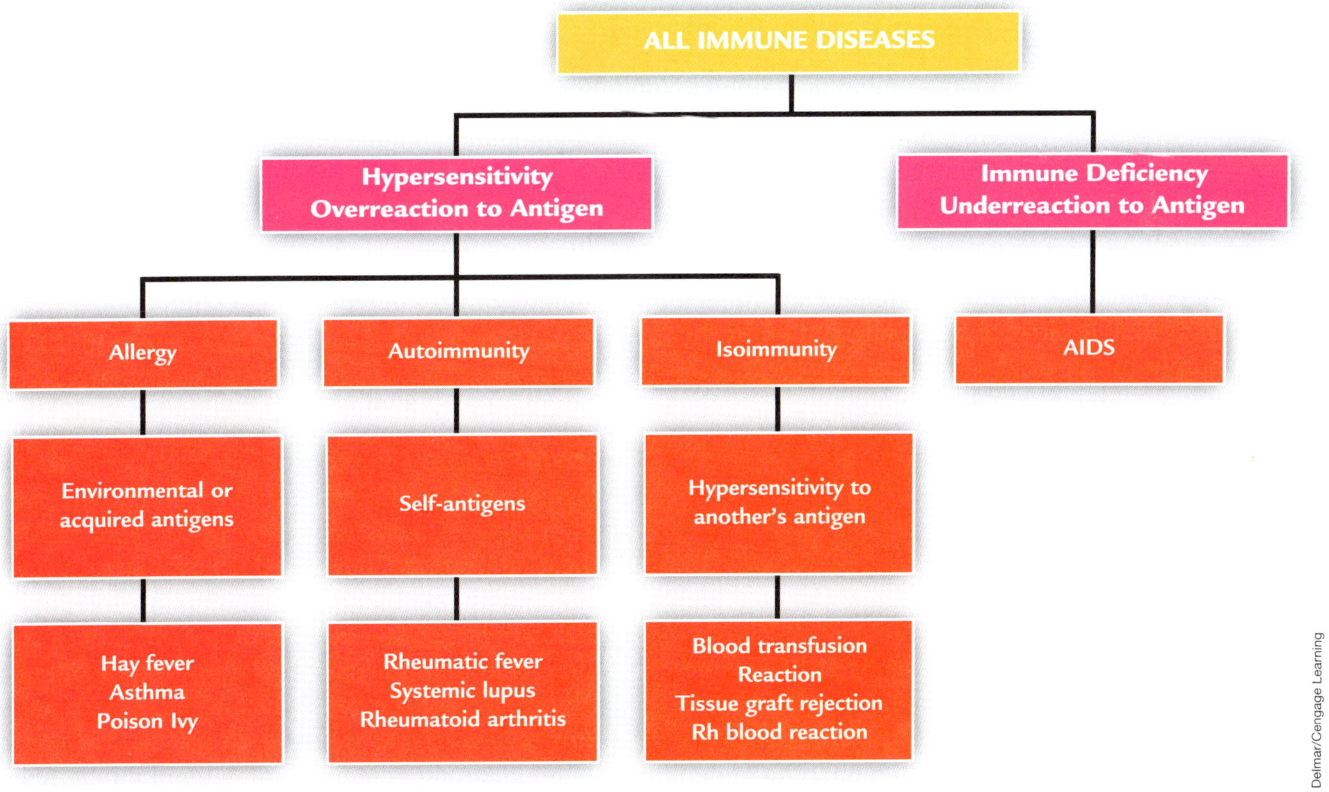

FIGURE 5–2 Classification of hypersensitivity disorders.

reaction characterized by intense wheals and itching), and contact dermatitis are common allergic reactions. These reactions are usually just bothersome, but they can be a serious health threat. Severe asthma, for example, may be life threatening. Food allergies are also common in some populations but may be difficult to diagnose.

■ ***ETIOLOGY.*** Allergy is an acquired hypersensitivity. The individual with an allergy must first be exposed or sensitized to the antigen. Subsequent or repeated exposure leads to a reaction, identified as an allergy or an allergic reaction, by the immune system. Allergens can cause an immediate response like those identified with hay fever, asthma, or food allergy. Delayed-response allergies are slower to react and are usually less harmful. An example of delayed response allergy would be contact dermatitis, caused by exposure to poison ivy.

■ ***SYMPTOMS.*** Most allergens are airborne. Respiratory symptoms can include runny nose, coughing, sneezing, wheezing, and nasal congestion. Other allergies can lead to redness, heat, swelling, and itching of the involved tissue.

■ ***DIAGNOSIS.*** Diagnosis of allergies is often made on the basis of history and physical exam along with testing. Positive skin sensitivity testing and blood testing, including an elevated blood eosinophil (a white blood cell that responds in allergic conditions) level, are indicative of allergies.

■ ***TREATMENT.*** Treatments include avoidance of the allergen, allergy desensitization injections, and antihistamine and steroid medications.

■ ***PREVENTION.*** Prevention of all hypersensitivity disorders is total avoidance of the allergen or, in the case of autoimmmue diseases, minimizing the hyperimmune symptoms.

HAY FEVER

■ ***DESCRIPTION.*** Hay fever is a reaction in the mucous membranes of the nose and upper respiratory tract to an allergen.

■ ***ETIOLOGY.*** The allergen is usually airborne and can be seasonal. Tree pollen, grasses, agricultural crops, and ragweed pollen can cause an increase in symptoms during the different seasons of the year. Nonseasonal hay fever can be the result of house dust, pet dander, or food allergies.

■ ***SYMPTOMS.*** Symptoms include sneezing, watery eyes, runny nose, and itching.

■ ***DIAGNOSIS.*** Skin testing is the most common method of allergy testing for hay fever.

■ ***TREATMENT.*** Treatment of hay fever includes removal of the allergen or separation of the allergen and the hay fever sufferer. Individuals who suffer from hay fever can choose to move permanently to a different climate or to vacation in a different area when the pollen count is high in their area. An air-conditioned environment is beneficial because it filters much of the allergen. Antihistamines and other drugs can be given orally—and in nose drops and sprays—in an effort to control symptoms. Allergy desensitization might be of benefit.

ASTHMA

■ ***DESCRIPTION.*** This chronic allergic condition is also known as bronchial asthma. It affects 5–10% of children, making it the leading cause of chronic illness in childhood. Male children have asthma twice as often as girls prior to puberty. After puberty, the ratio is more equal.

■ ***ETIOLOGY.*** When exposed to an allergen, the hypersensitive individual has episodes of wheezing due to **bronchospasm** (BRONG-ko-SPA-zm) or muscular constriction of the bronchi of the respiratory tract. The individual appears perfectly normal between episodes.

Asthma can be caused by allergens in the environment, such as pollen, dust, pet dander, smoke, or various fumes. Other causes of asthma are nonallergic and include events that produce stress. Triggers for nonallergic asthma include respiratory infections such as the common cold, changes in temperature and humidity, exercise, and emotional stress.

■ ***SYMPTOMS.*** Symptoms of an attack are extreme shortness of breath, difficulty breathing, wheezing, and anxiety. Attacks vary in severity from mild to almost suffocating. Coughing during the attack usually begins with a mild, dry cough, but progresses to production of large amounts of mucus as the attack continues. Skin might be pale and moist in mild attacks, with cyanosis of the nail beds and lips occurring in more severe attacks. During an attack, asthmatics often assume a sitting position, leaning forward with hands resting on the knees. This position helps the individual breathe by using all the respiratory muscles

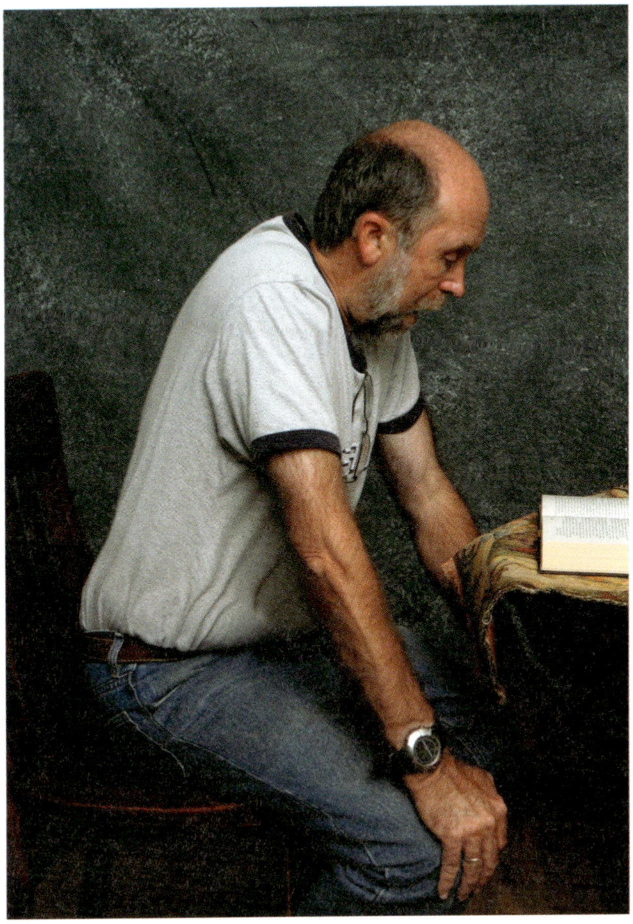

FIGURE 5–3 Positioning in an asthma attack.

(Figure 5–3). A severe attack that lasts for several days is called **status asthmaticus** (AZ-MAH-ti-kus) and is a life-threatening medical emergency.

■ ***DIAGNOSIS.*** Diagnosis is made after a complete history and physical exam along with lung function testing. A trial medication might be ordered. If the medication works, the diagnosis is probably asthma.

■ ***TREATMENT.*** Treatment includes avoidance of causative allergens, desensitization, education, and medications to treat symptoms. Deep breathing exercises, maintenance of proper posture, and relaxation techniques are beneficial. A regimen of medications to relax and open the bronchi (bronchodilators) and to thin the excessive mucus (mucolytics) is important. There is no cure for asthma, but it can be controlled by a combination of therapies including strict compliance to a medication regimen, relaxation techniques, exercise, and avoidance of allergens.

StudyWARE™ Connection

View an animation about asthma on your StudyWARE™ CD-ROM.

URTICARIA

■ ***DESCRIPTION.*** Commonly called hives or nettle rash, urticaria is a vascular reaction of the skin.

■ ***ETIOLOGY.*** This condition is caused by contact with an external irritant such as insect bites, pollen, drugs, food, or plants.

■ ***SYMPTOMS.*** The condition is characterized by slightly elevated lesions that are redder or paler than the surrounding skin and is associated with severe itching. The elevated areas are called wheals or hives. Scratching or rubbing the hypersensitive area can lead to formation of larger or additional wheals (Figure 5–4).

■ ***DIAGNOSIS.*** A physical examination will help diagnose this skin reaction. A history of recent exposure to plants, insect bites, pets, new foods or medications might assist in identifying the allergen.

■ ***TREATMENT.*** Treatment includes antihistamines and avoidance of the allergen.

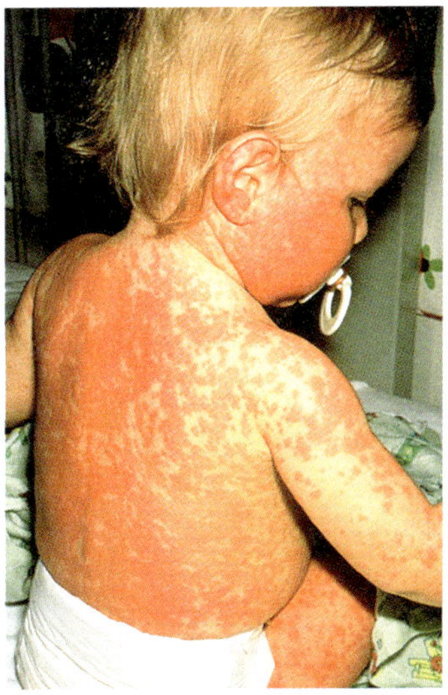

FIGURE 5–4 Urticaria.

ANAPHYLAXIS

■ ***DESCRIPTION.*** This is a severe allergic response to an allergen, often leading to anaphylactic shock.

■ ***ETIOLOGY.*** **Anaphylaxis** (AN-ah-fih-LACK-sis), also known as an anaphylactic reaction, is caused by absorption of the antigen into the blood directly or through the mucous membranes. Food allergy is believed to be the leading cause of anaphylaxis outside the hospital (Food Allergy Network, 2008). Other common causes of anaphylaxis include medications, insect stings, and latex.

■ ***SYMPTOMS.*** A local anaphylactic reaction might be mild and produce generalized itching, swelling, and urticaria. This reaction should be closely monitored because it might rapidly progress to systemic anaphylaxis. Systemic anaphylaxis is a true medical emergency involving the release of histamine throughout body tissues. Within minutes, the individual feels itching of the throat, tongue, and scalp. Edema or swelling of the face and airways leads to difficulty breathing. The individual suffers a huge drop in blood pressure (shock) and body temperature. Unconsciousness usually occurs with the drop in blood pressure. If these symptoms are not reversed with medical attention, death from respiratory and cardiac arrest can occur within 15 to 20 minutes.

■ ***DIAGNOSIS.*** Symptoms of anaphylaxis generally initiate within minutes and last less than 24 hours. A diagnosis is made rapidly, based on the presenting symptoms.

■ ***TREATMENT.*** Treatment during an attack might include performance of an emergency tracheostomy (TRAY-kee-OS-toh-me; trache = trachea, ostomy = new opening) or endotracheal (endo = within, trachea = windpipe) intubation with mechanical ventilation. Immediate administration of epinephrine medication is necessary. Epinephrine (adrenalin) is a vasoconstrictor and a smooth-muscle relaxant. Effects of epinephrine will raise the blood pressure, dilate the bronchi, and decrease laryngeal spasms. Antihistamines and **corticosteroids** (KORT-ti-ko-STEHR-oyds; powerful anti-inflammatory hormones) are given to limit histamine production, thus slowing the allergic reaction.

Follow-up treatment should include identifying the allergen. The individual is taught to identify and avoid the allergen and recognize the onset of a reaction. These individuals should wear an allergy identification necklace or bracelet. Individuals who experience this severe reaction should always carry an allergy kit containing Benadryl (an antihistamine), syringes, and vials of epinephrine. The individual and family members should understand and practice the appropriate steps in treatment of a reaction.

FOOD ALLERGIES

■ ***DESCRIPTION.*** Gastrointestinal food allergies are often difficult to diagnose. The process involves elimination of certain foods and then adding these to the diet one at a time.

■ ***ETIOLOGY.*** Chocolate and shellfish are common food allergies. Often, the allergy is not to a specific food but to additives or preservatives in the food. Allergy to milk might not be a true allergy but rather an intolerance to the lactose in the milk. Lactose intolerance can be treated by taking lactose enzyme (lactase) before consumption of dairy products.

■ ***SYMPTOMS.*** Symptoms of food allergies include cramping, diarrhea, and vomiting.

■ ***DIAGNOSIS.*** A thorough history from the patient and the patient's documented food diary aids in diagnosis. Testing, including skin tests, blood test, and food challenges, is also helpful.

■ ***TREATMENT.*** If the allergic reaction is mild, treatment with antihistamines might be sufficient. In a severe reaction, the first priority is to maintain the airway. Activation of the emergency medical system might be needed.

CONTACT DERMATITIS

■ ***DESCRIPTION.*** Contact dermatitis is an acute or chronic allergic reaction affecting the skin.

■ ***ETIOLOGY.*** Often the allergen is some type of cosmetic, laundry product, plant, jewelry, paint, drug, plastic, or a variety of other agents. Often, it is difficult to determine the causative agent and, once found, complete avoidance might not be possible.

■ ***SYMPTOMS.*** Allergic lesions can range from small, red, localized lesions to vesicular lesions that cover the entire body. A common example of contact dermatitis is poison ivy (Figure 5–5).

■ ***DIAGNOSIS.*** Skin patch testing helps determine the diagnosis of the allergen.

■ ***TREATMENT.*** Treatment is not available until the allergen is diagnosed. Avoiding the allergen is the most effective treatment.

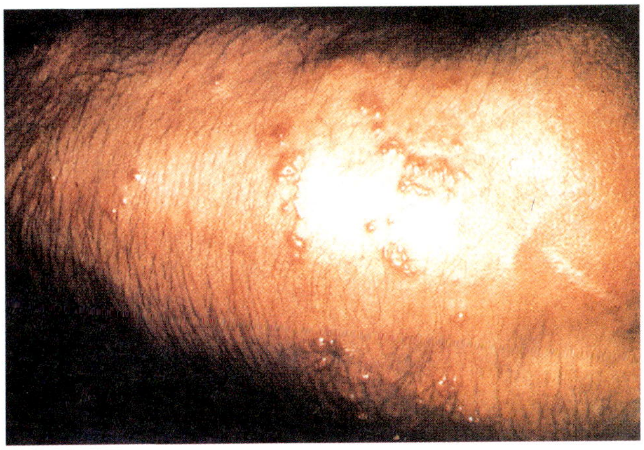

Courtesy of the Centers for Disease Control and Prevention, Atlanta, GA.

FIGURE 5–5 Contact dermatitis.

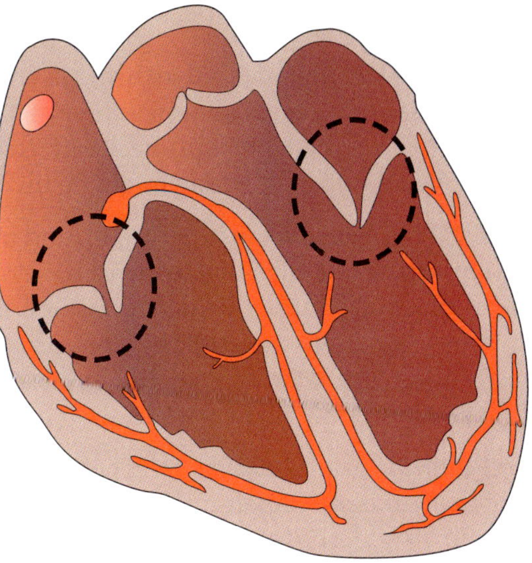

Delmar/Cengage Learning

FIGURE 5–6 Valves affected in rheumatic fever.

AUTOIMMUNE DISORDERS

Autoimmune disorders are hypersensitivities in which the body fails to recognize its own antigens or **self-antigen**. An individual's body cells have specific antigen on the cell surfaces. Failure to recognize this antigen as a self-antigen leads to the body attacking and destroying its own tissues. Several theories exist as to the cause of this type of disorder, but currently, the cause for autoimmune disorders is unknown. Autoimmune disorders include rheumatic fever, rheumatoid arthritis, myasthenia gravis, type 1 diabetes, lupus erythematosus, and scleroderma.

RHEUMATIC FEVER

DESCRIPTION. Rheumatic (ROO-MAT-ik) fever is an inflammatory disease that can affect the heart, joints, and skin.

ETIOLOGY. In a small number of individuals, rheumatic fever occurs following a group A **streptococcal** (STREHP-toh-KAHK-al) infection, usually strep throat. In this select number of individuals, the proteins in their hearts and other connective tissue is similar to the protein of the strep bacteria. For this reason, rheumatic fever tends to run in families. Exposure to strep bacteria causes the immune system to make antibodies to fight the bacteria. These antibodies also attack the tissues of the heart and joints because they cannot distinguish the differences in the proteins. Rheumatic fever is characterized by myocarditis (myo = muscle, cardi = heart, itis = inflammation) and arthritis.

SYMPTOMS. Rheumatic fever usually occurs 1 to 4 weeks after a streptococcal infection. Children and adolescents are most commonly affected. Onset of the disease can be sudden or gradual and includes symptoms of fever, malaise, and joint pain. The first occurrence of rheumatic fever might be mild and resolve without any permanent damage. Further episodes are usually more severe and might lead to permanent scarring and deformity of the heart valves (Figure 5–6). Deformity of the mitral and aortic valve can eventually lead to heart failure.

DIAGNOSIS. There is no definitive test for diagnosing rheumatic fever. Blood testing along with electrocardiogram to determine heart muscle damage are part of the diagnostic workup, and a positive throat culture for streptococcus bacteria is also indicative of the diagnosis.

TREATMENT. Culturing for strep infections and prolonged treatment (at least 10 days) with antibiotics is most effective. **Prophylactic** (pro-fil-LACK-tic; works to prevent) antibiotics can be given to susceptible individuals. Surgical replacement of the heart valves might be necessary for individuals with severe valve deformity.

PREVENTION. Prompt and accurate diagnosis and treatment of group A streptococcal infections is the best preventive measure against rheumatic fever.

RHEUMATOID ARTHRITIS

■ **DESCRIPTION.** Rheumatoid arthritis is an autoimmune disease that causes chronic inflammation of connective tissue. Joint tissue is primarily affected, but any connective tissue of the body might be involved.

■ **ETIOLOGY.** The exact cause of rheumatoid arthritis is unknown, but it is associated with the production of an abnormal antibody that attacks or attaches to the body's own cells and tissues. Presence of the antibody called *rheumatoid factor (RF)* in the affected individual's blood is indicative of the disease.

■ **SYMPTOMS.** Commonly, metacarpal-phalangeal joints of the hands are initially affected with rheumatoid arthritis. This leads to a classic sign of rheumatoid arthritis called ulnar deviation of the fingers (Figure 5–7). As the disease progresses, involvement of other synovial joints can occur. Joints affected can include those of the fingers, wrists, elbows, feet, ankles, and knees. Symptoms of rheumatoid arthritis can vary in severity from mild to severe and might go through periods of remission and exacerbation.

Rheumatoid arthritis begins with inflammation of the synovial lining of the joint, leading to pain, stiffness, and joint deformity. Eventually, the cartilage of the joint is destroyed and replaced with a granulation tissue called pannus (PAN-nus). As the disease progresses, the entire joint surface is destroyed and replaced with fibrous tissue, making the joint less movable. Fusion or total loss of joint function is called ankylosis (ANG-kih-LOH-sis) (Figure 5–8).

In addition to joint changes, the individual might also have lesions in the collagen of the lungs, blood vessels, heart, and eyes, leading to pleuritis (PLOO-RIGH-tis; pleura = pleura or lining of the lung, itis = inflammation), anemia, valvulitis (VAL-view-LYE-tis; valvu = valve, itis = inflammation), and glaucoma (glaw-KOH-mah), respectively. Rheumatoid nodules characteristically appear in the subcutaneous tissue around the fingers, toes, and elbows (Figure 5–9). Individuals with rheumatoid arthritis often appear frail and chronically ill. Anemia and infection are common secondary problems.

This chronic disease affects both sexes and all ages, but onset is most common in women between the ages of 20 and 40. Women are affected three times more often than men. Rheumatoid arthritis in children usually affects infants to children aged 16, can be very severe, and is called juvenile rheumatoid arthritis or Still's disease.

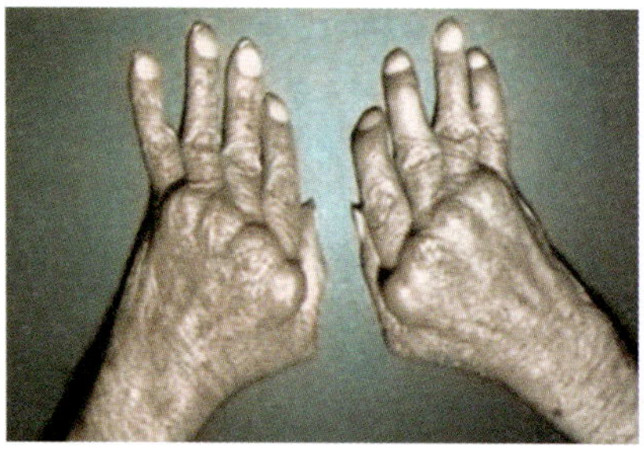

Delmar/Cengage Learning

FIGURE 5–7 Ulnar deviation from rheumatoid arthritis. *(Courtesy of Mark L. Kuss.)*

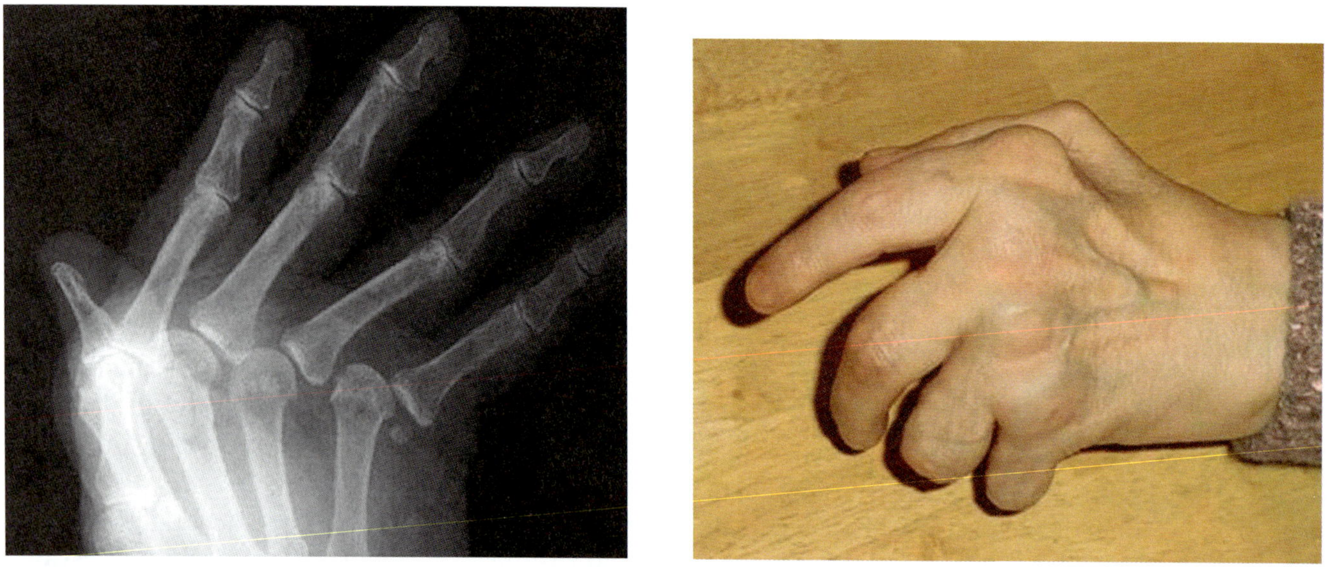

Courtesy of Mark L. Kuss

FIGURE 5–8 Joint changes from rheumatoid arthritis. (A) X-ray view (B) Ankylosis

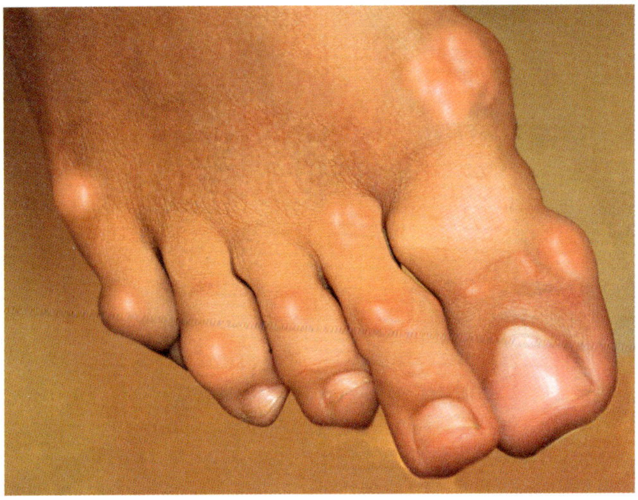

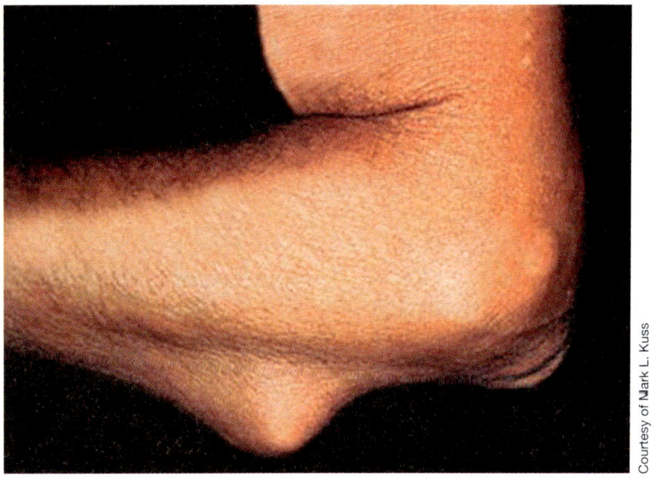

FIGURE 5–9 Rheumatoid nodules. (A) Foot (B) Elbow

■ ***DIAGNOSIS.*** No specific test exists that can confirm the diagnosis of rheumatoid arthritis. Diagnosis is based on physical examination, characteristic symptoms, and blood tests including positive rheumatoid factor and elevated erythrocyte sedimentation rate (ESR).

■ ***TREATMENT.*** Rheumatoid arthritis, like other autoimmune disorders, cannot be cured. Treatment includes use of anti-inflammatory medications and analgesics. An exercise and rest routine is developed to maintain joint function. Corticosteroids can be prescribed short term during periods of exacerbation. Surgical joint replacement might also be beneficial.

■ ***PREVENTION.*** There is no known way to prevent rheumatoid arthritis.

MYASTHENIA GRAVIS

■ ***DESCRIPTION.*** Myasthenia gravis (MY-uh-STHEE-nee-uh GRAV-iss) is characterized by severe muscle fatigue.

■ ***ETIOLOGY.*** This disease affects the transmission of nerve signals to muscle at the neuromuscular junction, but there is no muscle or nerve tissue disease. Nerve impulses are carried to the muscle by the neurotransmitter acetylcholine (ah-SEE-til-KOH-leen). These impulses are sent by the nerve but are not properly received by the muscle. This error in transmission is due to antibodies attacking the muscle receptors, which blocks the transmission by acetylcholine (Figure 5–10). This poor transmission of information to the muscle leads to weak muscle contractions and fatigue.

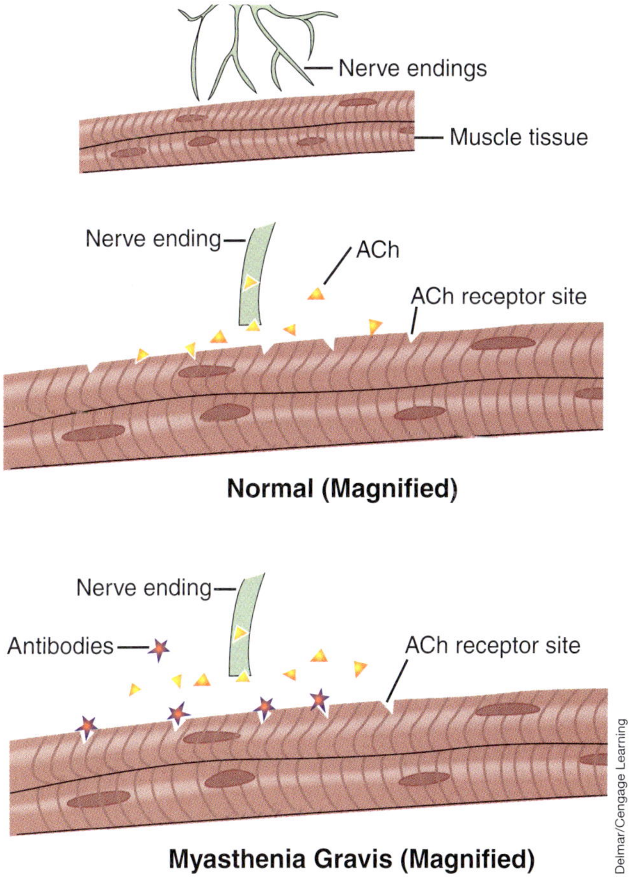

Nerves do not touch muscle tissue to stimulate movement. Nerve endings secrete a neurotransmitter, acetylcholine (ACh), that sticks to muscle tissue receptor sites causing muscle contraction.

Antibodies produced with myasthenia gravis block these receptor sites thus blocking muscle stimulus and movement.

FIGURE 5–10 Blocking of receptor sites in myasthenia gravis.

Myasthenia gravis is one of the less common autoimmune disorders with an estimated 200–400 cases per million people (Conti-Fine, 2006). Myasthenia can be categorized as an autoimmune, musculoskeletal, or neurologic disease because it has characteristics of problems in each of these systems.

■ **SYMPTOMS.** Onset of the disease is usually slow, and diagnosis might be difficult because it can affect any muscle of the body. Commonly, facial muscles are the ones initially affected, leading to diplopia (dip-PLOHP-ee-ah; double vision), ptosis (TOE-sis; drooping eyelids), dysphagia (dys-FAY-jee-ah; difficulty swallowing), dysphonia (dys-FOH-nee-ah; difficulty talking), and difficulty with facial expressions, which can leave the individual with an expressionless facial appearance. Other symptoms relate to fatigue of all voluntary muscles and include difficulty rising from a sitting position, lifting the arms, standing, and walking.

The degree of weakness varies with the time of day and activities. Generally, these individuals feel stronger in the morning due to a buildup of acetylcholine and become weaker as the day progresses because acetylcholine stores diminish. Short rest periods are necessary to help restore muscle function.

Periods of exacerbation and remission do occur. During exacerbation, complete bed rest might be necessary.

■ **DIAGNOSIS.** Myasthenia is difficult to diagnose because symptoms can be hard to distinguish from other neurological disorders. A thorough physical exam might reveal fatigue of the muscles; blood testing for antibodies against the acetylcholine receptor is also suggestive of myasthenia. Other tests include electromyography to test muscle fatigue and respiratory spirometry to assess respiratory function.

■ **TREATMENT.** Treatment can include cholinergic medications that do not allow the normal breakdown of the neurotransmitter acetylcholine, allowing a buildup of the neurotransmitter, thus improving neuromuscular transmission. Plasma exchange to remove the circulating antibodies provides some improvement in the condition. Recent advances in care and treatment have reduced the mortality rate to 3–4%. Death is usually due to muscle weakness leading to respiratory failure.

■ **PREVENTION.** Myasthenia gravis cannot be prevented, but avoiding stress, extremes in temperature, fever, illness, and overexertion can help prevent exacerbations.

TYPE 1 DIABETES MELLITUS (INSULIN-DEPENDENT DIABETES MELLITUS)

■ **DESCRIPTION.** Type 1 diabetes mellitus, formerly known as insulin-dependent diabetes mellitus (IDDM) is a disease that alters the body's carbohydrate or sugar metabolism.

■ **ETIOLOGY.** Type 1 diabetes mellitus is believed to be caused by an autoimmune disorder triggered by a viral infection. The most common viral infections that might lead to diabetes include rubella, mumps, and influenza. The infecting virus inflames insulin-producing beta cells of the pancreas, and the inflammatory process, for reasons that remain unclear, seems to stimulate the beta cells to produce an abnormal cell antigen. Lymphocytes recognize the abnormal antigen as non-self and destroy it along with the beta cells. Without insulin-producing beta cells, the individual becomes dependent on insulin injections to manage carbohydrate usage.

The normal antigens in the cells of the pancreas are histocompatibility locus antigens (HLAs). Individuals genetically inherit the HLAs of the pancreas. The tendency to develop an autoimmune response, and thus diabetes mellitus, is considered hereditary in nature.

There are other types of diabetes that are not caused by autoimmunity. Because all types of diabetes affect the endocrine system, they will be discussed and compared in detail in Chapter 14, "Endocrine System Diseases and Disorders."

LUPUS ERYTHEMATOSUS

■ **DESCRIPTION.** The term *lupus* originally referred to any chronic, destructive type of skin lesion. The Latin word *lupus* means *wolf*, and erythematosus refers to redness. The term *lupus erythematosus* has been used since the thirteenth century because physicians of that time thought the shape and color of the skin lesions resembled a wolf bite. The word *lupus* is often used to refer to lupus erythematosus, although used alone, this term truly has no meaning. There are several forms of lupus, including lupus pernio, lupus vulgarus, drug-induced lupus, and lupus erythematosus.

There are two types of lupus erythematosus: cutaneous (discoid) and systemic (diffuse). Cutaneous or discoid lupus erythematosus (DLE) is limited to skin or cutaneous involvement. DLE does not affect multisystems as does systemic lupus erythematosus (SLE).

DLE can be thought of as a type of systemic lupus because cause, testing, and treatment are similar for cutaneous involvement. DLE is the less serious type of lupus erythematosus.

SLE affects approximately 1 in 2,400 people. It primarily affects women, occurring 10 times more frequently in women than in men. Onset is usually between ages 30 and 40, but it can appear at any age. The disease is most severe among individuals of African-American descent.

ETIOLOGY. SLE is an autoimmune disorder in which B lymphocytes produce autoantibodies that attack body cells. Individuals with SLE have a high number of ANAs. These antibodies attack the body's own cell nuclei, destroying the RNA and DNA of the cell. Detection of ANA by microscopic immunofluorescence supports the diagnosis of SLE.

SYMPTOMS. SLE often affects the skin and a number of other organs or systems. A classic sign is the presence of a persistent, red, facial butterfly-shaped rash across the bridge of the nose and cheeks (Figure 5–11). Symptomatic individuals often complain of fever, joint pain, weight loss, and facial rash. Joint, kidney, and muscle involvement can lead to complaints of arthritis, glomerulonephritis (inflammation of the glomerulus, or filtering unit of the kidney), and atrophy, respectively. Heart valve deformities and abnormal blood composition are not unusual findings.

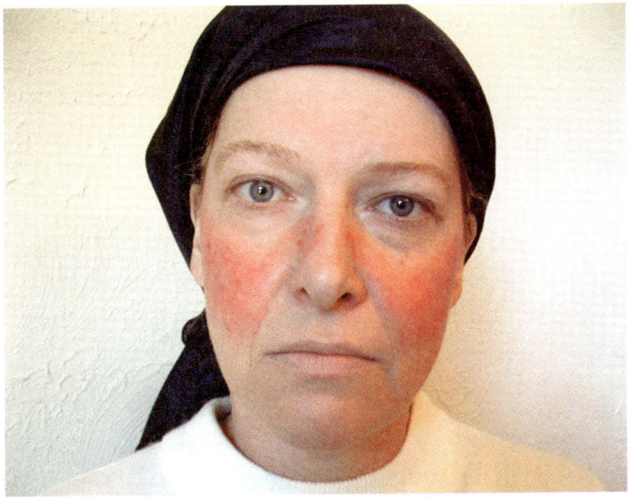
Delmar/Cengage Learning

FIGURE 5–11 Butterfly rash of systemic lupus erythematosus (SLE).

DIAGNOSIS. Diagnosis is often very difficult, but tests including electrolytes, renal function, liver enzymes, and complete blood count are helpful. The most definitive testing is a positive result on an antinuclear antibody test.

TREATMENT. SLE is a chronic disease that goes through periods of exacerbation and remission. Complete remission is very rare. Treatment is symptomatic. Nonsteroidal anti-inflammatory, antipyretic, and analgesic medications can be used to treat symptoms. Life-threatening exacerbations are often treated with corticosteroids. Prognosis depends on which organs are affected and the severity of the infection. Survival in patients with SLE in the United States, Canada, and Europe is approximately 95% at 5 years, 90% at 10 years, and 78% at 20 years (Harrison's, 2008). Renal insufficiency, bacterial endocarditis, cardiac failure, sepsis, and pneumonia commonly lead to death.

PREVENTION. SLE cannot be prevented or cured.

SCLERODERMA

DESCRIPTION. Scleroderma (skle-ro-DER-mah; sclero = hardening, derma = skin) is a chronic autoimmune disorder characterized by hardening, thickening, and shrinking of the connective tissues of the body, including the skin. Like many other chronic diseases, scleroderma might exhibit periods of remission and exacerbation. The generally slow progression of the disease allows the individual a reasonably long life, although if the disorder progresses rapidly, affecting vital organs, early death can result. Death is usually related to kidney failure.

ETIOLOGY. It is thought that this autoimmune reaction begins with the skin and connective tissues, attracting lymph cells. These lymph cells stimulate the production of collagen, leading to the disorder.

Milder forms of scleroderma commonly affect women 30–50 years of age and include those limited to the skin, face, and extremities. The more severe forms, called systemic or diffuse, usually affect men and older persons. This type not only affects the skin but also internal organs, including the heart, lungs, and kidney. These tissues become hardened, thickened, and often limited in function.

SYMPTOMS. Characteristically, individuals with scleroderma have thick, leather-like, shiny, taut skin and joint contractures. The first symptom is usually Raynaud's phenomenon, an episodic vasoconstriction affecting the hands. The mouth area often becomes wrinkled with a tight, purse-lipped appearance, leading to difficulty eating. Diagnosis can be confirmed by clinical examination and tissue biopsy.

■ ***DIAGNOSIS.*** Diagnosis is difficult because this disease initially mimics other disorders such as bursitis and arthritis.

Physical symptoms indicative of scleroderma include:

- Tight skin around the hands, face, and mouth.
- Changes in the capillaries at the base of the fingernails.
- Calcium deposits under the skin.

These physical symptoms, coupled with special blood testing for the presence of anticentromere antibodies, often yields a positive diagnosis.

■ ***TREATMENT.*** Currently, there is no treatment or cure to stop the progression of scleroderma. Treatment with anti-inflammatory medications, immunosuppressives, and antibiotics might be beneficial. Muscle stretching and strengthening exercises might also be beneficial to maintain muscle strength and joint mobility.

■ ***PREVENTION.*** No one really knows what causes scleroderma so at this time, there are no preventive methods identified.

Isoimmune Disorders

Isoimmunity refers to a hypersensitivity of one individual to another individual's tissues. Examples include blood type reactions, tissue rejections, and maternal–fetal reactions.

BLOOD TRANSFUSION REACTION

■ ***DESCRIPTION.*** As previously stated, all body cells have a specific antigen that identifies them. Red blood cells (RBCs) have surface antigens. Transfusion of blood from one individual to another is, in a sense, a type of tissue transplant. RBCs have to be typed and cross-matched to identify antigens properly and prevent rejection.

The blood types are identified by antigens and can be divided into four groups: A, B, AB, and O. Types O and A are the most common. Each RBC has an antigen and a corresponding antibody. Blood type A has an A antigen and anti-B antibody. B type has a B antigen and anti-A antibody. O has no antigen and both anti-A and anti-B antibodies. AB has an A and a B antigen and no antibody. These antigen-antibody patterns make type O the universal blood donor and type AB the universal blood recipient (Figure 5–12).

■ ***ETIOLOGY.*** If a blood type with an antigen is given to a type that has antibodies against that antigen, the antibodies will attack the antigen and break down the donor RBCs. For example, if type A (with antigen A and anti-B antibody) is given to type B (with antigen B and anti-A antibody), the anti-A antibody in the B type recipient's blood will attack the A antigen and break down the type A donor blood (see Figure 5–12).

As antibodies react with the antigen, they also cause clumping of the blood, leading to microthrombi (microscopic-sized blood clots). These microthrombi can lead to multiple organ emboli and have fatal consequences.

■ ***SYMPTOMS.*** Symptoms of transfusion reaction include chills, shivering, and fever.

■ ***TREATMENT.*** Reactions should be treated immediately by discontinuing the transfusion, contacting the director of the blood bank, medical physician, and nephrologist. Anticipation of complications such as hypotension, renal failure, disseminated intravascular coagulation (DIC), and possibly death should be expected and treated preventively or as symptoms arise.

■ ***DIAGNOSIS.*** Most transfusion reactions are diagnosed by watching for any significant change in a patient's condition during transfusion. Diagnosis depends on recognition of a significant change in vitals signs along with development of the signs and symptoms of a reaction.

■ ***PREVENTION.*** Prevention is aimed at by ensuring that the blood transfused is compatible by typing, cross-matching, and checking for antibody reaction.

ERYTHROBLASTOSIS FETALIS

■ ***DESCRIPTION.*** Erythroblastosis fetalis (eh-RITH-roh-blas-TOH-sis feh-TAH-lis) is an isoimmune condition in which antibodies in a mother's blood attack and destroy the antigen on the baby's RBCs ultimately killing the unborn fetus. This condition is also known

Type	Percent of Population with Type	Antigen	Antibody	Color Jar Example	Donate Blood To:	Reveive Blood From:
A	41	A	B	RED	A and AB	A and O
B	12	B	A	BLUE	B and AB	B and O
O	44	None	A and B	CLEAR	A, B, AB, O	O
AB	3	A and B	None	PURPLE	AB	A, B, AB, O

To understand the concept of transfusion reaction with antigen and antibodies, consider this example. The particular blood type can give blood to any type that does not change the color in the jar and receive blood from any type that does not change the color in the jar. For example, A can give blood to AB because adding red to purple will not change the purple color. However, A cannot give to B because giving red to blue will change the color. Since O is in the clear jar, it can give to all types but could not receive from anything but O or the clear color would change.

Delmar/Cengage Learning

FIGURE 5–12 Blood types for donors and recipients.

as hemolytic (hemo = blood, lytic = breaking or crushing) disease of the newborn.

Antigens on the RBCs give each type of cell a special identity. In addition to antigens that determine blood type, 85% of Americans have another antigen called the Rh factor. This group is collectively called Rh positive (Rh1) because they have the factor or antigen. Those who do not have the factor—approximately 15% of the population—are Rh negative (Rh2). Cross-matching for transfusions must not only match an appropriate type but also a compatibility factor. The common rule is, "those who don't have it don't want it; those who have it don't care." In other words, Rh2 individuals cannot receive Rh1 blood. On the other hand, Rh1 individuals "don't care," so they can receive Rh1 or Rh2 blood. Blood type and factor are genetically determined or received from an individual's mother or father.

Because blood type and factor is determined by one's mother or father, it is possible for a mother to be pregnant with a baby of different blood type and factor (received from the father) (Figure 5–13). Mothers pregnant with babies of different blood types do not have a problem because RBCs do not cross the placenta. Oxygen and nutrients simply diffuse across placental membranes to nourish the baby. RBCs do not normally exchange between the mother and the infant. Mothers who are Rh2 and "don't want" Rh1 factor might have difficulty with Rh1 babies.

■ ***ETIOLOGY.*** Rh2 mothers pregnant with Rh1 babies usually do not have a problem with the first baby. During the first pregnancy, the mother's blood has not had the opportunity to identify the antigen because there has been no exchange of blood cells or antigens. However, there may be some slight mixing of blood during the birthing process. As this blood intermingles, the Rh1 antigen is picked up by the mother's blood. The mother's immune system recognizes this antigen as a foreign invader and builds antibodies to destroy it. Subsequent Rh1 babies are not as fortunate as the first Rh1 baby.

■ ***SYMPTOMS.*** If this Rh2 mother becomes pregnant with another Rh1 baby, antibodies against the

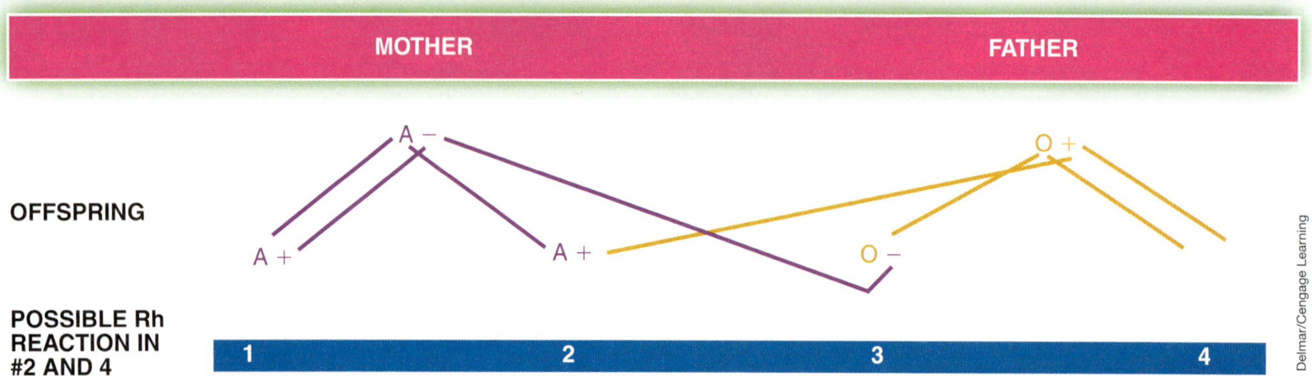

The offspring of this mother and father have the possibility of four different blood types. Since this is an RH– mother, there is a possiblility of an Rh reaction with the two Rh+ children. If the father was also Rh–, all offspring would be Rh– and no reaction would occur in any of the children. If the mother were Rh+ no Rh reaction could occur in any of the offspring since Rh+ mothers are not sensitive to the Rh antigen.

FIGURE 5–13 Blood type in inheritance patterns and identification of possible Rh reactions.

Rh factor that she has built up in her blood do cross the placental membranes. These antibodies attack the blood of the unborn child, breaking down the RBCs and leading to anemia and possible death of the baby.

This condition affects only Rh1 babies carried by Rh2 mothers. Rh1 mothers "don't care" about the factor. Rh1 mothers have the antigen, so they do not build up antibodies against it.

■ ***DIAGNOSIS.*** Prenatal diagnosis of erythroblastosis fetalis is accomplished by ultrasound. An abnormal or increased fluid accumulation might be noted in the abdomen, lungs, heart, skin, or all of these in the baby. There is also an increase in the amount of amniotic fluid along with thickening of the placenta.

■ ***TREATMENT.*** Treatment for erythroblastosis fetalis is exchange transfusion of the baby's blood with Rh2 blood at birth. This treatment stops the destruction of the baby's RBCs. Over a period of time, the transfused Rh2 blood is replaced by the baby's own blood. If erythroblastosis fetalis is a possibility in an Rh2 mother, the baby's condition can be monitored by amniocentesis. Babies who are mildly affected might be carried to full term. Severe cases, however, might indicate the need to induce labor and premature delivery of the baby to begin lifesaving treatment.

Historically, an Rh factor marital mismatch might have been the reason queens or wives of royalty were beheaded when unable to produce living heirs to the throne. If the king was Rh1 and the queen Rh2, every child after the first would have been at successively higher risk of fetal death. Erythroblastosis fetalis rarely occurs in the modern world. The development of RhoGAM, a special immune globulin, has halted this condition.

■ ***PREVENTION.*** RhoGAM is an injectable medication given to Rh2 females to prevent the development of antibodies against Rh1 factor. It is given prophylactically after the delivery of the first and any subsequent Rh2 fetuses to prevent development of Rh antibodies.

ORGAN REJECTION

■ ***DESCRIPTION.*** Organs such as the liver, kidney, heart, and lungs could be easily transplanted if not for the human immune system.

■ ***ETIOLOGY.*** The immune system recognizes transplanted tissue as foreign and attacks it. This attack by lymphocytes brings about donor tissue destruction recognized as tissue or organ rejection.

■ ***SYMPTOMS.*** Transplant rejection might be hyperacute in nature and actually occur during the surgical procedure. Acute rejection occurs within the first few weeks, whereas chronic rejection occurs over a period of time, usually months to years. Chronic rejection occurs slowly and is due to vessel damage that decreases blood flow to the donor tissue. Decreased blood flow causes chronic ischemia and, ultimately, death of the donor organ.

■ ***DIAGNOSIS.*** Diagnosis is made by physical examination and testing of the function of the newly transplanted organ. A biopsy of the organ can confirm rejection.

■ ***TREATMENT.*** Donated organs are matched to possible recipients. The closer the donor antigen matches that of the recipient, the less chance the organ will be rejected. Administration of immunosuppression medications also decreases the possibility of rejection.

■ ***PREVENTION.*** Immunosuppression medications must be taken prior to transplantation surgery and for the remainder of the organ recipient's life. This medication suppresses or decreases the body's ability to wage war against the donor tissue and thus prevents organ rejection.

Immune Deficiency Disorders

The last classification of immune disorders is immunodeficiency. These disorders represent an inability of the immune system to protect the individual against disease. This deficiency might be congenital due to a genetic disorder, or it might be acquired during the individual's lifetime. Acquired disorders are the most common type and can be due to disease therapies, such as chemotherapy and radiation treatments, by suppressing bone marrow, thus decreasing leukocyte production. Medications given to organ transplant recipients purposefully suppress the immune system. The most common and fatal disorder is acquired immunodeficiency syndrome (AIDS).

The classic clinical problem with immunodeficiency disorders is the development of unusual and severe infections such as pneumonia, meningitis, or septicemia, to name a few. Also, the development of infections by microorganisms that are not usually pathogenic (opportunistic infections) can be indicative of an immunodeficiency disorder. Other signs and symptoms are numerous and varied, depending on the organs or organ systems affected and the invading pathogen. Specific signs and symptoms will be included in the discussion of the disorder.

ACQUIRED IMMUNODEFICIENCY SYNDROME (AIDS)

■ ***DESCRIPTION.*** The name of this disease briefly describes its pathology. It is an acquired disease that causes the immune system to be deficient in protecting the body, leading to a syndrome of symptoms or secondary diseases.

AIDS was first diagnosed in the United States in the early 1980s. The first diagnosed cases were found in a group of homosexual men who became ill with a series of opportunistic diseases and eventually died. These individuals had surprisingly suppressed immune systems. Further research led to the discovery of the virus and mode of transmission.

■ ***ETIOLOGY.*** The cause of AIDS is a virus called human immunodeficiency virus (HIV). The wicked characteristic of HIV is its battle plan to wipe out the individual's lymphocytes, thus leaving the body defenseless against attack by all pathogenic organisms. The primary target is the T lymphocyte, but macrophages are affected as well. HIV is **cytotoxic** (cyto = cell, toxic = killing). Ultimately, the HIV-infected individual will have a low T lymphocyte cell count, indicative of a positive diagnosis of AIDS.

HIV is transmitted from one individual to another through intimate contact and sharing of body fluids. The virus must enter the body and bloodstream to infect the individual. HIV is fragile and easily killed by temperature changes. Many misconceptions and fears about the transmission of AIDS are still prevalent in society today. An individual cannot get HIV infection from toilet seats, doorknobs, furniture, water fountains, and other objects. An individual cannot get HIV from social kissing, coughing, sneezing, or even sharing eating utensils. HIV is not transmitted through air, food, urine, feces, or water. HIV is primarily transmitted in three ways:

1. **Sexual intercourse** Semen and vaginal secretions carry HIV. Transmission rate is higher from male to female because females might have microscopic vaginal tears during intercourse. Transmission rate is very high with anal intercourse because the internal lining of the rectum is very thin. Approximately 75% of infected individuals in the United States contract AIDS through sexual intercourse.
2. **Sharing of hypodermic needles** HIV-infected blood is injected into the body by sharing needles. This type of transmission accounts for 18–25% of infected individuals in the United States.
3. **In utero from infected mother to unborn child** HIV passes across the placenta to infect the baby. This accounts for 1–3% of AIDS cases.

Transmission of HIV through blood transfusions has been virtually eliminated by effective screening methods. Health professionals following appropriate precautions are at very little risk of contracting HIV.

■ ***SYMPTOMS.*** Previously, HIV was staged as four separate clinical presentations. Those stages were asymptomatic carrier, latency, AIDS-related complex (ARC), and full-blown AIDS. Currently, HIV infection is known to be a continuous disease process. Staging this disease might be helpful for medical intervention. The new stages of HIV infection are acute infection, asymptomatic HIV, symptomatic HIV, and advanced disease.

1. **Acute infection** This stage begins about 1 to 3 weeks after initial infection. During this time, the virus undergoes massive replication. Signs and symptoms include fever, sore throat, headache, and malaise. At this stage, HIV infection might be misdiagnosed as influenza.
2. **Asymptomatic HIV** No chronic signs or symptoms are displayed during this stage. Lymphadenopathy (lymph = lymphatic, adeno = gland, opathy = disease) and headache might occur intermittently. If blood testing is used during this stage, the T lymphocyte count can be dropping by 40–80 cells per microliter per year. (Normal T-cell count is 750–1000 cells per microliter.) T-cell count is a useful indicator of disease progression and is used in studying the effects of antiviral drugs and predicting the potential for opportunistic infections. This stage can last for 10–12 years, depending on drug therapy and individual resistance.
3. **Symptomatic HIV** This stage is divided into early and late phases. During the early phase, the individual becomes symptomatic with a variety of symptoms or diseases affecting any or all of the body organs. Fever is a common symptom along with oral Candida albicans, recurrent herpes simplex lesions, and night sweats. The chronic diarrhea of this phase leads to dehydration and cachexia. Individuals are considered to be in the late phase when T-cell count drops below 200 cells per microliter. Common diseases and disorders experienced during this phase include gastric ulcer, esophagitis, colitis, hepatitis, pancreatitis, fungal infections, neurologic disorders, herpes zoster, dermatitis, nausea, and vomiting, to name just a few. In this phase, the individual experiences severe weight loss, weakness, persistent diarrhea, and, usually, at least one opportunistic disease. These opportunistic infections include:

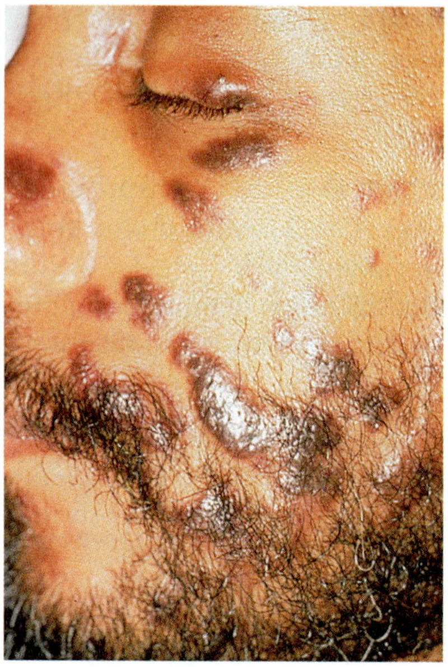

FIGURE 5–14 Kaposi's sarcoma.

   - **Pneumocystis carinii** (NEW-moh-SIS-tis kah-RYE-nee-eye) pneumonia, an infection of the lungs with a protozoan. This organism has never been documented as a cause of pneumonia in persons with normal immune systems.
   - **Kaposi's sarcoma** (KAP-oh-seez sar-KOH-mah), a blood vessel cancer that causes reddish-purple skin lesions (Figure 5–14).
4. **Advanced HIV** This stage is determined by a T-cell count of fewer than 50 cells per microliter. In this stage, mortality increases significantly. Commonly, more virulent and persistent infections occur that are more resistant to treatment. Symptoms at this stage include seizures, confusion, urinary and fecal incontinence, blindness, hemiparesis (hemi = one side, paresis = weakness), and coma.

■ ***DIAGNOSIS.*** When the T-cell count drops below 200 cells per microliter, the individual has met the criteria set by the Centers for Disease Control for a diagnosis of AIDS.

■ ***TREATMENT.*** When AIDS is diagnosed, life expectancy is approximately 3 to 5 years. Currently, AIDS is 100% fatal. Life can be extended by vigorous treatment of infections. In late-stage AIDS, every possible symptom or disease can be present because the individual's immune system is crumbling and

GLIMPSE OF THE FUTURE

Studying HIV/AIDS in Women

Historically, little research has been done on women who are HIV positive or who have AIDS. However, 50% of the individuals affected by the virus are women. In sub-Sarahan Africa, 60% are women, and many of them are adolesscent girls. Clinical trial research projects have virtually ignored women in the study protocols, but that is now changing. The United Nations AIDS division (UNAIDS) and the Global Coalition on Women and Aids (GCWA) have collaborated and developed some research goals that will help women affected by HIV in the future. They propose that more research is needed in the areas of sex differences and interventions. They also proposed that more advocacy is needed for women especially for the young adolescent women. Future research will be undertaken in these areas as well as looking at the effects of pregnancy and abortion on women with HIV, and how to best disseminate the new knowledge about the disease and treatments.

Source: Joint United Nations Programme AIDS Information Centre (2007).

incapacitated (Figure 5–15). Ultimately, super infections and massive diarrhea can be the cause of death. Antiviral medication such as zidovudine (AZT) might slow HIV replication and thus the progression of the disease to some extent.

PREVENTION. AIDS is currently a worldwide epidemic or pandemic. In 2007, the Joint United Nations Programme on HIV/AIDS estimated the number of people worldwide infected with HIV at 33.2 million. In that same year, approximately 2.5 million people were newly diagnosed and another 2.1 million people died. Although, these numbers are decreasing, they are still overwhelming. There were 21,000 deaths in North America but 1.6 million in sub-Saharan Africa (AIDS epidemic update, 2007). Costs for research, treatment, and prevention are escalating out of control.

AIDS can be stopped with preventive education and action. The only known method of prevention is avoiding exposure to the virus. However, an antiretroviral treatment, known as post-exposure prophylaxis, is believed to reduce the risk of infection if begun directly after exposure.

HEALTHY HIGHLIGHT

Preventive Strategies for HIV and AIDS

Preventive Strategies for HIV and AIDS

- Abstain from sexual intercourse or develop a monogamous relationship with a partner who is not infected and is not an intravenous drug user.
- Do not abuse alcohol or drugs in a manner that prevents you from being in control of your behavior.
- Do not use intravenous drugs. If you are an intravenous drug user, always use a sterile needle or one soaked in bleach, and do not share your needles.

Other Behaviors That Will Help Prevent the Spread of HIV

- Refrain from multiple sex partners or sex with intravenous drug users.
- Refrain from unprotected sex with homosexuals or bisexual men.
- Always use a latex condom with a spermicide and virucide if you are uncertain about your partner's sexual history.

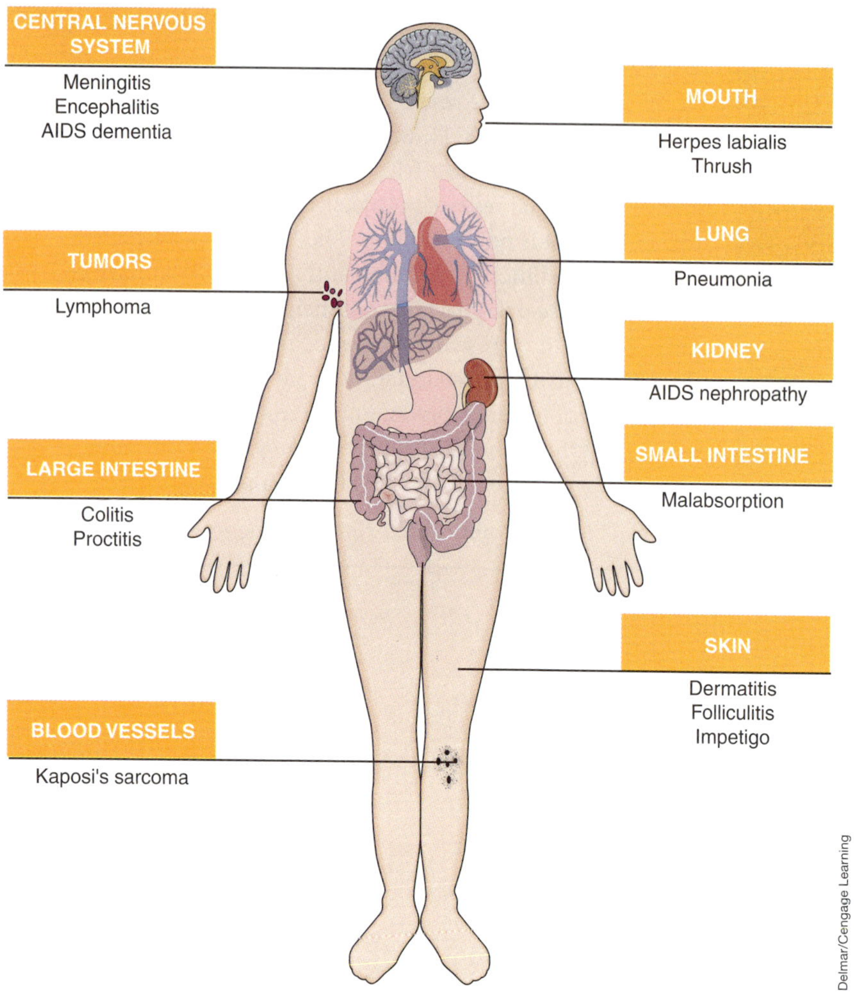

FIGURE 5–15 Pathologies associated with AIDS.

TRAUMA

Trauma to the immune system is generally limited to treatments or medications, such as chemotherapy and radiation treatments, that often lead to immunosuppression. Individuals on corticosteroid medications often have undetected infections because this medication suppresses the protective inflammatory response. Graft and organ recipients take immunosuppression medications to traumatize the system purposefully in hopes of protecting the transplanted graft or organ.

RARE DISEASES

Severe Combined Immunodeficiency Disease (SCID)

SCID is a group of inherited disorders in which there is partial or complete dysfunction of the immune system or complete deficiency. Untreated children usually die at a young age. Treatment can include a bone marrow transplant from a matched sibling and has restored complete immune function in some children. Protective isolation is necessary to prevent lethal infections. This protected environment has led to these children being called "bubble babies."

EFFECTS OF AGING ON THE IMMUNE SYSTEM

Presently, not all age-related changes in the immune system are well understood. It is known that the thymus gland degenerates with age. The thymus reaches its maximum size in early childhood and then slowly decreases in size after puberty. As the gland decreases in size, so does the number of T cells because they originate in the cortex of the thymus. The remaining T cells do not function as well, increasing the chance of developing invasive diseases, such as cancer, as an individual ages. Some defects in lymph cells also occur in the aging process.

The B-cell levels remain stable throughout life, but the antibodies in older persons might not function as well as in younger years. Thus, infections are common in the older population. The antibodies are more likely to attack the body's own tissue (autoantibodies) as a result of loss of tolerance to self-antigens. General resistance to disease seems to decrease with age, but this might be due to many other factors such as general nutrition, exercise, medications, and psychosocial influences rather than to changes in the immune system.

SUMMARY

The immune system consists of organs such as the thymus gland, bone marrow, lymph nodes, spleen, liver, and tonsils, and major cells such as the lymphocytes. The immune system is an important defense system for the body because a malfunctioning or compromised immune system weakens the body's defenses against invading microorganisms. Many secondary disorders such as infections are due to a compromised immune response. Primary diseases or disorders of the immune system are categorized as hypersensitivity disorders or immune deficiency disorders. Hypersensitivity disorders include allergies, autoimmune disorders, and isoimmune disorders. The immune deficiency disease, AIDS, is one of the most common and debilitating fatal conditions of the immune system. Diagnostic testing for immune disorders includes skin testing, complete blood cell counts, and some specific antibody studies. Treatment for immune disorders varies with the specific problem. Some immune disorders are quite mild, whereas others are severe and require long-term therapy.

REVIEW QUESTIONS

Short Answer

1. What are the functions of the immune system?

2. Which signs and symptoms are associated with common immune system disorders?

3. Which diagnostic tests are most commonly used to determine the type, cause, or both of an immune system disorder?

Matching

4. Match the disorders listed in the left column with the correct category of immune system diseases in the right column. (Right-hand column categories may be used more than once.)

_____ Hay fever	a. Allergies
_____ AIDS	b. Autoimmune disorders
_____ Anaphylaxis	c. Isoimmune disorders
_____ Rheumatic fever	d. Immune deficiency disorders
_____ Erythroblastosis fetalis	
_____ Organ rejection	

Multiple Choice

5. Which of the following behaviors might contribute to increased risk for HIV transmission?
   - a. Donating blood
   - b. Sharing intravenous needles
   - c. Failure to wash hands after toileting
   - d. Unprotected sex
   - e. Sharing eating utensils
   - f. Direct contact with body fluids
   - g. Frequent use of laxatives and enemas

True or False

6. T F The immune system is the body's only defense system against invading organisms.
7. T F Signs and symptoms of hypersensitivity disorders might include rash, redness, heat, swelling, nasal congestion, coughing, and sneezing.
8. T F The coombs test is used to detect certain antibodies in the blood.
9. T F Autoimmune disorders are hyposensitivities in which the body fails to recognize its own antigens.
10. T F The effects of aging put the older adult at an increased risk for immune system problems.

CASE STUDIES

■ Terry Stephens is a 26-year-old male who has been diagnosed as HIV positive. He has told you that he and his girlfriend have unprotected sex. You have been close friends for many years. What are some strategies you could use to inform Terry about the danger of this behavior? Should you also talk to his girlfriend? When Terry was hospitalized, you noticed his caregivers wore gloves when starting his IV and drawing blood. Was this because he is HIV positive? Would this be routine precautions?

■ Your friend, Janet, is suffering from a bout with the common cold. She asks you if she should use an over-the-counter preparation containing echinacea as a treatment. How would you answer her question? Can you safely say it is a good idea to try this treatment? Would it help boost her immune system? Is there strong evidence that it is beneficial? Does it prevent colds? What does the research say about the benefits of echinacea?

*Study*WARE™ Connection

To help you learn the content in this chapter, take a practice quiz or play an interactive game on your StudyWARE™ CD-ROM.

Workbook Practice

Go to your Workbook and complete the practice questions.

BIBLIOGRAPHY

AIDS epidemic update: 2007. (2007). Joint United Nations Programme AIDS Information Centre. 20 Avenue Appia, 1211 Geneva 27, Switzerland. *www.unaids.org* (accessed January 2008).

Bopp, C. M., Phillips, K. D., Fulk, L. J., Dudgeon, W. D., Sowell, R., & Hand, G. A. (2004). Physical activity and immunity in HIV-infected individuals. *AIDS Care 16*(3), 387–393.

Conti-Fine, B. M., Milani, M., & Kaminski, H. J. (2006). Myasthenia gravis: Past, present, and future. *Journal of Clinical Investigations 116*(11): 2843–54.

Franchi, L., Park, J., Shaw, M. H., Marina-Garcia, N., Chen, G., Yun-Gi, K., & Nunez, G. (2008). Intracellular NOD-like receptors in innate immunity, infection and disease. *Cellular Microbiology 10*(1), 1–8.

Franco, A. (2008). Glycoconjugates as vaccines for cancer immunotherapy: Clinical trials and future directions. *Anti-Cancer Agents in Medicinal Chemistry 8*(1), 86–91.

Frequently asked questions. The Food Allergy and Anaphylaxis Network. *www.foodallergy.org* (accessed May 2008).

Goldsobel, A. B. (2007). Use of complementary and alternative medicine by food-allergic patients. *Pediatrics 120*(supplement), S119–S120.

Harrison's Internal Medicine, 17th ed. Chapter 313. Systemic lupus erythematosis. *www.accessmedicine.com* (accessed May 2008).

Jay, F., Chantler, T., Lees, A., & Pollard, A. J. (2007). Children's participation in vaccine research: Parents' views. *Paediatric Nursing 19*(8), 14–18.

Kimura, K., Isowa, T., Ohira, H., & Murashima, S. (2005). Temporal variation of acute stress response in sympathetic nervous and immune systems. *Biological Psychology 70*(2), 131–139.

Kovaril, P., Sauer, I., & Schaljo, B. (2008). Molecular mecnanisms of the anti-inflammatory function of interferons. *Immunobiology 212*(9/10), 895–901.

Making HIV trials work for women. (2007). Joint United Nations Programme AIDS Information Centre. 20 Avenue Appia, 1211 Geneva 27, Switzerland. *www.unaids.org* (accessed January 2008).

Newburg, D. S. (2005). Innate immunity and human milk. *Journal of Nutrition 135*(5), 1308–1312.

Reviewing the evidence for cold fighters: Echinacea, vitamin C and zinc. (2007). *Tufts University Health & Nutrition Letter 25*(8), 6.

Taylor, R. M., Parke, A., & Day, H. (2004). Immunosupression for solid organ transplantation in children. *Paediatric Nursing 16*(2), 39–43.

Uniting the world against AIDS: 2007. (2007). Joint United Nations Programme AIDS Information Centre. 20 Avenue Appia, 1211 Geneva 27, Switzerland. *www.unaids.org* (accessed January 2008).

Vally, H. (2008). Allergic and asthmatic reactions to alcoholic drinks: A significant problem in the community. *Clinical & Experimental Allergy 38*(1), 1–3.

Whetzel, C. A., Corwin, E. J., & Klein, L. C. (2007). Disruption in Th1/Th2 immune response in young adult smokers. *Addictive Behaviors 32*(1), 1–8.

Wilson, H., & Vincent, R. (2006). Autoimmune connective tissue disease: Scleroderma. *British Journal of Nursing 15*(15), 805–809.

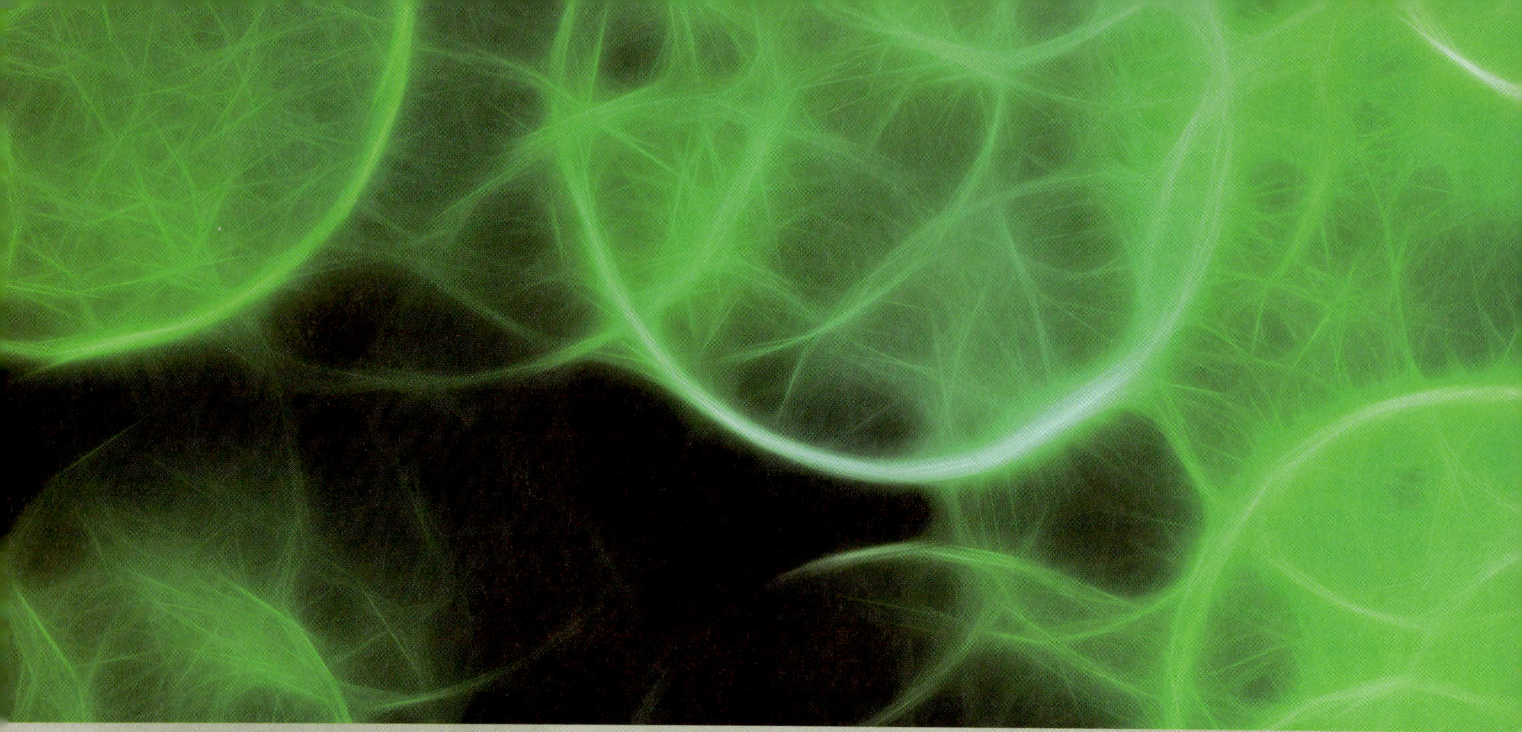

OUTLINE

- Anatomy and Physiology
- Common Signs and Symptoms
- Diagnostic Tests
- Common Diseases of the Musculoskeletal System
  - *Diseases of the Bone*
  - *Diseases of the Joints*
  - *Diseases of the Muscles and Connective Tissue*
  - *Neoplasms*
- Trauma
  - *Fracture*
  - *Strains and Sprains*
  - *Dislocations and Subluxations*
  - *Low Back Pain (LBP)*
  - *Herniated Nucleus Pulposus (HNP)*
  - *Bursitis*
  - *Tendonitis*
  - *Carpal Tunnel Syndrome*
  - *Plantar Fasciitis*
  - *Torn Rotator Cuff*
  - *Torn Meniscus*
  - *Cruciate Ligament Tears*
  - *Shin Splints*
- Rare Diseases
  - *de Quervain's Disease*
  - *Tuberculosis of the Bone*
  - *Paget's Disease*
  - *Myasthenia Gravis*
- Effects of Aging on the System
- Summary
- Review Questions
- Case Studies
- Bibliography

KEY TERMS

Anaerobic (p. 107)
Bone mass density (BMD) (p. 98)
Calcaneal (p. 116)
Computerized axial tomography (CAT or CT) (p. 98)
Densitometry (p. 101)
Diskectomy (p. 113)
Dowager's hump (p. 100)
Dual energy X-ray absorptiometry (DEXA) (p. 98)
Electromyography (p. 98)
Fascia (p. 116)
Interphalangeal (p. 104)
Laminectomy (p. 113)
Magnetic resonance imaging (MRI) (p. 98)
Meniscus (p. 117)
Metacarpophalangeal (p. 104)
Metatarsophalangeal (p. 105)
Mineralization (p. 103)
Myelogram (p. 113)
ORIF (p. 109)
Osteomyelitis (p. 102)
Radiologic (p. 98)
RICE (p. 112)
Sciatica (p. 115)
Spasms (p. 113)
Tetany (p. 108)
Tophi (p. 105)

Types of Fractures

articular (p. 104)
avulsion (p. 109)
closed (p. 109)
Colles' (p. 109)
comminuted (p. 109)
complete (p. 109)
compound (p. 109)
compression (p. 100)
displaced (p. 109)
extracapsular (p. 109)
femoral neck (p. 109)
greenstick (p. 109)
impacted (p. 109)
incomplete (p. 109)
intertrochanteric (p. 109)
intracapsular (p. 109)
longitudinal (p. 109)
nondisplaced (p. 98)
oblique (p. 109)
open (p. 109)
pathologic (p. 109)
Pott's (p. 109)
simple (p. 109)
spiral (p. 109)
stellate (p. 109)
stress (p. 109)
subcapital (p. 109)
transverse (p. 109)

6

Musculoskeletal System Diseases and Disorders

LEARNING OBJECTIVES

Upon completion of the chapter, the learner should be able to:

1. Define the terminology common to the musculoskeletal system and the disorders of the system.
2. Discuss the basic anatomy and physiology of the musculoskeletal system.
3. Identify the important signs and symptoms associated with common musculoskeletal system disorders.
4. Describe the common diagnostics used to determine type, cause, or both of a musculoskeletal system disorder.
5. Identify the common disorders of the musculoskeletal system.
6. Describe the typical course and management of the common musculoskeletal system disorders.
7. Describe the effects of aging on the musculoskeletal system and the common disorders associated with aging of the system.

OVERVIEW

The musculoskeletal system provides the structure and movement function for the individual. Because the muscles and bones run throughout the body, disorders of the system can affect any other system, and disorders of other systems frequently affect the musculoskeletal system. The system includes bones, joints, ligaments, muscles, and tendons; each of these has a unique function but also interacts with the other components of the system to support the person and provide for mobility. Problems with the musculoskeletal system frequently affect the individual's independence and, thus, the quality of life. ■

ANATOMY AND PHYSIOLOGY

The skeletal component of the musculoskeletal system is made up of bones and joints. The bones provide the framework to support the body. They also produce blood cells, store fat and minerals, protect soft tissues (such as the brain), and help create body motion. Bones are very vascular; blood circulates through them, picking up or storing body minerals such as calcium, phosphorus, magnesium, and sodium. Bones also contain osteoblasts, active bone-building cells; osteoclasts, cells that reabsorb bone; and osteocytes, mature bone cells.

Bones are often classified by shape and composition. For example, the skeletal system is composed of long bones such as the femur in the leg, short bones such as the metacarpal bones or bones in the fingers, flat bones such as the sternum or skull, and irregular bones such as the vertebrae or pelvic bones (Figure 6–1). The composition of bone is either cortical or cancellous. Cortical bone is dense, smooth, and compact, whereas cancellous bone is spongy, with many open spaces throughout. The ligaments are fibrous connective tissue that connect bones to other bones and joints.

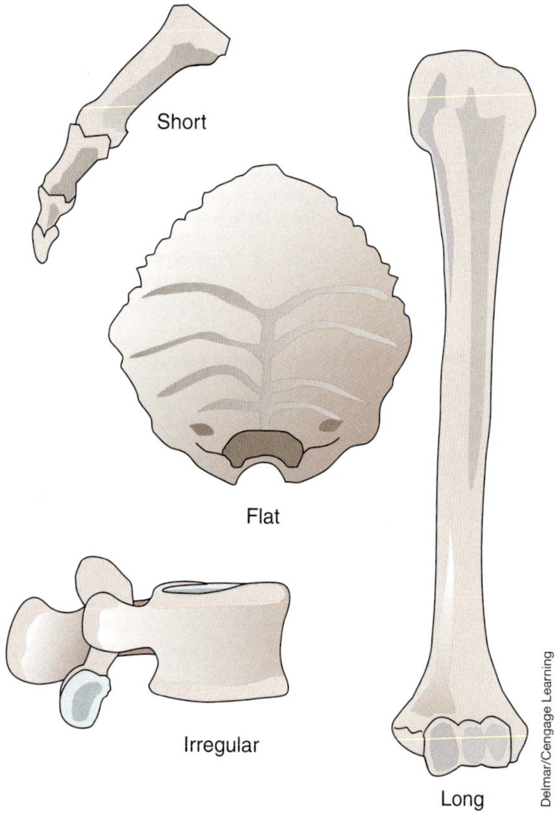

FIGURE 6–1 Examples of types of bones.

Bone can be damaged and repair itself. The steps of bone repair include (1) bleeding at the site of injury with clot and granulation tissue formation; (2) proliferation of cells at the site, forming a callus (soft bony deposit) over the injury or fracture; (3) cells becoming bone (osteoblasts) or cartilage at the site; (4) the bone calcifying (hardened) by the deposit of inorganic salts at the site; and (5) the remodeling of the bone to the shape necessary to complete its designated function. Bone repair is dependent on many factors such as the general health status of the individual, his or her age, the degree of injury, circulation to the site, and the presence of other diseases or infection.

The joints are where two or more bones meet. They are usually classified based on the amount of movement of the joint, as described in Table 6–1, but they also can be classified by their structure. Classification of joints by structure includes fibrous (such as the joints of the skull), cartilaginous (such as the joints of the vertebrae), and synovial (such as the joints of the knee). The synovial joints are those separated by a fluid-filled cavity.

The major movements of joints are flexion (bending), extension (reaching out or spreading out), abduction (away from the body), adduction (toward the body), rotation (turning on an axis), circumduction (circular movement), and elevation (lifting).

Cartilage is collagen tissue that supports articulating (adjoining) bones. It provides protection and a cushion to prevent friction between bones and acts like a shock absorber to reduce stress on the bone surface.

The functions of the muscles of the body are to provide structure and movement and to produce heat (Figure 6–2). The muscles of the musculoskeletal system are called striated because they look striped or banded under a microscope. They are also

TABLE 6–1 Classification of Joints by Movement

Classification	Amount of Movement	Example of Joint
Synarthrosis	No movement	Suture of the skull
Amphiarthrosis	Some movement but very limited	Pelvis
Diarthrosis	Complete movement	Knee, hip, elbow

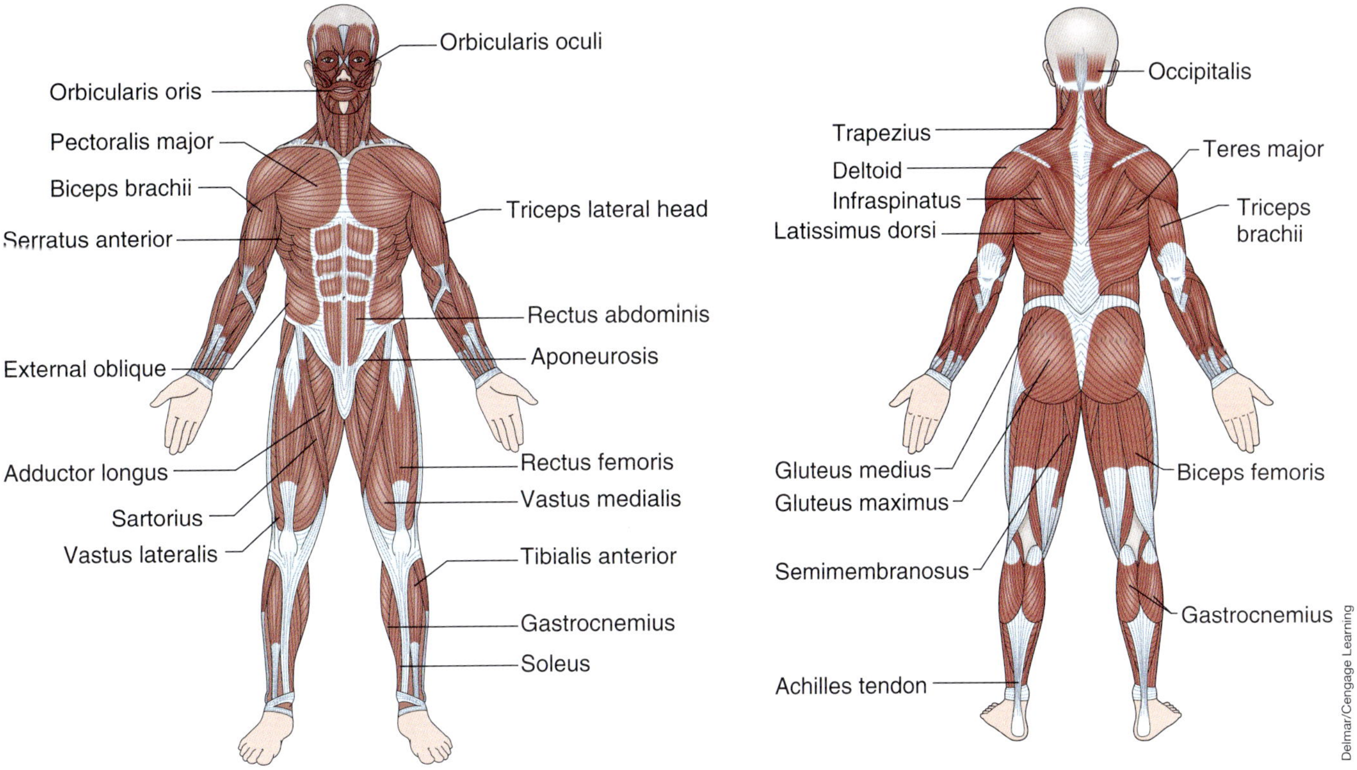

FIGURE 6–2 The skeletal muscles.

called voluntary muscles because most are moved by conscious control as opposed to other muscles, such as cardiac, that move involuntarily. Skeletal muscles move in response to signals from the central nervous system. Connective tissue holds the muscle fibers together, and tendons, long, fibrous, nonelastic connective tissues, attach muscle to bone.

Each muscle fiber in the body contains myofibrils, which are composed of sarcomeres that are the contracting and relaxing component of the muscle. This contracting and relaxing characteristic provides the smooth, elastic movement of the muscle.

The source of energy for the movement of muscles is the metabolism of adenosine triphosphate (ATP) in the cell. ATP is produced from available glucose and glycogen (stored glucose) in the cells, and oxygen as well as adequate stores of glucose are necessary for parts of this process.

COMPLEMENTARY AND ALTERNATIVE THERAPY

Herbal Medicine for Bone Diseases

The Korean preparation of *Gami-Honghwain* (HJ), which contains safflower seeds, has been tested for use in the treatment of bone diseases. In laboratory testing it was found to stimulate osteoblastic differentiation. The most important function of osteoblasts is to form mineralized bones. The differentiation of osteoblasts is important for this to occur. HJ also increased bone mineralization and bone proteins in cells. This herbal preparation has been used for centuries in Asian culture. New studies are determining how it really works.

Source: Kim, et al. (2008).

COMMON SIGNS AND SYMPTOMS

The most common signs and symptoms of bone and joint disease are pain, swelling, decreased mobility, and deformity. Most fractures are associated with pain due to a disruption of the periosteum and related sensory nerves. Many fractures are easy to recognize due to the obvious displacement and related deformity. **Nondisplaced** (not out of place or position) fractures are not as easy to recognize but can cause pain just the same.

Weakness is the most common sign or symptom of muscle disorders and can be related to a primary disease of the muscle or be secondary to a neurologic disorder. Muscle tissue will atrophy if weakness persists for an extended length of time. On the other hand, just the reverse can also occur, with muscle atrophy leading to muscle weakness.

DIAGNOSTIC TESTS

Radiologic examinations (X-rays) are the primary tool in diagnosing bone and joint disorders, but **computerized axial tomography (CAT or CT)** or **magnetic resonance imaging (MRI)** might be needed for more detailed studies.

CAT involves taking specialized X-rays of the affected individual in a special tube-like scanner. The individual must be able to lie still for approximately 30 minutes. The results are detailed X-ray pictures that appear to cut the area of consideration into slices, thus the name tomogram (tomo = cutting, gram = picture) (Figure 6–3).

MRI is another detailed X-ray type of examination; it uses a large magnet to make electromagnetic images. Here also, individuals must be able to lie still and must not wear any type of metal during the test. MRI is more expensive to perform but takes more detailed images of soft tissue than a CT scanner does.

Bone mass density (BMD) screening is used to confirm low bone mass and the diagnosis of osteoporosis. Bone **densiometry** testing techniques are simple radiology scans. The newest type, **dual energy X-ray absorptiometry (DEXA scan)**, takes measurements at the spine, hip, and wrist. A score above –1 is normal; a score between –1 and –2.5 reflects osteopenia (low bone mass); and a score below –2.5 is defined as osteoporosis.

Blood studies, including calcium, phosphorus, and an enzyme (alkaline phosphatase) also can prove helpful with metabolic disorders. Infectious disorders can be cultured. Often, the specimen for culture is obtained during surgical procedures such as débridement.

Muscle disorders are often evaluated by **electromyography** (EMG), accomplished by inserting a small needle into muscle tissue and recording the electrical activity. Electromyography can assist in determining whether the disorder is muscular or neurologic in nature. Muscle tissue biopsy can be performed on difficult cases. Biopsy is the most definitive means of determining cause of muscle disorder. Biopsy is also the most reliable test for tumors of the musculoskeletal system.

COMMON DISEASES OF THE MUSCULOSKELETAL SYSTEM

Diseases of the Bone

Diseases of the bone can range from mild to severe, with the most serious causing extreme deformity or disability. Many of the disorders are more common in the older adult because changes in the system can lead to increased risk for skeletal problems. Individuals with bone disease frequently need assistive devices such as crutches, walkers, or canes to maintain mobility. Internal devices such as artificial joints, pins, and braces also might be necessary.

SPINAL DEFORMITIES

DESCRIPTION. Deformities might be very obvious at onset, as with congenital defects, but more commonly, they progress slowly and are unnoticed until symptoms arise.

ETIOLOGY. Deformities can be caused by a variety of factors, including congenital defects, poor posture, bone disease, and growth disorders.

SYMPTOMS. Symptoms commonly include back pain and fatigue. Diagnosis is generally confirmed by X-ray and clinical examination.

DIAGNOSIS. Spinal deformities are diagnosed by thorough physical examination and a series of X-rays of the spine. A pulmonary function test might be needed if breathing is affected. MRI scans can assist in identifying tumor or infection.

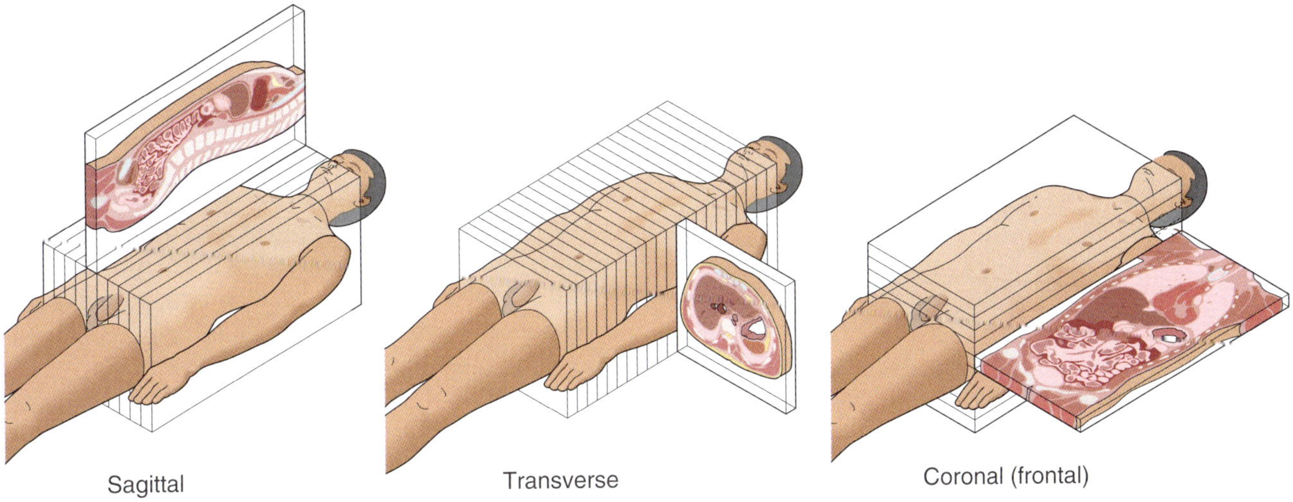

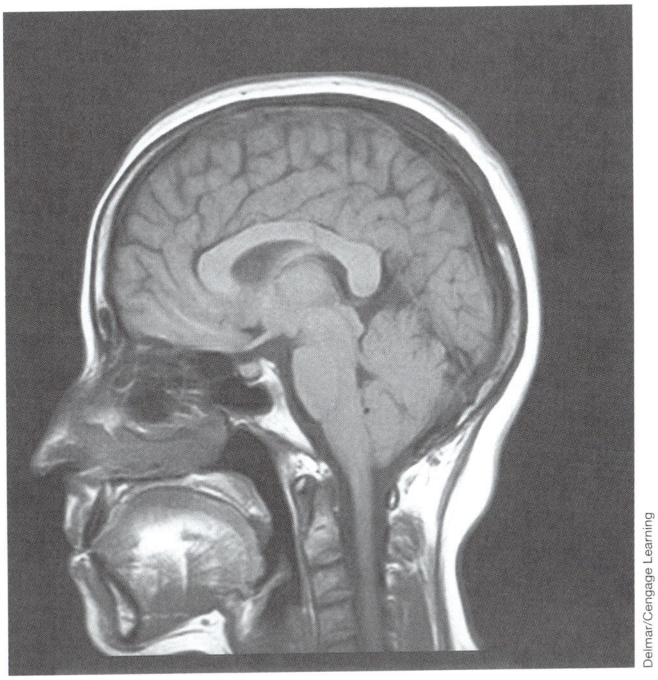

FIGURE 6–3 (Top) CT of chest and abdomen, (Bottom) MRI of head.

■ ***TREATMENT.*** Treatment includes eliminating or treating causative factors, bracing, and spinal surgery. Untreated spinal deformities can progress to life-threatening conditions when cardiac and respiratory function are compromised.

■ ***PREVENTION.*** There is no known prevention for spinal deformities.

KYPHOSIS

Kyphosis (kie-FOE-sis) is a humped curvature of the thoracic spine, commonly called humpback or hunchback. Kyphosis often appears in postmenopausal, osteoporitic females.

LORDOSIS

Lordosis (lor-DOE-sis) is an exaggerated anterior or inward curve of the lumbar spine, also called swayback. It normally occurs with pregnancy as the individual compensates for the increased size of the abdomen. When compared to the normal spine, lordosis results in a protruding abdomen and buttocks and a swayed lower back. Obesity is a common cause of lordosis.

SCOLIOSIS

■ ***DESCRIPTION.*** Scoliosis (SKOLE-lee-OH-sis) is a lateral curvature of the spine. It affects both sexes, but girls usually have more severe curvatures and account for approximately 90% of the cases. Scoliosis can occur at any age but is usually noticed during the early teen years, when growth rate is accelerated.

■ ***ETIOLOGY.*** The cause of scoliosis, in most cases, is unknown.

■ ***SYMPTOMS.*** Symptoms include (1) back pain due to muscles trying to conform to the spinal curving, (2) a rib or shoulder blade hump, and (3) uneven shoulders and hips.

Scoliosis is often noticed when dresses hang lower on one side or the other, and the brassiere straps need to be adjusted to different lengths.

■ ***DIAGNOSIS.*** Scoliosis screening in school-aged children was initiated in the 1960s and is now mandated by law in some states. Screening involves observation of the spine as the individual bends forward. Scoliosis is suspected if the spine curves to the side and the scapula shifts upward (Figure 6–4).

■ ***TREATMENT.*** Treatment is aimed at preventing a worsening of the condition and often includes bracing. Compliance with brace-wearing for female adolescents is often poor, leading to the need for further treatment. Most cases of scoliosis can be corrected if detected early and treated properly and promptly.

■ ***PREVENTION.*** Scoliosis cannot be prevented.

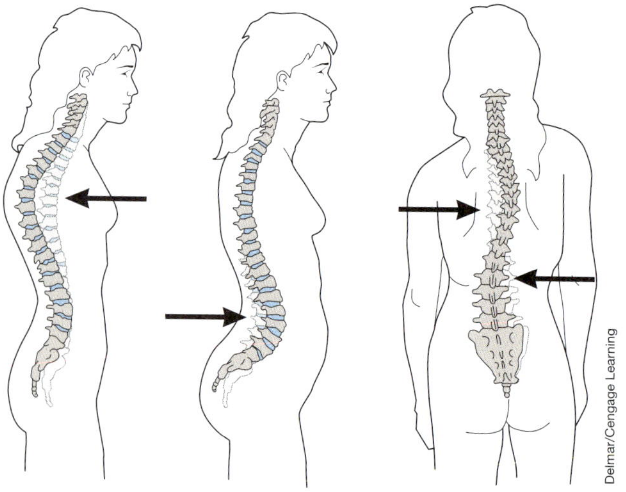

FIGURE 6–4 Spinal deformities: kyphosis, lordosis, and scoliosis (S curvature).

OTHER DISEASES OF THE BONE

OSTEOPOROSIS

■ ***DESCRIPTION.*** Osteoporosis (OS-tee-oh-por-OH-sis) is a metabolic bone disease that causes a porosity or Swiss-cheese appearance of the bone, leading to a decrease in bone mass. It is the most prevalent bone disease worldwide. It is estimated to cause major orthopedic problems in approximately one-third of the women in the United States.

■ ***ETIOLOGY.*** Many causative factors play a part in osteoporosis. Age-related osteoporosis affects both men and women equally and is due to normal age-related bone loss. Osteoporosis occurs secondary to diseases that affect mobility. For example, quadriplegia can lead to a loss of 30–40% of bone mass after 6 months of immobility. The most common type of osteoporosis is seen in women who are postmenopausal and estrogen-deficient. It is believed that this osteoporosis is due to a combination of factors, including a decrease in estrogen, calcium, and exercise.

Osteoporosis is a slow, progressive disease that robs skeletal bone of its mass and strength. It might be decades before the bone becomes weak enough to fracture. Most fractures in women over age 50 are related to osteoporosis.

■ ***SYMPTOMS.*** Early signs of osteoporosis include **compression** (bone mashed down on itself, common in vertebra) fractures of the spine and pathologic wrist fractures. Compression fractures of the spine lead to a decrease in height and pain in the thoracic and lumbar spine. Over a period of time, the individual might lose 4–5 inches of height, decreasing the thoracic and abdominal cavity size. This decrease in chest cavity size leads to decreased activity tolerance due to shortness of breath. A decrease in the abdominal cavity size leads to feelings of fullness after eating only small amounts of food and to a constant bloated feeling. Other symptoms are kyphosis and the appearance of a **Dowager's hump** (abnormal curvature in the upper thoracic spine; see Figure 6–5). Wrist fractures, especially of the distal radius, commonly occur in osteoporitic individuals with only a slight fall. As the disease progresses, the individual has an increased risk for fracturing a hip. More than one million hip fractures occur annually in the

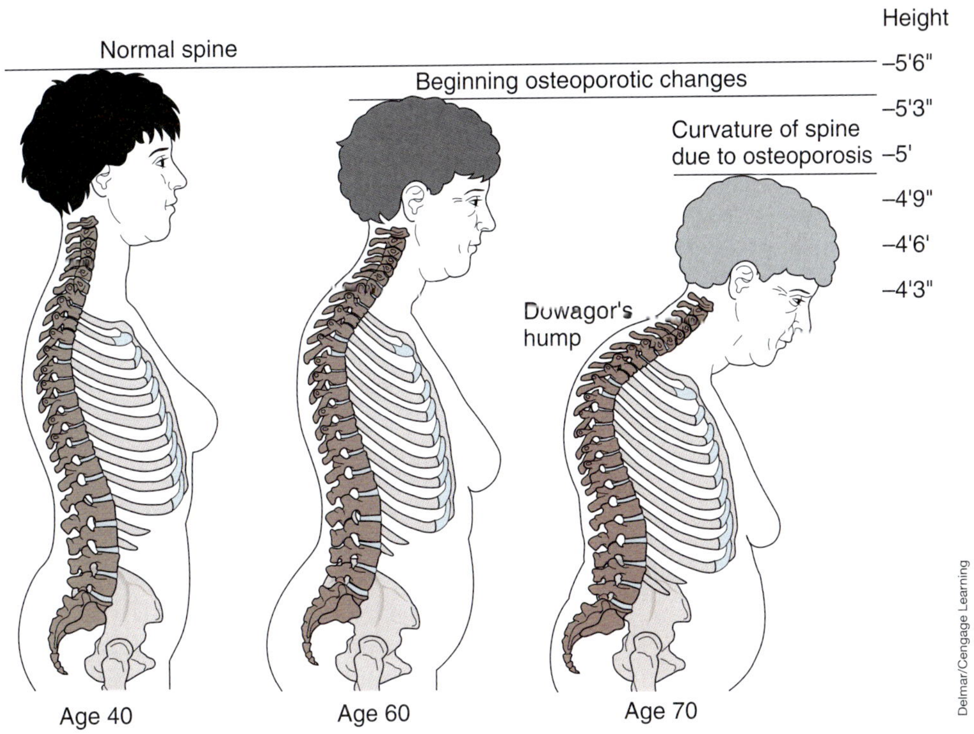

FIGURE 6–5 Osteoporosis: loss in height and the Dowager's hump.

United States. Hip fractures in frail, older women often lead to complications that result in mortality (Figure 6–6).

■ ***DIAGNOSIS.*** Diagnosis can be confirmed by clinical examination, X-rays, CT scans, and bone **densitometry** (measurement of bone thickness).

■ ***TREATMENT.*** Currently, there is no treatment to reverse osteoporosis, although the progression of osteoporosis can be slowed and bone mass levels maintained by a combination of therapies. Administration of the medications Fosamax®, Actonel®, Boniva®, and Reclast® appear to be helpful in preventing fractures.

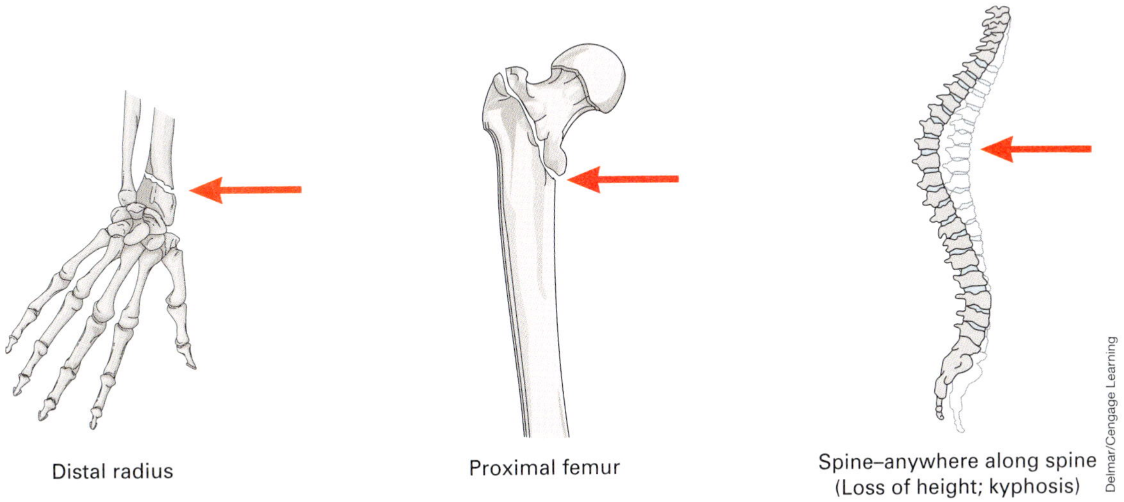

FIGURE 6–6 Fracture sites related to osteoporosis.

TABLE 6–2 Risk Factors for Osteoporosis

The following are considered factors that increase the risk of developing osteoporosis:

- Family history of osteoporosis
- Increased risk from aging
- Medications—tetracycline, corticosteroids, aluminum antacids, some diuretics, some anticonvulsants
- Female, white or Asian
- Lack of exercise
- Lack of calcium in diet or supplements
- Increased risk from postsurgery oophorectomy (removal of ovaries)

Reduction of risk factors includes decreasing alcohol and caffeine consumption and not smoking (Table 6–2). Other therapies include increasing estrogen, increasing calcium and vitamin D intake, and a daily exercise routine that includes weight-bearing exercise. Much controversy exists concerning the use of estrogen replacement therapy because it is associated with an increase in breast and gynecologic malignancies. An increase in calcium levels also might lead to the formation of kidney stones. These treatments must be considered on an individual basis. The one treatment that is agreed on by most practitioners is the need for daily exercise. Regular exercise has been shown to reduce the rate of hip fractures by 50%.

■ ***PREVENTION.*** Preventive measures for osteoporosis need to begin early because bone mass is built prior to age 30. Young women should be encouraged to exercise daily, eat a balanced diet, quit smoking, and limit caffeine and alcohol consumption. Entering menopausal years with good bone mass and maintaining as much of the bone as possible is the best weapon against osteoporosis.

OSTEOMYELITIS

■ ***DESCRIPTION.*** **Osteomyelitis** (OS-tee-oh-My-ull-LIE-tis; osteo = bone, myel = marrow, itis = inflammation) is an inflammation of the bone commonly caused by infection.

■ ***ETIOLOGY.*** *Staphylococcus aureus* is the responsible organism in approximately 90% of cases. This bacterium can enter the bone through a wound, spread from an infection nearby, or come from a skin or throat infection. Osteomyelitis usually affects the long bones of the arms and legs. It most often occurs in children and adolescents as a result of a throat infection. In severe cases, it can affect the growth plate of the bones, leading to shortening of the limb.

■ ***SYMPTOMS.*** Symptoms of osteomyelitis can include sudden onset of high fever, chills, tenderness over the affected bone, leukocytosis (leuko = white, cyto = cell, osis = condition of increase), and bacteremia (bacteria = microscopic organism, emia = blood, bacteria in the blood). In adults, osteomyelitis often occurs following a traumatic accident involving the bone or following bone surgery, especially when implants such as screws, plates, or other hardware are needed.

■ ***DIAGNOSIS.*** Physical examination revealing pain in a bone along with an elevated white blood cell count can suggest osteomyelitis. An indicative test is an elevated erythrocyte sedimentation rate (ESR), and an X-ray exam, an MRI scan, or a CT scan can also reveal abnormality. Diagnosis can be confirmed by taking samples of bone, pus, blood, or joint fluid to identify infective organisms.

■ ***TREATMENT.*** Treatment for osteomyelitis is aggressive intravenous antibiotic therapy. Affected bone is often débrided surgically to speed the healing process. Surgical hardware is often removed for this same reason. Acute osteomyelitis, if not treated effectively, can become chronic and lead to a lifetime of problems for the affected individual. Chronic osteomyelitis m can lead to large, gaping scar tissue and chronic wound drainage (Figure 6–7).

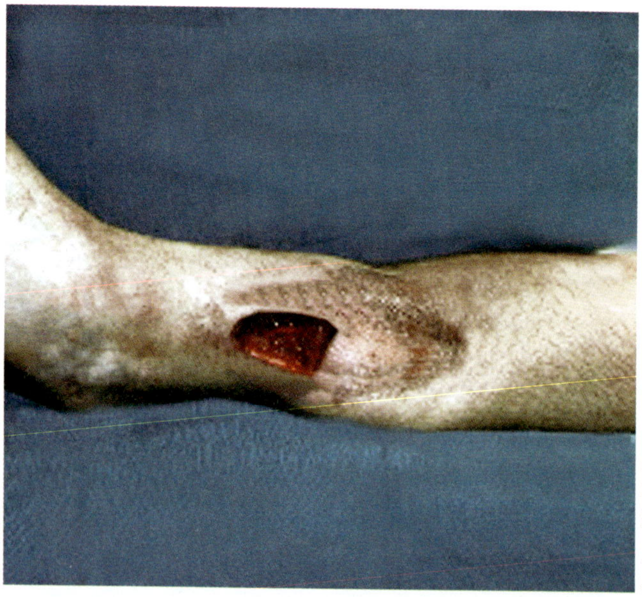

FIGURE 6–7 Chronic osteomyelitis scar of the lower leg.

PREVENTION. Cleansing and properly treating wounds, especially deep wounds, aids in the prevention of osteomyelitis. Blood-borne bacteria must also be promptly diagnosed and treated. Individuals with artificial joints or metal components should take preventive antibiotics prior to any surgery or dental procedure.

OSTEOMALACIA

DESCRIPTION. Osteomalacia (OS-tee-oh-muh-LAY-shuh; osteo = bone, malacia = softening) is the general term for softening of the bones due to defective **mineralization** and the general term for softening of the bones in adults; in children, it is called rickets.

ETIOLOGY. Osteomalacia is caused by a deficiency of vitamin D, which aids in the bone mineralization that causes their characteristic hardness. Without this process, the bone becomes soft and weak. To mineralize, bones need calcium, phosphorus, and vitamin D.

Vitamin D deficiency in adults can be due to inadequate nutritional intake, inadequate exposure to sunlight (skin exposed to sunlight synthesizes vitamin D), or a malabsorption problem.

SYMPTOMS. Symptoms and signs of osteomalacia include bone pain, loss of height, bending, and deformity in weight-bearing bones such as the spine, pelvis, and legs.

DIAGNOSIS. A thorough history of diet and amount of time in the sun is helpful in diagnosis, followed by blood testing to measure vitamin D levels and X-rays to look for cracks in the bone. A bone biopsy is quite definitive but often not needed for diagnosis.

TREATMENT. Correction of the deficiency potentially cures the problem. Administration of 200,000 IU weekly of vitamin D for 4 to 6 weeks, followed by an oral dose of 1,600 IU daily, is usually an adequate treatment. However, bones that have bowed, shortened, or flattened might not regain normal appearance and function.

PREVENTION. Vitamin D deficiency can usually be avoided by:

- Exposing arms and legs to sunlight for 5 to 10 minutes a day
- Eating foods high in vitamin D such as oily fish (salmon, sardines, mackerel) and egg yolks.
- Taking vitamin supplements if needed.

Diseases of the Joints

Most of the diseases of the joints occur as a slow, degenerative process, so they tend to be more common with age. As with diseases of the bones, diseases of the joints often result in the individual requiring assistive devices or artificial parts to maintain mobility. Frequently, damage to joints occurring during youth is not apparent until middle or older adulthood.

ARTHRITIS

Arthritis (arthro = joint, itis = inflammation) and *rheumatism* are terms commonly used to describe a variety of conditions that cause pain and stiffness in the musculoskeletal system. Both are terms that cover a broad group of conditions, but arthritis is a condition of inflammation in a joint, whereas rheumatism is a condition of stiffness. Arthritis is any inflammation of a joint. Everyone at some time or another has had arthritis; for example, a sprained ankle or jammed finger are arthritic conditions. Arthritis can be divided into two main groups: osteoarthritis and rheumatoid arthritis. Osteoarthritis is the most common form of arthritis, but rheumatoid arthritis is the more serious and debilitating type.

OSTEOARTHRITIS OR DEGENERATIVE JOINT DISEASE

DESCRIPTION. Osteoarthritis, a complex, degenerative process, or wearing out of a joint, is the leading cause of diability in the United States (Messier et al., 2007). It can begin in the early 20s with 90% of all adults showing some radiologic changes.

ETIOLOGY. The exact cause of osteoarthritis is unknown. The amount or degree of wear is associated with several factors (Table 6–3). Sports injuries speed the wear and tear on the joints, leading to osteoarthritis at a younger age.

TABLE 6–3 Risk Factors for Osteoarthritis

The following are considered factors that increase the risk of developing osteoarthritis:
Family history of osteoarthritis
Excessive wear and tear or injury to joints
Obesity
Increased risk with age
Female

■ ***SYMPTOMS.*** Older adults are usually symptomatic with this type of arthritis. It often affects frequently used joints, such as those in the hands, and joints that are weight-bearing such as those of the spine, hip, and knee. Affected joints of the hands often swell and become painful. The distal and proximal **interphalangeal** (inter = between, phalangeal = finger bones) joints are often affected and can acquire a crooked deformity of the fingers. The **metacarpophalangeal** (meta = beyond, carpo = wrist, phalangeal = finger bones) joints are usually not affected (Figure 6–8).

Osteoarthritis that affects weight-bearing joints often affects the spine, hips, and knees. As the joints of the spinal column are affected with arthritis, individuals can become symptomatic with back pain. Osteoarthritis affects the hips and knees by wearing away the **articular** (are-TICK-you-lar) cartilage at the end of the long bones where bones articulate, or meet. Eventually, the entire surface of the cartilage might be worn away, exposing areas of raw bone. When this occurs, new bone forms in and around the joint, causing the bone ends to thicken. Fragments of this new bone are called bone spurs and often lead to a decrease in joint motion. X-ray examination might reveal the spurs and only small patches of cartilage on the bone ends. This is called a bone-on-bone condition, and at this point, individuals are often candidates for total hip or knee replacement surgery. Osteoarthritis peaks in the fifth to sixth decade of life, with approximately 80% of individuals showing symptoms by age 70.

■ ***TREATMENT.*** Treatment for osteoarthritis includes rest, nonweight-bearing exercise such as swimming and biking, application of heat, and use of analgesics and anti-inflammatory medications. Severe osteoarthritis can be treated by steroid injections into the joint capsule to relieve pain. Total surgical joint replacement might be recommended.

■ ***DIAGNOSIS.*** The diagnosis is usually made based on history and physical exam because X-rays do not always correlate with symptoms.

■ ***PREVENTION.*** Maintaining a healthy body weight is the single best prevention. Excess weight strains joints, especially those of the knees and hips. It is estimated that every one pound of body weight places approximately three pounds of stress on the joints of the knees and even more on the hips.

RHEUMATOID ARTHRITIS

■ ***DESCRIPTION.*** Rheumatoid arthritis was discussed in Chapter 5, "Immune System Diseases and Disorders," as an autoimmune disorder that not only affects the joints but also the connective tissues of the

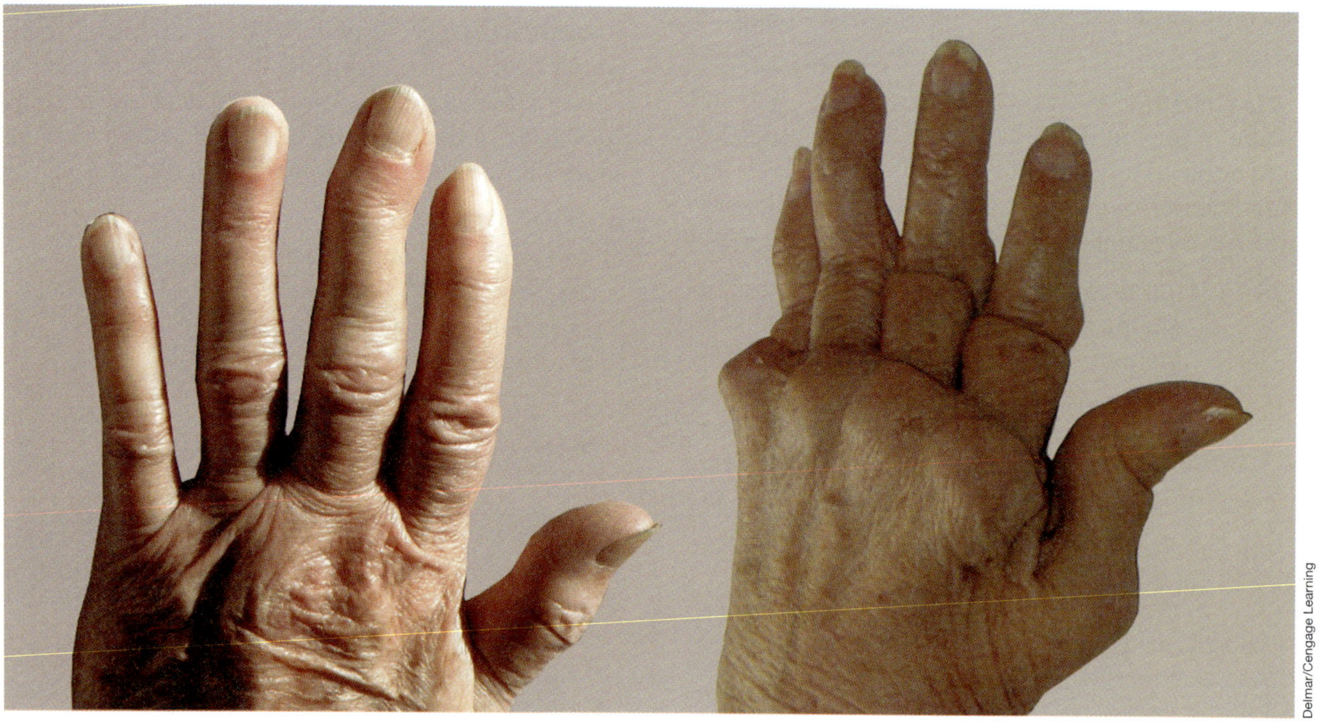

FIGURE 6–8 Comparison of (left) osteoarthritis and (right) rheumatoid arthritis: hands and joints.

HEALTHY HIGHLIGHT

Knuckle-Cracking

"Will knuckle-cracking cause arthritis in my joints?" This is a commonly asked question by those who have developed the habit of knuckle-cracking, the sound made by the rush of synovial fluid from one area of the joint to another as the joint is forcefully pulled apart. Research supports the fact that this action does not cause an increase in osteoarthritis, but it also supports the fact that individuals who crack their knuckles eventually have decreased grip and hand function. Research does not rule out the idea of knuckle-cracking causing joint damage. Knuckle-crackers might not have to worry about an increase in osteoarthritic pain due to chronic knuckle-cracking, but they might still develop long-term pain from chronic ligament inflammation. Some researchers feel that chronic joint pain, whether related to arthritis or not, is still chronic joint pain and thus recommend that knuckle-crackers stop this behavior. Interestingly, related research found that knuckle-crackers are also more likely to bite their fingernails, smoke, and drink alcohol.

entire body. Rheumatoid arthritis often affects the lungs, heart, and blood vessels, causing the individual to appear chronically ill. This type of arthritis often affects people in the prime of life and affects women more often than men. It is a debilitating, chronic disease that destroys the joints.

■ ***SYMPTOMS.*** A noticeable difference in the way osteoarthritis and rheumatoid arthritis affect the joints can be observed in joints of the hand. Osteoarthritis affects the working joints of the hand (primarily the distal and proximal interphalangeal joints), causing swelling and pain. All joints of the hand can be affected in rheumatoid individuals, often with noticeable deformity and destruction in the metacarpophalangeal joints (see Figure 6–8). Also, refer to Chapter 5 for more information on rheumatoid arthritis.

GOUT

■ ***DESCRIPTION.*** Gout is often called gouty arthritis because this condition leads to inflammation of the affected joints.

■ ***ETIOLOGY.*** Gout is caused by a metabolic alteration in the breakdown of certain protein foods. Individuals with gout deposit uric acid crystals in joints of the body.

■ ***SYMPTOMS.*** The primary joint affected is the **metatarsophalangeal** (meta = between, tarso = foot, phalangeal = toe bones) joint of the big toe. These uric acid crystals have razor sharp edges that irritate the joint, causing an acute inflammatory response. Symptoms are redness, heat, swelling, and pain in the joint.

Approximately 95% of gout patients are male, with onset usually after age 30. Chronic gout can be characterized by uric acid deposited in subcutaneous tissue as well as in the joint. These deposits appear as small, whitish nodules called **tophi** and are commonly seen around a joint and in the soft tissue of the ear (Figure 6–9). Kidney dysfunction and an increase in the occurrence of kidney stones are also common with chronic gout.

■ ***DIAGNOSIS.*** Diagnosis is based on finding uric acid crystals in joint, body fluids, tissues, or all of these.

■ ***TREATMENT.*** Treatment can include anti-gout medication (probenecid and allopurinol [Zyloprim®]) and dietary adjustments to decrease the amount of protein consumed. Weight loss in obese patients also can be beneficial.

■ ***PREVENTION.*** Avoiding foods high in purine such as meat, poultry, fish, and other seafood is helpful in preventing gouty attacks. Preventing dehydration by drinking plenty of fluids while avoiding diuretic drinks such as tea and alcohol is also helpful.

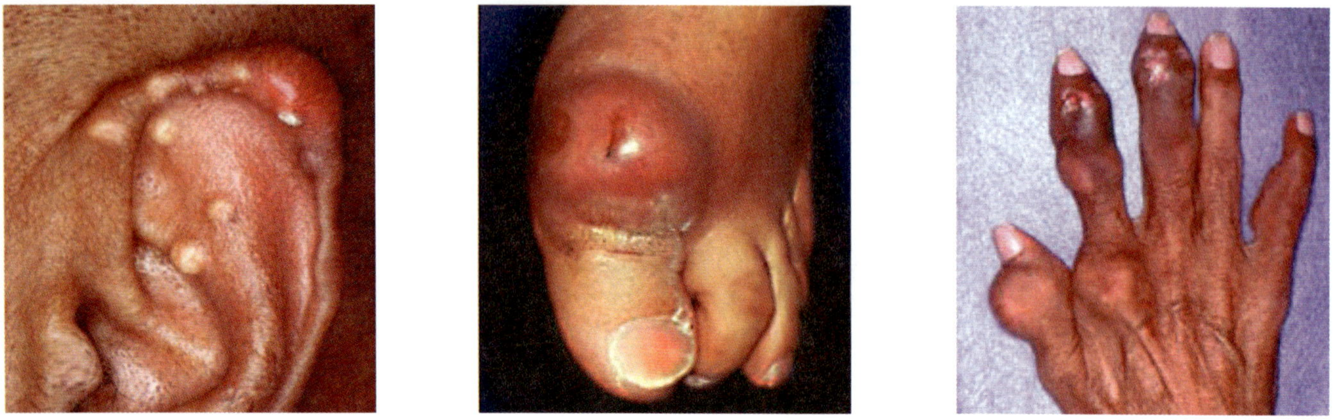

(A) (B) (C)

Courtesy of Mark L. Kuss

FIGURE 6–9 Common sites of tophi.

JOINT DEFORMITIES

HALLUX VALGUS

■ ***DESCRIPTION.*** Hallux (big toe) valgus (bent outward) is a deformity affecting the metatarsophalangeal joint of the big toe. It is more commonly called a bunion. This condition occurs more frequently in women and tends to run in families.

■ ***ETIOLOGY.*** The cause of bunions is controversial. Many experts think the cause is an inherited faulty foot formation that progresses over time and is irritated by poor or improper footwear. Others think the footwear actually causes the condition. Whatever the cause, all agree that wearing pointed-toe shoes, especially with high heels, aggravates the condition. This type of shoe forces the great toe into a valgus position and increases the pressure on the metatarsophalangeal joint. Over a period of time, this chronic irritation leads to a buildup of soft tissue and bone in the joint area (Figure 6–10).

■ ***SYMPTOMS.*** Symptoms and signs include redness, pain, and swelling in the area and, often, the inability to wear pointed-toe or high-heeled shoes.

■ ***DIAGNOSIS.*** Bunions are very visible and easily diagnosed by X-rays.

■ ***TREATMENT.*** Mild cases can be resolved by changing to a properly fitting, low-heeled shoe. Analgesic and anti-inflammatory medications can be beneficial in relieving pain. More severe cases might need surgical intervention with bunionectomy.

■ ***PREVENTION.*** Wearing proper footwear can prevent or at least slow the progression of bunion.

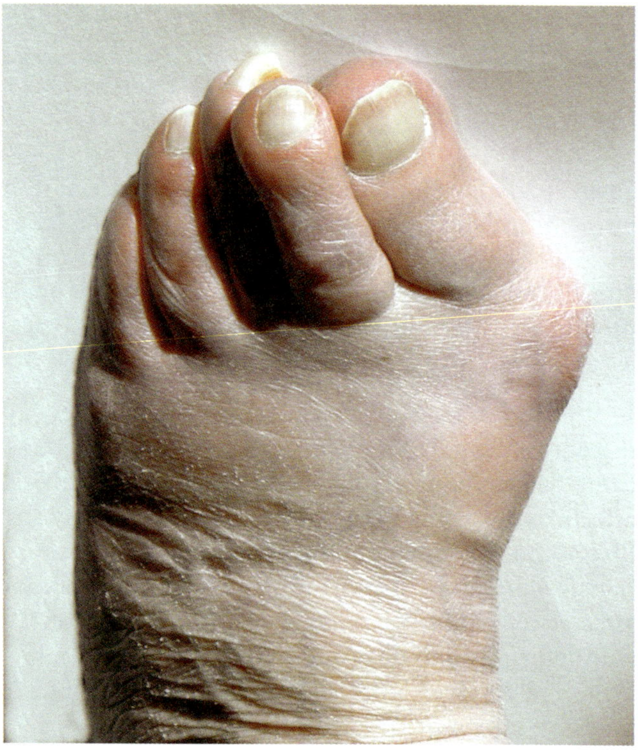

Delmar/Cengage Learning

FIGURE 6–10 Hallux Valgus (bunion).

TEMPOROMANDIBULAR JOINT SYNDROME (TMJ)

■ ***DESCRIPTION.*** TMJ is an inflammation of the temporomandibular joint, the joint that connects the lower jaw to the skull. This disorder can result in significant pain and impairment.

■ ***ETIOLOGY.*** TMJ might be due to joint tissue lesions, overbite, malocclusion, or improperly fitted dentures or dental work.

■ ***SYMPTOMS.*** Severe headaches and pain in the jaw joint might be indicative of TMJ. This pain can be made worse by chewing. Classic signs include marked decrease in the ability to open the mouth and a clicking sound made during chewing motion.

■ ***DIAGNOSIS.*** Examination of the mouth along with dental X-rays, CT scan, or MRI scan aids in diagnosis of TMJ.

■ ***TREATMENT.*** Treatment includes correction of the causative factors, often leading to surgical intervention.

■ ***PREVENTION.*** Controlling or eliminating causative factors aids in prevention of TMJ.

Diseases of the Muscles and Connective Tissue

Diseases of the muscles and connective tissue, unlike many of the bone disorders, are quite common in very young or young adult individuals. Some of these disorders, such as the muscular dystrophies, are chronic, progressive, and devastating to families because they usually result in early death. Other disorders of the muscles and connective tissue are considered to be rather minor and can be treated medically or surgically.

MUSCULAR DYSTROPHY (MD)

■ ***DESCRIPTION.*** Muscular dystrophy is an inherited genetic disorder that affects skeletal muscle. There are many types of dystrophies, but the most common type is Duchenne's MD, which primarily affects male children.

■ ***SYMPTOMS.*** Duchenne's MD is characterized by a wasting away of shoulder and pelvic girdle muscles. Survival beyond age 20 is rare. This disorder is discussed in detail in Chapter 19, "Genetic and Developmental, Childhood, and Mental Health Diseases and Disorders."

GANGLION CYST

■ ***DESCRIPTION.*** A ganglion cyst is a fluid-filled benign tumor that usually develops on a tendon sheath near the wrist area.

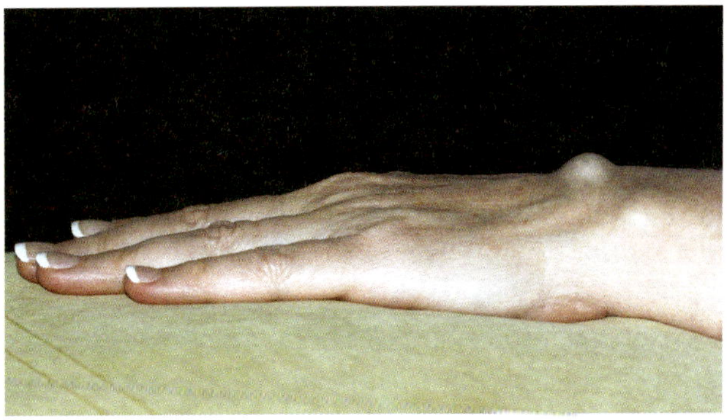

Courtesy of Mark L. Kuss.

FIGURE 6–11 Ganglion cyst.

■ ***ETIOLOGY.*** The cause of these cysts is unknown, although some feel that they might be associated with a repetitive injury.

■ ***SYMPTOMS.*** A cyst is commonly a single, smooth, round lump just under the skin (Figure 6–11). It can be quite small or grow to the size of a dime or quarter. Usually, these are painless but unsightly. Cysts can disappear gradually over a period of months.

■ ***DIAGNOSIS.*** A physical exam is often all that is needed to diagnosis this condition.

■ ***TREATMENT.*** If they are painful or unsightly, the physician might choose to rupture the cyst or drain it. Ganglionectomy, or surgical removal, also can be performed.

■ ***PREVENTION.*** There are no preventive measures for ganglion cysts.

TETANUS

■ ***DESCRIPTION.*** Tetanus, also called lockjaw, is an acute, infectious, life-threatening disease characterized by painful, uncontrolled contractions of skeletal muscle.

■ ***ETIOLOGY.*** A toxin produced by the bacillus bacterium, *Clostridium tetani*, causes tetanus. This bacterium is commonly found in animal feces and, when excreted, lives as spores in the soil. The number of these spores is especially high in barnyards, pastures, or garden areas fertilized with animal manure. When this infectious bacterium enters the body in an **anaerobic** (ana = without, erobic = air) wound such as a puncture, it grows and produces a dangerous toxin. This toxin travels in the blood and attaches to motor or muscle neurons. The toxin irritates the nerve, producing the stimulus for skeletal muscle contraction. Because of the neurological involvement, tetanus also may be categorized as a nervous system disorder.

■ ***SYMPTOMS.*** The bacterial toxin affects the nervous system rather slowly. The farther the distance between the wound and the spinal cord, the slower the progression. One to three weeks might pass before the onset of symptoms. The jaw muscles are often the first muscles affected with **tetany** (TET-ah-nee), or rigid muscle contraction, preventing the individual from opening the mouth, hence the term *lockjaw*. Eventually, muscles of the esophagus, neck, back, arms, and legs are affected. Other symptoms are a high fever, tachycardia (rapid pulse rate), dysphagia (difficulty swallowing), and intense pain.

■ ***DIAGNOSIS.*** Diagnosis is confirmed by a spatula test, which involves touching the posterior pharyngeal wall (the very back of the throat) with a soft-tipped instrument. A positive result is an involuntary contraction of the muscles causing the patient to bite down on the instrument.

■ ***TREATMENT.*** Treatment is a prompt and immediate cleansing of wounds with special consideration given to puncture-type wounds. Immunization might be needed, depending on the individual's immunization history. If the individual has not received a tetanus toxoid injection in the past 5 years, an antitoxin might be given to cause the immune system to build antibodies. Initially, tetanus toxoid should be administered to children as part of basic diphtheria, pertussis, and tetanus (DPT) immunization.

Tetanus antibodies must be boosted approximately every 7 to 10 years throughout life. Individuals with low tetanus antibody levels are susceptible to tetanus. An antitoxin can be given to prevent tetanus following an injury because the body does not have time to build up its own antibodies. Following this episode, it is usually recommended that the individual follow up with the proper tetanus toxoid booster.

Care of an individual with tetanus includes symptomatic treatment, often including respiratory, nutritional, and hydration support. Antibiotics and muscle relaxants also can be administered. Even with the best of care, tetanus is usually fatal due to respiratory failure. If the individual survives, the disease process usually lasts 6 to 8 weeks. Surprisingly, the disease usually does not leave any permanent disability, but it also does not confer any lasting immunity to tetanus.

■ ***PREVENTION.*** Tetanus can be prevented by vaccination. It is recommended that adults receive a booster vaccine every 10 years. Standard care practice in many places is to give the booster to any patient with a puncture wound who is uncertain of when he or she was last vaccinated or if he or she has had fewer than three lifetime doses of the vaccine.

SYSTEMIC LUPUS ERYTHEMATOSUS

■ ***DESCRIPTION.*** Systemic lupus erythematosus is an autoimmune disorder that affects the connective tissue throughout the body. One of the main characteristics is a butterfly-patterned rash across the nose and face. For more details, see Chapter 5.

Neoplasms

Primary neoplasms of the musculoskeletal system are uncommon. Typically, neoplasms of this system are secondary, metastasizing from the lungs, breast, and prostate. The most common primary tumor of bone is osteosarcoma, which affects the tibia, humerus, or femur. Ewing's sarcoma is also primarily a bone tumor, affecting long bones in children and teens. It is highly malignant and quickly metastasizes to nearly every organ of the body. Myeloma is the most common marrow tumor, commonly affecting the pelvis, vertebrae, and long bones of adults. Kaposi's sarcoma affects soft tissue of primarily immunosuppressed individuals. Rhabdomyosarcoma is a very rare but highly malignant tumor of skeletal muscle.

Symptoms of musculoskeletal tumors can include pathologic fracture and bone pain. Clinical examination followed by radiologic studies, CT scan, blood studies, and biopsy often confirm the diagnosis. Treatment of malignant tumors of the musculoskeletal system can include radiation, chemotherapy, and surgery. Surgical procedures often involve excision and amputation. Even with aggressive therapy, prognosis for these malignant neoplasms is often very poor.

TRAUMA

Trauma is the main cause of problems in the musculoskeletal system. Fractures are by far the most common and frequent injury to bone. Tennis elbow is the most frequent ailment of the upper body. Treatment for sprains and strains is among the top 10 reasons that patients seek medical attention for acute disease. Low back pain is in the top 10 for chronic disease.

Fracture

A fracture is any discontinuity of a bone. A fracture and a break are synonymous, although a **stress** (related to too much weight-bearing or pressure) fracture or incomplete fracture might not break the bone in two. Fractures can be caused by trauma (injury) or can be **pathologic** (caused by weakness from a disease).

Types of Fractures

Fractures may be classified in a number of ways. One method of classification is based on the condition of the overlying skin. If the bone has protruded through the skin or an object has punctured the skin, making an opening through the skin to the fracture site, it is an **open** fracture. Open fractures are also called **compound** fractures because the fracture, plus the open skin, is compounding the problem. An open fracture is always an emergency due to the high risk of bone infection. Patients with open fractures are taken to surgery for cleaning and débridement. If there is no opening in the skin, it is called a **closed**, or **simple, fracture**.

Another method of classification considers the condition of the bone. If the fracture goes completely through the bone, it is a **complete fracture**. If the bone is fractured but not in two, it is an **incomplete fracture**. A common incomplete fracture that occurs in children is called a **greenstick** fracture because it appears to have broken partially, like a sap-filled green stick.

Fractures also may be described by the number of fragments or the position of the fragments. A **displaced** fracture is one in which fragments are out of position, whereas nondisplaced means the fragments are still in correct position. If there are more than two ends or fragments, the break is a **comminuted** fracture. Bone appearing to be mashed down is a compression fracture. A common site of a **compression** fracture is in the vertebrae. An **impacted** fracture is one characterized as a bone end forced over the other end. **Avulsion** fracture describes a separation of a small bone fragment from the bone where a tendon or ligament is attached.

The position of the fracture line as compared to bone position might also describe the fracture. A **longitudinal** fracture runs the length of the bone; a **transverse** fracture runs across or at a 90-degree angle. **Oblique** fractures run in a transverse pattern, and **spiral** fractures twist around the bone. **Stellate** fractures form a star-like pattern.

Location may be used to describe the fracture. An articular fracture involves a joint surface. **Intracapsular** and **extracapsular** describe fractures inside or outside the joint capsule, respectively. **Intertrochanteric** describes fractures in the trochanter of the femur, and **femoral neck** and **subcapital** fractures describe fractures located on the femur. Finally, fractures may be named by the physician who first described them; for example, **Colles'** (Figure 6–12) and **Pott's** fractures are fractures of the wrist and ankle, respectively.

To be very specific, a fracture may be more clearly defined by using several descriptive names. For example, a diagnosis of a closed fracture is a broad diagnosis covering many kinds of fractures. A more descriptive diagnosis would be a closed, comminuted fracture. An even clearer diagnosis would be a closed, comminuted, femoral neck fracture.

Sites and causes of fractures vary by age and gender. Children commonly fracture their arms during falls. Teen males commonly have long bone fractures related to motor vehicle accidents (MVAs) or sports injuries. Older females suffer with hip fractures generally related to falls and osteoporosis.

Treatment of Fractures

Treatment of fractures often involves first aid at the site of the accident. First aid includes splinting the fracture site by immobilizing the area to decrease movement and prevent further injury. A splint should be applied in an as-is position. No attempt should be made to reduce the fracture or place the bone back in normal position at this time.

After medical assistance has been obtained, proper treatment might require reduction of the fracture. If this can be accomplished without a surgical incision, it is called a closed reduction, common in fractures of the extremities. Radiography can confirm proper position of the bones. If the fracture cannot be reduced without internal manipulation, the area is surgically opened, or incised, and an open reduction is performed. Open reductions commonly require some type of internal fixation or holding device such as pins, plates, screws, or rods in a procedure called an open reduction, internal fixation (**ORIF**). Open fractures require surgical intervention to clean and débride the involved tissue, usually by cleansing with copious (excessive) amounts of fluid to prevent infection and osteomyelitis.

Closed and open reductions can require the application of a splint or cast to immobilize the area during the healing process. Most fractures heal in 4

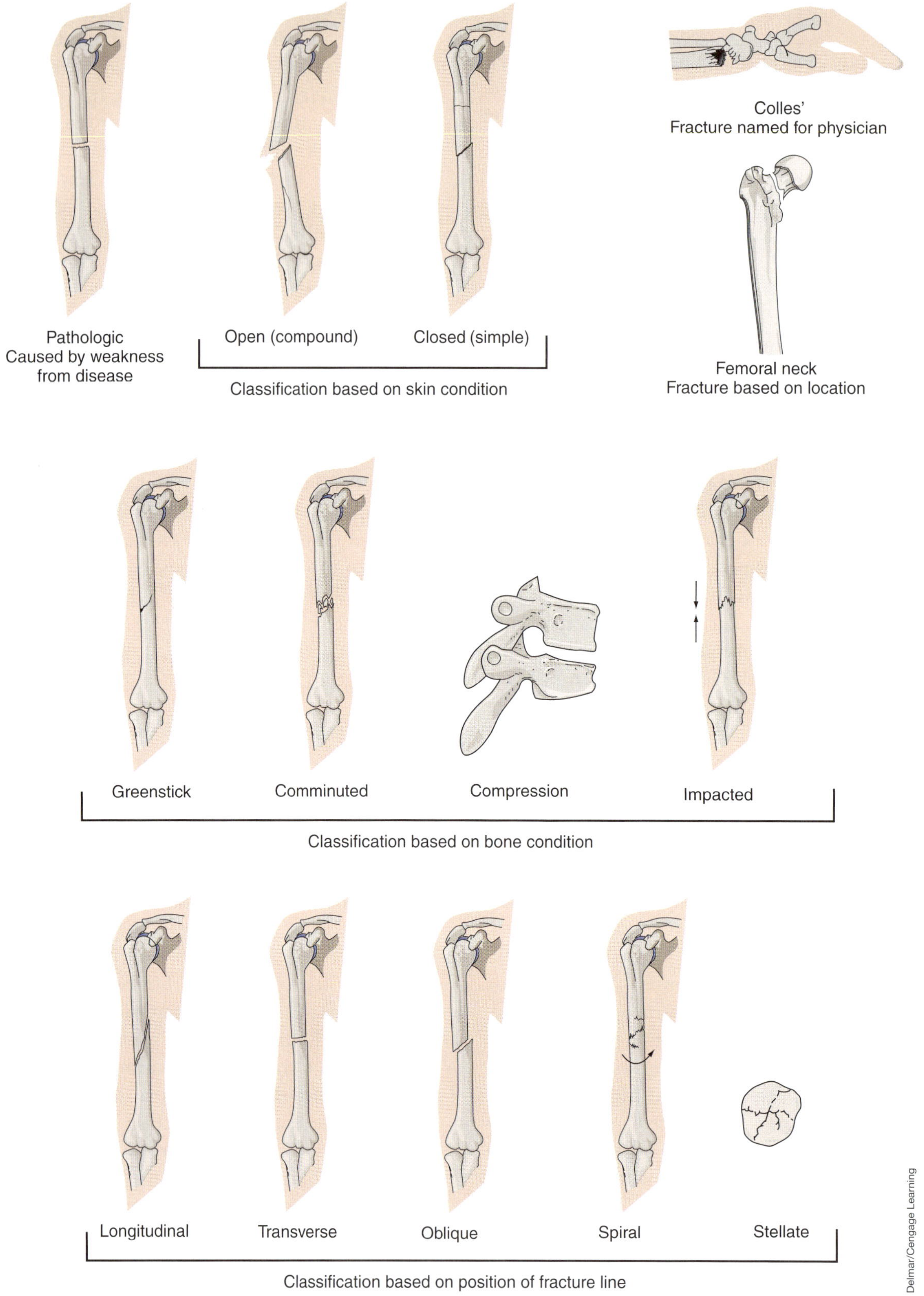

FIGURE 6–12 Types of fractures.

to 8 weeks, depending on the site of fracture, the type of fracture, and the age and nutritional status of the involved individual.

The application of traction might be beneficial to relieve muscle spasms, to hold a fracture in correct position, or to stretch the muscles, allowing bone fragment ends to separate, thus reducing pain and further tissue damage. Traction involves the application of a device to maintain alignment and apply a pulling force.

Traction may be classified by the type of application device, two basic types of which are skeletal and skin. Skeletal traction is used for long-term traction or when large muscle groups are involved such as for a femur fracture with resultant quadriceps spasm. Skeletal traction involves placement of a pin through the bone distal to the fracture, and then ropes, pulley devices, and weights apply traction or pull to the fracture site (Figure 6–13). Skin traction is used for short-term traction or when small muscle groups are involved. The traction device is applied to the skin with the use of adhesive or elastic wrapping. The same ropes, pulleys, and weights might be used for skin traction, but the amount of weight applied is usually less than with skeletal traction.

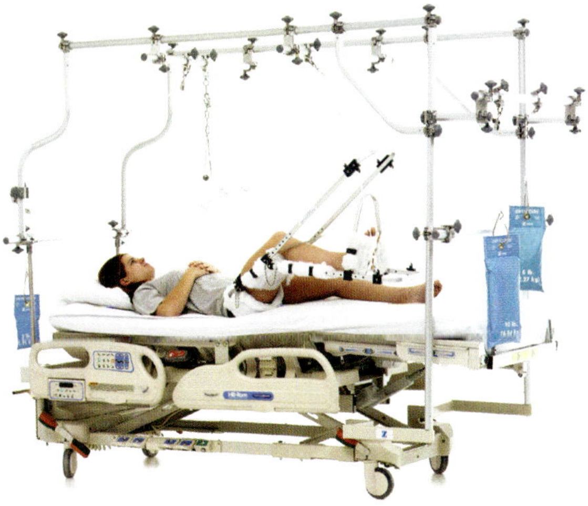

Courtesy of Thomas Balanced Suspension System, Zimmer Orthopaedic Surgical Products, Inc., Hill-Rom, A Hillenbrand Industry

FIGURE 6–13 Skeletal traction.

Complications of Fractures

Complications of fractures include mal-union, nonunion, avascular necrosis, and infection. Mal-union is healing of the fracture in an abnormal or nonfunctional position; nonunion is the failure of the bone to heal. The complication of avascular necrosis occurs when the blood supply to the bone is not adequate to maintain bone health and the bone tissue dies. Infection of the bone was discussed in detail under the section titled "Osteomyelitis" (see page 102).

*Study*WARE™ Connection

View animations on injuries, resulting from a twisting force and a direct force, on your StudyWARE™ CD-ROM.

HEALTHY HIGHLIGHT

Sports Injuries: When to See a Doctor

Participation in sports often results in numerous lumps, bumps, and bruises. Often, these injuries heal without medical treatment, but some injuries, left unattended, can lead to long-term difficulties. Often, individuals ask, "When should I see a doctor?"

The following may be used as general guidelines for seeking medical attention:

- Any injury in or near a joint
- Pain that does not subside after 10 days
- Any time there is obvious bone deformity
- Injury that has not improved in 5 to 7 days
- Any sign of infection: temperature of 101°F or greater, presence of pus, red streaks in the tissue, or swollen lymph glands

Strains and Sprains

STRAIN

DESCRIPTION. A strain is a very common over-stretching injury of a muscle.

ETIOLOGY. Individuals commonly have lumbar strains from lifting too much weight, lifting improperly, or lifting repetitively. Strained backs are common after a weekend of activity by an individual not in adequate physical condition.

SYMPTOMS. Symptoms include soreness, pain, and tenderness.

DIAGNOSIS. Strains, in most cases, are diagnosed based on a history and physical exam. Examination might reveal swelling and tenderness in the affected area.

TREATMENT. Treatment includes rest, moist heat, and the use of analgesics and anti-inflammatory medications. As pain subsides, physical therapy might be initiated to restore strength and flexiblity. A strain is less serious than a sprain.

PREVENTION. Avoiding extreme fatigue and warming up before exercise can help prevent strains.

SPRAIN

DESCRIPTION. A sprain is a traumatic injury to a joint with partial or complete tearing of ligaments.

ETIOLOGY. Sports activities commonly lead to sprains. The ankle joint is commonly affected and can become so painful that the joint cannot be used. The degree of ligament tearing, plus involvement of associated tendons, muscles, and blood vessels, determines the degree of injury. Severe sprains can exhibit complete tearing of the ligaments.

SYMPTOMS. Symptoms include varying degrees of swelling, pain, heat, and redness to purple or dark blue discoloration from blood vessel hemorrhage (Figure 6–14).

DIAGNOSIS. Physical examination is often all that is needed for diagnosis, although X-rays might be taken to rule out fracture. In extreme cases, MRI and arthroscopy can be used.

TREATMENT. Treatment depends on the severity of the sprain. Mild sprains are treated by implementing the concepts RICE: rest, ice, compression

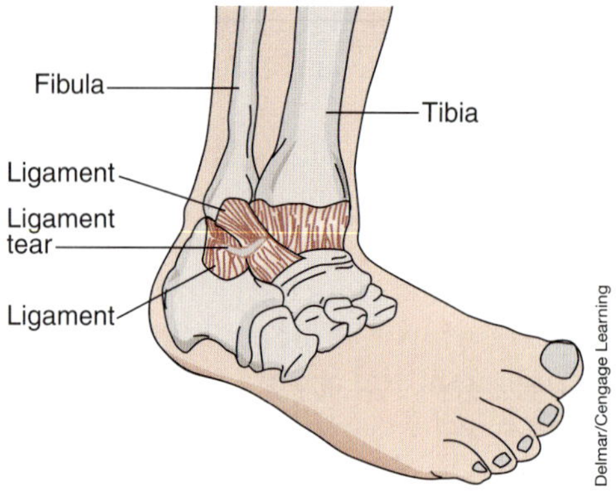

FIGURE 6–14 Sprained ankle.

(wrapping with an elastic bandage), and elevation. As the sprain heals and pain resolves, light exercise and gradual walking are recommended.

PREVENTION. Regular exercise, stretching, and strengthing to maintain good physical condition are the best preventions for sprains.

Dislocations and Subluxations

DESCRIPTION. Dislocation is the complete separation of a bone from its normal position in a joint. A subluxation is a partial separation (Figure 6–15).

ETIOLOGY. Dislocations occur with major traumatic injuries such as MVAs, contact sports, or falls and can cause a fracture as well. Dislocations can also be related to joint abnormalities or disease. In the case of disease, the dislocation might occur frequently and without cause.

SYMPTOMS. Dislocation causes acute pain and obvious joint deformity. In ball-and-socket joints, the ball can be totally anterior or posterior to the socket. The joint tissue rapidly swells, making reduction difficult.

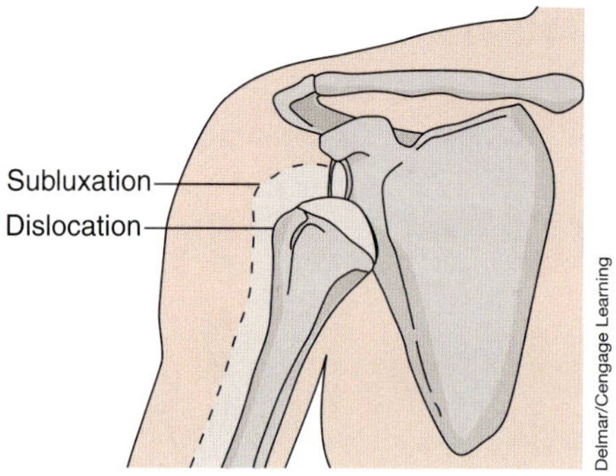

FIGURE 6–15 Dislocation and subluxation.

■ ***DIAGNOSIS.*** A history and physical exam by a physician is adequate for a diagnosis. An X-ray can be helpful in determining the extent of the injury.

■ ***TREATMENT.*** Because of the swelling, a dislocated joint should be reduced or repositioned by a physician immediately. Even with emergency treatment, general anesthesia might be needed for the reduction procedure.

Individuals who suffer with recurrent dislocations and subluxations can be taught how to reduce the joint. If the joint ligaments become weakened with repeated dislocations, surgery might be necessary to tighten the ligaments, thus strengthening the joint.

■ ***PREVENTION.*** Maintaining muscle strength around the joint will help prevent these conditions. Individual bandage wraps, braces, and special padding can also help.

Low Back Pain (LBP)

■ ***DESCRIPTION.*** The low back or lumbar area of the spine is very susceptible to stress or strain.

■ ***ETIOLOGY.*** This stress can be increased by such factors as obesity, poor posture, weak abdominal muscles, and constant or improper lifting. These factors are more likely to cause LBP in individuals who have spinal deformities or diseases affecting the spine.

Some disorders that affect the spine and often lead to LBP include spinal deformities, osteoarthritis, rheumatoid arthritis, osteoporosis, and bone cancer, to name just a few. X-ray examinations are usually helpful in determining the cause of LBP, but further detailed study with a CT scan or MRI might be needed.

■ ***SYMPTOMS.*** LBP is a very common disorder of the musculoskeletal system. It might be acute and resolve in a few days, or it might be a chronic discomfort that lasts a lifetime.

■ ***DIAGNOSIS.*** X-rays, CT, and MRI assist in the diagnosis of low back pain.

■ ***TREATMENT.*** Treatment of acute LBP is usually rest, warm moist heat, analgesics, and anti-inflammatory medications. Lumbar **spasms** (uncontrolled muscle contractions) are common and very painful. These spasms often twist the back out of normal position. Muscle relaxants might be prescribed for acute attacks, but rest and application of heat are usually adequate to control spasms. After the acute attack subsides, a daily exercise program including aerobic walking is very beneficial in building muscle tone and decreasing the risk of further attacks. One of the most common causes of LBP is a herniated intervertebral disk or herniated nucleus pulposus.

■ ***PREVENTION.*** Developing and maintaining a regular walking and exercise program are the best preventive measures for back pain prevention. Lifting properly is also an important preventive measure.

Herniated Nucleus Pulposus (HNP)

■ ***DESCRIPTION.*** HNP is commonly called herniated disk (or disc), ruptured disk, slipped disk, or bulging disk. All these terms are similar.

■ ***ETIOLOGY.*** HNP is the protrusion of the soft center (nucleus pulposus) of a disk in the spinal cord or spinal nerve (Figure 6–16).

■ ***SYMPTOMS.*** Pressure on the spinal nerve can cause pain in the sciatic nerve, called **sciatica**, which radiates down the back side of the leg.

■ ***DIAGNOSIS.*** Diagnosis involves physical examination, often confirmed by a CT scan, MRI, or **myelogram**. A myelogram involves injecting dye into the spinal canal and taking pictures to reveal compression on the spinal cord or spinal nerves.

■ ***TREATMENT.*** Treatment of HNP is often the same as for LBP. Extensive exercise therapy can reduce the size of the protrusion and relieve the associated LBP. If pain persists after therapy, or if the disk is found to be causing severe spinal cord or spinal nerve compression, surgery for disk removal might be needed. Surgery to remove the disk or to cut away vertebra to open the area around the nerve is called a **diskectomy** or **laminectomy**, respectively. A relatively new procedure to relieve the pain from osteoporotic compression fractures can also be performed. In this treatment, a large-bore needle is inserted with X-ray guidance into the compressed vertebra. A balloon is inserted into the bone through the needle and inflated, restoring the height of the vertebra. Sometimes, bone cement is injected into the bone to make sure it does not collapse again.

■ ***PREVENTION.*** Proper lifting, weight control, and maintaining a good exercise and walking program are all preventive measures.

HEALTHY HIGHLIGHT

RICE

RICE, an acronym for Rest, Ice, Compression, and Elevation, can be used effectively for almost all types of injuries from a sprained ankle to a broken bone. When an injury occurs, RICE should be followed for the first 24 hours.

- **REST** Immediate, nonweight-bearing rest will prevent further damage. Rest includes use of splints, slings, and crutches.
- **ICE** Application of ice slows bleeding and swelling by causing vasoconstriction. The more blood that collects in an area, the longer the healing time. Ice should not be applied directly to the skin; rather, wrap the ice pack in a towel before application. Alternating ice treatment—30 minutes on and 15 minutes off—is a general rule. Apply heat after 24 hours to improve vascular flow and carry away tissue debris.
- **COMPRESSION** Application of a compression stocking or ace wrap will provide support and limit swelling, thereby speeding healing time. Compression devices should be snug but not so tight they cut off circulation, which could lead to increased pain and numbness.
- **ELEVATION** Place the injured area at a height above the heart to allow gravity to assist venous flow to further reduce swelling.

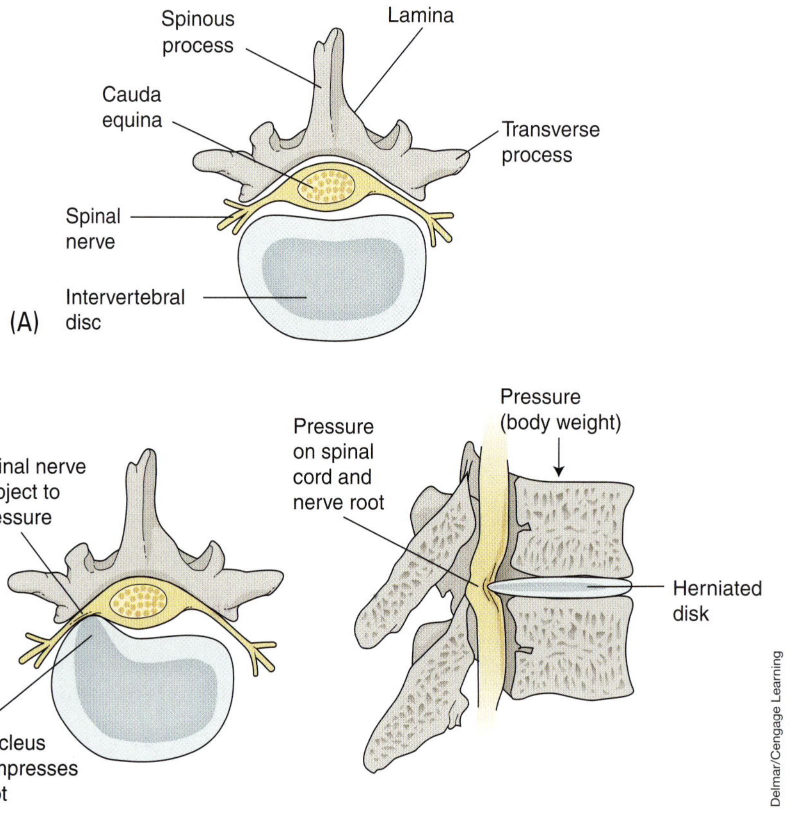

FIGURE 6–16 (A) Normal intervertebral disk. (B) Two views of a herniated disk.

Bursitis

■ ***DESCRIPTION.*** Bursitis (ber-SIE-tis) is the inflammation of a bursa or small, fluid-filled sac near joints. Bursae help reduce friction during movement.

■ ***ETIOLOGY.*** Repetitive motions often lead to irritation of the bursa, resulting in bursitis. Any joint can be affected, but bursitis of the shoulder is the most common type. Bursitis that occurs in the elbow is commonly called tennis elbow.

■ ***SYMPTOMS.*** Symptoms include severe pain that limits motion in the joint.

■ ***DIAGNOSIS.*** Bursitis is identified by location of pain or swelling and by pain with motion of the tissues in the affected area. X-ray testing can also help.

■ ***TREATMENT.*** Rest, application of moist heat, and use of analgesics and anti-inflammatory medications will usually resolve the condition. If bursitis persists, further treatment of the bursa includes injection with corticosteroids, draining, and surgical excision. Active range-of-motion exercises are needed after pain subsides to regain and maintain joint motion.

■ ***PREVENTION.*** Identifying and modifying activities that cause or aggravate the problem is the best prevention. Taking frequent breaks, especially from repetitive activities, is also helpful. Exercising and stretching to strengthen the muscle, ligaments, and tendons in the area of injury is important.

TENNIS ELBOW

■ ***DESCRIPTION.*** Tennis elbow is a type of bursitis that affects the elbow area.

■ ***ETIOLOGY.*** This bursitis is not always caused by playing tennis, as its name suggests. Tennis elbow is a repetitive-motion injury.

■ ***SYMPTOMS.*** The most commom symptom is a severe, burning pain on the outside of the elbow. Pain can be made worse by pressing on the outside surface of the elbow or by lifting or gripping objects. Lifting even the smallest object, such as a coffee cup, can lead to extreme pain.

■ ***DIAGNOSIS.*** Diagnosis can be confirmed by eliciting increased pain when the middle finger is pushed backward or extended against resistance.

■ ***TREATMENT.*** Treatment is the same as with bursitis. Application of a wide strap just below the elbow will change and support muscle movement in the forearm, thus reducing some of the pain.

■ ***PREVENTION.*** Stretching and strengthening the arm muscles so they are flexible and strong enough to support activities is the best prevention.

Tendonitis

■ ***DESCRIPTION.*** Tendonitis is inflammation of a tendon or connective tissue that attaches muscle to bone. Tendonitis can occur in any tendon, but most often, it affects the shoulder.

■ ***ETIOLOGY.*** Tendonitis is commonly a repetitive-motion injury but also can be caused by calcium deposits. Athletes in baseball, basketball, swimming, and tennis are often affected. Tendonitis also can occur in association with bursitis.

■ ***SYMPTOMS.*** Pain, gradual or sudden and severe, is the main symptom.

■ ***DIAGNOSIS.*** A physical examination revealing tenderness along the involved tendon along with pain when the muscle to which the tendon is attached is moved or worked against resistance will support the diagnosis.

■ ***TREATMENT.*** Treatment is rest, application of ice (which might irritate bursitis), and use of analgesics and anti-inflammatory medications. Active range-of-motion exercises can be initiated, after the pain subsides, to restore motion. If joint adhesions have developed, surgical intervention might be necessary to free the joint and restore mobility.

■ ***PREVENTION.*** Strengthening exercise, avoiding repetitive activities, and overuse of the of the arm or leg are preventive measures.

Carpal Tunnel Syndrome

■ ***DESCRIPTION.*** Carpal tunnel syndrome is a repetitive-motion injury affecting the hands and commonly seen in individuals who perform computer data entry, work at manufacturing jobs, or do any task that requires continuous, repetitive finger and wrist motions.

■ ***ETIOLOGY.*** The blood vessels, tendons, and nerves that feed or innervate the hands pass through a tunnel in the wrist area formed by the carpal tunnel ligament (Figure 6–17). The repetitive motion causes

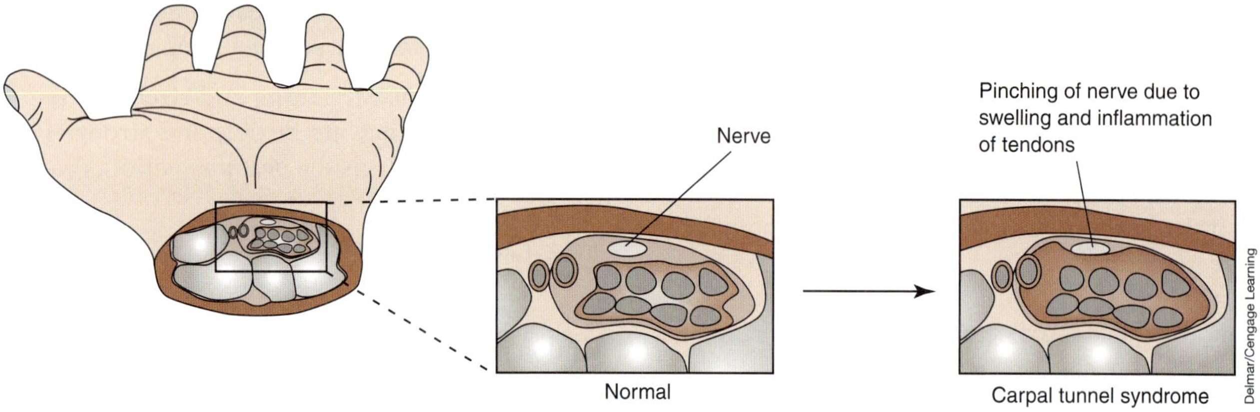

FIGURE 6–17 Carpal tunnel syndrome.

inflammation of the tendons, resulting in pressure on the medial nerve.

■ ***SYMPTOMS.*** Symptoms of carpal tunnel syndrome often include numbness, pain, swelling, coolness, and discoloration in the affected hand and fingers.

■ ***DIAGNOSIS.*** Diagnosis is confirmed by history, physical examination, and testing. Positive results of a Phalen's maneuver, performed by flexing the wrist as far as possible and watching for symptoms, is sufficient for diagnosis. A positive test is one that results in numbness in the median nerve area within 60 seconds of the maneuver.

■ ***TREATMENT.*** Treatment consists of stopping the repetitive motion, resting the hand, splinting, administration of anti-inflammatory medications, and physical therapy. Carpal tunnel syndrome not relieved by these measures might require surgery to split the carpal ligament, enlarging the tunnel and relieving pressure on the median nerve.

■ ***PREVENTION.*** Prevention of carpal tunnel syndrome is the best plan and can be accomplished by ergonomic principles and job rotation to improve hand positions and provide adequate rest periods, respectively.

Plantar Fasciitis

■ ***DESCRIPTION.*** Plantar fasciitis (FAS-ee-EYE-tis) is also called calcaneal spur or heel spur. The plantar **fascia** is a thick, fibrous, connective tissue that runs the length of the bottom or plantar surface of the foot. The plantar fascia attaches to the heel, or **calcaneal** area of the foot, and helps develop the arch of the foot (Figure 6–18).

■ ***ETIOLOGY.*** Plantar fasciitis is often seen in runners due to the repeated pressure placed on the fascia during running. This constant pressure causes inflammation and pain at the point of attachment to the calcaneus. It is not uncommon for individuals to have a small heel spur at this point of attachment, but it becomes more noticeable and more painful with this condition. Heel spurs do not cause the problem; they are the result of the problem.

■ ***SYMPTOMS.*** The common symptom of plantar fasciitis is an intermittent pain in the heel that is worse when taking the first few steps after sitting or standing for some time, when getting out of bed, or at the beginning of an exercise routine. Plantar fasciitis develops more often in individuals who have a sudden increase in activity or weight. Other sufferers include individuals who are flat-footed, toe runners, overweight and have high arches and poor shoe support.

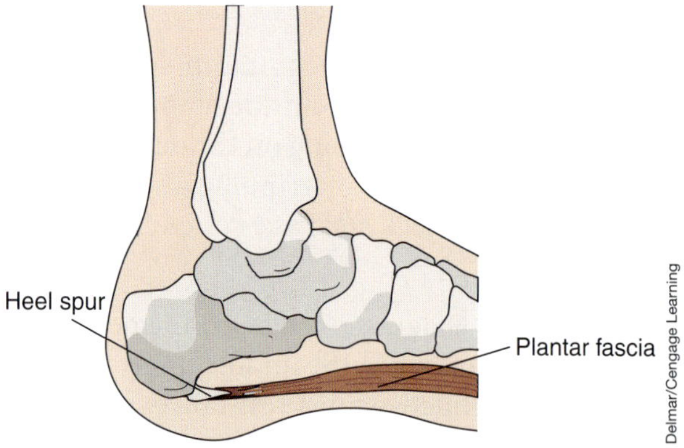

FIGURE 6–18 Plantar fasciitis.

■ ***DIAGNOSIS.*** History and physical exam is usually sufficient for diagnosis. The classic history is a complaint of pain in the foot during the first steps after getting out of bed or after sitting for a long period of time.

■ ***TREATMENT.*** Treatment includes rest, application of ice, use of analgesics and anti-inflammatory medication, and use of a heel pad or orthotic that relieves pressure on the heel. After pain subsides, exercises to strengthen the foot might help prevent reinjury. Surgery to remove the heel spur and release the plantar fascia has proven ineffective in most instances.

■ ***PREVENTION.*** Steps to prevent plantar fasciitis include wearing shoes with good arch support, exercising to stretch the Achilles tendon, maintaining proper body weight, and avoiding going barefoot.

Torn Rotator Cuff

■ ***DESCRIPTION.*** The rotator cuff comprises a group of muscles that hold the head of the humerus in the shoulder socket area.

■ ***ETIOLOGY.*** Tears are commonly caused by traumatic injuries of baseball, basketball, and tennis.

■ ***SYMPTOMS.*** Tears in the tendons that hold these muscles to the bone produce a snapping sound, followed by acute pain and the inability of the individual to abduct (move away from midline) or raise the arm.

■ ***DIAGNOSIS.*** Diagnosis is made by physical examination and can be confirmed with a CT scan or arthroscopy.

■ ***TREATMENT.*** Acute rotator cuff tears are surgically repaired to restore motion of the shoulder. Postoperatively, the individual is placed in a shoulder immobilizer for 3 to 4 weeks. Analgesics and anti inflammatory medications can be administered for acute pain. Active rehabilitation exercise is needed postoperatively to restore shoulder function.

■ ***PREVENTION.*** Daily exercise to maintain muscle strength and flexibility in the shoulder is the best preventive measure.

Torn Meniscus

■ ***DESCRIPTION.*** There are two semilunar cartilages in each knee joint, forming a lateral and medial meniscus. The **meniscus** (meh-NIS-cuss) is attached to the top of the tibia and provides cushioning for the distal femur.

■ ***ETIOLOGY.*** Athletes participating in football, baseball, soccer, and tennis commonly suffer with this injury. The tear usually results from a sudden twisting of the leg while the knee is flexed (Figure 6–19).

■ ***SYMPTOMS.*** Symptoms include acute pain with weight bearing on the affected knee. The individual might feel that the knee is locking or giving. Full flexion or extension of the knee might not be possible due to increased pain.

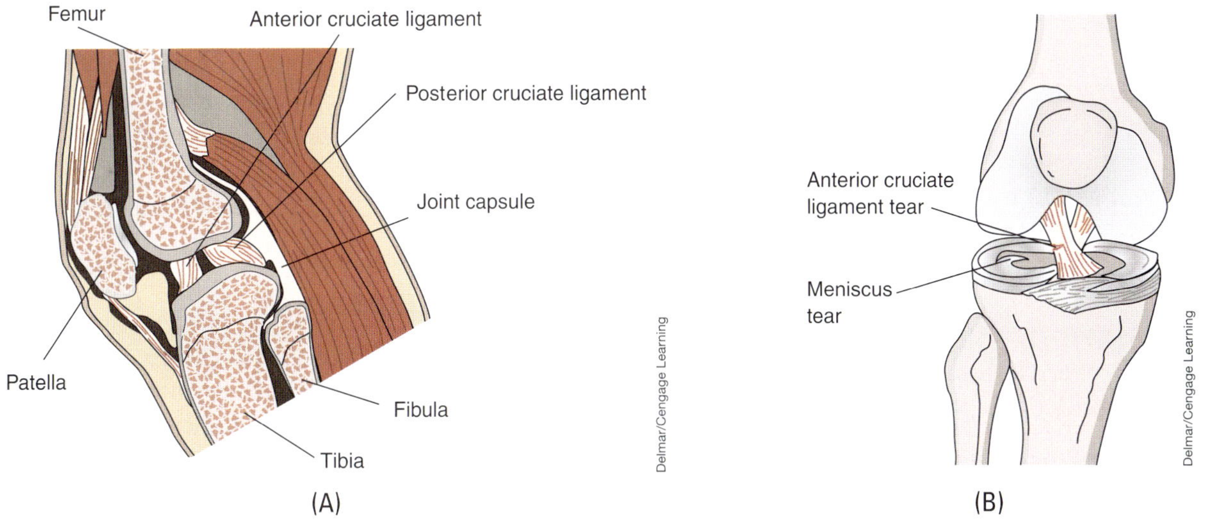

FIGURE 6–19 (A) Cruciate ligaments. (B) Meniscus and anterior cruciate ligament tear.

■ ***DIAGNOSIS.*** Physical examination of the knee along with X-ray or MRI confirm the diagnosis.

■ ***TREATMENT.*** Treatment is immobilization, elevation, and application of ice to decrease inflammation and pain. Analgesics and anti-inflammatory medications also can be needed. If surgical treatment is needed, it is commonly done arthroscopically or with the use of a scope to look into the knee. An extensive exercise rehabilitation program is begun postoperatively.

■ ***PREVENTION.*** Regular exercise,including strength training, aids in prevention of tears.

Cruciate Ligament Tears

■ ***DESCRIPTION.*** Cruciate (shaped like a cross) ligaments are located inside the knee joint (Figure 6–19a). They work as a pair (the anterior cruciate ligament and the posterior cruciate ligament) and form a cross, giving the knee front-to-back and rotary stability.

■ ***ETIOLOGY.*** These ligaments are often injured when the leg is twisted or hit from the front or back while in a planted or weight-bearing position (Figure 6–19b).

■ ***SYMPTOMS.*** A *popping* sound is commonly heard at the time of injury, followed by pain and swelling of the knee. Knee instability, front to back, is a primary sign of a cruciate ligament tear.

■ ***DIAGNOSIS.*** Diagnosis involves clinical examination, joint stability testing, and possible CT scanning.

■ ***TREATMENT.*** Treatment depends on the degree of injury and can vary from immobilization to surgical intervention.

■ ***PREVENTION.*** Maintaining excellent strength, flexibility, and endurance of the hamstrings and quadriceps muscles can prevent some anterior cruciate ligament (ACL) tears.

Shin Splints

■ ***DESCRIPTION.*** Shin splint is a term used to describe an overuse injury to the periosteum and extensor muscles of the lower leg.

■ ***ETIOLOGY.*** Shin splints occur routinely with a sudden increase in activity or a new exercise routine, commonly occuring in runners, joggers, and high-impact aerobics enthusiasts. Running on hard surfaces can also cause the problem.

■ ***SYMPTOMS.*** Pain and tenderness along the inner aspect of the tibia, worsening with exercise and disappearing with rest, are common symptoms.

■ ***DIAGNOSIS.*** Diagnosis is usually based on clinical examination, but X-ray examination can rule out a stress fracture.

■ ***TREATMENT.*** Rest, analgesics, anti-inflammatory medications, and alternating ice and heat treatments are usually beneficial.

■ ***PREVENTION.*** Proper conditioning, stretching exercises, and padded exercise shoes assist in preventing this disorder.

RARE DISEASES

de Quervain's Disease

de Quervain's disease is a repetitive-use tendonitis affecting the thumb. Pain can radiate up the forearm several inches and down into the thumb and increase if the individual attempts to pull the thumb and little finger together while the fingers are pointing upward. Physical examination and testing confirms the diagnosis.

Tuberculosis of the Bone

The bacterium *Mycobacterium tuberculosis* primarily affects the lungs, but it can also enter the bloodstream and travel to other organs of the body. Tuberculosis (TB) of the bone generally affects the arms and legs, and the knee is a common site for infection. Just as it does in the lungs, TB causes the development of cavities in the tissue, leading to bone weakness and pain. Antibiotic treatment is generally effective. A special form of TB in the vertebra or back of children is called Pott's disease.

Paget's Disease

Paget's (PAJ-ets) disease, also known as osteitis deformans, is a chronic metabolic bone disease that affects bone formation. Normally, bone is broken down and replaced at a consistent rate. Paget's is characterized by an overgrowth of new bone that outpaces the breakdown of old bone. The new bone is thicker than the old but much weaker, increasing the possibility of fracture. Radiologic examination reveals a mosaic bone pattern that is easily recognized as Paget's.

Paget's disease often affects the pelvis and long bones of the legs in individuals over age 40 and becomes more common with advancing age. Paget's can be asymptomatic, in which case, no treatment is necessary or beneficial. When symptomatic, individuals might complain of bone pain that becomes worse at night. Bones may fracture easily or become deformed, leading to bowed legs and curvature of the spine.

If the disease affects bones of the ear, hearing might become impaired. A secondary problem or complication of Paget's is the development of osteosarcoma, or bone cancer. The cause of Paget's is idiopathic. Treatment is primarily symptomatic, although a high-protein diet with calcium and vitamin D supplements can be beneficial.

Myasthenia Gravis

Myasthenia gravis (MY-us-THEE-nee-uh GRAV-iss) is an autoimmune disorder characterized by muscle weakness and fatigue that is somewhat relieved with rest. The problem is related to blocking of the acetylcholine neurotransmitter by antibodies in the neuromuscular junction. For more details about myasthenia gravis, see Chapter 5.

EFFECTS OF AGING ON THE SYSTEM

Normal changes that occur in bones, joints, and muscles cause a variety of problems in the older adult. Bone density decreases with age as calcium is reabsorbed from the bone. This causes greater brittleness of the bone with increased risks for fractures. Osteoporosis is a common problem in the older adult, especially in older females, because of its association with decreasing estrogen levels in the blood.

As the individual ages, muscles decrease in strength and mass. Some muscle cells atrophy and decrease in total number. Arm and leg muscles lose tone and become somewhat flaccid and flabby in appearance.

Changes in height and curvature of the spine occur from changes in the vertebral disks and compression of the vertebrae. As muscles waste and joints stiffen, some loss of flexibility and agility is also common, along with an overall decreased mobility. Research has demonstrated the benefits of weight training and exercise classes for the older adult to prevent some of the muscle wasting, decreases in bone density, and loss of flexibility.

Musculoskeletal diseases, especially the debilitating ones such as arthritis, are extremely difficult for the older adult. Healing, such as after a fracture, is slower and often impaired by other chronic disorders common to the older adult. Pain associated with these disorders and changes in the system tend to decrease the individual's mobility and independence even more. Safety issues are of utmost importance when musculoskeletal system disorders are present because falls are one of the most common causes of injury in the older adult.

GLIMPSE OF THE FUTURE

Vitamins and Exercise to Prevent Bone Loss

Antioxidant supplements and aerobic training may help prevent bone loss in the elderly. One recent study looked at a group of older adults who were given vitamin C and E supplements and participated in aerobic training programs. The researchers found that there was some benefit to using this therapy to prevent the age-related bone loss that occurs in most older adults. More research is needed to determine whether this therapy should be recommended to all elderly individuals in the future.

Source: Maimoun, et al. (2008)

SUMMARY

The musculoskeletal system consists of bones, joints, muscles, ligaments, and tendons. It is the body's main framework and is responsible for all movements, which are the result of contraction and relaxation of the muscle fibers. The muscles are stimulated by responses from the nervous system. Most muscle movements are voluntary movements. The most common symptoms of musculoskeletal system disorders are pain, immobility, and disability. Diagnosis of a musculoskeletal system problem is usually made by assessment and X-ray or magnetic resonance imaging. However, other specific tests such as bone scans or endoscopy also can be used. Although fractures are a major group of musculoskeletal system disorders, many other diseases are common to the system. Some of these are short term, but many are long-term, debilitating disorders. Individuals with musculoskeletal system diseases frequently need assistive devices such as crutches or walkers to maintain mobility. Changes in the musculoskeletal system in the older adult often leads to increased risk for fractures and disability.

REVIEW QUESTIONS

Short Answer

1. What are the major functions of the musculoskeletal system?

2. What are the common signs and symptoms associated with musculoskeletal system disorders?

3. What are the most common tests used to diagnose musculoskeletal system disorders?

Fill in the Blank

4. The musculoskeletal system is composed of ____________, ____________, ____________, ____________, and ____________.

5. ____________ attach muscle to bone.

6. ____________ joints are ones that have full movement.

7. The most common disorder of the system is ____________.

8. ____________ ____________ is the most serious form of arthritis, but ____________ is the most common type of arthritis.

Matching

9. Match the fracture-related term in the left column with the appropriate description in the right column.

_____ comminuted	a. Bone fragments are in correct position
_____ nondisplaced	b. One bone end is forced over another
_____ transverse	c. More than two ends or fragments are present
_____ greenstick	d. Bone has protruded through the skin
_____ stress	e. An incomplete fracture common in children
_____ impacted	f. Fracture runs across or at a 90-degree angle
_____ compound	g. Caused by too much weight-bearing or pressure

CASE STUDIES

■ Estella Gore is a 77-year-old resident of a local nursing home. She fell 4 weeks ago and fractured her left hip and is now in rehabilitation therapy and walking with the assistance of a physical therapy aide and a rolling walker. She states she is very frightened to walk and would rather use her wheelchair for mobility. What should you tell Ms. Gore about the importance of continuing to walk, even if she needs the assistance of a walker or personnel? Why is it important for her to be as mobile as possible? What are the overall effects of immobility? How does immobility affect other body systems?

■ Jeremy Dale is a 30-year-old recreational sports enthusiast and likes to play soccer and baseball on his days off from work. He mentions to you, his coworker, that he thinks he might have sprained his ankle over the weekend while playing soccer with some friends. He says it is swollen and very painful today and asks whether you think he should see a doctor or just wait for it to get better. What might be some good recommendations for you to give Jeremy about his sports injury? What could you tell him in general about minor sports injuries? How could he determine whether this is a sprain or a strain? Should he apply ice and elevate or compress the injuried ankle? Is it too late for that treatment to be helpful?

*Study*WARE™ Connection

To help you learn the content in this chapter, take a practice quiz or play an interactive game on your StudyWARE™ CD-ROM.

Workbook Practice

Go to your Workbook and complete the practice questions.

BIBLIOGRAPHY

Anders, M., Turner, L., & Wallace, L. S. (2007). Use of decision rules for osteoporosis prevention and treatment: Implications for nurse practitioners. *American Academy of Nurse Practitioners 19*(6), 299–305.

Arthritis Foundation Research Update. (May 2007). Are doctors advising their overweight patients to lose weight? *www.arthritis.org* (accessed May 2008).

Bainbridge, P. (2005). Fractured fortunes. *Nursing Standard 20*(1), 30–31.

Beraducci, A. (2007). Bone loss: An emerging problem following obesity surgery. *Orthopaedic Nursing 26*(5), 281–286.

Gardiner, A., El Miedany, Y., & Toth, M. (2007). Osteoporosis: Not only in women but in men too. *British Journal of Nursing 16*(12), 731–735.

Hanna, J., & Letizia, M. J. (2007). Kyphoplasty: A treatment for osteoporitic vertebral compression fractures. *Orthopaedic Nursing 26*(6), 342–348.

Hansberger, J. (2007). Osteoporosis: Review of disease, diagnosis and treatments for the advanced practice nurse. *Journal of Advanced Nursing Practice 8*(1), 5.

Ibandronate sodium. (2006). *Nursing 36*(8), 59.

Kim, K., Suh, S., Lee, T., Ha, K., Kim, J., Kim, D., Jeon, J., Moon, T., & Kin, C. (2008). Effect of safflower seeds supplementation on stimulation of the proliferation, differentiation and mineralization of osteoblastic MC3T3-E1 cells. *Journal of Ethnopharmacology 115*(1), 42–49.

Kuo, I., Ong, C., Simmons, L., Bliuc, D., Eisman, J., & Center, J. (2007). Successful direct intervention for osteoporosis in patients with minimal trauma fractures. *Osteoporosis International 18*(12), 1633–1639.

Maddalozzo, G. F., Widrick, J. J., Cardinal, B. J. Winters-Stone, K. M., Hoffman, M. A., & Snow, C. M. (2007). The effects of replacement therapy and resistance training on spine bone mineral density in early postmenopausal women. *Bone 40*(5), 1244–1251.

Maimoun, L., Simar, D., Caillaud, C., Perchon, E., Sultan, C., Rossi, M., & Mariano-Goulart, D. (2008). Effect of antioxidants and exercise on bone metabolism. *Journal of Sports Medicine 26*(3), 251–258.

Messier, S. P., Gutekunst, D. J., Davis, C., & DeVita, P. (2007). Weight loss reduces knee-joint loads in overweight and obese older adults wth knee osteoarthritis. *Arthtritis and Rheumatism 52*(7), 2026–2032.

Miller, N. C., & Askew, A. E. (2007). Tibia fractures: An overview of evaluation and treatment. *Nursing 26*(4), 224–225.

News and information. (2008). American College of Sports Medicine. *www.acsm.org* (accessed May 2008).

Osteoporosis "neglected" in nursing homes. (2006). *Pulse 66*(5), 17.

Suominen, H. (2007). Physical activity and health: Musculoskeletal issues. *Advances in Physiotherapy 9*(2), 65–75.

Sutcliffe, A. (2005). An overview of osteoporosis. *Nursing Standard 20*(2), 58–64.

Wright, R. M. (2007). Use of osteoporosis medications in older nursing facility residents. *Journal of the American Directors Association 8*(7), 453–457.

Yearly dose keeps bones strong. (2007). *Nursing 37*(7), 30.

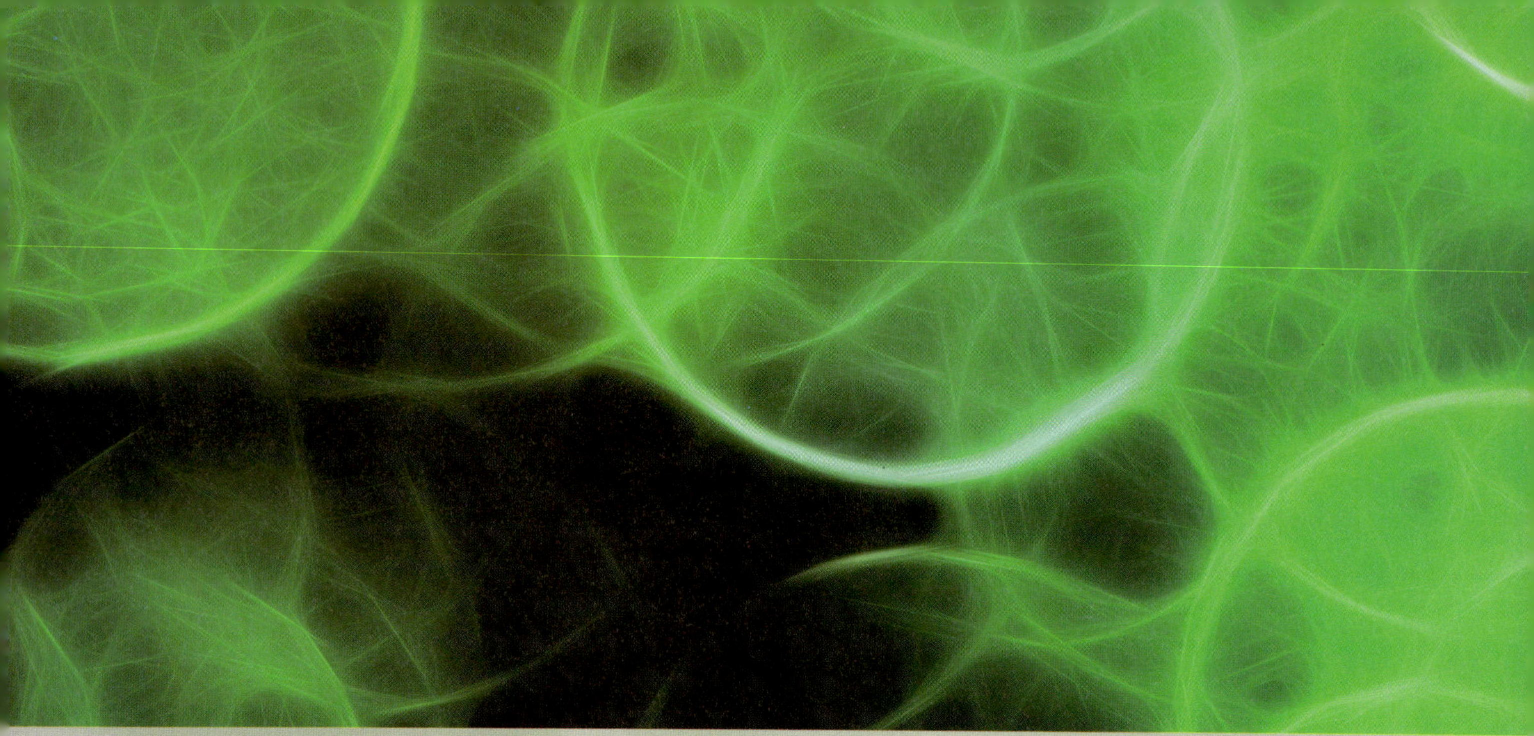

OUTLINE

- Anatomy and Physiology
- Common Signs and Symptoms
- Diagnostic Tests
- Common Diseases of the Blood and Blood-Forming Organs
  - *Disorders of Red Blood Cells*
  - *Disorders of White Blood Cells*
  - *Disorders of Platelets and Clotting*
- Trauma
- Rare Diseases
  - *Thalassemia*
  - *Von Willebrand's Disease*
  - *Lymphosarcoma*
- Effects of Aging on the System
- Summary
- Review Questions
- Case Studies
- Bibliography

KEY TERMS

Anemia (p. 127)
Bence Jones protein (p. 137)
Bleeding time (p. 129)
Complete blood count (p. 128)
Differential (p. 129)
Dyspnea (p. 130)
Ecchymoses (p. 128)
Epistaxis (p. 128)
Erythrocytopenia (p. 127)
Erythrocytosis (p. 128)
Hemarthrosis (p. 137)
Hematemesis (p. 138)
Hematocrit (p. 129)
Hematuria (p. 138)
Hemoglobin (p. 129)
Hemolyzed (p. 129)
Leukemia (p. 135)
Leukocytopenia (p. 128)
Leukocytosis (p. 128)
Lymphopenia (p. 128)
Neutropenia (p. 128)
Pallor (p. 130)
Pancytopenia (p. 133)
Petechiae (p. 128)
Purpura (p. 138)
Reed–Sternberg cell (p. 135)
Syncope (p. 130)
Tachycardia (p. 130)
Tachypnea (p. 130)
Thrombocytopenia (p. 128)
Thrombocytosis (p. 128)

7

Blood and Blood-Forming Organs Diseases and Disorders

LEARNING OBJECTIVES

Upon completion of the chapter, the learner should be able to:

1. Define the terminology common to the blood and blood-forming organs and the disorders of the blood and blood-forming organs.
2. Discuss the basic anatomy and physiology of the blood and blood-forming organs.
3. Identify the important signs and symptoms associated with common blood and blood-forming organ disorders.
4. Describe the common diagnostics used to determine the type and cause of blood and blood-forming organ disorders.
5. Identify the common disorders of the blood and blood-forming organs.
6. Describe the typical course and management of the common blood and blood-forming organ disorders.
7. Describe the effects of aging on the blood and blood-forming organs and the common disorders associated with aging of the system.

OVERVIEW

The blood and the blood-forming organs make up the individual's hematologic system. Blood is the body's life fluid, responsible for transporting nutrients to cells and removing wastes. The blood-forming organs are the lymph nodes, bone marrow, spleen, and liver. Disorders of the system can have severe effects on other systems because of the pervasive responsibilities of the blood and blood-forming organs. Altered nutrition, medications, and diseases of other systems, in turn, can greatly affect the functioning of the hematologic system. ■

ANATOMY AND PHYSIOLOGY

The blood and blood-forming organs are also called the hematologic system. The major function of the blood is to transport necessary nutrients to the cells and to aid in the removal of wastes. The blood also transports hormones secreted by the endocrine system. In addition, the white blood cells (leukocytes) are important in infection prevention. The blood is composed of a variety of substances of which plasma, a straw-colored liquid, makes up about 55% of the total. The formed elements constitute the other 45%. They include the erythrocytes (red blood cells, or RBCs), leukocytes (white blood cells, or WBCs), and platelets (clotting fragments) (Figure 7–1).

Descriptive properties of the blood include its color, volume, viscosity, and pH. Blood is bright red in the arteries due to its oxygen content; blood in the veins is a dark red (often depicted as blue) due to the absence of oxygen. The average adult has about 75 ml/kg of body weight of circulating blood (5–6 liters or approximately 1.5 gallons). The viscosity or density of blood is about three or more times greater than water. Blood is slightly alkaline (pH 7.35–7.45).

The erythrocytes transport oxygen from the lungs to the tissues. The normal erythrocyte count is 4.2 to 6.3 million. Erythrocytes formed in the bone marrow do not reproduce. Erythrocyte production increases when oxygen needs increase. During their life span, which is only about 120 days, red cells become worn and often ragged from bumping and bouncing into the vessel walls of the circulatory system. The worn RBCs are filtered out of circulation by the spleen and liver. These organs are responsible for breaking down the RBCs and saving the iron component for reuse in the development of new RBCs.

Hemoglobin, a component of the RBC, is important in the transport of oxygen. A low level of hemoglobin in the blood reduces the level of circulating oxygen. The normal level of hemoglobin for an adult male is 13.5–18g/100 ml, and 12–16g/100 ml for an adult female.

Leukocytes protect the individual from infections. The average white blood cell count for an adult is 4,500–11,000/cu mm. A count higher than

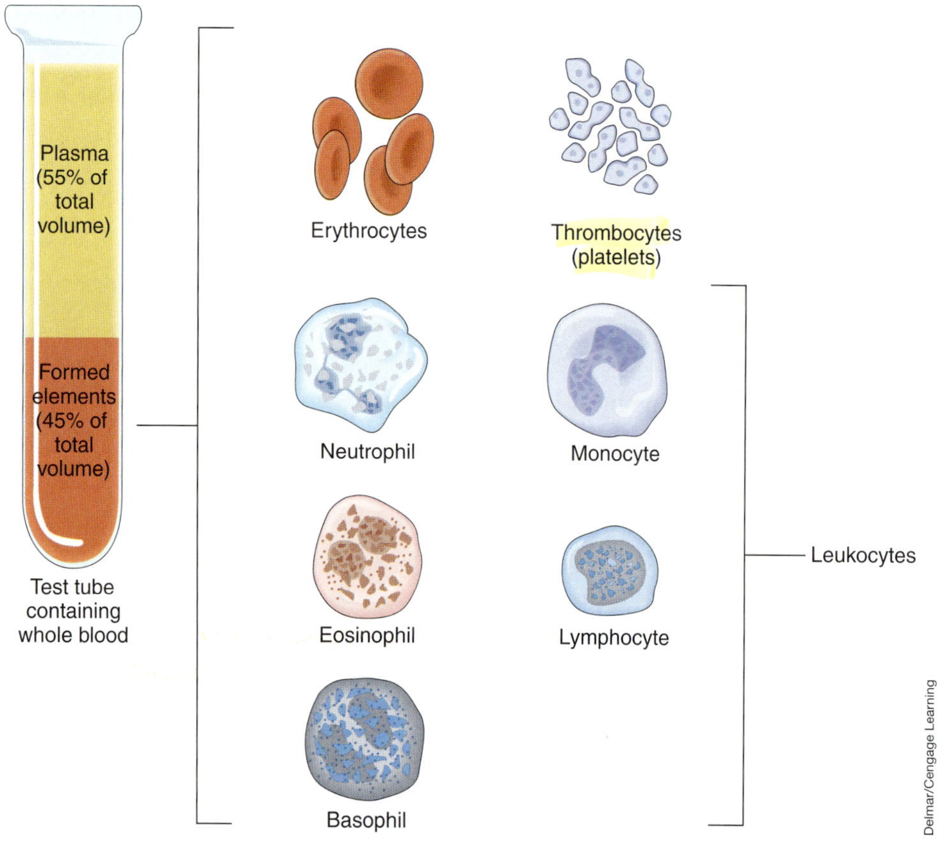

FIGURE 7–1 Blood components.

11,000 usually indicates the presence of an infection. See Chapter 4, "Inflammation and Infection," and Chapter 5, "Immune System Diseases and Disorders," for more information about leukocytes.

Platelets, also called thrombocytes, produce the thrombokinase used in the clotting process. The average number of platelets in adults is 150,000–350,000/mm^3 of blood.

The plasma portion of blood is composed of 91% water and 9% plasma proteins. The plasma proteins include (1) albumin, responsible for maintaining osmotic pressure; (2) globulin, responsible for infection fighting; (3) fibrinogen, responsible for part of the clotting process; and (4) prothrombin, also responsible for part of the clotting process.

Blood coagulation (clotting) occurs in phases. In the first phase, the platelets, in association with several plasma proteins, agglutinate (clump) at the site of injury or blood loss, and thromboplastin is formed. In the second phase, prothrombin is converted to thrombin in the presence of calcium. In the third phase, thrombin and fibrinogen form fibrin. With the presence of calcium, a fibrin clot is formed. In the fourth phase, the clot is removed through the process of fibrinolysis.

Blood is classified by the antigens in the RBCs and the antibodies in the plasma. The antigens are A and B, and the antibodies are anti-A and anti-B. In addition, a factor called Rh is used in the classification system. (See Chapter 5 under "Erythroblastosis Fetalis" and "Blood Transfusion Reaction" for more information.) Blood is typed as A, B, AB, and O. Type A blood has A antigens and anti-B antibodies, type B blood has B antigens and anti-A antibodies, type AB blood has A and B antigens and does not have anti-A or anti-B antibodies, and type O blood has neither A nor B antigens but has both anti-A and anti-B antibodies. The Rh designation is based on 12 distinct antigens. Rh positive blood contains this antigen, but Rh negative does not. Because of these designations and blood properties, blood transfusion recipients must have a type and cross-match of blood to be certain a reaction will not occur (Table 7–1).

The blood-forming organs include the lymph nodes, bone marrow, spleen, and liver. The lymph nodes are found throughout the body along the lymphatic vessels. The lymph nodes filter the lymph and produce the lymphocytes and antibodies important for protection from pathogens.

Bone marrow is found in the center part of long bones and in the spongy part of other bones. It is the major blood cell–producing organ in the body.

TABLE 7–1 RBC Blood Donor and Recipient Chart

	RBC Recipient (Receiver)			
	O	A	B	AB
RBC Donor (Giver)				
O	YES	YES	YES	YES
A	NO	YES	NO	YES
B	NO	NO	YES	YES
AB	NO	NO	NO	YES

YES = This type can receive the donated RBCs.
NO = This type cannot receive the donated RBCs.

The spleen is found in the upper left quadrant of the abdomen. It produces lymphocytes, plasma cells, and antibodies and filters microorganisms from the blood. It also removes old blood cells from the body.

The liver is a large organ found in the right upper quadrant of the abdomen. It has multiple responsibilities for many body systems. The liver functions as a blood-forming organ in intrauterine life and is active the rest of the individual's life as a producer of prothrombin and fibrinogen for blood clotting.

StudyWARE™ Connection

View an animation on the blood on your StudyWARE™ CD-ROM.

COMMON SIGNS AND SYMPTOMS

Signs and symptoms of this system include those related to increases and decreases in the number of blood cells. Diseases affecting the blood-forming organs (primarily spleen, bone marrow, and lymph nodes) can lead to decreased or increased production of cells. Diseases that hemolyze, destroy, or use up the cells lead to a decrease in cell number and volume.

Erythrocytopenia (erythro = red, cyte = cell, penia = decrease) leads to **anemia** (an = without, emia = blood). Anemia does not mean without any blood; it means low or decreased RBC volume. Signs and symptoms of anemia can be minor or major, asymptomatic to life-threatening, depending on cause. Common signs and symptoms include a low erythrocyte count, headache, fatigue, pallor, and shortness of breath.

Erythrocytosis (erythrocyte = red cell, osis = condition) is a condition of increased RBCs. Common signs and symptoms include a high RBC count, reddened skin tones, bloodshot eyes, increased blood volume and pressure, and an increase in the workload of the heart.

Leukocytopenia (leuko = white, cyte = cell, penia = decrease) is a decrease in white cell count. Leukocytopenia weakens the immune system because these cells are primary players in the defense system. **Neutropenia** (neutrophil decrease) and **lymphopenia** (lymphocyte decrease) can be associated with chronic infection because the numbers are used up during a long-term battle. Signs and symptoms are related to the particular type of infection.

Leukocytosis (leukocyto = white cell, osis = condition of) is an increase in white cell count. This condition is a normal response to acute infection. If leukocytosis is related to a tumor, these numbers can be extreme, as in the case of leukemia (leuk = white, emia = blood).

Thrombocytopenia (THROM-boh-SIGH-toh-PEE-nee-ah; thrombocyte = platelet, penia = decrease) is a decrease in platelets, leading to a coagulation problem. Signs and symptoms include small hemorrhages in the skin called **petechiae** (pee-TEE-kee-eye), large areas of bruising or hemorrhage called **ecchymoses** (ECH-ih-MOH-ses), and **epistaxis** (EP-ih-STACK-sis; nosebleeds). Bleeding lesions in the mouth, gums, and mucous membranes are also common.

Thrombocytosis (THROM-boh-sigh-TOE-sis; thrombocyte = platelet, osis = condition of) is an increase in platelets. This condition is uncommon and usually has no serious side effects (Table 7–2).

TABLE 7–2 Blood Cell Abnormalities and Associated Symptoms

Red Blood Cells	Condition	Symptoms
INCREASED	Erythrocytosis	Reddened skin, increased blood pressure, increased workload on the heart
DECREASED	Erythrocytopenia	Anemia
White Blood Cells		
INCREASED	Leukocytosis	Usually asymptomatic
DECREASED	Leukocytopenia	Weakened immune system
Thrombocytes		
INCREASED	Thrombocytosis	Increased clotting
DECREASED	Thrombocytopenia	Increased bleeding

DIAGNOSTIC TESTS

Diagnostic tests for blood and blood-forming organ disorders include complete blood count with differential and indices. Biopsy of the blood-forming organs also can be helpful in diagnosing disorders of the spleen, lymph nodes, and bone marrow.

A **complete blood count** (CBC) identifies the number of RBCs, WBCs, and platelets per cubic millimeter (Table 7–3) and can be used in the determination

TABLE 7–3 CBC Normal Values

Cells	Values
Erythrocytes	**Males** 4.6–6.3 million/mm^3 **Females** 4.2–5.4 million/mm^3
Hematocrit	**Males** 40–54% **Females** 38–47%
Hemoglobin	**Males** 13.5–18 g/dl **Females** 12–16 g/dl
RBC Indices	
MCV	80–96 mm^3
MCH	27–31 pg
MCHC	32–36%
Leukocytes	4,500–11,000 million/mm^3
Differential	
Myelocytes	0/mm^3
Band neutrophils	1,500–3,000/mm^3
Segmented neutrophils	300–500/mm^3
Lymphocytes	50–250/mm^3
Monocytes	15–50/mm^3
Eosinophils	15–50/mm^3
Basophils	15–50/mm^3
Platelets	150,000–350,000/mm^3
Reticulocytes	25,000–75,000/mm^3

Key:
mm^3 = cubic millimeter
g/dl = grams per deciliter
pg = picograms

of most blood diseases. RBC count and indices can assist in the determination of the different anemias, polycythemia, and erythrocytosis. A **differential** is a more detailed count, identifying the number of each type of leukocyte. A WBC count and differential can assist in determination of inflammation and infection or tumors of white cells. **Hematocrit** (Hct) reflects the amount of red cell mass as a proportion of whole blood. **Hemoglobin** (Hgb) reflects the amount of hemoglobin or oxygen-carrying potential available in the blood. Special measurements of red cells are called indices and include:

- **MCV** Mean corpuscular volume; reflects average size of the red cell
- **MCH** Mean corpuscular hemoglobin, or average hemoglobin content
- **MCHC** Mean corpuscular hemoglobin concentration, or average hemoglobin concentration

The morphology of each of the cells and platelets can be observed by performing a blood smear. A blood smear is performed by placing a drop of blood on a glass slide, smearing it to spread the cells to a thin layer, and staining and examining it microscopically for abnormal cell morphology or shape. Adding a staining solution to the slide helps in the identification of granular and agranular WBCs. A blood smear can be helpful in determining the cause of anemia, especially sickle cell disease.

A **bleeding time** test can assist in determining blood disorders such as hemophilia, thrombocytopenia, and disseminated intravascular coagulation. This test is performed by making minor cuts in the forearm of the involved individual and measuring the amount of time it takes for the area to clot or stop bleeding. Prothrombin time (PT) and partial thromboplastin time (PTT) are both blood tests that measure the ability of the blood to clot related to clotting factors. The international normalized ratio (INR) is also commonly used to measure bleeding time. It measures the time it takes for blood to clot and compares it to an average.

Biopsy of blood-forming organs can be helpful in diagnosing diseases and disorders. For instance, bone marrow biopsy is performed by boring a needle into the bone of the iliac crest of the hip to obtain tissue that is prepared and microscopically examined. Lymph node biopsy can be performed to determine functioning of the marrow, detect anemias, and diagnose neoplasms.

COMMON DISEASES OF THE BLOOD AND BLOOD-FORMING ORGANS

The most common problem related to this system is anemia, a decrease in RBC mass that can be caused by a number of different disease processes. Anemia is generally a sign of a disease but is commonly used as a diagnosis until the cause is discovered. Anemia can be serious if the cause is not determined or cannot be corrected.

Disorders of WBCs are usually secondary to other diseases rather than as a primary disease. Infections demand an increased need for WBCs because they are used up while fighting the invader. This can lead to leukocytopenia, a decrease in WBC number.

Any disorders of the blood-forming organs (spleen, bone marrow, and lymph nodes) can lead to secondary disorders of this system. Leukemias, lymphomas, and myelomas are the primary tumors affecting the system.

Disorders of Red Blood Cells

Any increase or decrease in number or size of RBCs will affect the mass or volume. Red cell mass is important because it directly affects the amount of hemoglobin available (oxygen-carrying potential). Commonly, the problem is not enough red cell mass leading to anemia. Too much red cell mass is called erythrocytosis, the most common type of which is a condition called polycythemia.

ANEMIA

DESCRIPTION. Any decrease in oxygen-carrying ability of the RBC is anemia. There are more than 400 types of anemia (HealthSource, 2008), but the three most common types are related to deficiency of iron, folic acid, and vitamin B_{12}.

ETIOLOGY. Anemia is commonly due to a low number of RBCs or a decrease in hemoglobin in RBCs. Acute hemorrhage or chronic bleeding can lead to a low number of circulating RBCs and, thus, anemia.

Any disease of the liver, spleen, or bone marrow can also lead to anemia. For instance, if the cells are broken down (**hemolyzed**) too soon, this can lead to a decrease in cell number; if cells are not formed quickly enough to replace the worn cells, the number of circulating cells will be low. If cells are formed abnormally, their ability to carry oxygen can be impaired because although the number of cells might be adequate, their oxygen-carrying ability is not. Dietary deficiencies often lead to an inadequate supply of nutrients to make RBCs.

■ ***SYMPTOMS.*** Despite the cause, the symptoms of anemia are fairly common. The individual suffering from anemia commonly is pale or has a condition of **pallor**. Facial paleness can be difficult to determine, but further examination of the mucous membranes of the mouth and conjunctiva of the eyes will reveal definite paleness. The nail beds also might be noticeably pale in color.

Anemic individuals are weak and suffer from fatigue due to poor oxygenation of muscle tissue. Shortness of breath, **dyspnea** (DISP-nee-ah; dys = difficult, pnea = breathing), **tachycardia** (TACH-ee-KAR-dee-ah; tachy = fast, cardia = heart), and **tachypnea** (TACK-ip-NEE-ah; tachy = fast, pnea = breathing) are common as the heart and lungs attempt to meet the body's oxygen need. Headache, irritability, and **syncope** (SIN-koh-pee; fainting) can also be symptoms.

■ ***DIAGNOSIS.*** Anemia can be very simple or related to a complicated or chronic disease. For simple cases, a history and physical exmaination along with blood tests measuring the level of hemoglobin, hematocrit, iron, folic acid, and vitamin B_{12} assist in diagnosis. Microscopic examination of the size and shape of the red cells also provides futher clues to the type of anemia.

More complicated anemias, or those caused by chronic disease, might need further testing, including urine analysis, stool sampling, endoscopy, colonoscopy, and bone marrow biopsy.

■ ***TREATMENT.*** Determining the cause of anemia is very important because treatment is directed at the cause. Therefore, treatment for anemia varies, depending on cause or type of anemia. Some anemias can be cured, whereas others, such as sickle cell anemia, are not curable.

■ ***PREVENTION.*** Eating a healthy diet including foods high in iron and B complex vitamins will prevent deficiency anemias. More complicated types might not be preventable or treatable.

IRON DEFICIENCY ANEMIA

■ ***DESCRIPTION.*** Iron deficiency anemia arises when there is insufficient iron for the body to produce the oxygen-carrying component, hemoglobin, within RBCs.

■ ***ETIOLOGY.*** Iron deficiency anemia can be due to a loss of iron, such as from chronic blood loss, or to an inadequate intake of iron such as from low dietary intake of iron. Chronic blood loss can be due to bleeding hemorrhoids, gastrointestinal bleeding, and heavy or prolonged menstrual flow. Iron deficiency anemia is commonly seen in females during times of increased iron demand as occur during pregnancy and breastfeeding. During their menstrual years, females often have iron loss due to a combination of menstruation and inadequate dietary intake of iron.

■ ***SYMPTOMS.*** Those previously described in the anemia section pertain here as well, but, briefly, include pallor, weakness, fatigue, and dyspnea.

■ ***DIAGNOSIS.*** History and physical examination along with blood tests indicating low levels of hemoglobin, iron, or both assist in diagnosis of an iron deficiency. For cases caused by bleeding, further tests include looking for the presence of blood in urine and stool samples. Gastroscopy and colonoscopy also can help determine the origin of the bleeding.

■ ***TREATMENT.*** Treatment is aimed at the cause and can include resolving a bleeding problem or increasing dietary intake of iron. Foods high in iron include fruits, green vegetables, lean meat, and whole grain breads.

■ ***PREVENTION.*** Deficiency anemia can be prevented by eating a healthy diet high in iron. Anemia related to blood loss can be prevented by seeking medial help at the first sign of excessive bleeding.

FOLIC ACID DEFICIENCY ANEMIA

■ ***DESCRIPTION.*** Folic acid is a B complex vitamin necessary for the maturation of RBCs. A deficiency in folic acid leads to this type of anemia.

■ ***ETIOLOGY.*** Deficiency of folic acid can be related to poor diet, overcooking vegetables, or alcoholism. Deficiency can also occur during times of high folic acid need such as those associated with infancy and pregnancy.

■ ***SYMPTOMS.*** Symptoms can include fatigue, weight loss, abdominal pain, black or bloody stools, and chest pain.

■ ***DIAGNOSIS.*** Blood testing aids in the diagnosis. CBC will show anemia and abnormally large RBCs.

The blood folate level will also be low. Bone marrow biopsy is seldom needed but also will show abnomally large red cell size.

■ ***TREATMENT.*** Treatment is aimed at increasing dietary intake of foods high in folic acid such as green leafy vegetables, mushrooms, lima beans, and kidney beans.

■ ***PREVENTION.*** Consumption of a diet high in folic acid aids in prevention.

VITAMIN B_{12} DEFICIENCY ANEMIA

■ ***DESCRIPTION.*** Vitamin B_{12} anemia results from dietary deficiency in B_{12} or inability of the digestive tract to absorb it. Vitamin B_{12} is essential for the body to produce RBCs as well as to maintain a healthy nervous system.

■ ***ETIOLOGY.*** Inability to absorb B_{12} can be due to several factors, including (1) removal of the small intestine, where B_{12} is absorbed, (2) having a disease that affects the small intestine, such as Crohn's disease, that interferes with absorption, (3) consumption of a diet deficient in B_{12}, or (4) loss or lack of intrinsic factor. This last cause of deficiency is the most common and is also called pernicious anemia.

PERNICOUS ANEMIA

Pernicious anemia usually affects older individuals and has an unusual cause. The mucosa, or lining, of the stomach normally secretes a protein called intrinsic factor. This factor is necessary for vitamin B_{12} absorption in the small intestine. Those affected have had an autoimmune disorder (a disorder caused by the person's own immune system) that blocks production or destroys the cells that produce this intrinsic factor.

■ ***SYMPTOMS.*** Common symptoms include pallor, fatigue, weakness, confusion, depression, and numbness in the hands and feet.

■ ***DIAGNOSIS.*** Vitamin B_{12} deficiences are diagnosed by a thorough history and physical, CBC, and blood testing for vitamin B_{12}. A history of small-intestine surgery or chronic disease of the small intestine can be recognized easily and diagnosed. Dietary deficiency and pernicious anemia can be more difficult to diagosis and might need further testing, including a gastroscopy (looking through a scope into the stomach) to view the cells that produce intrinsic factor.

■ ***TREATMENT.*** Treatment depends on the cause of the deficiency. Absorption and diet deficiency anemia can be treated with oral vitamin tablets, injectable vitamin B_{12}, or consumption of a diet high in vitamin B_{12}. Meat, fish, poultry, and milk are all sources of B_{12}.

Pernicious anemia cannot be treated with a change in diet because without intrinsic factor, no amount of B_{12} can be absorbed. Treatment is a monthly injection of vitamin B_{12} for the life of the individual.

■ ***PREVENTION.*** Anemias related to poor diet can be prevented by eating a diet high in vitamin B_{12}. Pernicious anemia, at this time, is not preventable.

HEMOLYTIC ANEMIA

■ ***DESCRIPTION.*** Hemolytic anemia is characterized by increased destruction of RBCs.

■ ***ETIOLOGY.*** This type of anemia can be related to an antigen–antibody reaction as with Rh factor in blood transfusion reaction or erythroblastosis fetalis. (See Chapter 5 for detailed information.) Hemolytic anemia also can occur due to a disorder of the immune system leading to destruction of one's own erythrocytes. This type of anemia can be severe and lead to death of the individual. Hemolytic anemia can be brought on by exposure to chemicals such as benzene; medications, including aspirin and penicillin; and bacterial toxins.

■ ***SYMPTOMS.*** Symptoms include pallor, weakness, fatigue, and tachycardia, the last of which can lead to heart failure.

■ ***DIAGNOSIS.*** A thorough history and physical along with blood testing will aid in diagnosis. CBC will reveal anemia. A blood smear will reveal an increased number of immature and fragmented red cells.

■ ***TREATMENT.*** Treatment can include prompt exchange transfusion (removal of the individual's blood and replacement by donor blood). Steroid medication along with splenectomy can also help.

■ ***PREVENTION.*** Hemolytic anemia due to genetic inheritance is not preventable. Acquired hemolytic anemias such as transfusion reactions can be prevented with proper screening.

SICKLE CELL ANEMIA

■ ***DESCRIPTION.*** Sickle cell anemia is a hereditary anemia, found in the African-American race, that causes an abnormal sickle shape of the erythrocyte.

Interestingly, sickle cell disease is thought to have developed as a defense mechanism against malaria. The parasite that causes malaria does not grow in cells that sickle, giving these individuals a health advantage in countries where malaria is prevalent.

■ ***ETIOLOGY.*** The sickle cell has abnormal hemoglobin that causes it to elongate or sickle when deoxygenated (as it loses the oxygen load). The cell regains its normal shape after it is reoxygenated (picks up an oxygen load) (Figure 7–2). The sickle shape causes a problem because it does not allow the cell to travel smoothly through small blood vessels. Sickle cells tend to stick and clump together in small vessels, leading to occlusion of the vessel, ischemia, and infarction. This occlusion can occur in any vessel, causing multiple thrombi (clots) and emboli (traveling clots) formations that can lead to infarctions throughout the body, including the vital organs.

■ ***SYMPTOMS.*** Symptoms of the disease can vary from mild to severe. Pain in the back, legs, and abdomen are the most common symptoms. Other symptoms include fatigue, irritability, swollen joints, leg sores, and gum disease. A classic mark of sickle cell anemia is a group of symptoms called sickle cell crisis, marked by episodes of pain in two or more locations. The pain is often compared in severity to cancer pain. This crisis generally occurs any time the body has an increased need for oxygen, so increased activity, physical stress, and illness can lead to a crisis. The crisis itself increases the body's need for oxygen and often sets off a vicious cycle of oxygen demand and sickling of more cells. Individuals suffering severe symptoms often die in infancy or childhood. Few severely affected individuals live beyond age 20, and even mildly affected individuals usually die before age 50.

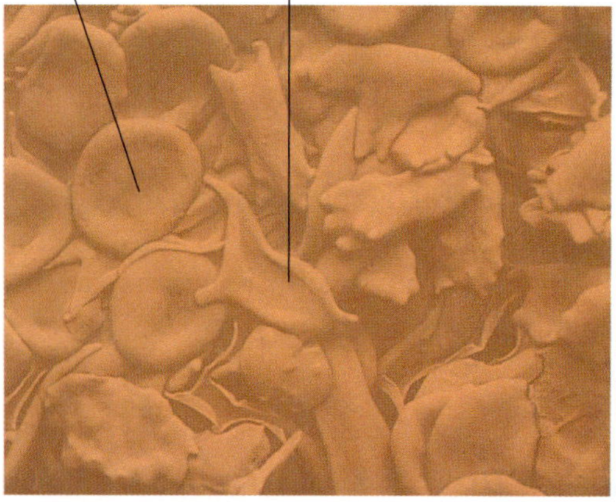

FIGURE 7–2 Sickled erythrocytes.

■ ***DIAGNOSIS.*** Diagnosis is made after history and blood testing. Two blood tests determine sickle cell disease. The first is hemoglobin electrophoresis, which measures the amount of normal and abnormal hemoglobin in the blood. The second is the Sickledex test, which measures the percent of red sickle cells after mixing a small drop of blood with a deoxygenating agent. A positive test is one in which 25% or more of cells sickle.

■ ***TREATMENT.*** There is no cure for sickle cell disease, and treatment is symptomatic. An increase in fluid intake to twice the normal amount can help by increasing blood volume and improving sickle cell movement.

■ ***PREVENTION.*** Because sickle cell anemia is a hereditary disorder, the only prevention is through genetic counseling and decision by potential carriers to avoid childbearing.

HEMORRHAGIC ANEMIA

■ ***DESCRIPTION.*** This anemia is caused by the loss of whole blood and can also be called blood loss anemia. A common complication of losing large amounts of blood is hypovolemic shock.

■ ***ETIOLOGY.*** Acute loss of large amounts of blood, which can be caused by such activities as surgery and any trauma or accident involving blood loss, leads to hemorrhagic anemia. Accidents such as motor vehicle accidents and accidental amputations of arms or legs can easily lead to hemorrhagic anemia.

■ ***SYMPTOMS.*** Symptoms include pallor, cool clammy skin, tachypnea, and tachycardia. If large amounts of blood have been lost, other symptoms can arise, including dizziness, fainting, and an extreme thirst as a result of dehydration.

■ ***DIAGNOSIS.*** Hemorrhagic anemia is easily diagnosed when the blood loss is external. Internal bleeding also leads to hemorrhagic anemia but is often more difficult to diagnosis. A history and physical are necessary, and a CBC showing low cell mass, hemoglobin, and hematocrit is indicative of hemorrhagic anemia.

■ ***TREATMENT.*** Treatment depends on the severity of the condition. In an acute blood loss, controlling or stopping the bleeding is the primary concern. Applying oxygen immediately to increase the oxygen-carrying capacity of the remaining blood supply is also important. Intravenous fluids and liquids taken by mouth help restore fluid volume. In severe cases of blood loss, a blood transfusion might be needed.

In chronic or slower blood loss anemia, finding the cause and stopping the bleeding is again the primary focus. If the blood loss is not severe, blood fluid will be replaced within a few hours. The decreased number of circulating erythrocytes will stimulate the bone marrow to step up production of them. Bone marrow can replace large numbers of blood cells, thus correcting this type of anemia. Consuming a healthy diet especially high in protein and iron will help restore the body's blood reserves and return it to a healthy state.

■ **PREVENTION.** Accident prevention and controlling chronic bleeding are helpful in preventing hemorrhagic anemia.

APLASTIC ANEMIA

■ **DESCRIPTION.** Aplastic anemia is characterized by failure of the bone marrow to produce blood components. A severe decrease or total absence of erythrocytes, leukocytes, and thrombocytes, called **pancytopenia** (pan = all, cyto = cell, penia = decrease), is common.

■ **ETIOLOGY.** This anemia is due to injury or destruction of the blood-forming area of the bone marrow. Causes include chemotherapy, radiation, viruses, and chemical toxins.

■ **SYMPTOMS.** This decrease in blood cells leads to anemia, infection, and hemorrhage, respectively.

■ **DIAGNOSIS.** Aplastic anemia is diagnosed by using a history and physical examination with blood testing. A CBC will show a low hemoglobin and hematocrit, indicative of anemia. Blood can also be tested for iron and folic acid levels to rule out these types of anemia.

A reticulocyte count test measures reticulocytes, or immature RBCs, and helps determine whether the bone marrow is producing RBCs as it should. In aplastic anemia, the reticulocytes numbers will be low.

Because blood cells are formed inside bone, a bone marrow aspiration or biopsy can also be used. In both of these tests, a large-bore needle or surgical instrument removes small pieces of marrow and bone, respectively. The cells are then examined under a microscope to look for abnormal cells. In aplasic anemia, the red cell production and numbers are low.

Other tests that can be helpful in diagnosis include X-ray, CT scan, and ultrasound. These tests help rule out cancer, infection, and other types of anemia.

■ **TREATMENT.** Severe cases of aplastic anemia have a poor prognosis, with 50% fatality. Treatment includes discontinuing or avoiding the causative agent. Other treatment might include bone marrow transplantation and blood transfusions.

■ **PREVENTION.** Avoiding causative agents is helpful in prevention, but too often, the causative agent is unknown or unavoidable, making prevention impossible.

POLYCYTHEMIAS

POLYCYTHEMIA (PRIMARY OR VERA)

■ **DESCRIPTION.** Polycythemia is also called primary polycythemia or polycythemia vera. It is a condition of too many blood cells.

■ **ETIOLOGY.** Primary polycythemia is caused by hyperplasia (hyper = excessive, plasia = growth) of the cell-forming tissues of the bone marrow, leading to an increase in the production of erythocytes, leukocytes, and thrombocytes. This disease has an unknown etiology.

■ **SYMPTOMS.** The increase in erythrocytes leads to an increase in blood volume, which raises blood pressure and causes an increase in the workload on the heart. The spleen, an organ of blood cell storage, is enlarged. The mucous membranes are reddened in color and the eyes often appear bloodshot. The palms of the hands are noticeably a deeper red color.

■ **DIAGNOSIS.** Polycythemia can be accidentally discovered through routine blood testing before a person has any symptoms. Hemoglobin (the protein that carries oxygen in RBCs) will be abnormally high as will the hematocrit (the percentage of RBCs in the total blood volume). Platelets and WBCs might also be increased.

■ **TREATMENT.** Treatment is to reduce the red cell count and, thus, blood volume. Phlebotomy or blood removal at regular intervals will reduce the volume and is a common treatment.

■ ***PREVENTION.*** Polycythemia cannot be prevented. With treatment, symptoms and complications can be prevented or delayed.

SECONDARY POLYCYTHEMIA (ERYTHROCYTOSIS)

■ ***DESCRIPTION.*** Secondary polycythemia, or erythrocytosis (erythocyte = red cell, osis = condition of), differs from primary polycythemia in that only red cell numbers are increased.

■ ***ETIOLOGY.*** Erythrocytosis is a protective mechanism of the body to meet the need for extra oxygen, a normal compensatory mechanism for people who are not getting enough oxygen. It is seen as a positive change in people in high altitudes where oxygen content of air is low. Also, highly trained athletes can have erythrocytosis to meet the high oxygen demands of the body's muscle tissue. Certain respiratory conditions and circulatory conditions cause a decrease in oxygen supply to the tissues and thus stimulate erythrocytosis also. When the conditions calling for extra oxygen are returned to normal, the erythrocytosis disappears. For example, if people living in high altitudes move to a lower altitude, the red cell count will return to a normal level. Smoking, which impairs RBCs' ability to deliver oxygen to body tissues, can cause secondary polycythemia.

■ ***SYMPTOMS.*** Headaches, weakness, and fatigue are often the first symptoms of secondary polycythemia; lightheadedness and shortness of breath are also common. If the polycythemia is due to disease of the lungs, the face might be reddened and become blue during exercise or other exertion.

■ ***DIAGNOSIS.*** Following a history and physical exam, diagnosis of secondary polycythemia is assisted by blood testing. Arterial blood gases (ABGs) testing shows the concentration of oxygen in an artery, and low oxygen levels in this test can be indicative of secondary polycythemia. Blood levels of erythropoietin, a hormone that stimulates the bone marrow to produce RBCs, can also be measured. Normal or low erythropoietin levels can indicate secondary polycythemia. X-ray and CT imaging studies also can rule out liver, kidney, or spleen disorders or tumors.

■ ***TREATMENT.*** Secondary polycythemia is treated by addressing the cause of the disorder. For example, lung disorders such as those caused by cigarette smoking can cause secondary polycythemia; not smoking helps treat the lung condition and improve the secondary polycythemia.

■ ***PREVENTION.*** In some cases, secondary polycythemia can be prevented by stopping the causative factor or by not doing the things that deprive the body of needed oxygen. Living in high altitudes and smoking, for example, can be avoided or stopped.

Disorders of White Blood Cells

Disorders of WBCs are common problems of the hematologic system, especially among certain age groups. For example, mononucleosis is common in teenage populations. The common symptom of WBC disorders is a compromised immune response, leaving the individual susceptible to infections.

MONONUCLEOSIS

■ ***DESCRIPTION.*** Infectious mononucleosis, sometimes called kissing disease or mono, is often joked about, but the real disease can be quite serious. This infection primarily affects children and young adults. It is somewhat contagious and often will cause illness for several weeks.

■ ***ETIOLOGY.*** This infection is caused by an Epstein-Barr virus (EBV), which is very common. Many people have been exposed and are lifetime carriers of the virus but might never develop the illness.

The most common way to become infected with mononucleosis is by kissing someone who has been infected. Any activity involving direct contact with the saliva, such as sharing eating utensils or drinking straws, can spread the virus.

■ ***SYMPTOMS.*** Symptoms usually begin 4 to 7 days after infection and include fatigue, sore throat, fever, swollen lymph glands, and splenomegaly (spleen enlargement).

■ ***DIAGNOSIS.*** Diagnosis is confirmed by history and physical examination and a WBC count showing a marked elevation in monocytes.

■ ***TREATMENT.*** Treatment is symptomatic and includes rest, analgesics, and throat gargles. If there are no complications, symptoms of mononucleosis are usually resolved in 3 to 4 weeks. To prevent potential injury to the spleen, sports activities should be avoided for 1 month following the illness.

■ **PREVENTION.** Slowing the spread of the virus can be accomplished by frequent hand washing, covering mouth and nose when sneezing or coughing, and not sharing drinks or eating utensils.

LEUKEMIA

■ **DESCRIPTION.** Leukemia is a malignant neoplasm of the blood-forming organs (bone marrow, lymph nodes, and spleen). It is characterized by an abnormally high production of immature leukocytes that function abnormally and cause a decrease in the production of erythrocytes and platelets.

Leukemia may be classified as acute or chronic. Acute forms commonly affect children, progress rapidly, and can be fatal. Chronic forms occur more commonly in older adults, are often asymptomatic, and might not be the cause of death. Leukemia is also classified as myelogenous (affecting the bone marrow) and lymphocytic (affecting the lymph nodes).

■ **ETIOLOGY.** The cause of leukemia is unknown.

■ **SYMPTOMS.** Symptoms of leukemia include fatigue, headache, sore throat, dyspnea, bleeding of the mucous membranes of the mouth and gastrointestinal system, bone and joint pain, and enlargement of lymph nodes, liver, and spleen. Infections are common because white cells are not functioning properly. Bleeding disorders and anemia are due to erythrocytopenia and thrombocytopenia, respectively.

■ **DIAGNOSIS.** Leukemia is usually diagnosed by clinical history and blood studies. A bone marrow biopsy is the most definitive test for confirming the diagnosis.

■ **TREATMENT.** Treatment includes aggressive chemotherapy using several neoplastic agents. When the illness is in remission, a bone marrow transplant to replace the neoplastic tissue with normal tissue can be performed. Pain from enlargement of lymph nodes, spleen, and liver can be treated with analgesics. Complete remission occurs approximately 50% of the time, depending on the type of leukemia and the individual's tolerance of the treatment.

■ **PREVENTION.** There is no known way to prevent leukemia, although avoiding toxic chemicals, cigarette smoking, and radiation might prevent some types of leukemia.

LYMPHOMAS

Lymphoma refers to several types of neoplasms that affect lymphoid tissue (lymph nodes, tonsils, spleen, and lymph fluid). There are many types of lymphoma, but all affect normal lymphocyte production, leading to impaired immunity. Lymphoma is the most common type of blood cancer in the United States.

HODGKIN'S DISEASE

■ **DESCRIPTION.** Hodgkin's disease is the most common lymphoma. It is characterized clinically by the orderly spread of disease from one lymph node group to another.

■ **ETIOLOGY.** The cause is thought to be viral in nature.

■ **SYMPTOMS.** Lymphoma is characterized by painless enlargement of the lymph nodes in the neck, weight loss, and fever. Hodgkin's primarily affects young adults with an average age of 35 years. Men are affected with Hodgkin's at a slightly higher rate than women.

■ **DIAGNOSIS.** Diagnosis is made when a large connective tissue cell called Reed–Sternberg cell is present in lymphatic tissue. The diagnosis can be confirmed by lymph node and bone marrow biopsy.

■ **TREATMENT.** Treatment with radiation and chemotherapy is usually effective in bringing about remission. If the disease is kept in remission for 5 years or longer, complete cure might be possible. The cure rate is about 93%, making it one of the most curable forms of cancer—if it is detected in the early stages. Mortality rate is approximately 20%.

■ **PREVENTION.** Because the cause of Hodgkin's is unknown, there are no known preventive measures.

NON-HODGKIN'S LYMPHOMA

■ **DESCRIPTION.** Non-Hodgkin's lymphoma (NHL) is a group of lymphomas not containing the Reed–Sternberg cell characteristic of Hodgkin's and more widespread than Hodgkin's. NHL affects more older adults than Hodgkin's disease, with the average age of 50 years. Men are affected one and a half times more often than women.

■ **ETIOLOGY.** The cause of NHL is unknown, but individuals receiving, or who have received, immunosuppressive medications have more than a 100-times greater chance of developing NHL.

GLIMPSE OF THE FUTURE

New Treatments on the Horizon for Sickle Cell Anemia Complications

Sickle cell anemia affects thousands of people in the United States. Blood transfusion, a frequently used treatment, can lead to iron overload (the deposition of iron in organs). The liver is one organ affected by the iron overload. A liver biopsy is used to diagnose the problem but this often leads to bleeding and infection. Now, an MRI is being used to detect the iron overload and prevent the complications of a liver biopsy. New treatements for the iron overload complication are also being researched. Recently the FDA approved using an iron chelator, called deferasirox. A chelator is a substance that binds particular ions, removing them from solution. In addition, new clinical trials are ongoing to assess the benefit of therapeutic phlebotomy (removing blood for treatment purposes) for treating the complication of iron overload. This may be the teatment of choice in the future.

Source: Hankins, J. S. (2007).

■ ***SYMPTOMS.*** Usually, there is painless enlargement of lymph nodes in the neck, axilla, and inguinal areas. Other symptoms include fever, night sweats, and weight loss.

■ ***DIAGNOSIS.*** Diagnosis is made when there is the absence of the Reed–Sternberg cell in lymphatic tissue. The diagnosis is confirmed by lymph node and bone marrow biopsy.

■ ***TREATMENT.*** Treatment and prognosis depends on the type of NHL, but some combination of radiation and chemotherapy is usually beneficial.

■ ***PREVENTION.*** Although the cause of NHL is unknown, those at increased risk include those exposed to pesticides, solvents, and fertilizers. Avoiding these risk factors might assist in prevention of the disease.

MULTIPLE MYELOMA

■ ***DESCRIPTION.*** Multiple myeloma is a malignant neoplasm of plasma cells, or B-lymphocytes, in which the plasma cells multiply abnormally in the bone marrow, causing weakness in the bone and leading to pathologic fractures and bone pain (Figure 7–3).

■ ***ETIOLOGY.*** The cause of multiple myeloma is unknown. It occurs increasingly with age, peaking in the 70s, and is more common in men. It is one of the most common neoplasms affecting the bone.

■ ***SYMPTOMS.*** Overgrowth of plasma cells leads to a decrease in other blood components, causing anemia, leukocytopenia, and thrombocytopenia. The breakdown of bone leads to hypercalcemia (hyper = excessive, calc = calcium, emia = blood), excessive blood calcium levels. Antibodies secreted by the plasma cells attach to kidney tubules, causing tissue damage leading to kidney failure.

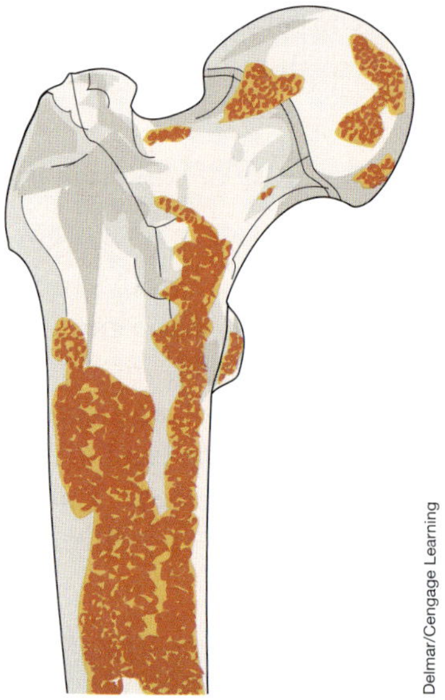

FIGURE 7–3 Multiple myeloma—extensive bone destruction caused by disease.

■ ***DIAGNOSIS.*** Diagnosis is confirmed by:

- X-ray exhibiting a honeycombed bone pattern due to tumor involvement.
- Hypercalcemia due to the tumor breaking down bone.

COMPLEMENTARY AND ALTERNATIVE THERAPY

Using Alternative Therapies in Sickle Cell Disease

A study looked at the use of a variety of alternative treatment strategies for patients with sickle cell anemia. The purpose of the study was to determine which complementary and alternative therapies are presently being used. The various therapies used included bioenergic therapies (praying, spiritual healing), lifestyle-mind-body therapies (relaxation, exercise, imagery, diet), biochemical therapies (herbal products, vitamins, medicines), and biomechanical therapies (massage). Most of the participants reported alternative therapies were helpful. Prayer and spiritual healing were used most frequently. There has been some research that reported positive effects from relaxation practices and spiritual healing. More reserch is need to determine whether relaxation and spiritual practices are effective.

Source: Sibinga, et al. (2006).

- Evidence of **Bence Jones protein** (a special protein) in the blood and urine.
- A bone marrow biopsy confirming the presence of an excessive number of plasma cells.

■ ***TREATMENT.*** Prognosis is poor for multiple myeloma. Chemotherapy and radiation are not very effective, and death is usually within 2 to 3 years as the result of infection and kidney failure.

■ ***PREVENTION.*** Risk factors have been identified as herbicides, petroleum products, heavy metals, and radiation. Avoidance of these risk factors might aid in prevention of this disease.

Disorders of Platelets and Clotting

Platelet disorders are varied in terms of cause, severity, treatment, and prognosis. However, they all share the common symptom of bleeding, which might be mild or severe, depending on the particular condition. Many of these disorders are inherited diseases.

HEMOPHILIA

■ ***DESCRIPTION.*** Hemophilia refers to a group of bleeding disorders characterized by abnormally slow clotting and long bleeding times. These characteristics make hemophiliacs "love blood" or, more realistically, need transfusions. There are several types of hemophilia, but the most common is Type A.

■ ***ETIOLOGY.*** Hemophilia (hemo = blood, philia = lover) is an X-linked hereditary bleeding disorder. Hemophilia commonly occurs in male children and is passed on to these children, often, by their mother, who is usually asymptomatic and unaffected. Hemophiliacs lack a blood protein that plays a part in clot formation.

■ ***SYMPTOMS.*** Symptoms of frequent epistaxis (nosebleeds), bruising, and prolonged bleeding in a male child might be indicative of hemophilia. This condition can vary from mild to severe—a hemophiliac might experience severe and prolonged bleeding with a minor injury. Severe hemophilia often leads to **hemarthrosis** (hem = blood, arthro = joint, osis = condition) or bleeding into joints, which is extremely painful, and recurrent episodes often lead to joint deformity.

■ ***DIAGNOSIS.*** Diagnosis is confirmed by obtaining a detailed medical history, physical examination, and blood testing. Blood tests include measurement of clotting time and the presence of clotting proteins. An extended or lengthy clotting time and low levels or absence of clotting proteins can be indicative of hemophilia.

■ ***TREATMENT.*** There is no cure for hemophilia. Treatment is aimed at prevention of injury and treatment of symptoms. Whole blood transfusions can be needed along with a concentrated form of the necessary clotting protein.

■ ***PREVENTION.*** Because hemophilia is an inherited genetic disease, the only way it can be prevented is by genetic testing of possible carriers with the decision not to have children.

THROMBOCYTOPENIA

■ ***DESCRIPTION.*** Thrombocytopenia, also known as thrombocytopenia purpura, is a decrease in platelets that leads to an inability to clot blood normally.

■ ***ETIOLOGY.*** Thrombocytopenia can be due to inadequate or abnormal platelet production or destruction. In the case of abnormal destruction, platelet life might be reduced to hours instead of days. The cause of this disorder is frequently unknown. In these cases, the condition may be called idiopathic thrombocytopenia purpura.

■ ***SYMPTOMS.*** This condition is characterized by abnormal bleeding in the skin, mucous membranes, and internal organs. The skin might exhibit small hemorrhagic spots called petechiae or larger purplish hemorrhagic spots called ecchymoses. This purple coloring of the skin leads to another descriptive term, **purpura** (PUR-pew-rah; purplish color of the skin caused by hemorrhaging). Symptoms of thrombocytopenia include gastrointestinal hemorrhages, frequent epistaxis (nosebleeds), and **hematuria** (HEM-ah-TOO-ree-ah; hema = blood, uria = urine, blood in the urine).

■ ***DIAGNOSIS.*** Diagnosis is made from individual clinical history along with platelet count and bleeding time. A low platelet count and an extended or longer than normal bleeding time can be indicative of the disease.

■ ***TREATMENT.*** Treatment includes avoiding tissue trauma to reduce the potential for bleeding, administration of vitamin K to improve clotting, and transfusion of platelets. If the disorder persists, a splenectomy might alleviate symptoms because the spleen is the main site of platelet destruction. Splenectomy is usually the last treatment of choice but is very effective.

■ ***PREVENTION.*** Certain cases of thrombocytopenia might be preventable, but most are not. Two steps that can be taken to prevent complications include:

- Avoiding medications that decrease platelet aggregation or stickiness, thus making them less likely to clot. This includes but is not limited to aspirin and ibuprophen
- Avoiding heavy drinking because alcohol slows platelet production.

DISSEMINATED INTRAVASCULAR COAGULATION (DIC)

■ ***DESCRIPTION.*** DIC is a condition of abnormal clotting followed by abnormal bleeding. It is a disease process by which blood starts to coagulate or clot throughout the entire body. This overall clotting depletes platelets and clotting factors, allowing the body then to bleed freely. These two activities set up a potentially catastrophic situation in which the body can have clotting (thrombosis) and massive bleeding (hemorrhage) at the same time.

■ ***ETIOLOGY.*** DIC usually follows some major trauma such as blood transfusion reaction, surgery, septicemia, complicated childbirth, trauma involving massive tissue destruction, shock, malignancy, or snakebite.

■ ***SYMPTOMS.*** The individual with DIC might initially have microthrombi in the fingers and toes, turning these extremities blue to black in color, or larger thrombus formation, often leading to life-threatening pulmonary embolism. Lodging of clots in the small and large blood vessels and in body organs slows blood supply, often resulting in organ damage. As platelets and clotting factors are used, other symptoms appear, including oozing of blood, resulting in petechiae; ecchymosis; hematoma and hematuria; gastrointestinal bleeding that causes **hematemesis** (HEM-ah-TEM-eh-sis; hema = blood, emesis = vomiting); blood in the stool, and symptoms associated with anemia.

■ ***DIAGNOSIS.*** Diagnosis is made on the basis of history of trauma and blood studies. Important blood studies include CBC showing platelet levels, bleeding time, and fibrinogen level (a clotting factor). A positive test for DIC will reveal a decreased number of platelets, increased or long bleeding time, and low fibrinogen levels.

■ ***TREATMENT.*** Identifying and treating the underlying cause usually stops DIC. In addition to treating the cause, other treatment includes heparin, an anticoagulant medication, to halt the formation of thrombi, and platelet administration to stop hemorrhage or increase clotting ability. This disorder is very difficult to manage because one administers agents both to clot and to prevent clotting at alternating intervals. The condition is usually life-threatening and leads to death; hence, it is known colloquially as "Death Is Coming."

PREVENTION. A preventive measure includes getting prompt medical treatment for any condition that might bring on this disorder.

TRAUMA

Any traumatic injury to the bone marrow, spleen, or lymph nodes can lead to a decrease in the production of blood cells. Enlargement of the spleen or splenomegaly can lead to premature breakdown of blood cells, and chemotherapy and radiation treatments affecting bone marrow often lead to symptoms of anemia and infection related to decreased production of red cells and white cells, respectively.

RARE DISEASES

Thalassemia

Thalassemia is a hereditary hemolytic anemia that primarily affects people of Mediterranean descent. The RBCs are fragile and thin and form defective hemoglobin. These RBCs do not function normally and lead to symptoms of anemia. One form of thalassemia is called Cooley's anemia, or thalassemia major. This is the most severe form of the disease and presents in childhood.

Von Willebrand's Disease

Von Willebrand's disease is a hereditary, congenital bleeding disorder caused by a deficiency in clotting factor and platelet function. It is also called angiohemophilia and affects females as well as males.

Lymphosarcoma

Lymphosarcoma is a type of lymphoma also known as NHL. Symptoms are similar to those found in Hodgkin's disease and occur more frequently in males of all age groups. Prognosis is good if treatment leads to remission. Without remission, the prognosis is poor.

EFFECTS OF AGING ON THE SYSTEM

Older adults might be more prone to developing diseases of the hematologic system because of the age-related changes occurring in other systems such as the immune or digestive system, leaving them more susceptible to infections and nutritionally related blood disorders. However, total serum iron, total iron-binding capacity, and intestinal iron absorption all decrease with age. Aging does not change the number of lymphocytes, but their functioning decreases to some degree over time.

The most common disorder of the blood in the older adult is anemia. This is not usually due to a defect in the system but rather to poor nutrition (iron deficiency anemia) or inability to absorb the needed nutrients (pernicious anemia). The anemia problem often complicates other chronic diseases of the affected individual.

Some types of leukemia are more common in the older adult. Problems can arise during treatment for the condition due to decreased gastric motility and impaired circulation. These age-related changes can reduce the effectiveness of some therapies and increase the chance of experiencing side effects of the treatment.

SUMMARY

The blood and blood-forming organs (hematologic system) form the body's life fluid by transporting oxygen and nutrients to cells, removing wastes, and helping prevent infection. The main components of the system include the blood, lymph nodes, bone marrow, spleen, and liver. Common signs and symptoms of diseases of the blood and blood-forming organs are fatigue, shortness of breath, bleeding, lesions, pain, and increased susceptibility to infections. The most common disorder of the system is anemia. Although there are several types of anemia, they all have some common symptoms. WBC disorders include mononucleosis and leukemia as the most common. Disorders of platelets include the major bleeding diseases of the blood and blood-forming organs, such as hemophilia. The older adult can develop problems of the hematologic system such as anemia, but it is usually due to other problems or disorders in other systems.

REVIEW QUESTIONS

Multiple Choice

1. Which of the following are major functions of blood? (Select all that apply.)
   a. transportation of nutrients
   b. metabolism of nutrients
   c. removal of wastes
   d. protection from infection
   e. production of lymphocytes
   f. production of erythrocytes

2. Which of the following are common signs and symptoms of disorders of the blood and blood-forming organs? (Select all that apply.)
   a. inflammation
   b. fatigue
   c. shortness of breath
   d. paralysis
   e. urinary frequency
   f. bleeding
   g. pain
   h. lesions

3. The individual with a bleeding disorder should avoid which of the following activities?
   a. shaving with a straight razor
   b. using mouthwash
   c. eating solid foods
   d. jogging

4. The purpose of the screening test for sickle cell anemia is to determine:
   a. whether the individual is a carrier of the sickle cell trait.
   b. the presence of the sickled hemoglobin.
   c. the severity of the disease.
   d. whether the individual will eventually develop sickle cell anemia.

5. Bone marrow biopsies are performed to:
   a. determine the presence and number of platelets.
   b. diagnose cancers, anemias, and bone marrow functional disorders.
   c. diagnose vitamin B_{12} deficiency.
   d. test for antigens to prevent antigen–antibody reactions.

6. Foods recommended for the individual with a folic acid deficiency would include:
   a. milk and cheeses.
   b. beef and chicken.

c. green and yellow vegetables.
d. breads and grains.

7. In which of the following ways does primary polycythemia differ from secondary polycythemia (erythrocytosis)?
   a. The most common symptom of the primary type is shortness of breath, and fatigue is the most common symptom of the secondary type.
   b. The primary type responds to phlebotomy, whereas the secondary type does not.
   c. The primary form of the disease is considered to be a type of cancer, but the secondary form is not.
   d. Both red and white cell numbers are increased in the primary type, but just red cell numbers are increased in the secondary type.

8. Which of the following statements is true about hemophilia?
   a. It is most common in the older adult.
   b. It results in continuous minor bleeding internally.
   c. It is caused by a deficiency of clotting factor.
   d. It is found in male children of mothers who carry the defective gene.

9. Which of the following statements is true about leukemia?
   a. It is considered to be a group of disorders with a cancerous development occurring in the bone marrow.
   b. It is the most common cause of death in young children.
   c. Chemotherapy is ineffective against leukemia.
   d. There are several types of leukemias, but most types are diagnosed in the young or middle-aged adult.

Short Answer

10. List some of the common tests used to diagnose disorders of the blood and blood-forming organs.

11. List some diseases of the blood or blood-forming organs that are transmitted through an inherited trait.

12. Describe the common effects of a hemorrhagic disorder on an individual.

13. Why would an individual with Hodgkin's disease be instructed to avoid individuals with coughs, colds, and fever?

14. What diagnostic test would probably be used to diagnose leukemia?

15. Why are older adults with hematologic disorders more susceptible to infections?

CASE STUDIES

- Ms. Sloan is a 27-year-old who is complaining of fatigue, shortness of breath, stomach pain, and overall weakness. She is diagnosed with iron deficiency anemia. What could you tell her about this condition? What specific nutritional needs does she have, based on her diagnosis, gender, and age?

- Joe Butler has a friend who is having surgery and wants to donate blood for his friend in case he needs a transfusion during the surgery. Joe knows his blood type is O positive but does not know his friend's blood type. He asks you to explain to him some details about donating and receiving blood. What should you tell him? Will his blood be compatible with his friend's blood type? Which blood type is considered the universal recipient? Which blood type is considered the universal donor?

StudyWARE™ Connection

To help you learn the content in this chapter, take a practice quiz or play an interactive game on your StudyWARE™ CD-ROM.

Workbook Practice

Go to your Workbook and complete the practice questions.

BIBLIOGRAPHY

Anderson, N. (2006). Hydroxyurea therapy: Improving the lives of patients with sickle cell disease. *Pediatric Nursing 32*(6), 541–543.

Anglin, S. (2007). New challenges and new thinking in sickle screening. *British Journal of Nursing 16*(15), 914–915.

Anionwu, E. (2007). Menace in my blood: My affliction with sickle cell anaemia. *Nursing Standard 21*(17), 31.

Aplastic anemia. (2008). National Organization for Rare Disorders, Inc. *www.rarediseases.org* (accessed June 2009).

Barr, P., Fisher, R., & Friedberg, J. (2007). The role of bortezomib in the treatment of lymphoma. *Cancer Investigation 25*(8), 776–775.

Branson, R. (2007). Life blood. *Nursing Standard 21*(38), 26–27.

Brown, E., & Bennett, M. (2007). Survey of blood transfusion practice for palliative care patients in Yorkshire: Implications for critical care. *Journal of Palliative Medicine 10*(4), 919–922.

Dennison, C. A. (2008). Transfusion-related acute lung injury: A clinical challenge. *Dimensions of Critical Care Nursing 27*(1), 1–7.

Disease information. (2008). The Leukemia & Lymphoma Society. *www.leukemia.org* (accessed June 2009).

Educational material. (2008). American Sickle Cell Anemia Association. *www.ascaa.org* (accessed June 2009).

Fullbroock, S. (2007). Death by denomination. *British Journal of Nursing 16*(21), 1306–1307.

Hampson, F. A., & Shaw, A. S. (2008). Response assessment in lymphoma. *Clinical Radiology 63*(2), 125–135.

Hanks, J. S. (2007). Iron overload and sickle cell anemia: monitoring and treatment. *FASEB Journal* 21(5), A92.

HealthSource Network. (2008). Health Encyclopedia – Anemia. *www.healthsource.com* (accessed June 2009).

Hurley, G. (2007). Anemia: Overview and management. *Primary Health Care 17*(6), 25–30.

Hurter, B., & Bush, N. J. (2007). Cancer-related anemia: Clinical review and management. *Clinical Journal of Oncology Nursing 11*(3), 349–359.

Long, J. M. (2007). Treatment approaches and nursing applications for non-Hodgkin lymphoma. *Clinical Journal of Oncology Nursing 11*(Supplement), 13–21.

Norman, K. (2004). Alternative treatments for disseminated intravascular coagulation. *Drug News Perspect 17*(4), 243–250.

Pharmacy corner. (2007). *Oncology Nursing Forum 34*(3), 737.

Potera, C. (2007). Too much of a good thing. *American Journal of Nursing 107*(4), 20.

Prasomsuk, S., Jetsrisuparp, A., Ratanasiri, T., & Ratanasiri, A. (2007). Lived experiences of mothers caring for children with thalassemia major in Thailand. *Journal for Specialists in Pediatric Nursing 12*(1), 13–23.

Sibinga, E. M., Shindell, D. L., Casella, J. F., Duggan, A. K., & Wilson, M. H. (2006). Pediatric patients with sickle cell disease: Use of complementary and alternative therapies. *Journal of Alternative and Complementary Medicine 12*(3), 291–298.

Thalassemia. (2008). National Organization for Rare Disorders, Inc. *www.rarediseases.org* (accessed June 2009).

Thomas, C. M., Coleman, R., & Taub, L. M. (2007). A case study of an older adult with severe anemia refusing blood transfusion. *Journal of the American Academy of Nurse Practitioners 19*(1), 43–48.

Whelton, S. (2007). Radioimmunotherapy in treatment of non-Hodgkin's lymphoma. *Nurse Practitioner 32*(12), 35–38.

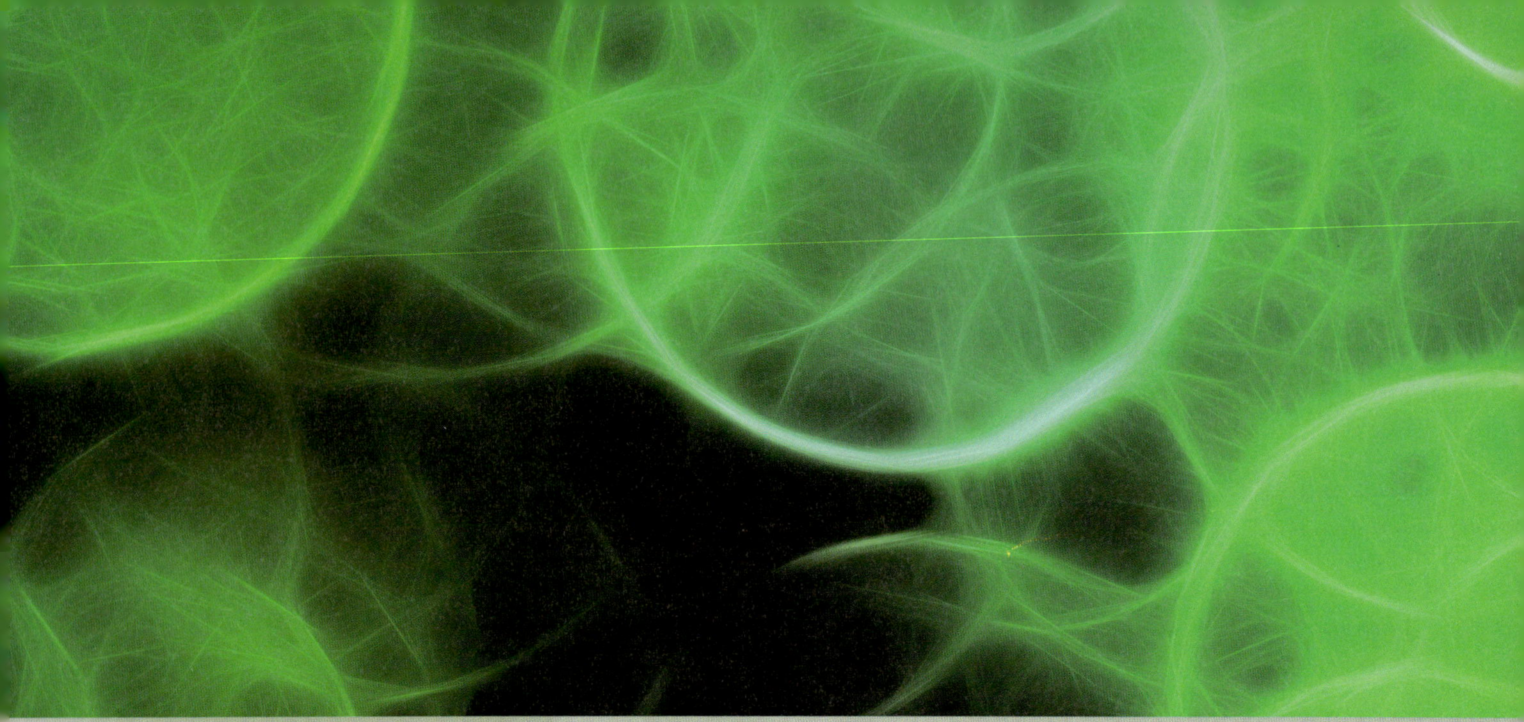

OUTLINE

KEY TERMS

Angioplasty (p. 159)
Ankle-brachial index (ABI) test (p. 150)
Auscultation (p. 148)
Cardiac catheterization (p. 150)
Cardiac palpitations (p. 148)
Cyanosis (p. 148)
Diastolic (p. 150)
Doppler (p. 150)
Electrocardiogram (p. 150)
Embolus (p. 154)
Endarterectomy (p. 157)
Exsanguination (p. 167)
Fibrillation (p. 165)
Hemothorax (p. 167)
Intermittent claudication (p. 157)
Ischemia (p. 148)
Lumen (p. 152)
Murmur (p. 164)
Patency (p. 150)
Perfusion (p. 168)
Plaque (p. 154)
Systolic (p. 150)
Tachycardia (p. 148)
Thrombus (p. 159)

8

Cardiovascular System Diseases and Disorders

LEARNING OBJECTIVES

Upon completion of the chapter, the learner should be able to:

1. Define the terminology common to the cardiovascular system and the disorders of the system.
2. Discuss the basic anatomy and physiology of the cardiovascular system.
3. Identify the important signs and symptoms associated with common cardiovascular system disorders.
4. Describe the common diagnostics used to determine the type and cause of the cardiovascular system disorders.
5. Identify the common disorders of the cardiovascular system.
6. Describe the typical course and management of the common cardiovascular system disorders.
7. Describe the effects of aging on the cardiovascular system and the common disorders associated with aging of the system.

OVERVIEW

The cardiovascular system is often regarded as the major body system because the individual cannot live without a functioning heart and circulatory system. The heart is responsible only for pumping blood, whereas the vascular system transports the blood throughout the body. Disorders of the system often share common symptoms and problems. Other systems are affected when the cardiovascular system is malfunctioning because it is responsible for delivering necessary nutrients and oxygen to the body. Diseases of the cardiovascular system are a major cause of morbidity and mortality in all ages but especially in older adults. Heart disease is also the number one cause of death overall in women. ■

ANATOMY AND PHYSIOLOGY

The heart, arteries, and veins, along with the blood, make up the cardiovascular system. The heart is a four-chambered muscular structure. It is about the size of a man's fist and weighs about 300 grams. The heart is situated approximately in the middle of the chest, slightly to the left, behind the sternum (breastbone). The heart is composed of the pericardium, the chambers, and the valves. The pericardium is a two-layered sac with fluid between the layers. The wall of the heart is divided into three layers. The epicardium is the outermost layer, the myocardium is the middle layer, and the endocardium is the innermost layer.

The four chambers in the heart are the right atrium, right ventricle, left atrium, and left ventricle. The tricuspid valve is between the right atrium and ventricle; the mitral valve is between the left atrium and ventricle; the pulmonary valve is between the right ventricle and pulmonary artery; and the aortic valve is between the left ventricle and the aorta.

Blood enters the heart from the superior vena cava and then passes through the right atrium and the tricuspid valve into the right ventricle. It then passes through the pulmonary valve into the pulmonary artery and travels to the lungs, where carbon dioxide is exchanged for oxygen. The oxygenated blood returns to the heart through the pulmonary vein and is pumped into the left atrium through the mitral valve and into the left ventricle. It then passes through the aortic valve into the aorta and to the body (Figure 8–1). The heart itself is supplied with blood by the coronary arteries.

Cardiac muscle normally contracts continually throughout one's lifetime. Designated areas of the heart produce electrical stimulation, causing the heart muscle to contract and pump the blood to the body. This sequence of events is termed the cardiac cycle and begins in the sinoatrial (SA) node, then passes to the atrioventricular (AV) node to the bundle of HIS and the Purkinje fibers (Figure 8–2).

One sequence of the conduction pathway is one cardiac cycle. This is represented on the electrocardiogram as the PQRST segment. The P wave represents the electrical stimulation beginning and passing over the atria (depolarization). The QRS wave is caused by the stimulation passing over the ventricles. The T wave represents the recovery of the ventricles

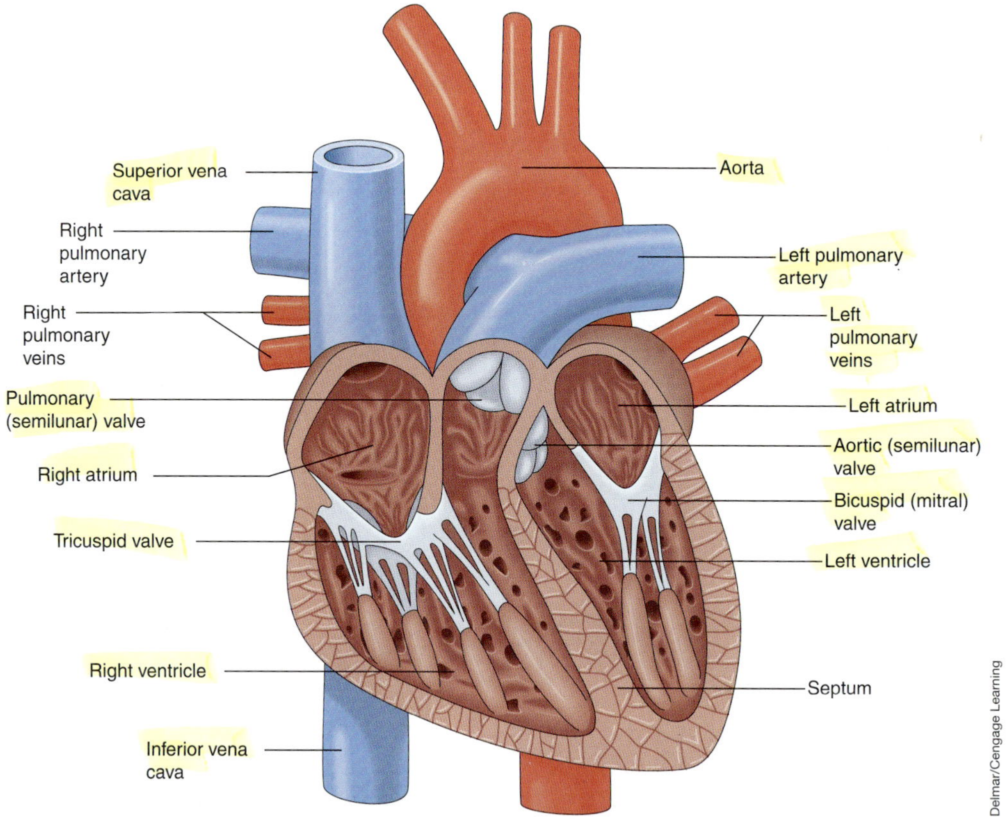

FIGURE 8–1 The heart: four chambers and great vessels.

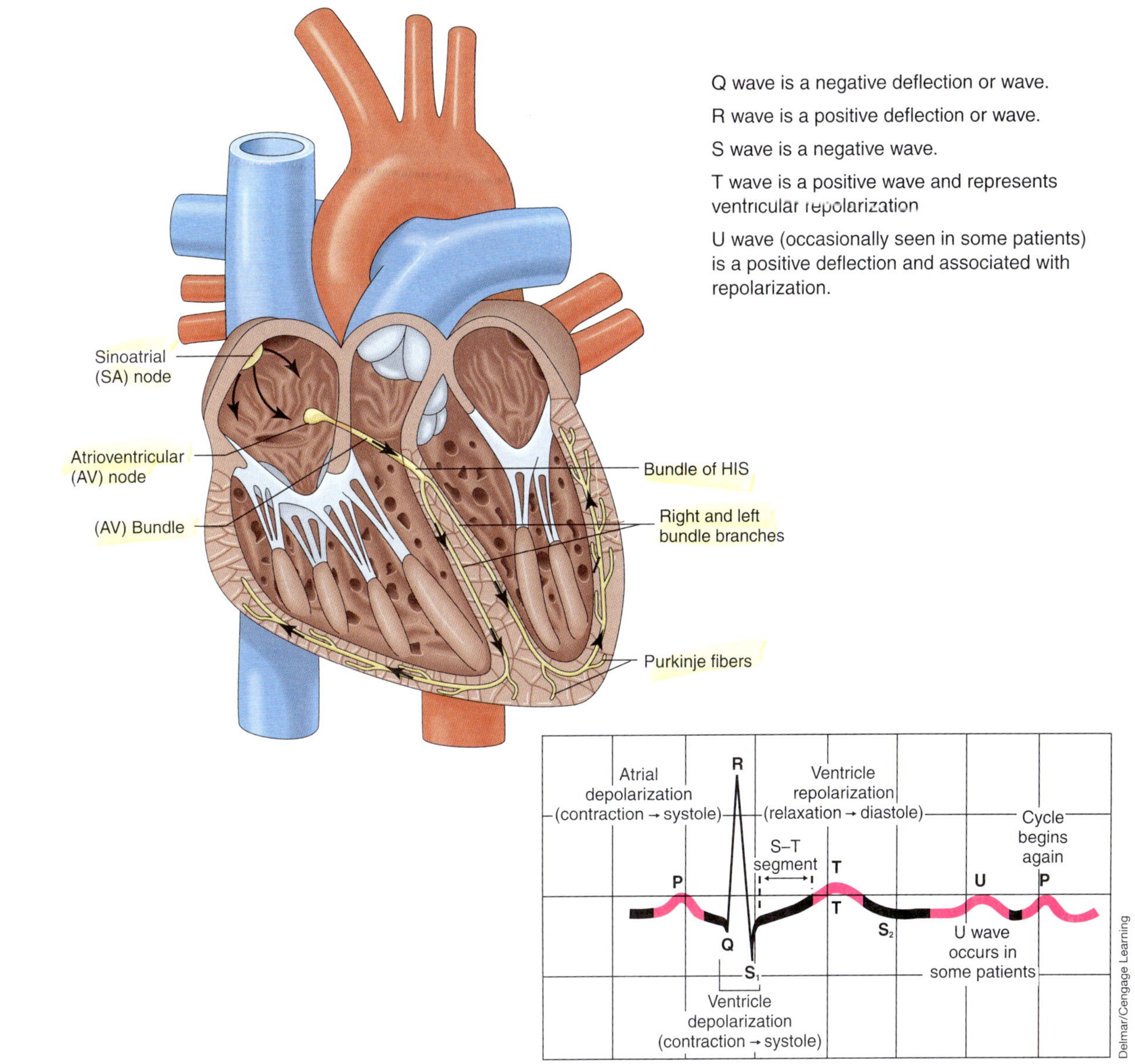

FIGURE 8–2 The conduction system.

(repolarization). The cardiac cycle repeats itself approximately 60–100 times per minute in the average adult. One cycle is one heartbeat. The pulsation (heartbeat) felt with the hand over the chest or the fingertips placed over an artery (such as at the wrist or neck) is called the pulse (Figure 8–3). The pulse rate is the number of pulsations felt in a minute. The closing of the heart valves produces the sounds heard when listening with a stethoscope over the heart.

The circulatory component of the cardiovascular system includes the arteries and veins (Figure 8–4). The three major subsystems include the portal unit, the pulmonary unit, and the systemic unit. Each of these circulatory subsystems has special functions in addition to delivering blood to the body. The portal unit, or subsystem, includes the circulation to the stomach, spleen, intestine, and pancreas. Blood from these organs goes through the liver before returning to the heart. The pulmonary subsystem includes the pulmonary artery and its divisions, leading from the heart to the lungs, the circulation through the lungs, and the pulmonary vein leading from the lungs back to the heart. In this subsystem, nonoxygenated blood from the systemic circulation passes through the lungs, where an exchange of carbon dioxide for oxygen occurs. The oxygenated blood returns to the heart to be pumped throughout the body. The systemic subsystem includes all the arteries and veins

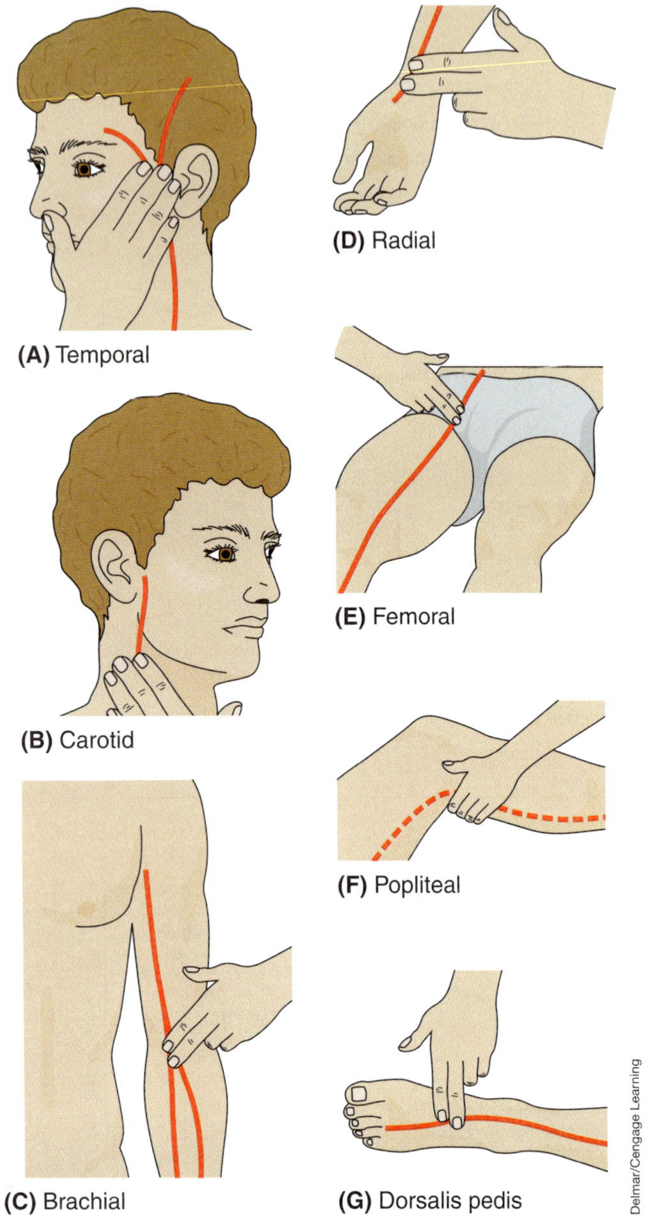

FIGURE 8–3 Pulse points of the body.

and their capillaries not already included in the previously mentioned subsystems. This subsystem carries the oxygen and nutrients to the body cells and removes waste products.

The level of pressure of the blood pushing against the walls of the vessels as it is delivered throughout the body is referred to as blood pressure. Most individuals are familiar with the arterial blood pressure taken with a sphygmomanometer on the arm over the brachial artery. The pressure measured with this instrument is divided into two parts. The systolic pressure, caused by the contraction of the ventricles, is the first number recorded. The second number is the diastolic pressure, reflecting the relaxation of the ventricles. The average adult pressure is 120/80 mm Hg (millimeters of mercury).

> ***Study*WARE™ Connection**
>
> View an animation on the heart on your StudyWARE™ CD-ROM.

COMMON SIGNS AND SYMPTOMS

Common symptoms of heart disease include chest pain, shortness of breath, fatigue, and **tachycardia** (TAK-ee-KAR-dee-ah; tachy = rapid, cardia = heart). Chest pain might be described as a severe, crushing pressure as though someone is crushing the chest, or the pain might be milder and described as a constant feeling of indigestion. Pain also can radiate down the left arm or into the jaw. Shortness of breath is also a common symptom because a lack of oxygen to the tissues stimulates the respiratory system. Individuals with heart disease often feel fatigued and experience episodes of tachycardia. Other symptoms include **cardiac palpitations** (an unusually strong, rapid, or irregular heart rate that is so abnormal that the individual "can feel" it), sweating (diaphoresis), edema in the extremities, and nausea and vomiting.

Pain, edema, and cyanosis are symptoms of diseases of the vascular system. Pain is often associated with poor blood perfusion to the tissues, leading to **ischemia** (iss-KEE-me-ah; lack of oxygen) of the organ. Edema of the extremities is commonly due to poor venous return, leading to congestion of blood and fluids in the tissues. Tissues that lack oxygen often exhibit a characteristic blue color called **cyanosis** (SIGH-ah-NO-sis; cyano = blue, osis = condition).

DIAGNOSTIC TESTS

Noninvasive procedures of the cardiovascular system involve listening to the heart and movement of blood in the vessels with a stethoscope in a procedure called **auscultation** (AUS-kul-TAY-shun). During auscultation, the stethoscope may be placed

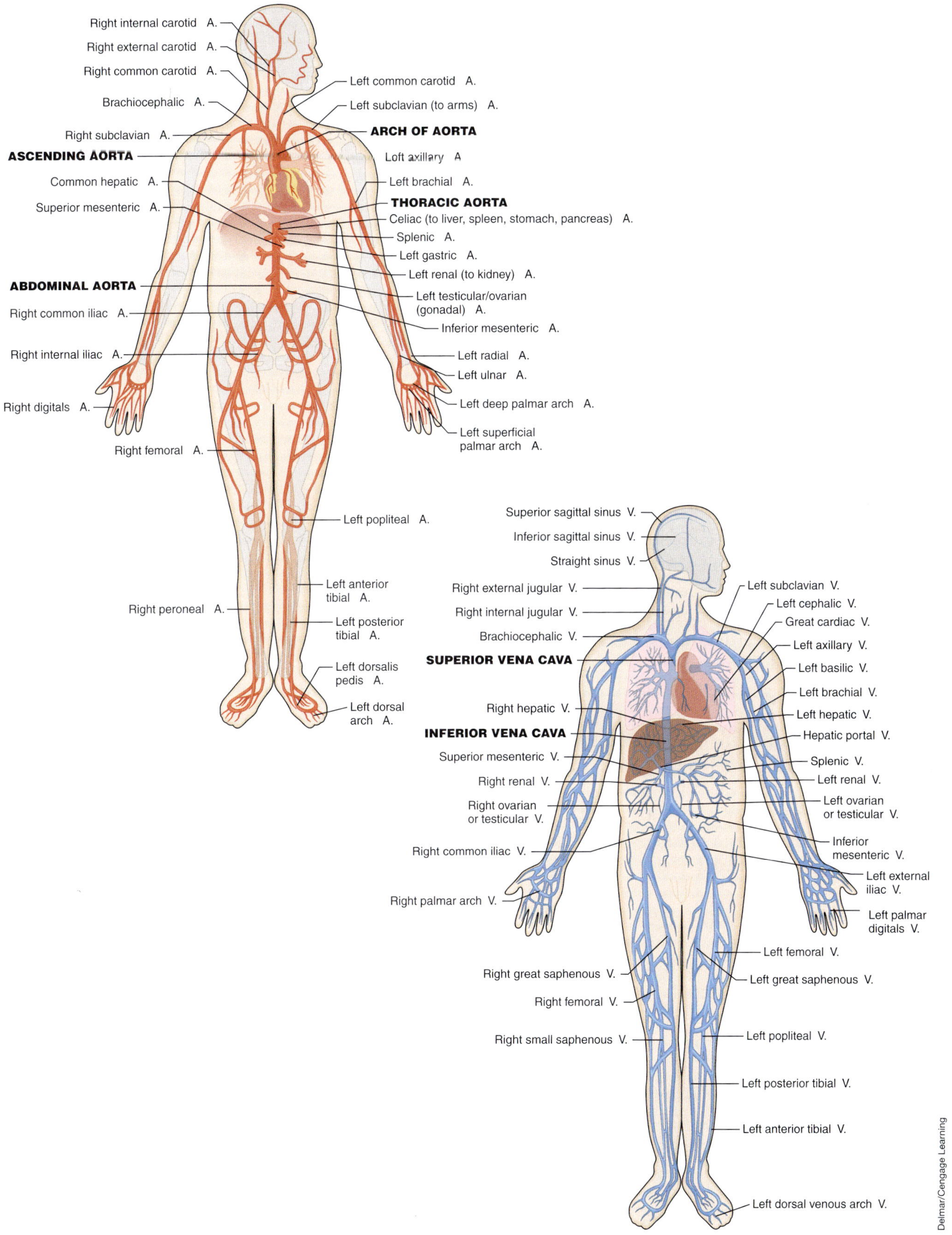

FIGURE 8–4 The circulatory system.

on the chest to listen to the heart and over various arteries to listen for blood flow. Murmurs can be auscultated in the heart area and indicate abnormal flow through the heart valves. A **Doppler** device can be placed over arteries to magnify the sound of blood flow. Decreased blood flow can be due to heart disease, vessel disease, or both.

Arterial blood pressure is simply referred to as blood pressure and is measured by a sphygmomanometer, a cuff and pressure gauge used to measure pressure when the heart beats (**systolic**; sis-TALL-ick) and when it rests (**diastolic**; dye-as-TOL-ick). Venous blood pressure is an important measure of the heart's pumping ability and can be determined by examining the individual for edema. Edema in the extremities and distention of the jugular veins in the neck are common indicators of increased venous pressure.

The action of the heart may be drawn or graphed by an electrocardiograph, a machine that receives electrical information and draws a graph of heart action. The picture produced is an **electrocardiogram** (ECG or EKG) (ee-LECK-troh-KAR-dee-oh-GRAM; electro = electrical, cardio = heart, gram = picture). The procedure involving use of a machine to make this picture is called electrocardiography. ECG or EKG is also used as an abbreviation to name the machine and the procedure. ECG is helpful in determining most cardiac diseases.

Use of ultrasound for diagnostic purposes is valuable for both heart and vessel diseases. Echocardiography (ECK-oh-KAR-dee-OG-rah-fee) and ultrasound arteriography (AR-tee-ree-OG-rah-fee) both use sound waves to produce pictures of the heart and arteries, respectively. These procedures are noninvasive.

Positron emission tomography (PET) scanning is a diagnostic test that involves imaging of radioactive positron emission. Prior to testing, a radioactive substance is administered as an intravenous injection. During imaging, different levels of tissue activity and function can be determined, and these images of the body developed by PET scanning can be used to evaluate a variety of diseases. PET scans of the heart assist in determining heart muscle function and blood flow to the heart muscle.

Cardiac catheterization (KATH-eh-ter-eye-ZAY-shun) is an invasive procedure used to sample the blood in the chambers of the heart to determine the oxygen content and blood pressure in the chambers.

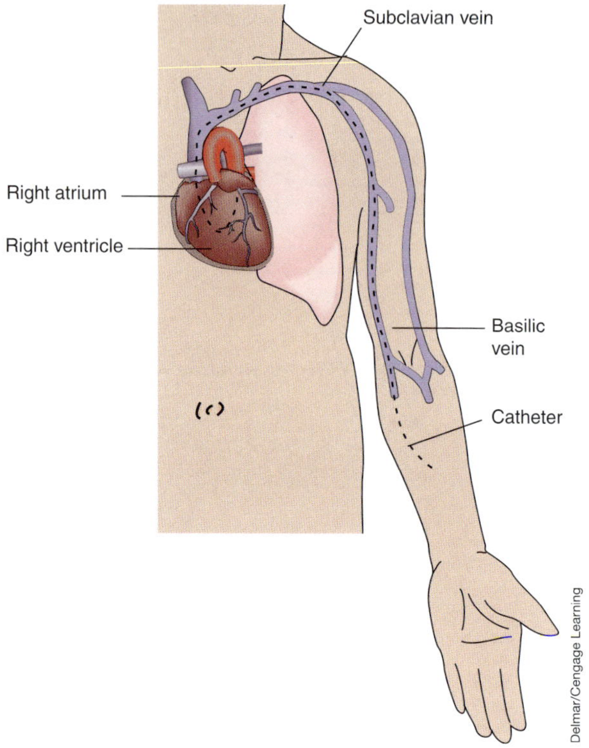

FIGURE 8–5 Cardiac catheterization.

Cardiac output also can be checked this way. This procedure involves passing a small plastic catheter into the heart through a vein or artery. A vein is used for right-sided catheterization, and an artery is used for a left-sided approach. Vessels of the arms and legs are commonly used (Figure 8–5).

X-rays of the heart and vessels can be beneficial in determining normal structure, size, and **patency** (openness). These procedures involve injecting dye into the system and taking pictures of the heart and vessels. Common X-ray procedures include angiocardiography (AN-jee-oh-KAR-dee-OG-rah-fee; angio = vessel, cardio = heart, graphy = procedure), arteriography (arterio = artery, graphy = procedure), and venography (veno = vein, graphy = procedure). The X-ray pictures produced are called angiocardiograms, arteriograms, and venograms, respectively (Figure 8–6).

The **ankle-brachial index (ABI) test** screens for peripheral arterial disease (PAD) by measuring the blood pressure at the ankle and in the arm. The result is calculated by dividing the systolic blood pressure in the ankle by the systolic blood pressure in the arm. The normal ABI is 1.0. The blood pressure

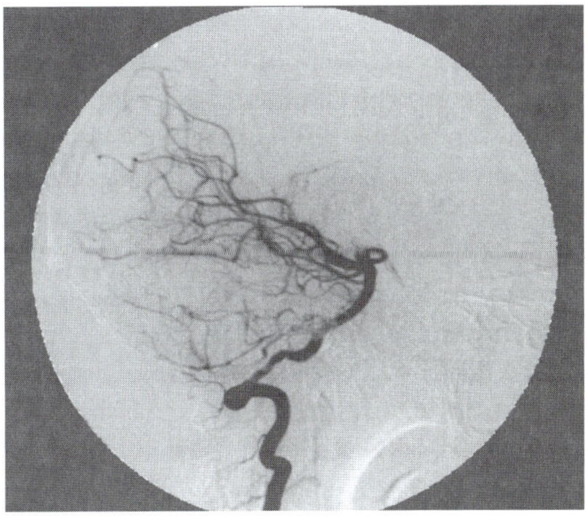

FIGURE 8–6 Arteriogram.

in the ankle should be the same or greater than the pressure in the arm. Less than 0.9 indicates some narrowing of the blood vessels in the legs, which can lead to PAD.

Blood tests of this system include enzyme studies that assist in determining whether the individual has had a myocardial infarction (MI) (heart attack). As the heart muscle dies, enzymes are released. The enzyme levels help determine the time and degree of the infarction. Common enzyme studies measure the levels of creatinine phosphokinase (CPK) and the protein troponin (TnL) lactic dehydrogenase. In the past, lactate hydrogenase (LDH) was usually measured, but research has shown that cardiac troponin and CPK are more specific.

COMMON DISEASES OF THE CARDIOVASCULAR SYSTEM

Cardiovascular disease (CVD) is the leading cause of death in the United States today (Figure 8–7), with more than 80,700,000 people in the United States having one or more forms of cardiovascular disease. One in every 2.8 deaths is related to CVD. In 2004, 869,724 people died with CVD (American Heart, 2005). High blood pressure accounts for most of these cases, but coronary heart disease, rheumatic heart disease, and other forms of cardiovascular disease also contribute to these staggering numbers. Education about lifestyle behavioral changes has helped decrease some individuals' risk for CVD.

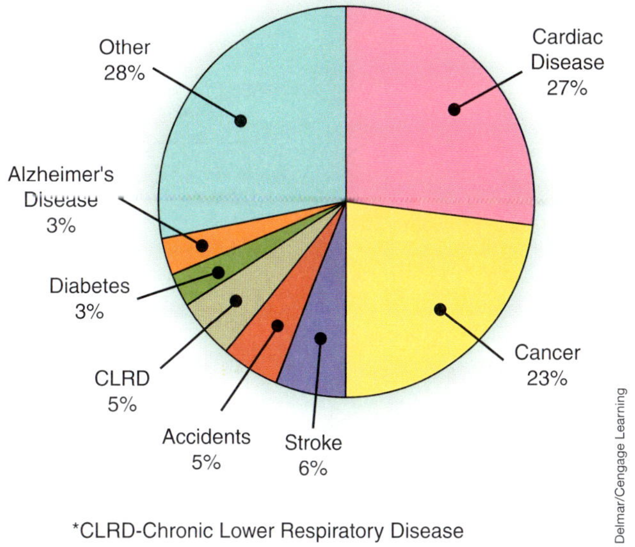

FIGURE 8–7 Mortality statistics comparing cardiac disease to other diseases.

Diseases of Arteries

Arterial disorders are the most common among all the CVDs. High blood pressure (hypertension) accounts for the largest incidence of arterial disorders, but coronary artery disease (coronary heart disease) is the leading cause of death overall.

HYPERTENSION

■ ***DESCRIPTION.*** Most people are familiar with the basic concept that hypertension is high arterial blood pressure. Other concepts include the fact that hypertension is not only a disease process but also serves as an indicator of the development of cerebrovascular, cardiovascular, and kidney disease. Hypertension is a chronic disease and is the leading cause of stroke and heart failure. Life expectancy in all individuals, regardless of age or sex, is reduced when diastolic hypertension is greater than 90 mm Hg.

Blood pressure varies from individual to individual, but average adult blood pressure is considered to be less than 120/80 mm Hg. The top number (120) is the systolic pressure and measures the highest amount of pressure in the artery when the ventricles of the heart contract. The lower number is the diastolic pressure and measures the artery pressure when the ventricles relax. If one could view the arteries as the heart beats, one would see a wavelike pattern of

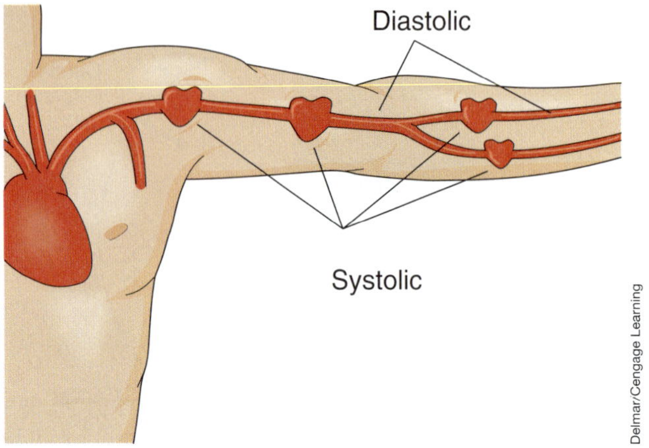

FIGURE 8–8 Systolic and diastolic blood pressure.

blood flow related to the heart beating and resting (Figure 8–8). Medical parameters for diagnosing high blood pressure start with pre-hypertension at levels above 120/80. Stage I hypertension is recognized when the level reaches 140/90 and greater.

In addition to heartbeat, blood vessel resistance also helps determine blood pressure. One might compare the heart and vessels to a water pump and hose: the amount of water the pump pumps and the width of the hose help determine the amount of water flow or water pressure. In the same way, the amount of blood the heart pumps and the resistance of the vessel, or size of the **lumen** (LOO-men; inner open space or width), will help determine blood pressure. The larger the lumen or the more patent the vessel, the easier it is for the heart to pump blood and, generally speaking, the lower the blood pressure.

Specialized nerve receptors in the body help control pressure by bringing about vasoconstriction and vasodilation at appropriate times. For example, when an individual stands up suddenly, the blood pressure to the head drops, often causing momentary dizziness. To correct this situation, nerves react and constrict blood vessels, raising blood pressure and restoring normal pressure in the head. If blood pressure is too high, these nerve receptors dilate vessels leading to the kidneys. This increased blood flow leads to greater urine formation and output. Increased urine production decreases blood volume and thus lowers blood pressure. In this way, the kidneys play a vital role in blood pressure. If pressure is too low—as often occurs in shock—blood flow to the kidneys is diminished, urine output is minimal, blood fluid is maintained, and blood pressure is maintained or restored.

■ ***ETIOLOGY.*** Because blood pressure and the kidneys have such a close relationship, any disease of the kidneys can cause an alteration in blood pressure, and any change in blood pressure can have an adverse effect on the kidneys. The kidneys play a vital role in elimination of salt and water, two substances that also have a great effect on blood pressure. Retention of salt and water increases blood pressure, whereas elimination of these substances reduces blood pressure. Hypertension caused by kidney disease or some other type of disease process is called secondary hypertension. Only 10% of all hypertensive cases are due to secondary problems.

Primary or essential hypertension accounts for approximately 90% of all hypertensive cases. This type

COMPLEMENTARY AND ALTERNATIVE THERAPY

Grape Seed Extract

Grape seed extract had been used historically to improve diseases of the heart and blood vessels such as hypertension, atherosclerosis, and peripheral vascular disease. Research shows that grape seed extract counteracts free radicals, which are atoms or molecules that have unpaired electrons in their outer ring. Free radicals have been linked to damage in the cell membrane leading to several disorders and diseases. Antioxidants are molecules which can safely interact with free radicals and terminate the chain reaction before vital molecules are damaged. The most common antioxidants are vitamin E, beta-carotene, and vitamin C. Grape seed extract has been shown to have antioxidant effects, which may be why it has been used for treating heart and blood disorders.

Herb at a Glance, (2007).

of hypertension is idiopathic, or due to an unknown cause, and usually has a gradual onset over a number of years.

Some identified genetic and environmental risk factors are known to cause primary hypertension. These include:

- **Heredity** Hypertension affects black individuals twice as often as whites.
- **Diet** High salt and fat intake increases the risk of hypertension.
- **Age** Blood pressure tends to rise with age.
- **Obesity** Obesity causes an increased workload on the heart.
- **Smoking** Nicotine causes vasoconstriction.
- **Stress** Stress causes a rise in blood pressure due to vasoconstriction.
- **Type A personality traits** This type of personality tends to experience more stress.

SYMPTOMS. Symptoms usually do not occur until significant heart and vessel damage has already occurred. If left untreated, high blood pressure overworks the heart. Because the left ventricle works harder to pump blood, it is the area most often affected, leading to left ventricle hypertrophy (muscle enlargement). The vascular system, or blood supply, to the left ventricle does not increase with this enlargement of muscle, so this extra tissue does not have adequate blood supply, often leading to bouts of angina or chest pain due to ischemia. This condition often leads to MI, or heart failure, and death.

Hypertension not only affects the heart but also adversely affects the vessels. Over a period of years, the vessels become hardened (sclerotic) and lose elasticity, a contributing factor in arteriosclerosis (arterio = artery, scler = hardened, osis = condition of). Sclerotic (hardened) vessels are also more likely to form thrombi and to rupture, which can cause damage or death to the involved organs.

DIAGNOSIS. Blood pressure screening is very important in diagnosing hypertension before the cardiovascular system is damaged. A random blood pressure of greater than 140/90 might be physiologic; thus, screening with frequent blood pressure readings under varied conditions is needed to confirm the diagnosis.

Further evaluation for hypertension consists primarily of:

1. Taking a medical and family history because hypertension tends to run in families.
2. Completing a physical examination.
3. Testing blood for:
   - Cholesterol: should be under 200
   - LDL (low-density lipo—bad cholesterol): should be under 100
   - HDL (high-density lipo—good cholesterol): should be over 45.
   - Triglycerides (tri-GLISS-er-ides—stored energy in the cells): should be under 200.
4. EKG to test the action of the heart.

Several other blood tests can be used to check kidney dysfunction, which can also cause high blood pressure.

TREATMENT. Treatment of hypertension depends on the degree of hypertension and the number of risk factors involved. If blood pressure is extremely high, antihypertensive medications might be prescribed immediately. If hypertension is discovered in a milder form, lifestyle changes or reduction of risk factors might be the initial treatment. A low-salt, low-fat diet; stress-reducing exercise; and smoking cessation might solve the problem. (See Healthy Highlight on page 154.)

If this treatment is ineffective or inadequate, the individual might be placed on diuretic medications. Diuretics increase urine output, thus lowering blood pressure. If further control is needed, other antihypertensive medications can be prescribed. Patient compliance with hypertension treatment is often a factor in addressing this chronic disease. Difficulty with lifestyle changes and following the medication regimen for the rest of one's life is often difficult for the individual to manage.

PREVENTION. WebMD suggests that lifestyle changes, which include the following, can help prevent hypertension:

- Do not smoke.
- Reduce sodium (salt) intake to about 2 grams per day, which equals about 1 teaspoon of salt.
- Maintain a normal body weight.

HEALTHY HIGHLIGHT

Prevention of Cardiovascular Disease

To help reduce the risk of developing CVD, practice the following lifestyle behaviors:

- Decrease intake of fats, especially saturated fats.
- Decrease intake of salt.
- Participate in a regular program of moderate exercise at least three times weekly.
- Keep weight within normal limits for age and body structure.
- Have blood pressure checked routinely. If necessary, take prescribed medications to reduce hypertension.
- Do not smoke.
- Decrease stress by participating in stress reduction activities.
- Limit alcohol intake to two drinks per day for men and one drink per day for women.
- Exercise for 30 minutes daily.
- Get a daily intake of approximately 3,500 mg of potassium daily.

ARTERIOSCLEROSIS AND ATHEROSCLEROSIS

DESCRIPTION. Arteriosclerosis is a group of diseases that are characterized by a loss of elasticity and a thickening of the artery wall. Atherosclerosis is the most common form of arteriosclerosis. For this reason, these terms are often used interchangeably; *hardening of the arteries* is a lay term describing this condition. The common result of arteriosclerosis is the gradual narrowing of the vessel lumen (Figure 8–9). This narrowing leads to a slowing or complete stoppage of blood flow to the organs supplied by those vessels. Without proper blood supply, these organs become ischemic and eventually might die if blood supply is not restored.

An artery has a very smooth endothelium (inner lining), like a nonstick finish. As with nonstick cookware, food particles normally do not stick to the surface. If the endothelium is damaged, however, blood material begins sticking to the inner lining of the artery just as food particles begin sticking to scratched cookware. The artery wall surrounds this endothelium. Atherosclerosis is a condition characterized by deposits of fatty or lipid material in the wall of the artery (see Figure 8–9). These fatty, cholesterol-containing deposits, called **plaque**, damage the artery and interrupt blood flow by:

- Pushing into the endothelium, thus damaging the inner lining. Damage to this lining allows blood material to stick to the inner lining and occlude the lumen.
- Causing the artery wall to harden or lose elasticity. This loss of elasticity increases blood pressure and increases workload on the heart. A hardened vessel is not able to expand and accommodate the surge of blood caused by the beat of the heart.
- Thickening the artery wall to the point that the lumen is partially or completely occluded.
- Leading to formation of plaque that often ulcerates or breaks loose, forming an **embolus** (EM-boh-lus; material floating in the blood) that can stick in a vessel and occlude or stop blood flow, leading to ischemia or death of the organs supplied by that vessel.

Narrowing of the lumen of the artery in all the aforementioned ways increases blood pressure, increases workload on the heart, and decreases blood supply to the organs. Increased blood pressure stretches the hardened arteries, causing further artery damage and further increasing workload on the heart.

Atherosclerosis can affect all arteries in the body, but four major areas are often affected by atherosclerosis, many times leading to disability or mortality (Figure 8–10).

These major areas affected are the following:

1. **Coronary arteries** These arteries feed the muscle tissue of the heart. Atherosclerosis of these arteries leads to coronary artery disease, also

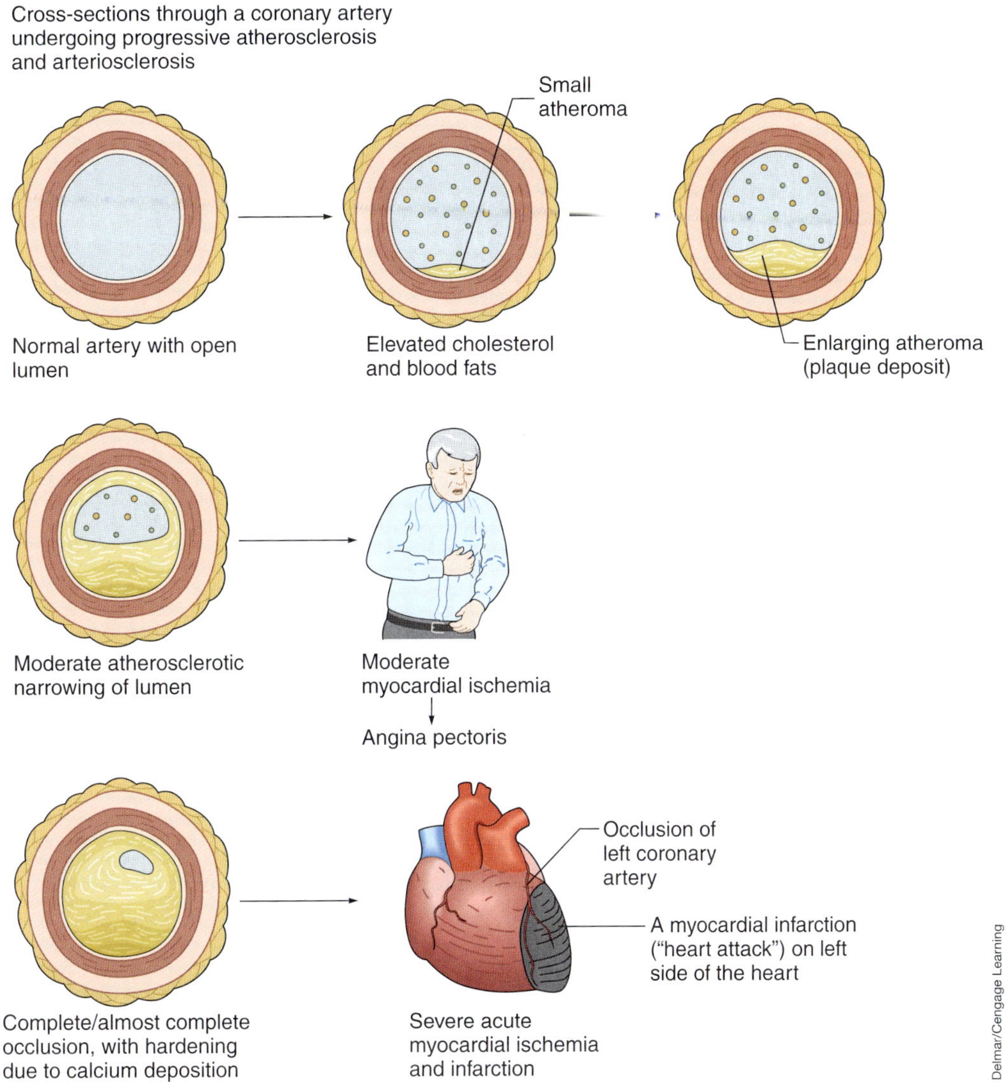

FIGURE 8–9 Atherosclerosis: narrowing of arterial lumen.

called coronary heart disease. Consequences of coronary artery disease can include MI (heart attack).

2. **Cerebral arteries** These arteries feed brain tissue. Atherosclerosis of these arteries can lead to a cerebrovascular accident (CVA), commonly called a stroke.

3. **Aorta** This artery is the largest artery in the body and is responsible for carrying blood to the general circulatory system. Atherosclerosis of this artery in any area can lead to aneurysms.

4. **Peripheral arteries** Peripheral arteries primarily feed the extremities (arms and legs). Atherosclerosis of these arteries can lead to peripheral vascular disease.

ETIOLOGY. The cause of atherosclerosis is unknown, but it is thought to be the result of a combination of factors, some of which are not controllable, but many are and can be altered by a change in lifestyle. Important risk factors include the following:

NONCONTROLLABLE FACTORS

- **Heredity** Atherosclerosis appears to run in families. This might be related to common diet or, in some instances, a clear genetic tendency to develop hypercholesterolemia (hyper = increased, cholesterol, emia = blood).
- **Age** Atherosclerosis is considered a degenerative disease because all adults over the age of 30 have some degree of plaque formation. In general, the older the person, the more atherosclerosis is present.

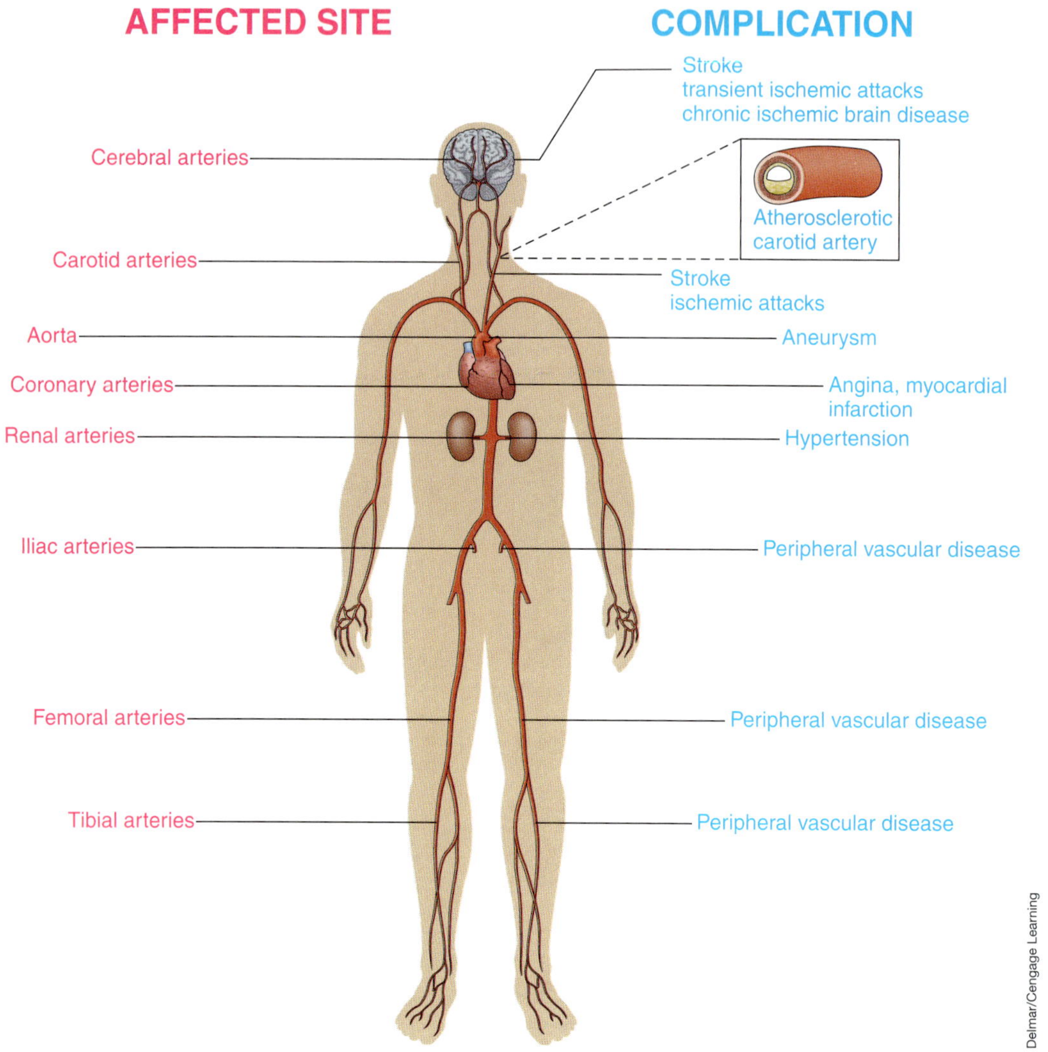

FIGURE 8–10 Atherosclerosis: major areas affected.

- **Sex** Men have more atherosclerosis present than women until after female menopause, at which time, the incidence becomes more equal.
- **Diabetes** Individuals with diabetes have more existing atherosclerosis than those who do not have diabetes. However, if their diabetes is Type 2 and related to obesity, it is considered to be a controllable factor.

CONTROLLABLE FACTORS

- **Diet** Obese individuals have more atherosclerosis present than individuals in the normal weight range. The higher the diet in carbohydrates and fats, the higher the incidence of atherosclerosis.
- **Sedentary lifestyle** Lack of exercise increases the risk of development of atherosclerosis.
- **Cigarette smoking** This is one of the most important risk factors. Stopping smoking is 10 times more effective in reducing risk than a combination of exercise and diet control.
- **Stress** Stress increases blood pressure, but research does not support the idea that stress increases atherosclerosis.
- **Hypertension** The higher the blood pressure, the greater the risk for development of atherosclerosis. It is difficult to determine which of these diseases occurs first. Atherosclerosis causes an increase in blood pressure, and hypertension leads to an increase in atherosclerosis. Often, hypertension

and atherosclerosis occur simultaneously, each complicating the treatment of the other.

■ ***SYMPTOMS.*** Symptoms of atherosclerosis appear late in the disease process and vary, depending on the area affected.

■ ***DIAGNOSIS.*** Diagnosis of atherosclerosis is by blood pressure measurement, arteriograms, and X-ray. Doppler studies to determine blood flow also can be used.

■ ***TREATMENT.*** Treatment is aimed at treating symptoms as they arise. Surgery to bypass occluded arteries and remove plaque is commonly used. Prevention of atherosclerosis includes exercise, estrogen medication postmenopause, and changing lifestyle to reduce risk factors.

■ ***PREVENTION.*** Preventive methods are discussed in the Healthy Highlight titled "Prevention of Cardiovascular Disease."

PERIPHERAL VASCULAR DISEASE (PVD)

■ ***DESCRIPTION.*** PVD refers to any disease of the arteries, veins, or lymph vessels. The most common type of PVD is peripheral artery disease (PAD). Disease of the arteries (PAD) affects more than 8 million Americans. It becomes more common with age and affects about 12–20% of the population (American Heart Association, 2008).

■ ***ETIOLOGY.*** PVD is caused by atherosclerotic plaque, primarily in the arteries supplying blood to the legs. The occlusion by the plaque can be chronic or acute. Chronic occlusion is generally related to a progressive narrowing of the femoral and popliteal arteries. As these arteries become occluded, the blood supply to the leg muscles is decreased.

■ ***SYMPTOMS.*** Individuals with PVD have adequate blood supply to leg muscles during minimal activity such as sitting or slow walking. If activity is increased to brisk walking or running, blood supply becomes inadequate, causing leg muscle cramps. Resting the legs will relieve the muscle cramps and allows the muscles once again to receive the needed amount of blood flow. This condition of developing muscle cramps that are relieved with rest and increase with activity is called **intermittent claudication** (KLAW-dih-KAY-shun).

■ ***DIAGNOSIS.*** Diagnosis is critical because people with PVD have four to five times the risk of heart attack and stroke (American Heart Association, 2008). The classic symptom of PVD is intermittent claudication. Other tests include:

- Feeling for a pulse in the foot. A Doppler flow probe can quickly pick up a pulse if one is present.
- ABI (the measurement of the blood pressure in the arm compared to the blood pressure in the leg).
- A treadmill test to attempt to induce intermittent claudication.
- Angiography and magnetic resonance imaging (MRI) to determine location and thickness of the atherosclerosis (plaque).

■ ***TREATMENT.*** Treatment of chronic PVD often involves opening the artery and cleaning out the plaque. This surgical treatment is called **endarterectomy** (END-ar-ter-ECK-toh-me; endo = inside, arter = artery, ectomy = excision). If the artery is damaged, it might be bypassed with a graft. A femoral popliteal graft might be used to treat the symptoms of chronic occlusion.

■ ***PREVENTION.*** Risk can be reduced by following the guidelines in the Healthy Highlight, "Prevention of Cardiovascular Disease."

Acute occlusion of the peripheral arteries often involves smaller arteries supplying blood to the feet and toes. This type of PVD often leads to necrosis and gangrene. Amputation or resection might be needed to treat acute occlusion.

ANEURYSM

■ ***DESCRIPTION.*** Aneurysm (AN-you-rizm) is a weakening in the wall of an artery that allows the vessel to bulge or rupture (Figure 8–11).

■ ***ETIOLOGY.*** This weakening is often due to atherosclerosis but also might be due to a congenital defect or injury.

■ ***SYMPTOMS.*** Aneurysms are usually asymptomatic and are often discovered accidentally during physical examinations or X-rays. The most common area affected is the abdominal aorta. Rupture of an aneurysm is a medical emergency, often causing death due to massive hemorrhage and shock.

■ ***DIAGNOSIS.*** A thorough physical examination can lead to the discovery of an aortic aneurysm. Placing a stethoscope on the abdomen allows a physician to hear the abnormal blood flow through the artery. Smaller

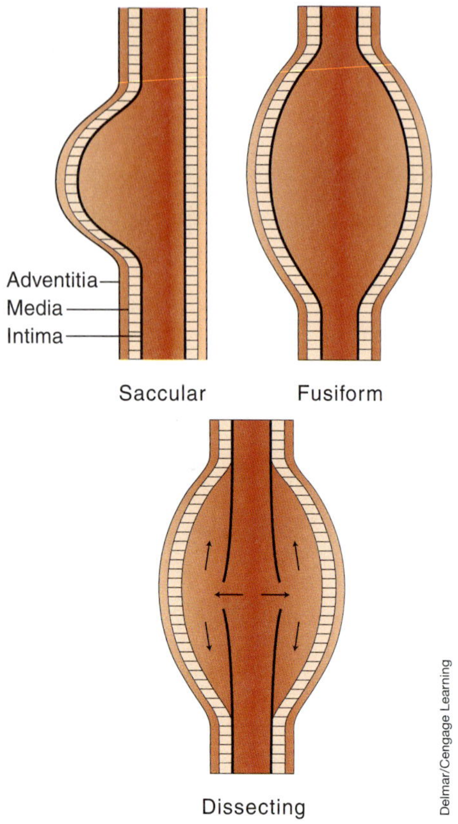

FIGURE 8–11 Three types of aneurysm.

aneurysms and those located in other areas are more difficult to hear and might be discovered by angiogram. Other diagnostic tests include computerized tomography (CT) and MRI scans.

■ ***TREATMENT.*** Treatment is aimed at repairing the aneurysm before rupture. Surgical resection and grafting is commonly performed (Figure 8–12).

■ ***PREVENTION.*** Preventing atherosclerosis and hypertension aid in prevention of aneurysm. Congenital aneurysms cannot be prevented.

CORONARY ARTERY DISEASE

■ ***DESCRIPTION.*** Coronary artery disease (CAD), often called coronary heart disease, is the narrowing of arteries that supply blood to the myocardium, the heart muscle. It is the leading cause of death in the United States today.

■ ***ETIOLOGY.*** This disease is commonly due to atherosclerosis.

■ ***SYMPTOMS.*** Progressive or slow narrowing of the arteries leads to ischemia of the heart muscle and symptoms of angina. Some muscle cells can actually die and be replaced with scar tissue. This scar tissue cannot function like muscle tissue, causing an increase in the workload of the remaining heart muscle. Congestive heart failure often results.

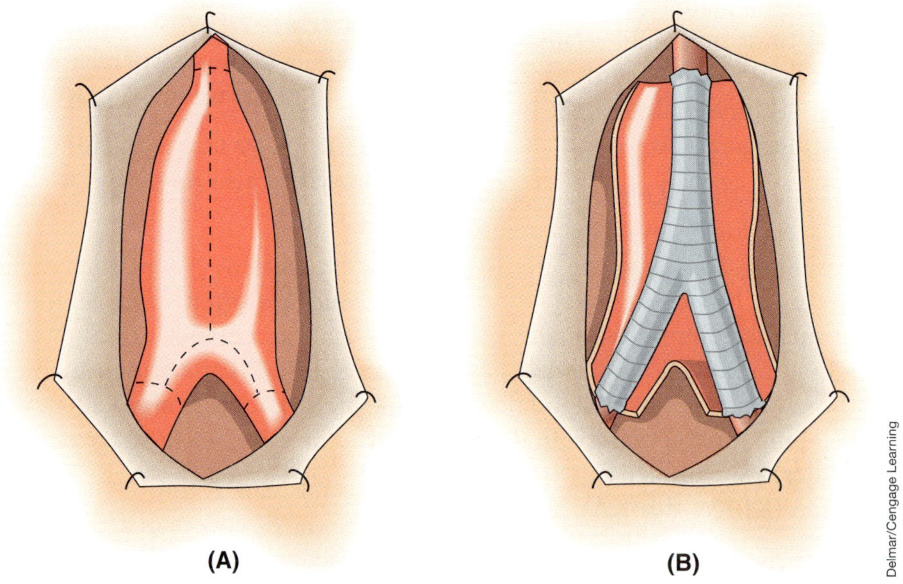

FIGURE 8–12 Abdominal aneurysm surgical resection (A) and grafting (B).

If a coronary artery becomes blocked to the point that heart muscle oxygen demands cannot be met, the heart muscle dies. Occlusion can progress slowly as plaque builds up in the vessel, or it can develop suddenly as the result of a **thrombus** (THROM-bus; a blood clot attached to a vein or artery) or embolus (traveling blood clot, free in the circulatory system, more dangerous than a thrombus). This dead muscle is called an infarct or myocardial infarct. The process of the myocardium dying is called MI.

Slow, progressive occlusion of the arteries often leads to development of collateral arteries that extend into ischemic tissue. Collateral circulation provides some protection against ischemia and infarction. For this reason, infarction caused by slow occlusion oftentimes has a better outcome than infarction caused by sudden occlusion of a vessel.

■ ***DIAGNOSIS.*** Diagnosis of CAD is made from a history of symptoms, EKG, and angiograms. Symptoms usually do not develop until the vessels are at least 70% occluded.

■ ***TREATMENT.*** Treatment of CAD is aimed at increasing blood flow or decreasing oxygen needs. Angina is often treated with rest and vasodilators. A coronary artery **angioplasty** (AN-jee-oh-PLAS-tee; angio = vessel, plasty = surgical repair) might be attempted to open the vessel by passing a catheter into the artery and inflating a balloon on the catheter to push the plaque against the vessel wall, thus widening the lumen of the vessel (Figure 8–13). Another common surgical treatment for CAD is a coronary artery bypass graft, commonly called a CABG (pronounced cabbage). This procedure bypasses the occlusion (Figure 8–14). Mammary vessels from the breast area and saphenous vessels from the legs are often used for the bypass.

■ ***PREVENTION.*** It is very important for individuals with CAD to reduce atherosclerotic risk factors. Diet, exercise, and a no-smoking regimen are prescribed to slow the progression of the disease.

Diseases of the Heart

Diseases of the heart are frequently due to the atherosclerotic narrowing of the coronary arteries. The result of this is usually angina, a heart attack (MI), or both. Decreasing lifestyle behaviors that contribute to the development of atherosclerosis decreases one's risk for heart disease.

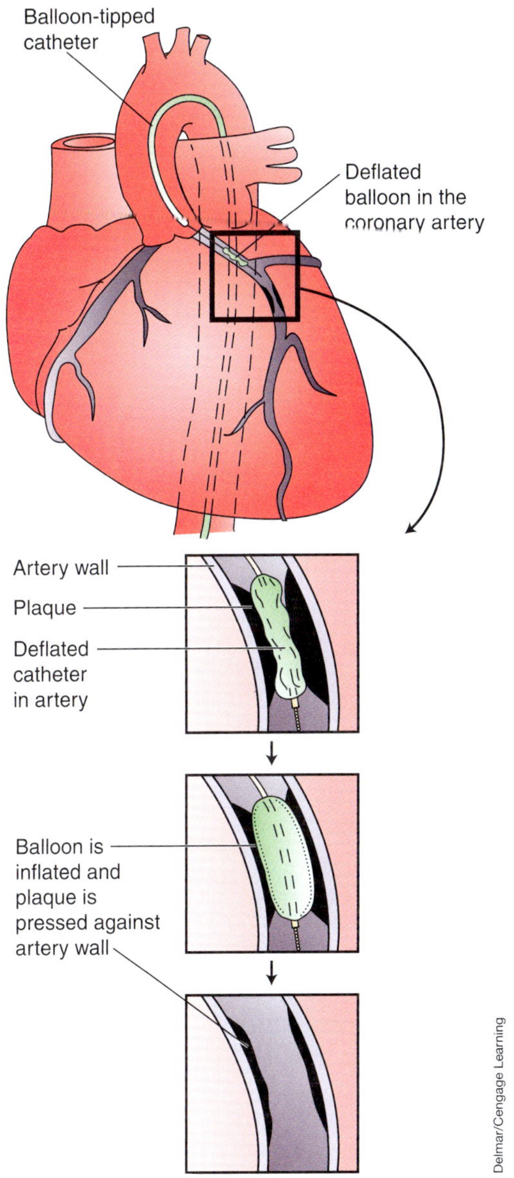

FIGURE 8–13 Coronary artery angioplasty.

■ CORONARY HEART DISEASE ■

Coronary heart disease, CAD, and arteriosclerotic heart disease are all one and the same. This disease was previously discussed as CAD. Coronary heart disease is the most common type of heart disease in the United States. The risk of this disease rises rapidly with increased age.

ANGINA PECTORIS

■ ***DESCRIPTION.*** Angina pectoris (an-JIGH-nah PECK-toh-riss) is commonly called chest pain.

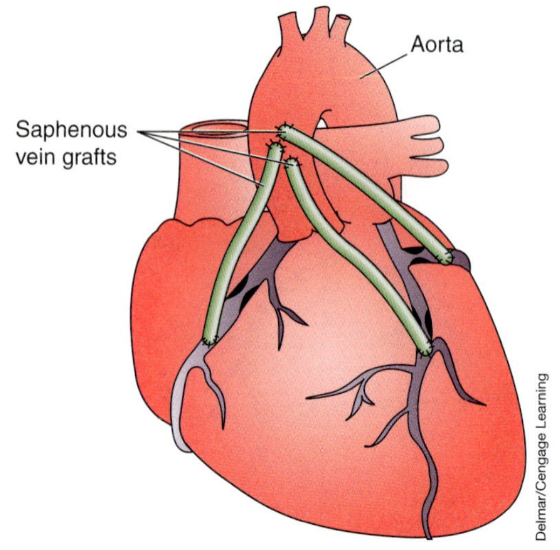

FIGURE 8–14 Coronary artery bypass graft (CABG).

■ ***ETIOLOGY.*** Angina pectoris is caused by lack of oxygen to the myocardium (heart muscle). Atherosclerosis is the leading cause of angina, although in some cases, it can be brought on by a spasm of the muscles in the arteries that restricts blood flow to the heart. Angina is commonly a symptom of impending MI.

■ ***SYMPTOMS.*** During an attack, the individual might complain of a suffocating tightness in the chest that radiates to the left arm, neck, and jaw (Figure 8–15). Angina usually occurs during periods of increased workload on the heart such as those experienced with physical exercise, emotional stress, or digestion of a large meal.

■ ***DIAGNOSIS.*** A thorough physical exam, along with blood test, electrocardiogram, and cardiac catheterization, assist in diagnosis. Blood tests include cholesterol and triglyceride blood levels. An electrocardiogram can assist in recognizing abnormal heart function. A cardiac catheterization is the most definitive procedure to discover the cause of angina.

■ ***TREATMENT.*** Treatment of angina is to decrease workload on the heart by stopping the aggravating activity and increasing blood flow to the heart muscle. Vasodilatation of the coronary arteries or those that supply the heart muscle, will improve blood flow and help relieve the oxygen deficit. Nitroglycerin is a vasodilator that is commonly used. It is administered sublingually (under the tongue) and usually provides immediate relief. Individuals suffering with angina need medical attention.

■ ***PREVENTION.*** Angina can be prevented or controlled by making healthy lifestyle choices as previously listed.

MYOCARDIAL INFARCTION

■ ***DESCRIPTION.*** The term *myocardial infarction* (MY-oh-KAR-dee-al in-FARK-shun) comes from the meanings of the words *myocardium* (heart muscle) and *infarction* (tissue death from lack of oxygen). It is commonly called a heart attack and often leads to cardiac arrest—stopping of the heartbeat.

■ ***ETIOLOGY.*** MI occurs when the heart muscle does not get adequate oxygen due to a decrease in blood supply, an increase in oxygen need, or a combination

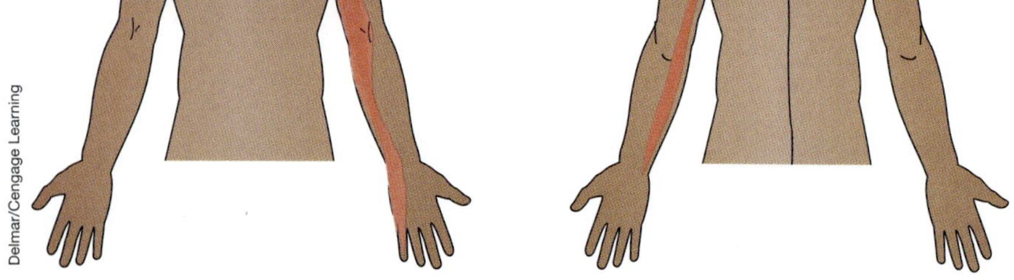

FIGURE 8–15 Patterns of angina.

of both. The decrease in blood supply is most commonly caused by the atherosclerotic plaque of CAD. Any activity that increases the oxygen need of the heart beyond the supply level can lead to a myocardial infarct. Such activities can include shock, hemorrhage, stress, or excessive physical exertion.

■ ***SYMPTOMS.*** Classic symptoms of a MI include severe chest pain with diaphoresis (sweating) and nausea. Often, the symptoms are not as obvious and can include referred pain in the left arm, neck, and jaw along with a discomfort similar to bad or unrelieved indigestion. Severity of symptoms can depend on the size of the infarction. If the area is small, symptoms might be mild, and the infarction can be labeled a silent MI. If the infarcted area is large, symptoms can include cardiogenic shock and death. Mortality from MI is approximately 35%.

■ ***DIAGNOSIS.*** The diagnosis of MI is made by history and physical examination along with electrocardiogram and blood testing. Two specific cardiac blood tests indicative of MI are creatine phosphokinase (CPK) and troponin.

■ ***TREATMENT.*** Treatment of a MI involves immediate attention to prevent shock, relieve respiratory distress, and decrease workload on the heart. The individual should be assisted into a lying position. Tight or restrictive clothing should be loosened to improve respiratory function. If cardiac arrest has occurred, appropriate cardiopulmonary resuscitation (CPR) should be administered immediately, and the individual should be transported immediately to a medical facility.

Medical treatment involves the administration of oxygen and pain medication, and medication to treat arrhythmias is often needed. Intravenous thrombolytic, or clot-busting, therapy using a tissue plasminogen activator (TPA) or streptokinase might be used to open the occlusion and restore blood flow. Education following a MI is aimed at prevention by possible changes in lifestyle to reduce risk factors. Smoking cessation, dietary changes, and exercise are usually recommended.

The main site involved in a MI is the left ventricle. This is the hardest working area of the heart and has the greatest need for oxygen. Tissue changes that appear with an infarction depend on the degree or extent of oxygen deprivation suffered by the cells. Under microscopic examination, the infarcted area might take on a bull's eye appearance (Figure 8–16). The central core is made up of cells that are dead or necrotic with severely damaged cells surrounding this core. These cells might regain function within a few weeks, or they might die, thus extending the infarcted area. On the outer border of the bull's eye pattern are cells that suffered from ischemia. These cells usually live and can regain function.

Death of myocardial cells brings about a release of certain enzymes and proteins (CPK and troponin) into the general circulation. Blood tests to measure these levels assist in determining the amount of dead or necrotic tissue and the severity and time of the attack.

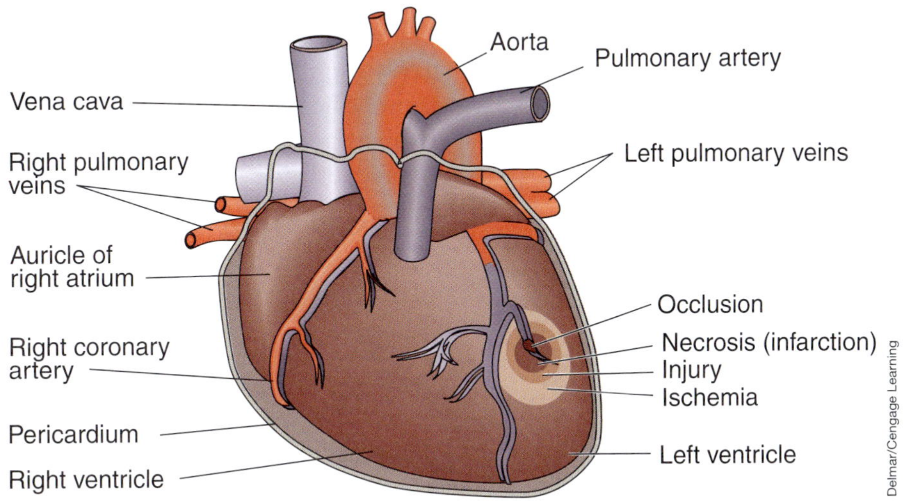

FIGURE 8–16 Myocardial infarction: areas of ischemia.

Blood levels, along with an EKG, history, and physical examination, often confirm the diagnosis of MI.

Tissue infarction and injury naturally cause the inflammatory response. With this response comes an outpouring of PMNs and macrophages. Within the first five to seven days, macrophages phagocytize the dead tissue, often leaving a thin, weak myocardial layer. Possibility of rupture and sudden death is greatest at this time. Any activity that increases the workload of the heart or increases blood pressure should be avoided. Rest is essential during this time.

Within two weeks, the infarcted area is healing with granulation tissue. This tissue is not made of muscle tissue; it is scar tissue. This scar will not stretch or contract like normal muscle, and it will never function as normal heart tissue. The inability of this scarred area to function increases workload on the remaining heart muscle cells for the rest of the individual's life.

■ ***PREVENTION.*** Risk factors for MI are the same as for CAD and primarily include hypertension, cigarette smoking, a sedentary lifestyle, obesity, and a high-cholesterol diet. Controlling risk factors is the primary way to prevent MI.

HYPERTENSIVE HEART DISEASE

■ ***DESCRIPTION.*** Hypertensive heart disease is a group of disorders cause by hypertension. It is the number one cause of death associated with hypertension and is the result of long-term hypertension.

■ ***ETIOLOGY.*** Any disease or disorder that causes a chronic elevation in blood pressure can lead to hypertensive heart disease. Essential hypertension, arteriosclerosis, atherosclerosis, and kidney diseases are common causes.

■ ***SYMPTOMS.*** As previously discussed, chronic hypertension leads to increased workload on the heart, causing cardiac hypertrophy and, eventually, heart failure.

■ ***DIAGNOSIS.*** Diagnosis is made by thorough history and physical examination. X-rays revealing enlargement of the heart along with abnormal heart function as determined by an echocardiogram is indicative of this disease. Late in the course of the disease, there can be pulmonary (lung) congestion as a result of heart failure.

■ ***TREATMENT.*** Treatment of hypertensive heart disease is related to treating the cause of hypertension. If the hypertension cannot be cured, as with essential hypertension, then controlling blood pressure is necessary. Hypertensive heart disease, like hypertension, is not cured, only controlled.

■ ***PREVENTION.*** Preventing hypertensive heart disease is achieved by preventing or controlling hypertension.

RHEUMATIC HEART DISEASE

■ ***DESCRIPTION.*** Rheumatic heart disease refers to the cardiac symptoms related to rheumatic fever. Rheumatic fever was discussed in Chapter 5, "Immune System Diseases and Disorders," as an autoimmune disorder.

■ ***ETIOLOGY.*** Recall that rheumatic fever is commonly caused by a streptococcal throat infection. The immune system in a select group of individuals builds antibodies that attack the bacteria and the heart tissue. All layers of the heart might be affected, along with the valves of the heart.

■ ***SYMPTOMS.*** All the symptoms of rheumatic fever might be present, including joint pain and shortness of breath. Another symptom is valvular damage leading to stenosis (narrowing) of the mitral and aortic valves and then to heart murmurs.

■ ***DIAGNOSIS.*** A history of rheumatic fever along with a positive tropomyosin (a cardiac antibody) blood test is indicative of this disease. A chest X-ray showing an enlarged heart, lung congestion, and abnormal electrocardiogram are also positive indicators.

■ ***TREATMENT.*** Treatment is aimed at prevention and proper treatment of streptococcal infections. Valvular stenosis increases the workload of the heart and can cause further heart disease. During acute carditis, treatment includes bed rest, to reduce the workload on the heart, and other symptomatic treatment. Severe valve damage can lead to the need for valve surgery to correct the deformity or replace the valve.

■ ***PREVENTION.*** The best defense is to prevent rheumatic fever. Rapid diagnosis and proper antibiotic treatment can often prevent rheumatic fever from developing.

CONGESTIVE HEART FAILURE (CHF)

■ ***DESCRIPTION.*** CHF is a condition in which the heart fails to pump an adequate amount of blood to meet the body's needs. The cardiopulmonary and general vascular system gradually become congested.

■ ***ETIOLOGY.*** CHF develops slowly and usually follows any type of cardiac condition that increases the workload of the heart. Such diseases include MI, hypertension, CAD, and rheumatic heart disease, to name a few.

■ ***SYMPTOMS.*** The individual experiences a gradual increase in shortness of breath. Tachycardia (tachy = rapid, cardia = heart) and rapid breathing occur as the body tries to compensate for decreased blood flow. As CHF progresses, fluid builds up in the vascular system, leading to neck vein distention and edema in the ankles and lower legs. Right-sided heart failure leads to congestion of the liver and spleen. Left-sided failure leads to congestion and edema of the lungs (pulmonary edema) (Figure 8–17).

■ ***DIAGNOSIS.*** A history and physical examination, coupled with the symptoms of shortness of breath and edema, are enough for a basic diagnosis of CHF. Further testing includes chest X-ray to show enlargement of the heart, electrocardiogram to check for irregular heart rate, and echocardiogram to view valve function.

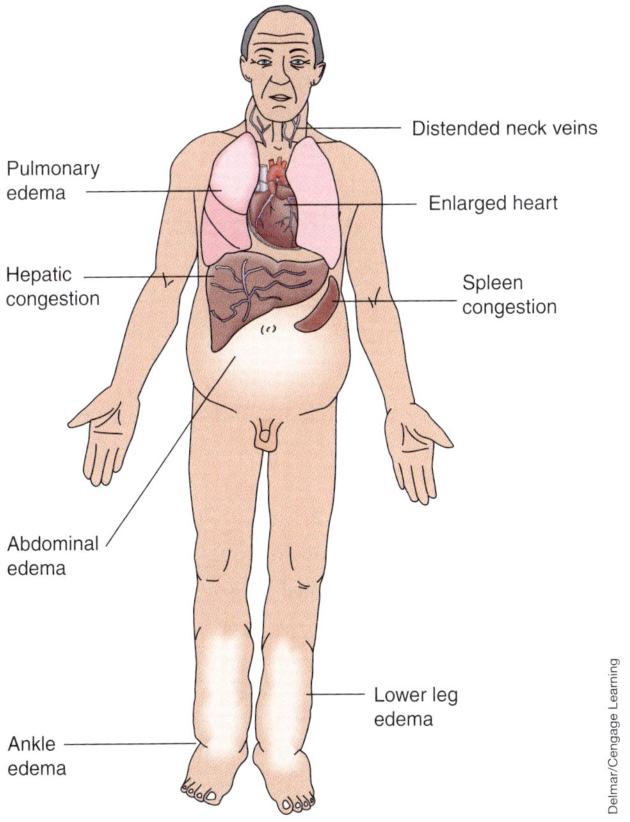

FIGURE 8–17 Signs of congestive heart failure.

■ ***TREATMENT.*** Treatment is aimed at decreasing the workload of the heart. Diuretic medications, low-salt diet, and fluid restrictions might be prescribed to increase urine output and limit fluid retention, thus reducing blood fluid volume. Cardiac medications, such as digitalis, can be prescribed to strengthen and slow the heartbeat.

■ ***PREVENTION.*** Adopting preventive lifestyle habits such as smoking cessation, weight control, diet modification, and regular exercise help prevent this disease.

> ***Study*WARE™ Connection**
>
> View an animation on congestive heart failure on your StudyWARE™ CD-ROM.

CARDIOMYOPATHY

■ ***DESCRIPTION.*** Cardiomyopathy (KAR-dee-oh-MY-OP-ah-thee; cardio = heart, myo = muscle, opathy = disease) literally is heart muscle disease. It is a deterioration of the function of the myocardium. Cardiomyopathy can be classified as primary or secondary.

■ ***ETIOLOGY.*** Primary cardiomyopathy is idiopathic, but a high number of cases are seen in association with alcoholism. Secondary cardiomyopathy is due to a specific cause often associated with other diseases. There are three main types of secondary cardiomyopathy: dilated, hypertrophic, and restrictive.

Dilated cardiomyopathy is the most common form. The heart is enlarged (dilated), is weak, and does not pump properly, leading to heart failure. Hypertrophic cardiomyopathy is inherited and characterized by heart muscle enlargement (hypertrophy), often causing the heart valves to leak. The least common type is restrictive cardiomyopathy, characterized by rigid muscle tissue, making it difficult for the heart to fill with blood. This type is usually seen in the elderly.

■ ***SYMPTOMS.*** Common symptoms for all types of cardiomyopathy include those associated with heart failure, including weakness, fatigue, shortness of breath, and swelling of the feet and legs.

■ ***DIAGNOSIS.*** Diagnosis of all types of cardiomyopathy is dependent on history and physical examination along with electrocardiogram and chest X-ray.

■ ***TREATMENT.*** Cardiomyopathies are incurable and often lead to CHF, MI, and death. Treatment is based on relieving symptoms and can include diuretic medications, heart medications, and change of lifestyle behaviors.

■ ***PREVENTION.*** Cardiomyopathy, in most cases, cannot be prevented. If diagnosed early, treatment can prevent worsening of the disease.

CARDITIS

■ ***DESCRIPTION.*** Carditis (kar-DYE-tis) is a general term describing inflammation of the heart. Forms of carditis include pericarditis, myocarditis, and endocarditis, depending on the area of the heart involved. Pericarditis affects the serous membrane on the outside of the heart as well as the pericardial sac. Myocarditis affects the heart muscle layer, and endocarditis affects the inside of the heart.

■ ***ETIOLOGY.*** All these inflammatory states can be due to unknown causes, bacteria, and viruses or as a result of rheumatic fever. Carditis is often secondary to a respiratory tract, urinary tract, or skin infection. It also can be related to dental infections or diseases of other systems.

■ ***SYMPTOMS.*** Symptoms vary, depending on the site and cause, but a common symptom includes varying degrees of chest pain.

■ ***DIAGNOSIS.*** Diagnosis is often difficult, but a thorough history and physical examination along with EKG, chest X-ray and blood cultures can be helpful.

■ ***TREATMENT.*** Treatment of carditis generally includes bed rest to decrease the workload on the heart. Other treatments depend on the cause of the disease and can include antibiotics, analgesics, and antipyretics (anti = against, pyro = heat, or against fever).

■ ***PREVENTION.*** Depending on cause, many of the cases of carditis are preventable with accurate diagnosis and treatment of the cause.

VALVULAR HEART DISEASE

■ ***DESCRIPTION.*** Valvular heart disease is related to malfunction of the heart valves. The purpose of a valve in the heart and the vascular system is to prevent backflow of blood. Backflow causes extra workload on the heart because the heart has to re-pump the blood.

■ ***ETIOLOGY.*** Common causes of valvular disease can be congenital anomalies or malformations, rheumatic fever, or endocarditis. Malfunction of a valve can be due to the valvular opening being too narrow (stenotic) or being too large to close properly (valvular insufficiency). Both of these problems can affect all the heart valves and lead to heart murmurs. A heart **murmur** is an abnormal sound in the heart or vascular system. One complication of all valve defects is the vascular tendency to form clots (thrombi) on the affected areas. If the thrombus breaks loose and becomes an embolus, it might occlude arteries leading to major organs such as the lungs, brain, liver, or kidneys. Another common problem of valvular heart disease is CHF due to the increased workload on the heart.

■ ***SYMPTOMS.*** Symptoms include chest pain, edema (swelling) in the ankles, heart palpitations, dizziness, and weakness. The severity of the symptoms might not reflect the severity of the disease. In other words, some individuals have severe symptoms with mild disease, whereas others with severe disease might have only mild symptoms.

■ ***DIAGNOSIS.*** Physical examination can reveal a murmur and lung congestion. Chest X-ray showing an enlarged heart and an EKG revealing arrhythmias are indicative of this disease.

■ ***TREATMENT.*** Treatment depends on the cause and severity of the disease. Minor problems might not require treatment, but those with serious disease can be treated successfully with medications. Typical medication treatments include anti-arrhythmics, antibiotics to prevent or treat infection, anticoagulants to prevent blood clot formation, and diuretics to assist in removal of excess fluid.

■ ***PREVENTION.*** Prevention is aimed at controlling heart disease by not smoking, eating a healthy diet, and daily exercise. Diseases caused by infection are prevented by quickly treating any infection. If medications are not effective, open heart surgery to repair or replace heart valves might be performed.

ARRHYTHMIAS

■ ***DIAGNOSIS.*** Arrhythmias (ah-RITH-me-ahs) are abnormalities in heart rhythm due to a disturbance in the conduction system of the heart.

■ ***ETIOLOGY.*** Often, the cause of these is unknown. Known causes include medications, ischemia of the heart muscle, and a previous MI. Auscultation and electrocardiography can diagnose arrhythmias.

■ ***SYMPTOMS.*** Normal heart rhythm is often called normal sinus rhythm and indicates that the rate is between 60 and 100 beats per minute, is regular, and is originating normally from the SA node. An unusually fast (up to 350 beats per minute) but regular heart rate is called flutter. If the rhythm is wild and uncoordinated, it is an arrhythmia called **fibrillation** (FIH-brih-LAY-shun). Fibrillations affect the atria or the ventricles. Atrial fibrillations are usually not serious in nature. However, ventricular fibrillations, commonly abbreviated as V fib, are serious cardiac arrhythmias that require emergency defibrillation by electrical shock.

Heart block is another group of arrhythmias caused by an interruption in the conduction system. Heart block is divided into first, second, and third degree, depending on the seriousness of the blockage. Third-degree block is treated with insertion of an artificial pacemaker.

Premature or early contractions can affect the atria or the ventricles. Premature ventricular contractions are commonly abbreviated as PVCs.

■ ***DIAGNOSIS.*** After physical examination, the first diagnostic test will usually include an EKG. If this shows an abnormal rhythm, the next step is often wearing a Holter monitor, a small portable EKG machine that performs a continuous monitor strip of the heart. An exercise stress test can also be useful in diagnosis.

■ ***TREATMENT.*** Treatment is usually unnecessary as long as the number of beats per minute is minimal and the individual is otherwise asymptomatic.

■ ***PREVENTION.*** Prevention is aimed at preventing heart disease in general with health lifestyle behaviors and by quickly treating any known heart disease.

StudyWARE™ Connection

View an animation on ventricular fibrillation on your StudyWARE™ CD-ROM.

DISEASES OF THE VEINS

Diseases of the veins are more common in older adults. Age-related changes in the vessels and valves, along with other changes in the circulatory system, contribute to the overall general weakness of the vessels. Fluid often pools in the extremities, causing edema. Disorders of the veins are usually more serious in individuals with other chronic disorders such as diabetes mellitus.

PHLEBITIS

■ ***DESCRIPTION.*** Phlebitis (fleh-BYE-tis; phlebo = vein, itis = inflammation) is relatively common, especially in the veins of the arms and lower legs. Phlebitis commonly refers to inflammation of superficial (near the skin surface) veins (Figure 8–18).

■ ***ETIOLOGY.*** The cause of phlebitis is often unknown, but known causes can include injury, obesity, poor circulation, prolonged bed rest, and infection. Injury to a vein is often a known cause of phlebitis. Intravenous medications and catheters can cause vein injury in the arms. Pooling of blood, as occurs with varicose veins or physical injury to the vessel, might lead to phlebitis in the legs.

■ ***SYMPTOMS.*** Symptoms of phlebitis include pain, swelling, and, often, the appearance of a red cord-like hardening that extends along the vein from the area of injury upward toward the heart. Occasionally,

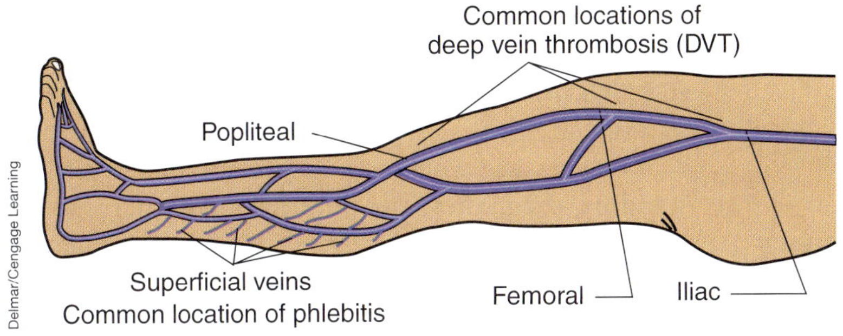

FIGURE 8–18 Superficial versus deep veins in development of phlebitis and thrombus.

phlebitis in the lower leg of the mother occurs after childbirth in association with the onset of milk production. This form of phlebitis is commonly called "milk leg."

■ ***DIAGNOSIS.*** Phlebitis is commonly diagnosed by physical examination of veins in the legs. An ultrasound is useful to determine the extent of the disease and to look for clots and blockage of blood flow.

■ ***TREATMENT.*** Treatment of superficial phlebitis often includes analgesics and warm compresses to reduce pain and improve circulation. Elevation of the area above heart level will improve venous return and decrease edema. To improve venous return in the lower extremities, the use of elastic or compression stockings and exercise can be prescribed.

■ ***PREVENTION.*** To prevent phlebitis, participate in moderate physical exercise to maintain circulation and muscle tone and avoid smoking and sitting for long periods of time.

THROMBOPHLEBITIS

A complication of phlebitis is the development of a clot in the inflamed vessel, a condition called thrombophlebitis. Clots in superficial veins rarely embolize (break loose and travel), but clots in deep veins often do, making this condition of serious concern in a deep vein. Thrombophlebitis in the deep veins is called deep vein thrombosis.

DEEP VEIN THROMBOSIS (DVT)

■ ***DESCRIPTION.*** DVT primarily occurs in the lower legs, thighs, and pelvis (see Figure 8–18). Clots occurring in the femoral and pelvic veins commonly embolize.

■ ***ETIOLOGY.*** Risk factors for DVT include:

- **Immobility** Early postoperative ambulation (walking) is encouraged. Prolonged bed rest greatly increases risk.
- **Dehydration** Dehydration increases blood viscosity (thickness) and increases risk of thrombus formation.
- **Varicose veins** Veins already weakened with disease are more likely to develop a thrombus.
- **Leg or pelvic surgery, obesity, and pregnancy** These conditions alter venous blood flow and increase risk.

■ ***SYMPTOMS.*** These clots are generally asymptomatic until embolization occurs, often causing a pulmonary embolism. Pulmonary embolism is often fatal.

■ ***DIAGNOSIS.*** A positive Homan's test is very commonly performed as an initial indication of DVT. Homan's is performed by pulling the toes toward the knee; a positive test will cause pain in the posterior calf. If squeezing the posterior calf also elicits pain, this indicative of DVT and is called a Pratt's sign. Ultrasonography, or ultrasound imaging of the veins, is the most widely used test to evaluate the disease.

■ ***TREATMENT.*** Treatment of DVT is aimed at reducing the formation of more clots and preventing embolization. Bed rest with elevation of the affected area is essential to improve blood flow. Anticoagulants are given to decrease potential thrombus formation; they will not dissolve clots, only prevent formation of new ones.

■ ***PREVENTION.*** Prevention is aimed at healthy lifestyle behaviors, including maintaining proper body weight, exercising, and not smoking. Wearing graduated elastic compression stockings during times of prolonged standing or sitting is also a preventive measure.

VARICOSE VEINS

■ ***DESCRIPTION.*** Varicose veins (VAR-ih-kohs VAYNS) are dilated, tortuous, and elongated veins commonly found in the legs. Blood in the legs must move upward against the pull of gravity. Leg muscles are primarily responsible for this movement by contracting and relaxing. This action pushes against the vessel wall and pushes blood upward. Valves are necessary to prevent backflow of blood. With varicose veins, the flow of blood is slowed, collects in the veins, or both, causing increased pressure on the vessel walls and the valves and eventually leading to incompetent valves (Figure 8–19). Prolonged pooling of blood in the veins stretches the vessel wall and leads to the formation of varicosities.

■ ***ETIOLOGY.*** Development of varicosities can be due to any activity that slows return flow and increases venous pressure. Such activities as prolonged sitting, standing, pregnancy, and obesity tend to increase the risk of developing varicose veins. Heredity also plays a part in this disorder; there appears to be an inherited vessel wall weakness.

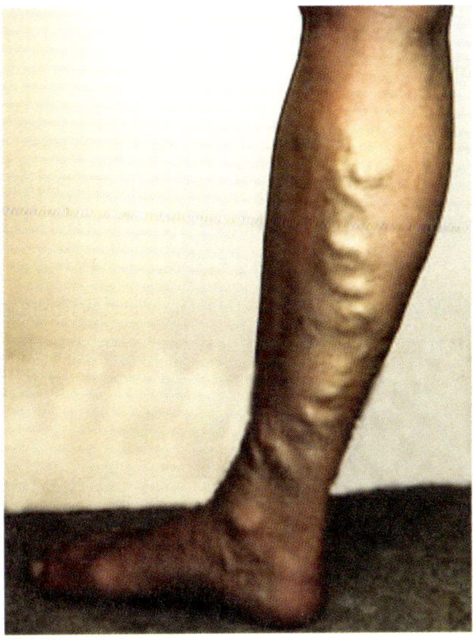

FIGURE 8–19 Varicose veins.

■ ***SYMPTOMS.*** Varicose veins develop gradually. Initial symptoms might include leg fatigue and leg cramps, and veins often become thick, hardened, and unsightly. Poor venous blood flow causes edema and congestion of fluid in the extremities. This congestion slows arterial flow, leading to stasis dermatitis and ulceration. Stasis dermatitis is characterized by edema, dry and scaly skin, and small pinpoint hemorrhages. The skin also turns brown in color as blood pigment accumulates in the connective tissue. Stasis ulcers do not heal well and can necessitate amputation of the affected area.

■ ***DIAGNOSIS.*** Simply looking at the veins in the legs is often enough for a simple diagnosis. A Doppler ultrasound to evaluate blood flow can provide a more definitive diagnosis.

■ ***TREATMENT.*** Treatment includes improving vascular flow by elevating legs, walking, and using support or elastic hose. Surgery might be indicated to relieve discomfort and avoid recurrent thrombosis. Surgical treatment involves tying off the vessel and removing it, a procedure commonly called vein stripping. There are numerous superficial veins, so blood return to the heart from this area is through alternate venous routes.

■ ***PREVENTION.*** Wearing compression stockings, regularly elevating the legs above heart level, avoiding prolonged standing or sitting, controlling weight, and not smoking are activities that help prevent varicose veins.

TRAUMA

Hemorrhage

■ ***DESCRIPTION.*** Hemorrhage (hemo = blood, orrhage = burst forth) is an abnormal loss of blood. Hemorrhagic blood loss can be external or internal, and blood loss can be acute (sudden onset) or chronic.

■ ***ETIOLOGY.*** Acute blood loss is usually related to trauma, whereas chronic loss is more often related to disease processes.

External and internal blood loss, if severe enough, can lead to **exsanguination** (loss of circulating blood volume) and death. Internal blood loss can cause filling of body cavities such as **hemothorax** (hemo = blood, thorax = chest, blood in the chest cavity). Internal bleeding might not be noticeable until a large amount of blood has been lost and the individual begins to show signs and symptoms of shock.

■ ***SYMPTOMS.*** Hemorrhage can affect different vessels and have varying results. Hemorrhage of low-pressure vessels (the capillaries and veins) into the tissues leads to reddish to dark-purple spots on the skin and mucosa. These discolorations are called petechiae, ecchymosis, or purpura, depending on the size or cause of the discoloration. Petechiae (pee-TEE-kee-ee) are pinpoint hemorrhages. Ecchymosis (ECK-ih-MOH-sis) is a larger area of purplish color commonly called a bruise. Purpura (PUR-pew-rah) is spontaneous bleeding into the tissues related to a hemorrhagic disease that might be characterized by both petechiae and ecchymosis. Hemorrhage of the high-pressure vessels (the arteries) leads to forceful squirting of bright red (highly oxygenated) blood. The squirting of arterial blood is directly related to the beat of the heart.

Large venous and arterial hemorrhages, if not controlled, can be fatal. Blood volume varies with body size; the average adult has about 5 liters (approximately 5 quarts) of blood. Adults may lose approximately 500 ml (approximately 1 pint) of blood without any problems. This amount is equal to the amount given during a blood donation. Loss of 1 liter of blood, however, can result in hypovolemic shock. Greater losses, 1,500 ml or more, are usually lethal. Hemorrhaging in a closed cavity also can cause organ damage due to increased pressure. For example, bleeding in the head can lead to brain tissue damage or death from the resulting increase in intracranial pressure.

Chronic hemorrhages, such as those occurring in the gastrointestinal tract and female reproductive tract, commonly lead to anemia. Normal menstrual bleeding is approximately 70–80 ml. As discussed in Chapter 7, "Blood and Blood-Forming Organs Diseases and Disorders," replacement of the lost iron also can lead to iron deficiency anemia.

■ ***DIAGNOSIS.*** Hemorrhage is often diagnosed by a complete blood count revealing a low hemoglobin count and hematocrit. Although external hemorrhage is easy to recognize, determining the location of internal bleeding is much more difficult. Stool testing can help determine bleeding in the gastrointestinal tract. A CT scan might be needed to determine the location of internal sites.

■ ***TREATMENT.*** Treatment is focused on stopping the bleeding and replacing the blood volume, if needed, with blood transfusions.

■ ***PREVENTION.*** Although not all hemorrhages can be prevented, avoiding the causes of hemorrhage will prevent many of the occurrences.

Shock

■ ***DESCRIPTON.*** Shock can be defined in many ways, but basically, it is extremely low blood pressure that leads to decreased tissue **perfusion** (to pour through or supply with blood).

■ ***ETIOLOGY.*** This low blood pressure can be caused by one of three mechanisms:

- Not enough blood volume
- Inadequate pumping of blood by the heart
- Vasodilatation that allows blood to pool in the vessels, thereby reducing circulating blood volume

Remember, the vascular system is composed of thousands of miles of vessels. If all these vessels were to open at the same time, the circulating volume of blood would be zero.

Shock can be caused by a variety of situations. Every injury brings about some degree of shock and should be treated appropriately. No matter the cause, shock leads to inadequate perfusion of tissues with blood. Inadequate perfusion can cause tissue hypoxia, anoxia, ischemia, and necrosis as discussed in Chapter 2, "Mechanisms of Disease." Types of shock include:

- **Cardiogenic shock** The leading cause of death due to shock. This type of shock results from the inability of the heart to pump blood adequately, often due to MI. Treatment can involve CPR and administration of cardiotonic and vasoconstrictor medications. (Vasoconstrictor medications cause muscle contraction of vessels, increasing blood pressure.)
- **Septic shock** The second most common cause of death due to shock. Septic shock usually results from an overwhelming septicemia (bacteria or microorganisms in the blood). Treatment can involve administration of antibiotics and vasoconstrictor medications.
- **Hypovolemic shock** Results from low fluid volume and can be due to hemorrhage (often called hemorrhagic shock), severe burns leading to loss of blood plasma, severe vomiting, and diarrhea. Treatment can involve blood transfusions and intravenous fluid volume replacement.
- **Neurogenic shock** Results from generalized vasodilatation and can be due to highly emotional situations such as fear, surprise, pain, and unpleasant sights. Medications and spinal anesthesia also can lead to neurogenic shock. Treatment can involve vasoconstrictor medications.
- **Anaphylactic shock** Results from severe allergic reactions and might be due to allergens such as contrast dyes for diagnostic tests, bee stings, medications, and blood transfusion reaction. Treatment can involve removing the allergen and administering antihistamines and bronchodilators.

■ ***SYMPTOMS.*** Signs and symptoms of shock vary, depending on the degree of the situation, and can include facial pallor, cool and clammy skin, cyanosis, tachycardia, tachypnea, altered mental status, syncope (fainting), unconsciousness, oliguria, and anuria.

■ ***DIAGNOSIS.*** Diagnosis is most often established through a thorough medical history and physical exam. Blood pressure less than 90/50 is recognized as shock.

■ ***TREATMENT.*** Treatment depends on the type of shock. Other treatment measures include laying the individual in a supine (on the back) position, keeping the individual warm and quiet, and elevating the feet and legs above heart level to improve vascular return.

■ ***PREVENTION.*** Preventing the conditions that cause shock is the best way to prevent it. Monitoring and managing these conditions can prevent progression of symptoms thus prevent shock.

RARE DISEASES

Malignant Hypertension

Malignant hypertension is a form of essential hypertension that is considered a medical emergency. Diastolic blood pressure can reach 130–170 mm Hg. Symptoms include headache, blurred vision, and dyspnea. Without treatment, malignant hypertension is fatal.

Cor Pulmonale

Cor pulmonale is right-sided heart failure related to acute or chronic pulmonary disease. Increased pulmonary blood pressure causes hypertrophy of the right ventricle, leading to decreased pumping ability. Polycythemia develops as the body tries to compensate for hypoxemia. This increase in red blood cell number increases the viscosity of the blood, further increasing workload on the heart. Treatment involves treating the lung disease and can also include phlebotomy to decrease blood viscosity.

Raynaud's Disease

Raynaud's disease is a vasospastic disorder primarily affecting the fingers and toes. This idiopathic disease occurs most frequently in young women and is usually related to cold temperature and emotional stress. During vasospasm, the extremities can turn pale and then cyanotic before returning to normal color. As the disease progresses, small ulcers might develop on the extremities and can lead to contractures and chronic disability of the hands. Treatment is avoidance of cold and application of warmth to the extremities. Cigarette smoking is discouraged because nicotine causes further vasoconstriction.

Buerger's Disease

Buerger's disease is also known as thromboangiitis (thrombo = clot, angi = vessel, itis = inflammation) obliterans and is an inflammation of the peripheral vessels with clot formation. The affected individual often has pain in the legs and feet that is made worse with activity and improves with rest. Progression of the disease leads to muscle atrophy, ulcers, and gangrene. The primary cause of Buerger's disease is cigarette smoking. Treatment involves cessation of smoking, exercises to improve circulation, and vessel bypass surgery.

Polyarteritis Nodosa

Polyarteritis nodosa is a vasculitis that is characterized by inflammatory, necrotizing lesions in many vessels. This rare autoimmune disease is usually fatal as a result of occlusion and rupture of the involved vessels.

EFFECTS OF AGING ON THE SYSTEM

Heart and blood vessel diseases are a significant cause of death and disability in the older adult. As the individual ages, the heart muscle loses some of its contractility, causing a decreased cardiac output, an increased heart rate to compensate for the changes, or both. The vessels lose elasticity and become more rigid and narrowed. The valves also lose some functioning and become thick and sclerotic. These changes add to the workload of the heart by increasing the heart rate and the blood pressure, and the older adult can become tachycardic with minimal exercise. Although many of the changes in the system are due to the normal aging process, other changes observed in the older adult are directly due to lifestyle. Many individuals have smoked for years, been overweight, eaten a high-fat diet, endured a stressful job, and lived a fairly sedentary life. These modifiable behaviors contribute to the adverse changes in the cardiovascular system and increase the risk of chronic and acute problems in the system over time. Most older adults are at risk for hypertension, MI, angina, arrhythmias, CHF, varicosities, and other cardiovascular problems.

With age, the arteries become more rigid, causing decreased blood flow to organs and distal body tissues. The vein valves lose some of their competency, reducing good blood flow even further. Decreased peripheral circulation often results in cool or pale extremities, improper healing, and pooling of fluid

GLIMPSE OF THE FUTURE

New Drugs for Treating Hypertension

There are many research projects now studying the effects of various new drugs for treating hypertension. The hope is to develop new and more effective cardiac therapies. The new drugs are formulated differently than the ones most commonly used at this time. These new drugs have an entirely different mechanism of action in the body. The goal is to improve the effectiveness of the medication with fewer side effects. Aggressive new treatments and drug combinations might be recommended in the near future. These drug therapies will have greater potential for keeping the patient's blood pressure at normal limits.

Source: Balsamo, et al. (2008).

(edema) in the legs and feet. Medications might not be as efficiently transmitted to the body with these changes in circulation, which can affect the therapeutic regimen for the individual.

Many older adults have postural hypotension, which can be a significant safety problem. Postural hypotension is the decrease or drop in blood pressure that occurs when the individual rises to a sitting or standing position from a reclining position. The individual usually feels very dizzy on rising and might fall. Prevention strategies should be in place to prevent injuries from postural hypotension.

SUMMARY

The cardiovascular system is responsible for pumping the blood throughout the body, delivering nutrients and oxygen to cells, and removing waste products. CVD affects over 64 million Americans. It is a significant cause of mortality, especially in the older adult. The risk for developing many diseases of the system can be reduced by lifestyle behavioral changes. Common symptoms of CVD include pain, fatigue, difficulty breathing, tachycardia, cyanosis, and edema. Some of the most common disorders of the system include hypertension, CAD, arteriosclerosis, and varicosities. Older adults are at greatest risk for developing heart disease, the number one cause of death in the older population.

REVIEW QUESTIONS

Multiple Choice

1. Which of the following risk factors are controllable or modifiable?
   - **a.** Heredity
   - **b.** Diet
   - **c.** Age
   - **d.** Stress
   - **e.** Smoking
   - **f.** Exercise

2. Which of the following statements are correct in relation to CAD?
   a. It is often called coronary heart disease.
   b. Slow, progressive occlusion of arteries often leads to development of collateral arteries that extend into ischemic tissue, providing some protection against infarction.
   c. It will always lead to a MI.
   d. Diagnosis of CAD is made by evaluating the history, EKG, and angiograms.
   e. CAD is not usually diagnosed in the older adult.
   f. The disease is commonly due to atherosclerosis.

3. Define the following terms related to hemorrhage.
   a. Petechiae
   b. Ecchymosis
   c. Purpura

Short Answer

4. What are the functions of the cardiovascular system?

5. Which signs and symptoms are associated with common cardiovascular system disorders?

6. Which diagnostic tests are most commonly used to determine the type, cause, or both of cardiovascular system disorders?

7. What symptoms are usually seen in CHF?

8. What is the difference between phlebitis and thrombophlebitis?

9. What are the most common signs and symptoms of shock?

10. What are some of the changes that occur in the cardiovascular system with age?

CASE STUDIES

■ Mr. Winston is a 72-year-old who has been diagnosed with CHF. He is a middle-class gentleman with a fairly broad educational background. He is a college graduate who has managed a business for 30 years. He asks you to explain his condition to him and his wife. How would you explain CHF to them? In addition, he wants to know why he is so short of breath at times, why he has edema in his ankles in the evenings, and why the physician ordered a low-sodium diet. How would you answer those questions?

■ Mrs. Marconi is a 68-year-old retired woman who volunteers 3 days per week at the hospital. A group of nursing students from the local college were holding a health fair and invited her to participate. One station was set up to check the ankle-brachial index (ABI) on the participants. Mrs. Marconi asked the students to explain what an ABI is and why she needs this test. How would you answer this question? Describe how the test is done. When should someone be referred for further testing after having the ABI checked?

*Study*WARE™ Connection

To help you learn the content in this chapter, take a practice quiz or play an interactive game on your StudyWARE™ CD-ROM.

Workbook Practice

Go to your Workbook and complete the practice questions.

BIBLIOGRAPHY

Albert, N. M. (2007). Heart failure with preserved systolic function. *Critical Care Nursing Quarterly 30*(4), 287–298.

Alcalai, R., Seidman, J. G., & Seidman, C. E. (2008). Genetic basis of cardiomyopathy: From bench to clinics. *Journal of Cardiovascular Electrophysiology 19*(1), 104–110.

American Heart Association. (2005). Cardiovascular disease statistics. American Heart Association. *www.*Americanheart .org (accessed May 2008).

American Heart Association. (2008). Diseases and conditions. American Heart Association. *www.Americanheart .org* (accessed May 2008).

Artinian, N. (2007). Effects of nurse-managed telemonitoring on blood pressure at 12-month follow-up among urban African-Americans. *Nursing Research 56*(5), 312–322.

Assessing leg ulcers. (2007). *Nursing Standard 22* (14–16), 59.

Ayer, J., Almafragy, H. S., Anushka, A., Hellyer, R. L., & Clelrmajer, D. S. (2008). Body mass index is an independent determinant of left atrial size. *Heart, Lung & Circulation 17*(1), 19–24.

Backris, G., Hill, M., Mancia, G., Steyn, K., Black, H. R., Pickering, T., DeGeest, S., Ruilope, L., Giles, T. D., Morgan, T., Kjeldsen, S., Schiffrin, E. L., Coenen, A., Mulrow, P., Loh, A., & Mensah, G. (2008). *Journal of Human Hypertension 22*(1), 63–70.

Balsamo, A., Calderone, V., & Rapposelli, S. (2008). New emerging prospects in the pharmacotherapy of hypertension. *Cardiovascular & Hematological Agents in Medicinal Chemistry 6*(1), 1–19.

Chen, E. H., & Hollander, J. E. (2007). When do patients need admission to a telemetry bed? *Journal of Emergency Medicine 33*(1), 53–60.

Cork, A. (2007). Theory and practice of manual blood pressure measurement. *Nursing Standard 22*(14–16), 47–50.

Covelli, M. M. (2007). Prevalence of behavioral and physiological risk factors of hypertension in African-American adolescents. *Pediatric Nursing 33*(4), 323–332.

Doering, L. V., Cross, R., Vredevoe, D., Martinez-maza, O., & Cowan, M. J. (2007). Infection, depression, and immunity in women after coronary artery bypass: A pilot study of cognitive behavioral therapy. *Alternative Therapies in Health & Medicine 13*(3), 18–21.

DVT threatens both legs. (2007). *Nursing 37*(9), 34.

Energy drinks may pose risks for people with high BP and heat disease. (2008). *Journal of Cardiovascular Nurisng 23*(1), 2.

Fink, A. M. (2006). Endocarditis after valve replacement surgery. *American Journal of Nursing 106*(2), 40–51.

Gardetto, N. J., & Carroll, K. C. (2007). Management strategies to meet the core heart failure measures for acute decompensated heart failure. *Critical Care Nursing Quarterly 30*(4), 307–320.

Herb at a glance: Grape seed extract. (2007). *Nursing 37*(10), 29.

Iqbal M. B., Fisher, N. G., Lyne, J. C., & McDonagh, T. A. (2008). Thiazolinediones and heart failure: The potential to precipitate irreversible cardiac dysfunction. *International Journal of Cardiology 123*(2), 35–37.

Kelechi, T. J., & Michel, Y. (2007). A descriptive study of skin temperatures, tissue perfusion, and tissue oxygen in patients with chronic venous disease. *Biological Research for Nursing 9*(1), 70–80.

Mackin, P. (2008). Cardiac side effects of psychiatric drugs. *Human Psychopharmacology: Clinical & Experimental 23*(S1), S3–S14.

Male, S., Coull, A., & Murphy-Black, T. (2007). Preliminary study to investigate the normal range of ankle-brachial pressure index in young adults. *Journal of Clinical Nursing 16*(10), 1878–1885.

Nemer, M. (2008). Genetic insights into normal and abnormal heart development. *Cardiovascular Pathology 17*(1), 48–54.

Older people who are active fare better after angioplasty. (2007). *Nursing Standard 22*(2), 15.

Putney, L. J. (2007). Bloodless cardiac surgery. *Critical Care Nursing Quarterly 30*(3), 263–270.

Radiological Society of North America, Inc. (RSNA). Positron emission topography (PET) imaging. (2008). *www.radiologyinfo.org* (accessed May 2008).

Rupert, R. A. (2007). Superior vena cava syndrome. *American Journal of Nursing 107*(10), 72C–72G.

Wang, Y., & Streicher, J. M. (2008). The role of COX-2 in heart pathology. *Cardiovascular & Hematological Agents in Medicinal Chemistry 6*(1), 69–79.

WebMD Medical Reference from Healthwise. Hypertension and high blood pressure. *www.webmd.com* (accessed May 2008).

Whitson, B. A., Heddleston, S. J., Savik, K., & Shumway, S. J. (2007). Bloodless cardiac surgery is associated with decreased morbidity and mortality. *Journal of Cardiac Surgery 22*(5), 373–378.

Women who eat whole grains reduce risk of high blood pressure. (2007). *Nursing Standard 22*(7), 19.

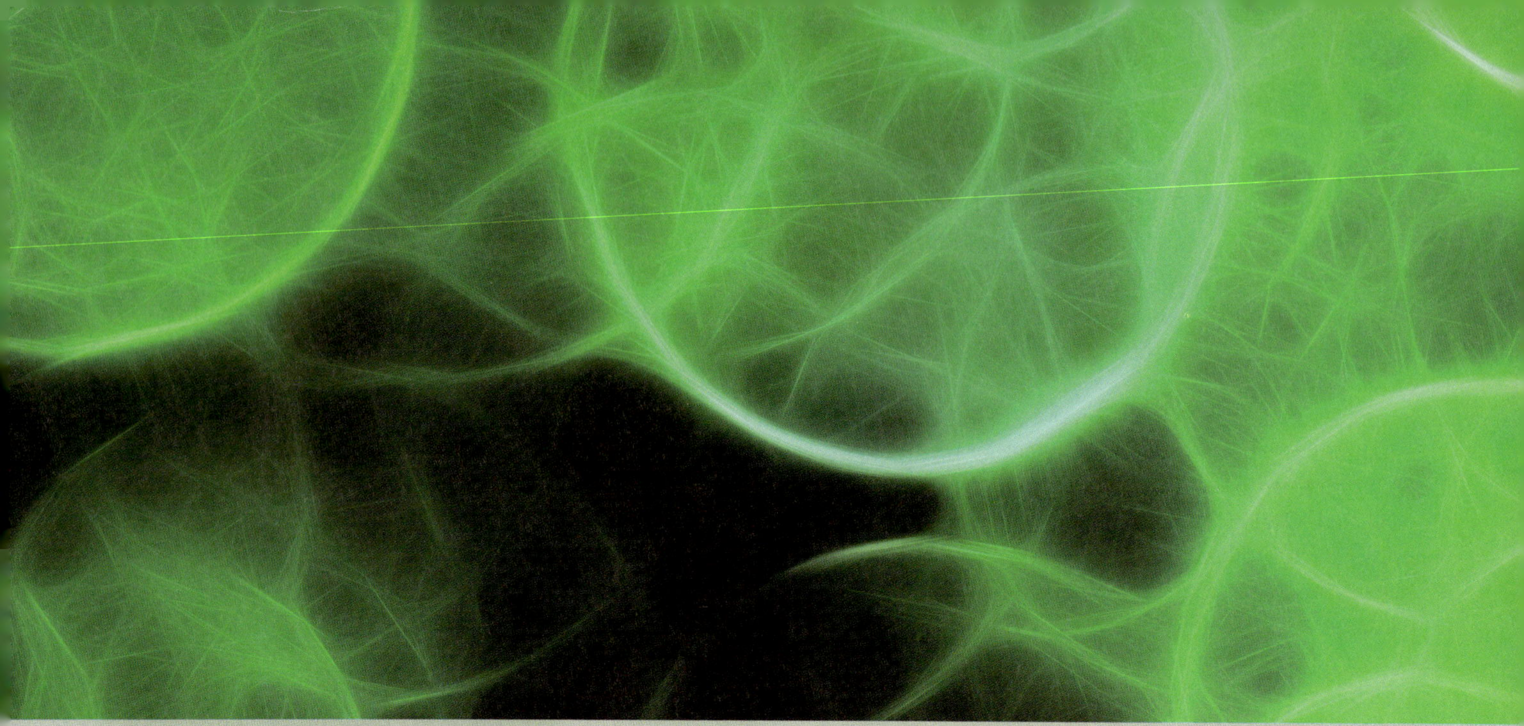

OUTLINE

- Anatomy and Physiology
- Common Signs and Symptoms
- Diagnostic Tests
- Common Diseases of the Respiratory System
  Diseases of the Upper Respiratory Tract
  Diseases of the Bronchi and Lungs
  Diseases of the Pleura and Chest
  Diseases of the Cardiovascular and Respiratory Systems
- Trauma
  Pneumothorax and Hemothorax
  Suffocation
- Rare Diseases
  Pneumoconiosis
  Fungal Diseases
  Legionnaires' Disease
- Effects of Aging on the System
- Summary
- Review Questions
- Case Studies
- Bibliograhy

KEY TERMS

Analgesics (p. 180)
Antipyretics (p. 180)
Apnea (p. 177)
Arterial blood gases (p. 179)
Bronchiectasis (p. 185)
Bronchoscopy (p. 179)
Clubbing (p. 178)
Cyanosis (p. 177)
Dyspnea (p. 177)
Hemoptysis (p. 177)
Hypoxemia (p. 177)
Hypoxia (p. 185)
Orthopnea (p. 177)
Productive cough (p. 177)
Rales (p. 179)
Rhinorrhea (p. 181)
Rhonchi (p. 179)
Sputum (p. 177)
Tachypnea (p. 178)
Thoracentesis (p. 192)
Wheezing (p. 177)

9

Respiratory System Diseases and Disorders

LEARNING OBJECTIVES

Upon completion of the chapter, the learner should be able to:

1. Define the terminology common to the respiratory system and the disorders of the system.
2. Discuss the basic anatomy and physiology of the respiratory system.
3. Identify the important signs and symptoms associated with common respiratory system disorders.
4. Describe the common diagnostics used to determine type and cause of the respiratory system disorders.
5. Identify the common disorders of the respiratory system.
6. Describe the typical course and management of the common respiratory system disorders.
7. Describe the effects of aging on the respiratory system and the common disorders associated with aging of the system.

OVERVIEW

The respiratory system includes the chest, lungs, and internal airway structures. To maintain life, the individual must breathe and have a continuous exchange of oxygen for carbon dioxide. Breathing and the exchange of gases that takes place within the system are complex processes involving the respiratory system as well as the neurological and circulatory systems. Diseases of the respiratory system include some of the most well-known disorders such as the common cold, pneumonia, and influenza. Public health officials are worried about new strains of influenza becoming widespread. Respiratory diseases affect all ages, but older people are the most susceptible to both chronic and acute disorders of the system. ■

ANATOMY AND PHYSIOLOGY

The respiratory system consists of the chest (thorax), lungs, and conducting airways. The chest, or thorax, is the structure that houses the lungs and the mediastinum (heart and major vessels). The respiratory system structures in the thorax include the lungs, 12 pairs of ribs, part of the vertebral column, and the sternum. The diaphragm, a large muscle of respiration, separates the thorax from the abdomen (Figure 9–1). The lungs are two spongy organs divided into three lobes in the right lung and two lobes in the left lung. They lie in the pleural cavity, which is lined with a membrane called the pleura, in the thorax. The lungs are also covered with a second membrane or pleura. Between the two pleural membranes is a lubricating liquid that prevents friction as the process of breathing and lung expansion occurs.

Usually, the airways of the respiratory system are divided into two parts. The upper respiratory system includes the nose (nasal cavities), mouth, sinuses, pharynx, and larynx. The lower respiratory system includes the trachea, bronchi, and bronchioles. The alveoli, grape-like clusters of air sacs that are surrounded by capillaries (Figure 9–2), are found at the distal end of the terminal bronchioles. This is where the oxygen–carbon dioxide gas exchange in the lungs occurs.

The mechanism of ventilation, the movement of air into and out of the respiratory system, and gas exchange is a complex process that requires both inhalation and exhalation to occur. Ventilation is controlled by chemosensory receptors in spinal fluid and by arterial carbon dioxide tension and oxygen deficiency in the carotid and aortic arteries. As the receptors detect increases or decreases in carbon dioxide, oxygen, or both, ventilation is increased or decreased as needed to meet body requirements. Because the respiratory control center is located in the medulla of the brain, this process can be altered by respiratory or neurologic disease.

The exchange of gases occurs both in the lungs and throughout the body at the tissue level. In the lungs, carbon dioxide is released from the capillary beds into the alveolar spaces by the process of diffusion. In the same way, oxygen moves from the air spaces into the capillaries for transport to the tissues. This process is reversed at the tissue level throughout

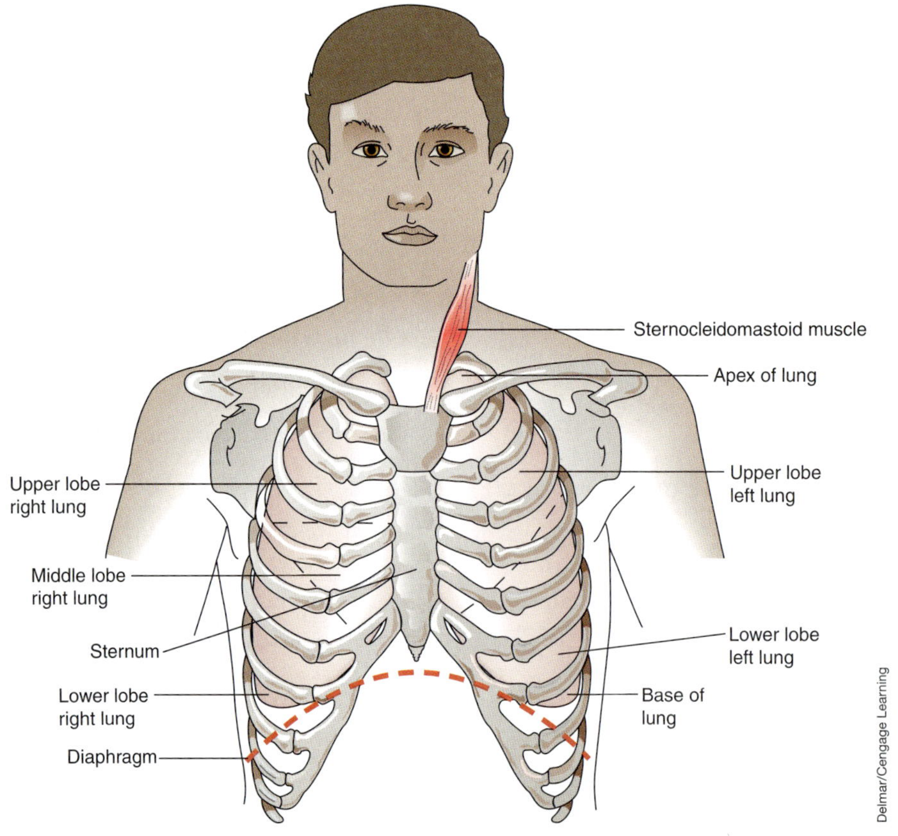

FIGURE 9–1 The respiratory system.

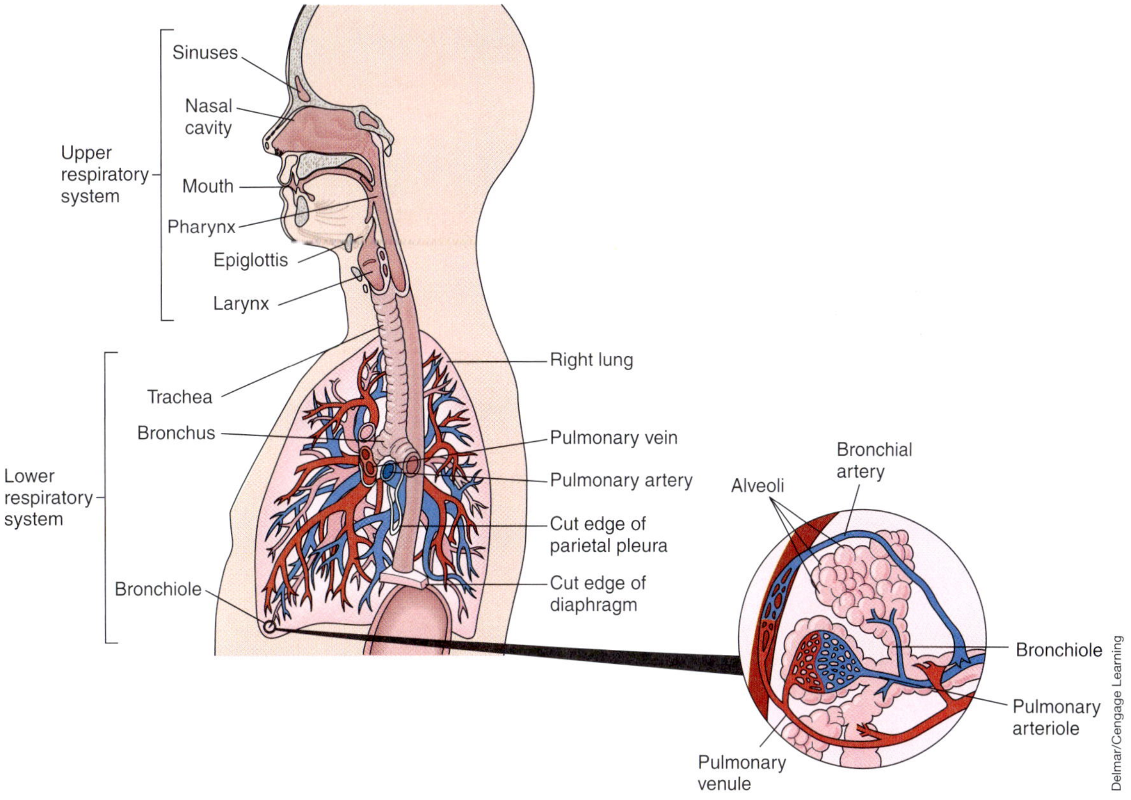

FIGURE 9–2 Airway divisions and terminal bronchiole/alveoli.

the body, where oxygen moves from the bloodstream into the tissues, and carbon dioxide moves from the tissues into the blood for transport to the lungs and removal from the body (Figure 9–3).

StudyWARE™ Connection

View an animation on respiration on your StudyWARE™ CD-ROM.

COMMON SIGNS AND SYMPTOMS

There are many common signs and symptoms of respiratory disease, ranging from mild (the common cold) to severe (pneumonia). Dyspnea, orthopnea, apnea, wheezing, coughing, and nasal discharge are some of the most common symptoms.

Dyspnea (DISP-nee-ah; dys = difficulty, pnea = breathing) is a common sign of respiratory disease. It can be in the form of **orthopnea** (or-THOP-nee-ah; ortho = straight, pnea = breathing), in which an individual has difficulty breathing in a lying position or is able to breathe with less difficulty when standing or sitting straight up. **Apnea** (ap-NEE-ah; a = without, pnea = breathing) for an extended length of time is a life-threatening emergency. Dyspnea caused by a partial obstruction of the airways will produce **wheezing**. Severe dyspnea can lead to **hypoxemia** (high-POX-SEE-me-ah; hypo = not enough, ox = oxygen, emia = blood), low blood oxygen level. A common sign of hypoxemia is **cyanosis** (SIGH-ah-NO-sis; cyano = blue, osis = condition), a blue color often observed in the nail beds and lips.

Coughing is another common symptom, caused by irritation of the airways or a buildup of fluid in the lung tissue. **Sputum** (SPYOU-tum) is fluid or secretions coughed up from the lungs, not to be confused with saliva or spit from the digestive system. A **productive cough** is one in which sputum or excessive mucus is brought up and expelled. Coughing up blood is called **hemoptysis** (he-MOP-tih-sis; hemo = blood, ptysis = saliva) and can be a sign of serious respiratory disease.

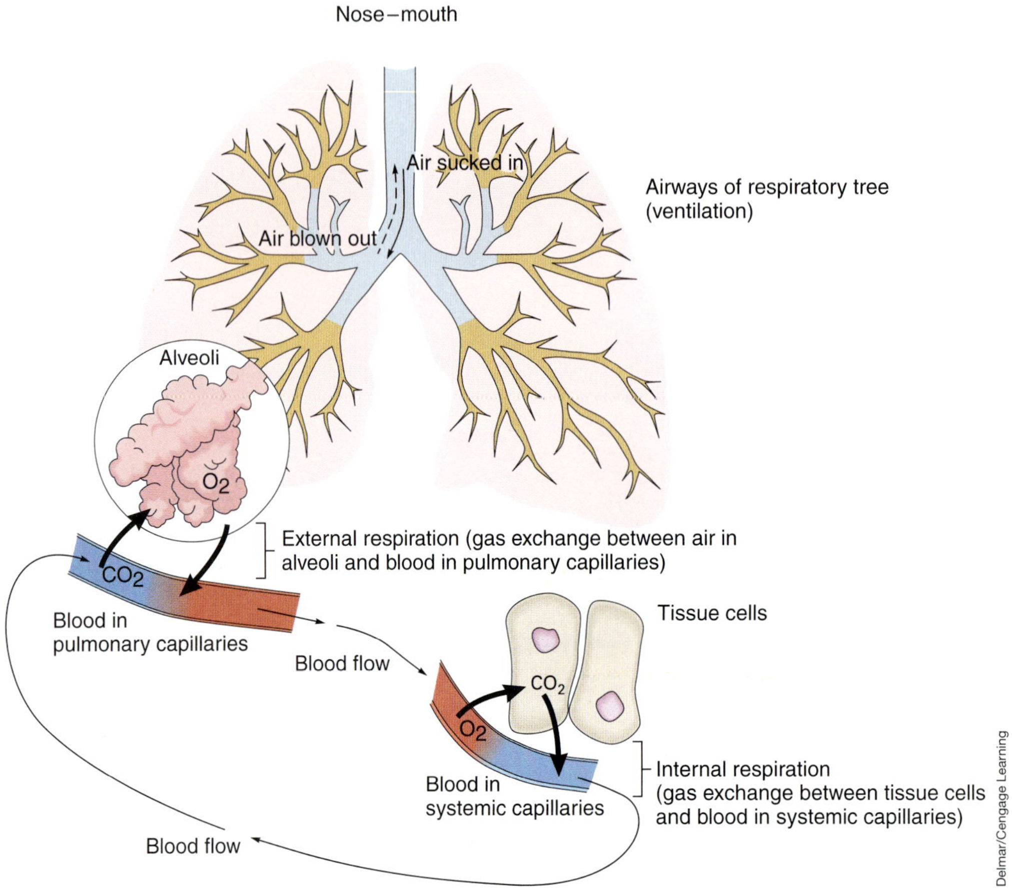

FIGURE 9–3 Gas exchange in the lungs and tissues.

Nasal discharge is frequently present in infections, inflammation, and allergic respiratory reactions. It is the most frequent symptom of the common cold, but it is also present in other respiratory disorders and can be a serious symptom of a chronic problem.

Hiccoughs, commonly called hiccups, are the result of a sudden spasm of the diaphragm. They commonly occur after eating or drinking and can be stopped by a variety of techniques, including holding the breath and drinking water through a straw. Hiccoughs might accompany disease and, in such an instance, are more difficult to eliminate.

Chronic respiratory conditions often lead to abnormal, permanent signs such as clubbing and barrel-chested appearance. **Clubbing** is a condition of unknown pathogenesis, but it usually is related to poor distal circulation and oxygenation. It affects the distal portion of the fingers and is characterized by soft tissue enlargement and an abnormal curvature of the nail (Figure 9–4). A barrel chest appears because the individual uses accessory chest muscles over a long period of time in an effort to improve breathing.

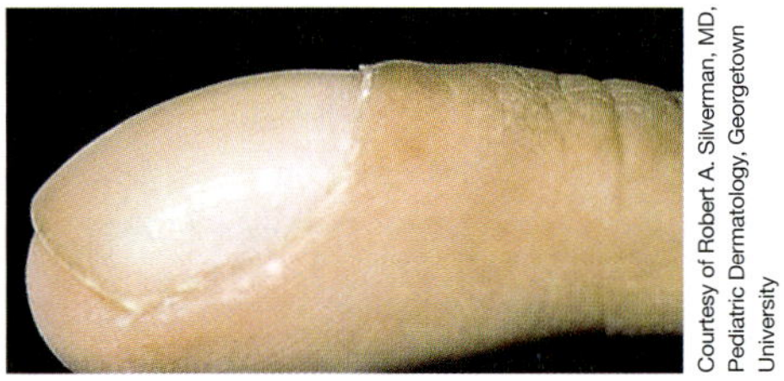

FIGURE 9–4 Clubbing.

DIAGNOSTIC TESTS

A physical examination including auscultation (listening to the chest with a stethoscope) should be completed to assess for abnormal breathing quality and rate. **Tachypnea** (TACK-ihp-NEE-ah; tachy = rapid, pnea = breathing), or rapid breathing, and abnormal breath sounds, including wheezes, rales, and rhonchi, are common with respiratory diseases. **Rales** are abnormal musical sounds heard on inspiration and are often called crackles. **Rhonchi** are dry rattling sounds in the bronchi due to obstruction of the airways.

A chest roentgenogram (X-ray) is a major diagnostic tool used to diagnose lung diseases such as tumors, tuberculosis, abscesses, and pneumonia. Sputum cultures are effective in determination of infectious disease. A tissue biopsy can be obtained as a definitive test for lung disease. Tissue biopsy is often obtained during a **bronchoscopy** (brong-KOS-koh-pee; broncho = bronchus or lung passageways, oscopy = procedure to look into the bronchus) (Figure 9–5). Lung tissue can be biopsied by using a fine-needle technique.

The best indicator of lung function is measurement of the amounts of carbon dioxide (waste) and oxygen in the blood. These measurements are done on arterial blood and are called **arterial blood gases (ABGs)**. Normal arterial blood gases should be high in oxygen and low in carbon dioxide. Parameters for normal ABGs are oxygen (PaO_2) 70–100 mm Hg and carbon dioxide ($PaCO_2$) 35–45 mm Hg. The reverse of these readings is indicative of poor pulmonary function. Another important ABG is oxygen saturation (O_2Sat) with normal levels of 95–100%.

Pulmonary function tests (PFTs) are a group of tests that measure volume and flow of air by using a spirometer (Figure 9–6) and are valuable in the diagnosis of a respiratory problem. PFTs can also be performed before and after brochodilation treatment to measure treatment effectiveness. PFTs are measured against a norm for the individual's age, height, and sex.

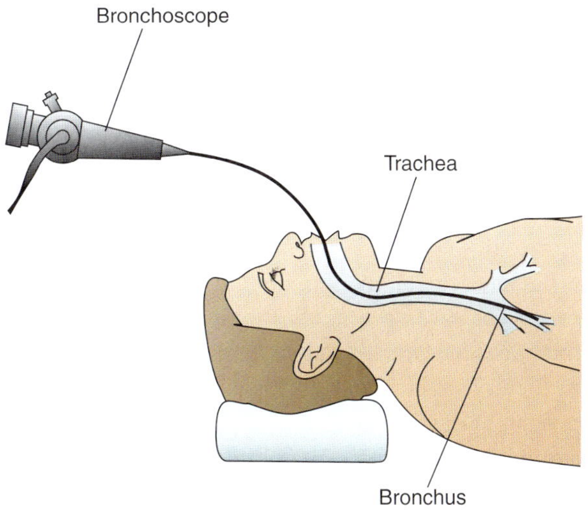

Delmar/Cengage Learning

FIGURE 9–5 Bronchoscopy.

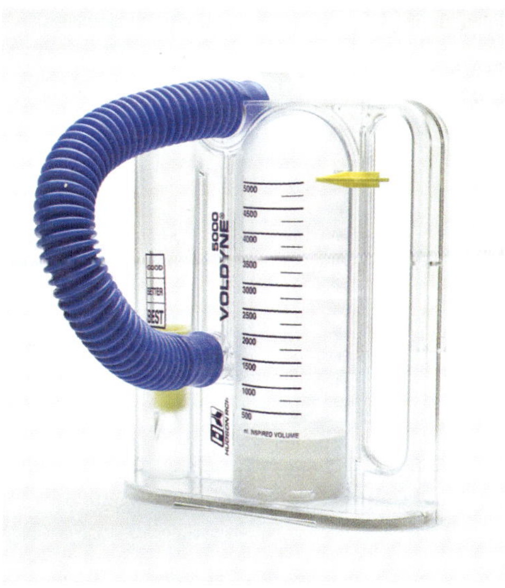

Courtesy of Teleflex Medical. Voldyne is a registered trademark of Teleflex Incorporated

FIGURE 9–6 Spirometer: used for pulmonary function tests. *Voldyne 5000 Incentive Spirometer.*

COMMON DISEASES OF THE RESPIRATORY SYSTEM

Diseases of the respiratory system range from simple to very serious. The symptoms of the various disorders are often similar in the early stages, with most conditions manifesting in shortness of breath and coughing, wheezing, or both, although some disorders might not present symptoms until late in the disease development. Smoking is the number one risk behavior for developing chronic respiratory disease. Although influenza and other communicable respiratory diseases have been common for centuries, epidemics in the United States have not been as devastating as they were historically. Now public health officials are seeing new strains of respiratory viruses emerge and the threat of an epidemic is cause for concern.

Diseases of the Upper Respiratory Tract

Respiratory illnesses, which are mostly viral infections, account for approximately 50% of all acute illnesses, and respiratory infections account for more than 80%

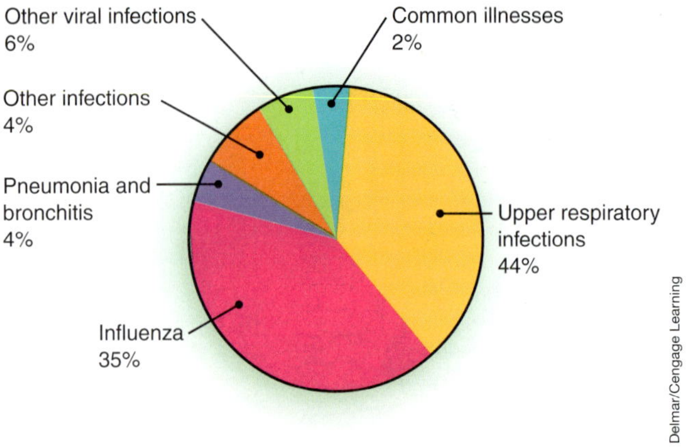

FIGURE 9–7 Frequency of infectious diseases.

of all infections (Figure 9–7). Most disorders of the upper respiratory tract are not life threatening.

UPPER RESPIRATORY INFECTION (URI)

DESCRIPTION. URI is a broad term referring to several infectious diseases of the upper respiratory tract. These infections are the most common cause for lost days of work for adults.

ETIOLOGY. Most URIs (not to be confused with UTI, urinary tract infection) are caused by viruses. The most common is a group called rhinovirus.

SYMPTOMS. Symptoms commonly include nasal congestion, runny nose, sore throat, ear pain or fullness, sneezing, coughing, mild fever, headache, and generalized aches. Symptoms usually resolve in 7–10 days.

DIAGNOSIS. Diagnosis is usually made on the basis of a history and physical examination revealing the common signs and symptoms.

TREATMENT. General treatment for viral diseases includes rest, drinking increased amounts of fluids, and taking **antipyretics** (anti = against, pyretic = fever) and **analgesics** (an = without, algesic = pain). Antibiotics are not effective with viral infections but might be needed for secondary bacterial infection. The common cold is the most frequent URI and often leads to secondary infectious diseases.

PREVENTION. Prevention is often difficult because viruses are easily spread by droplet infection such as sneezing or coughing. These microscopic droplets are then picked up on the hands and carried to the membranes of the respiratory tract by touching or wiping the eyes and nose. The greatest preventive measure is regular hand washing. Other preventive activities include avoiding crowds, avoiding smoking, and maintaining general health.

COMMON COLD (ACUTE RHINITIS)

DESCRIPTION. The common cold is an acute inflammation of the mucous membranes of the upper respiratory tract. There are several hundred virus strains that cause a cold. Developing immunity to one strain does not provide immunity to others.

ETIOLOGY. A cold is very contagious and is usually passed from one individual to another through touch and air droplets. Many individuals believe that getting chilled or wet is the cause of a cold. In actuality,

COMPLEMENTARY AND ALTERNATIVE THERAPY

Vitamin Preparations for Asthma and Allergic Rhinitis

The traditional therapies for asthma and allergic rhinitis might include corticosteroids and antihistamines. These medications often cause a variety of side effects. The use of vitamin preparations and other herbal remedies for treating pulmonary disorders is increasing, but the value of these treatments has not been well established. Vitamin E (tocopherol) has been promoted as a therapy for asthma and allergic rhinitis. Some research studies have reported that a form of tocopherol, called α-tocopherol, found in many dietary supplements, is not as effective as y-tocopherol, which is the primary form of dietary vitamin E. This type has been shown to reduce the systemic inflammation in allergic reactions. It also has some effect on the mucus-producing cells, inhibiting their function.

Source: Wagner, et al. (2008).

these actions do not directly cause a cold; they merely lower an individual's resistance to invasion by a cold-causing virus. Children, older people, and individuals in generally poor health are at increased risk of contracting a cold.

■ ***SYMPTOMS.*** Most individuals are very familiar with the symptoms of runny nose, or **rhinorrhea** (rye-nor-REE-ah; rhino = nose, orrhea = run through), watery eyes, stuffy head, sore throat, sneezing, and fever.

■ ***DIAGNOSIS.*** Diagnosis is usually determined by physical examination and presence of signs and symptoms.

■ ***TREATMENT.*** Treatment involves basic comfort care, including rest, drinking increased fluids, and taking antipyretics and analgesics as prescribed.

■ ***PREVENTION.*** Good hand washing is the best preventive measure against a cold.

HAY FEVER (ALLERGIC RHINITIS)

Allergic rhinitis is an inflammation of the mucous membranes due to allergies. This sensitivity to an allergen tends to run in families. Ragweed and grasses are two common allergens. Hay fever was discussed in detail in Chapter 5, "Immune System Diseases and Disorders."

SINUSITIS

■ ***DESCRIPTION.*** Sinusitis is an inflammation of the mucous membrane lining the sinuses. The sinuses are air-filled cavities in the bony tissue of the head. The membranes that line the nose extend into the sinuses.

■ ***ETIOLOGY.*** Acute rhinitis often leads to sinusitis. It is also believed that blowing the nose too hard actually spreads infection into the sinuses. As mucous membranes become swollen, the drainage system becomes blocked. Mucus accumulates in the sinuses, causing increased pressure and often leading to sinus headaches, dizziness, and difficulty breathing. Other causes of sinusitis include tooth infections, air pollution, and nasal deformities.

■ ***SYMPTOMS.*** Pain in the area of the affected sinus is common. Headaches upon awakening is most common with sinus involvement, and pain in the forehead area can be related to frontal sinus inflammation. Other symptoms include tiredness, a night cough, runny nose, nasal congestion, and sore throat.

■ ***DIAGNOSIS.*** Diagnosis is based on clinical history, physical examination, computed tomography (CT) scan or magnetic resonance imaging (MRI), and laboratory tests to help identify the allergies.

■ ***TREATMENT.*** Treatment often includes antibiotics and decongestants. Because sinusitis can lead to more serious infections such as mastoiditis and encephalitis, aggressive treatment is necessary.

■ ***PREVENTION.*** Sinusitis in many cases cannot be prevented, although there are measures that might reduce frequency of attacks, such as use of a humidifier, avoiding cigarette smoke and other air pollutants, avoiding alcohol because it causes nasal membranes to swell, and avoiding swimming in pools due to the chlorine.

PHARYNGITIS

■ ***DESCRIPTION.*** Pharyngitis is an inflammation of the throat (pharynx = throat, itis = inflammation) commonly called a sore throat.

■ ***ETIOLOGY.*** The most common cause is viral infection. Bacterial infection by streptococcus can also occur and is more common in children. Irritation to the mucous membranes, such as breathing extremely hot or cold air, chemical fumes, or smoke, can also lead to pharyngitis.

■ ***SYMPTOMS.*** Symptoms include sore throat, fever, headache, swollen lymph glands in the neck, and pain with swallowing.

■ ***DIAGNOSIS.*** Physical examination, including viewing the pharynx (throat), eyes, skin, and lymph nodes is useful. A streptococcal throat swab culture might be taken to diagnosis strep infection.

■ ***TREATMENT.*** Treatment depends on the cause. Viral infections are treated with comfort care and throat lozenges, antiseptic or salt-water gargles, and analgesics. Bacterial infections, such as strep throat, also need antibiotic treatment. Chronic pharyngitis due to tonsillitis and adenoiditis can be treated by surgical removal of the tonsils and adenoids, called a tonsillectomy and adenoidectomy (T&A), respectively.

■ ***PREVENTION.*** Good handwashing, maintaining general health, and avoiding close contact with anyone who is contagious aid in prevention of pharyngitis.

Using a new toothbrush after the symptoms disappear also aids in prevention.

LARYNGITIS

DESCRIPTION. Laryngitis is an inflammation of the larynx (LAR-inks) and vocal cords.

ETIOLOGY. Laryngitis can be caused by viral or bacterial infections or by breathing irritants such as extremely hot or cold air, chemical fumes, and smoke. Laryngitis frequently follows other URIs such as the common cold, pharyngitis, and sinusitis. Another cause can be overuse of the voice for an extended time.

SYMPTOMS. Most individuals are familiar with the hoarse voice quality caused by laryngitis. Other symptoms include difficulty swallowing (dysphagia), throat pain, and fever.

DIAGNOSIS. A history of a recent cold or flu followed by hoarseness is a common clue for diagnosis. A harsh wheezing sound in the throat area is usually indicative of laryngitis. A laryngoscope can be used to view the airway and vocal cords for other signs of disease.

TREATMENT. Treatment can include voice rest, increased fluid intake, analgesics, throat lozenges, and removal of causative factors.

PREVENTION. Frequent hand washing, avoiding those with infections, and avoiding breathing irritants aid in prevention.

Diseases of the Bronchi and Lungs

Diseases of the bronchi and lungs are usually more severe than diseases of the upper respiratory system. Many of these can be life threatening, such as influenza, especially in the older population.

ASTHMA

DESCRIPTION. Asthma is a hypersensitivity reaction that causes constriction of the bronchi, leading to difficulty breathing.

ETIOLOGY. Asthma, also called bronchial asthma, was discussed in detail as a hypersensitivity disorder in Chapter 5.

SYMPTOMS. Asthma is characterized by episodes of wheezing and dyspnea.

DIAGNOSIS. A diagnosis of asthma usually is based on the patient's symptoms, medical history, a physical examination, and laboratory tests that measure pulmonary (lung) function.

TREATMENT. Treatment includes avoidance of causative allergens, desensitization, education, and medications to treat symptoms.

PREVENTION. Prevention is aimed at identification and control of allergic factors and use of bronchodilators.

ACUTE BRONCHITIS

DESCIPTION. Acute bronchitis is inflammation of the mucous membrane lining of the bronchus. It often involves the trachea (tracheobronchitis).

ETIOLOGY. Acute bronchitis is a short-term disorder commonly following a URI. Other causes include inhaling fumes, smoke, dust, cold air, and other irritants.

SYMPTOMS. Symptoms include fever, a tight feeling behind the sternum, and a dry cough that later progresses to a productive cough (coughing up or expectorating mucus or sputum).

DIAGNOSIS. Tests are usually unnecessary in diagnosis because this disease is easy to determine from a history and physical examination including X-ray can be ordered.

TREATMENT. Treatment consists of drinking increased amounts of fluids to help liquefy secretions, rest, cough syrup, analgesics, and antipyretics. Antibiotics are helpful only if secondary bacterial infections occur. Prognosis is generally good for most individuals. Infants and small children can become seriously ill because the bronchioles are very small and can become obstructed by swollen tissue or mucus plugs. Older people and the chronically ill might have a poor prognosis because they have an increased risk for developing secondary bacterial infections such as pneumonia.

PREVENTION. Preventive activities include:

- Washing hands frequently
- Not smoking and avoiding secondhand smoke
- Avoiding allergens such as dust and household fumes
- Not sharing eating utensils with others
- Maintaining a healthy lifestyle

INFLUENZA (FLU)

■ *DESCRIPTION.* Influenza is an acute, highly contagious respiratory infection. Influenza is a serious disease. In the United States alone, each year more than 200,000 people are hospitalized from flu complications and approxmately 36,000 people die from the flu. The elderly, young children, and people with certain health conditions are at high risk for serious flu complications (CDC, 2008).

■ *ETIOLOGY.* Influenza is a viral infection commonly spread by coughing of respiratory secretions. There are many strains of influenza virus, the primary of which are identified as A, B, and C. Substrains, or subtypes, include H0N1, H1N1, H2N2, H3N2, and several others. Avian (bird) flu is an influenza A virus that usually does not affect humans. However, recent diagnosed cases in humans have caused concern among public health workers. Although the cases have been found outside the United States, with the mobility of people, it is a concern. Deaths have been attributed to avian influenza in children and adults. Most human infections have occurred following direct contact with infected poultry.

The flu virus has great genetic variation, and the number of strains and variations help explain how this virus causes epidemics year after year. Unfortunately, like the common cold, immunity to one viral strain does not provide immunity to another, so an individual can have the flu multiple times. Flu epidemics commonly occur in the winter and early spring.

■ *SYMPTOMS.* Influenza is characterized by sudden onset of fever, chills, headache, and back muscle pain. Other symptoms can include cough, runny nose, sore throat, sneezing, hoarseness, nausea, vomiting, and diarrhea.

■ *DIAGNOSIS.* Flu can be difficult to distinguish from many other types of common cold viruses and bacterial infections. A history and physical exam that reveals a sudden onset of symptoms can assist in diagnosis. Rapid diagnostic tests are available that can detect influenza viruses in 30 minutes.

■ *TREATMENT.* Treatment of influenza is symptomatic and can include bed rest, analgesics, and antipyretics. Oseltamivic (Tamiflu) and zanamivir (Relenza) are Food and Drug Administration (FDA)–approved antiviral medications recommended for treatment of both influenza A and B viruses. These medications must be started within 2 days of symptoms to be effective. Antibiotics are not indicated unless secondary bacterial infections occur.

HEALTHY HIGHLIGHT

Influenza Immunization (Flu Shots)

Because influenza is a viral infection, antiviral medications can be given, but there is no major treatment other than supportive treatment of symptoms in most cases. An individual is dependent on the immune system to build antibodies to kill the virus. Antibiotics can be helpful for secondary bacterial infections but do not kill the influenza virus.

The best course in dealing with flu is prevention, which includes frequent hand washing, avoiding crowds of people during flu season or when there is a local epidemic, avoiding individuals infected with influenza, and leading a healthy lifestyle to keep resistance high.

An immunization is available and is recommended for all individuals but especially for older people, those with chronic diseases, pregnant women, children, and health care workers. Reactions to the flu immunization are rare but do occur. Individuals allergic to eggs should not take the immunization because the virus is grown in eggs. Allergic hypersensitivity reactions usually occur immediately after receiving the injection, although a reaction to the antigen can occur 6 to 12 hours after the injection. Reaction symptoms mimic the flu and include fever, muscle pain, and malaise.

■ ***PREVENTION.*** Vaccination is the best way to prevent influenza. Antiviral medications are also effective in prevention.

CHRONIC OBSTRUCTIVE PULMONARY DISEASE (COPD)

■ ***DESCRIPTION.*** COPD is the name for two distinct diseases characterized by the inability to get air into or out of the lungs. Chronic bronchitis and ephysema frequently coexist, hence the preference to call them, collectively, COPD. There can be pure forms of either, but usually, the individual has predominantly one or the other coexisting with the second. This term does not include other obstructive diseases such as asthma.

Both chronic bronchitis and emphysema cause excessive inflammation that leads to abnormalities in the lung that permanently obstruct airflow (thus the term *chronic obstructive*). With COPD, the loss of normal respiratory response is not unusual.

Normally, individuals are stimulated to breathe by an increase of carbon dioxide in the blood. A secondary or backup stimulus is a decrease of oxygen in the blood. Individuals with COPD commonly have high levels of carbon dioxide in the blood. Initially, the body attempts to correct this by increasing breathing in an effort to blow out excessive CO_2. When this effort fails, the respiratory system adapts to the high CO_2 levels and begins responding to the secondary stimulus of low blood oxygen levels. Giving oxygen to these individuals can be fatal because high oxygenation removes the stimulus to breathe.

Approximately 24 million people suffer from this disease, fourth most significant cause of death in United States (American Lung Association, 2007).

■ ***ETIOLOGY.*** Ninety percent of the time, these diseases are due to cigarette smoking. Other causes include air pollution and chronic respiratory infections. Exposure to certain industrial pollutants can also increase the risk of developing COPD.

■ ***SYMPTOMS.*** Symptoms of COPD occur due to lung damage. In smokers, it might take 40 to 50 years for symptoms to occur. Symptoms can occur many years after the individual actually quits smoking, quite simply because the lungs have a large amount of reserve capacity.

As we age, we normally lose lung function, but not enough to cause symptoms unless our lungs are damaged or diseased. Smokers lose function at a rate approximately five times faster than normal. Even at this rate, it commonly takes decades for a smoker to lose enough lung function to experience symptoms.

If an individual quits smoking, the loss of function slows back to approximately normal. However, if smoking has already destroyed a large portion of the lung tissue, symptoms of COPD will appear as the individual ages and continues to lose function at a normal rate. If one continues to smoke, decline continues at an accelerated rate. Quitting smoking at any time in one's life can slow loss of function and improve quality of life.

Common symptoms include:

- Dyspnea (difficulty breathing) is the most common symptom. Onset is usually gradual and often noticed only with exercise. As the disease progresses and the individual ages into his or her 60s and 70s, dyspnea becomes increasingly prominent as lung function declines.
- Chronic cough usually begins in the morning but slowly progresses to an all-day cough. This progression can be so slow the individual does not even recognize the fact that he or she is coughing all the time.
- Wheezing appears and is due to air passing through tight or narrow airways.
- Hemoptysis, or coughing up blood, usually occurs during acute attacks. This hemoptysis is usually blood-streaked sputum, not active bleeding. Bloody sputum in an individual with COPD also can be indicative of lung cancer.
- Cyanosis, or a bluish discoloration of the skin, nail beds, and lips is common, especially during acute attacks. Cyanosis indicates a low blood oxygen level.
- Weight loss is common because individuals with COPD work hard and burn increased calories in the activity of breathing. Shortness of breath caused by the activity of eating often interrupts meals, leading to malnutrition.
- Pursed-lip breathing is an acquired breathing pattern that forces air out of the lungs. By pursing the lips together during exhalation, the back pressure or positive pressure holds airways open to allow forced exhalation of the air through narrowed passageways. This breathing pattern is hard work, burns increased calories, and weakens the already damaged airways.

- Barrel chest describes a bulging, rounded chest that resembles the shape of a barrel. This is a symptom of late stage COPD. The lungs are chronically overinflated with air, causing the rib cage to stay partially expanded. This change in physical structure of the chest makes breathing less efficient and leads to more shortness of breath.

DIAGNOSIS. Diagnosis of COPD is made by history and physical examination and by ruling out other pulmonary diseases. Chest X-rays, pulmonary function tests (PFTs), and arterial blood gases (ABGs) help confirm the diagnosis.

TREATMENT. Symptomatic treatment includes use of bronchodilator medications, inhalers, mucolytics, and cough medications. Avoiding exposure to individuals with respiratory tract infections is important because these diseases aggravate COPD. Influenza vaccination is recommended. Cessation of smoking can slow or reverse the disease in the early stages and will ease symptoms in the later stages.

There is no cure for end-stage COPD. Individuals often become debilitated in the final stages of the disease, and prognosis is poor due to progressive deterioration of pulmonary function, often leading to respiratory failure and death.

PREVENTION. Not smoking is the best preventive action. Other preventive measures include avoiding respiratory irritants and infections and maintaining a healthy lifestyle.

CHRONIC BRONCHITIS

DESCRIPTION. Chronic bronchitis is a long-term inflammation and scarring of the lining of the bronchial tubes. It is characterized by increased mucus production with a productive cough. Chronic inflammation leads to hypertrophy of the mucus-secreting glands, thickening of the mucous membrane, and **bronchiectasis** (BRONG-kee-ECK-tah-sis), a chronic dilatation of the bronchus.

SYMPTOMS. Bronchiectasis allows mucus to pool in the bronchus, producing a foul-smelling cough. This cough is commonly called smoker's cough and occurs primarily in the morning hours. As the disease progresses, obstruction of the bronchi and bronchioles becomes more pronounced, leading to difficulty getting air into the lungs. Coughing, dyspnea, and **hypoxia** (HIGH-POCK-see-ah; hypo = low, oxia = oxygen) occur. During bouts of hypoxia, the individual often becomes cyanotic (blue condition). In the final or end stage, the symptoms are more continuous, causing lung damage, debilitation of the individual, and eventual death.

EMPHYSEMA

DESCRIPTION. Emphysema comes from the Greek word *emphysana*, meaning "to inflate." This chronic disease is characterized by an increased production of mucus, causing trapping of air in the tiny alveoli or air sacks of the lung. As air becomes trapped in the alveoli, they become overinflated, leading to destruction of the alveoli wall. Destruction of the alveoli wall allows the alveoli to fuse with another alveoli, forming a larger air sack and trapping more air (Figure 9–8).

SYMPTOMS. The individual with emphysema is able to get air in, but the air becomes trapped and must be forced out before more air can be taken in. These enlarged alveoli have a decreased surface area, thus decreasing oxygenation of the blood. Air trapping and decreased oxygen exchange lead to dyspnea, tachypnea, wheezing, and coughing.

Individuals with emphysema often lean over a table or chair to use accessory respiratory muscles to blow out the trapped air more effectively. Pursing the lips also helps hold the alveoli open while pushing the

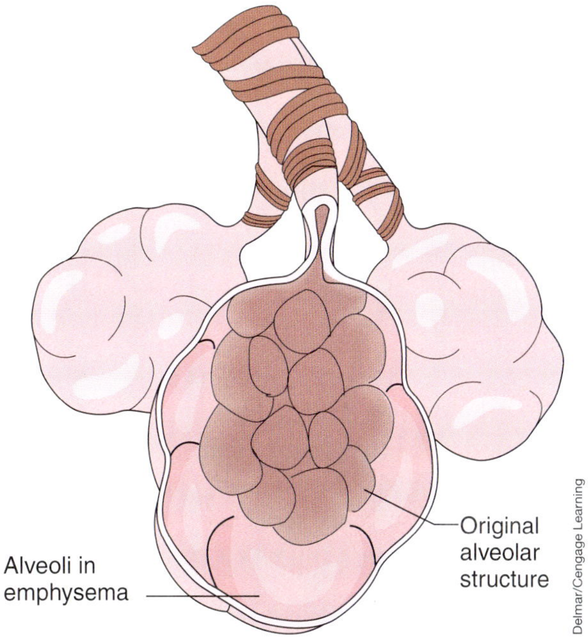

FIGURE 9–8 Normal versus emphasematous alveoli.

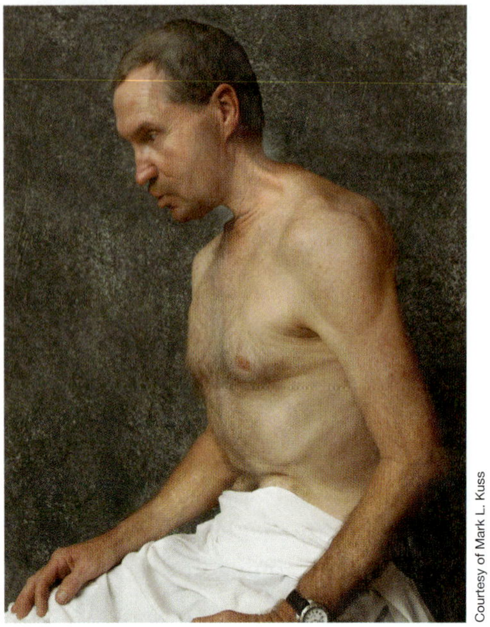

FIGURE 9–9 Pursed lips and barrel chest of emphysema.

air out (Figure 9–9). This extra pressure often causes the face and skin to become reddened. Extra pressure on the chest muscles also produces a characteristic barrel-chested appearance.

Individuals with emphysema use large amounts of energy in their respiratory efforts, so a supplemented diet is often needed. Food is eaten in small, frequent feedings to allow time for respiratory efforts. Even with a supplemented diet, these individuals are often unable to get adequate nutrition and commonly are quite thin.

ATELECTASIS

■ ***DESCRIPTION.*** Atelectasis (Ah-tel-EK-teh-sis) is the collapse or airless state of part or all of a lung. More commonly, it affects only a small section of the lung.

■ ***ETIOLOGY.*** Atelectasis is often related to inadequate breathing patterns related to pain. Surgical pain and fractured ribs often cause inadequate breathing, leading to atelectasis. Blockage of the airway by a mucus plug can also cause atelectasis.

■ ***SYMPTOMS.*** Dyspnea, cyanosis, and anxiety are common symptoms.

■ ***DIAGNOSIS.*** Diagnosis is confirmed after a positive chest X-ray and physical examination.

■ ***TREATMENT.*** Ambulation (walking), frequent deep breathing and coughing, and analgesics for pain help open the airway, expand the alveoli, and avoid atelectasis. Prognosis is good if complications do not occur. Pneumonia is a common complication.

■ ***PREVENTION.*** Prevention is aimed at relieving the cause if possible.

PNEUMONIA

■ ***DESCRIPTION.*** Pneumonia is an inflammation of the bronchioles and alveoli due to infection by bacteria, virus, or other pathogens. Pneumonia is the term specifically related to infection. Inflammation without infection is termed *pneumonitis*. Pneumonitis is inflammation generally caused by a hypersensitivity to dusts and chemicals.

Pneumonia can be identified in several ways. The cause might be included in the name, as in "pneumococcal," "aspiration," and "tuberculous pneumonia." The location might be identified in the name, as in "lobar," "bilateral," and "double pneumonia." Secondary pneumonia indicates a connection to another cause. Often, the location and cause can be combined to describe the pneumonia, as in "bilateral pneumococcal pneumonia."

Bacterial pneumonias tend to be the most serious, whereas viral pneumonias are the most common. People who have difficulty swallowing, as is common in those with throat surgery or stroke, are at risk for aspiration pneumonia.

Pneumonia affects millions of individuals each year and can range from mild to life threatening. It occurs more often among older people, the chronically ill, and those who are immunosuppressed and is a significant cause of death in these individuals.

■ ***ETIOLOGY.*** Actions that inhibit the normal protective mechanisms of the respiratory system, such as smoking, immobility, general anesthesia, and endotracheal intubation, allow the invasion of pathogens into lung tissue.

Pathogens that cause pneumonia can reach the lung tissue through the respiratory system or through the blood as a result of septicemia. Invasion of pathogens into the alveoli leads to inflammation of the alveolar tissue, causing the classic outpouring of blood fluid and white cells from the capillaries into the tissues, filling the alveolus. This causes a decrease in gas exchange, leading to hypoxia (Figure 9–10). This inflammation and infection of the lungs is pneumonia.

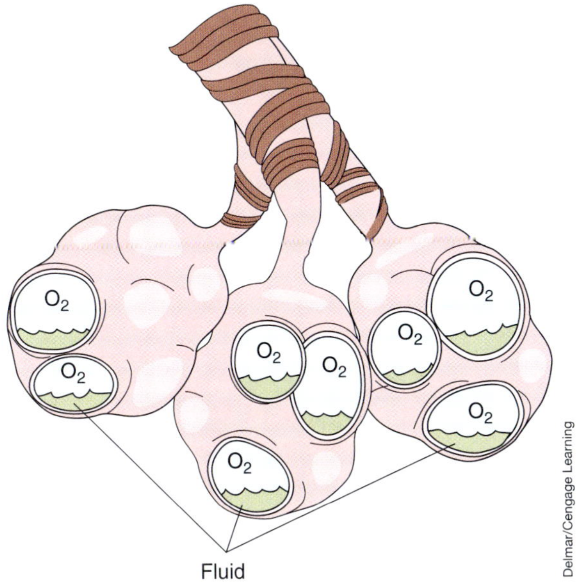

FIGURE 9–10 Pneumonia: alveoli filling with fluid.

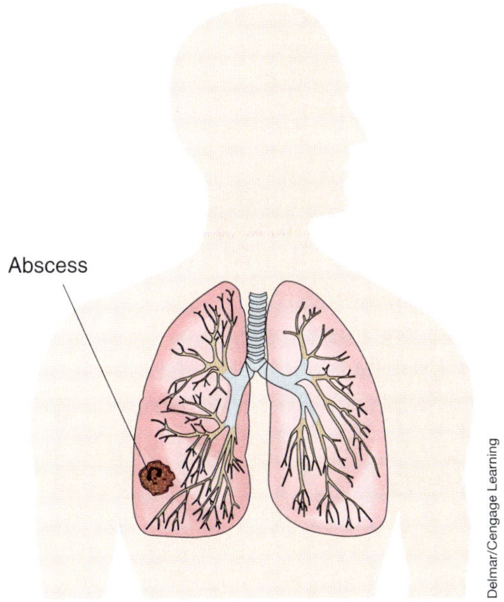

FIGURE 9–11 Pulmonary abscess.

■ ***SYMPTOMS.*** Symptoms of pneumonia are related to the area involved and the amount of tissue involved. Symptoms include dyspnea, weakness, fever, chills, chest pain, and cough.

■ ***DIAGNOSIS.*** Diagnosis is made after completion of a chest X-ray, history, physical examination, and sputum culture to determine the infective pathogen.

■ ***TREATMENT.*** Treatment depends on cause. Bacterial infection is treated with antibiotics. Viral infection is treated symptomatically. Rest, analgesics, oxygen therapy, increased fluid intake, and high-calorie diet are common treatments for all types of pneumonia.

■ ***PREVENTION.*** Preventive activities include not smoking, frequent hand washing, and wearing a mask when working with fumes, dust, or mold. Vaccines can also prevent pneumonia. Pneumococcal, flu, and Haemophilus influenza type B (Hib) (for children) vaccines are all effective. Taking deep breaths and use of a breathing device aid in prevention of pneumonia after surgery.

PULMONARY ABSCESS

■ ***DESCRIPTION.*** Pulmonary abscess, also called lung abscess, is a collection of infectious material contained within a capsule (Figure 9–11). Abscess formation was discussed in detail in Chapter 4, "Inflammation and Infection."

■ ***ETIOLOGY.*** Lung abscess is often related to a number of other diseases, including pneumonia, tuberculosis, and lung cancer. It can also be caused by aspiration of food or foreign objects.

■ ***SYMPTOMS.*** Symptoms include chills, fever, chest pain, and cough. Coughing of bloody or foul-smelling sputum and foul-smelling breath can also be indicative of a pulmonary abscess.

■ ***DIAGNOSIS.*** Diagnosis is made by completion of a history and physical examination, chest X-ray, and sputum cultures.

■ ***TREATMENT.*** Pulmonary abscesses are commonly treated with long-term antibiotic therapy. Surgical resection might be indicated if the abscess is quite large or if antibiotic therapy is unsuccessful.

■ ***PREVENTION.*** Preventing aspiration is the most important preventive measure.

PULMONARY TUBERCULOSIS

■ ***DESCRIPTION.*** Pulmonary tuberculosis is often called tuberculosis (TB). It is a contagious bacterial infection that mainly involves the lungs but can spread to other organs such as the kidneys, bones, and brain.

According to the World Health Organization (WHO), one third of the world's current population has been infected by TB, and new infections occur at the rate of one per second. Recently, WHO declared TB a global health emergency and developed a global plan to stop TB that aims at saving 14 million lives by the year 2015 (WHO, 2006).

ETIOLOGY. TB is a bacterial infection caused by *Mycobacterium tuberculosis*. It is acquired by breathing air that is infected with the bacteria and is spread by coughing and sneezing.

Mycobacterium tuberculosis is protected in a strong coating that enables it to live outside the body for a lengthy amount of time. Infected droplets that are coughed or sneezed can dry up and remain on inanimate objects as dust but can be killed by bactericidal solutions or by direct sunlight.

TB is often prevalent in areas of overcrowding and poor sanitation. The incidence of TB was greatly reduced decades ago with the introduction of effective antibiotics. More recently, however, the number of TB cases in the United States has seriously risen due to the influx of high numbers of infected immigrants, the homeless, individuals with AIDS who have poor resistance to infection, and the development of drug-resistant bacteria.

The infection begins with a primary lesion in the lungs. *Mycobacterium tuberculosis* does not attract polymorphic nuclear cells (PMNs) and thus does not cause an acute inflammation. Lymphocytes and macrophages are attracted to these encapsulated bacteria. These immune cells begin producing antibodies and walling off the infection by forming a type of granuloma called a tubercule, hence the name, tuberculosis. The inside of the tubercule contains dead bacteria, lung tissue, and immune cells that together exhibit a cheesy appearance called caseous necrosis.

After necrosis, the tubercules change by fibrosing and calcifying. If the immune system is effective in walling off the bacteria, the disease can be arrested or rendered inactive for a long period of time (months to years). During this time, the individual is often asymptomatic and not aware that he or she has TB. If the disease is not arrested, the individual will become symptomatic with progressive primary TB. The antibodies that are produced during this time circulate in the blood for the remainder of the infected individual's life in readiness to attack future TB bacteria. These circulating antibodis are the basis for the positive reaction to a TB skin test.

Secondary TB occurs when an individual is reinfected with *Mycobacterium tuberculosis*, or the primary disease is reactivated due to a decline in the individual's resistance. Antibodies formed during the primary stage of the disease activate quickly and lead to larger areas of necrosis in the lung tissue. During secondary TB, the individual becomes symptomatic. The tubercule mass becomes liquified and is coughed up, leaving a cavity in the lung tissue (Figure 9–12). Frequent coughing often ruptures capillaries in the lung tissue, leading to hemoptysis (coughing, spitting of blood, or both). Coughing by the infected individual fills the surrounding air with disease.

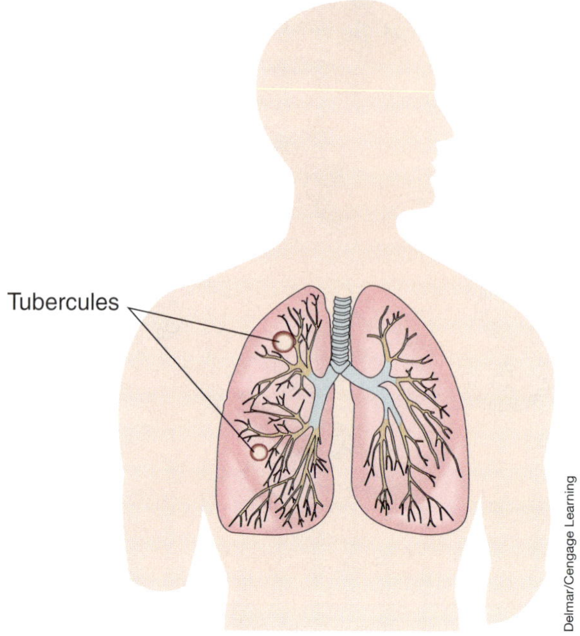

FIGURE 9–12 Tuberculosis.

As large cavities are formed in the lung tissue, the ability of the tissue to oxygenate the blood is decreased. The individual becomes dyspneic and cachectic with a general appearance of being consumed by the disease. For this reason, historically, this disease was called consumption. During that time, individuals were placed in sanitariums to prevent the spread of TB and to provide much-needed rest. Without effective treatment, many infected individuals died from TB.

SYMPTOMS. Tuberculosis in an otherwise healthy individual is often asymptomatic, so testing is needed to determine the presence of the disease. If symptoms appear, they are often vague and include loss of weight, energy, and appetite. As the disease progresses, the individual might become symptomatic

HEALTHY HIGHLIGHT

Tuberculosis Skin Test

TB skin testing works on the principle that after an individual is exposed to *Mycobacterium tuberculosis*, the immune system will develop antibodies. These antibodies will be present in all cells of the body (cellular immunity) from that point on. Introduction of the bacillus or a derivative, through injection or re-exposure, will cause a cellular reaction. The Mantoux (man-TOO) test uses this principle. A small amount of purified protein derivative (PPD) is injected intradermally. PPD contains modified tuberculin bacteria that are no longer infectious. If the individual has been exposed to TB and has developed antibodies, the immune system will react. A reaction will also occur if the individual has been previously immunized with Bacille-Calmette-Guerin (BCG) tuberculin vaccine. A reaction is shown by the formation of an intradermal wheal. An 8–10 mm wheal within 48–72 hours of injection is considered a positive, now called significant, reaction. The Centers for Disease Control and Prevention (CDC) recommend using the QuantiFERON-TB test to detect TB in health care workers and suspected cases (see Glimpse of the Future box).

After an individual has a positive skin test (significant reaction) once, that individual will always have a reaction, so a skin test is no longer beneficial in determining whether the individual has active TB. Individuals exhibiting a positive skin test need to be educated in the symptoms of TB, which include unexpected weight loss, persistent cough, night sweats, and malaise. If these symptoms occur and persist, the individual will need a chest X-ray and possible sputum culture to determine the presence of disease.

with a chronic productive cough, dyspnea, fever, and night sweats.

■ ***DIAGNOSIS.*** TB is diagnosed by skin testing, chest X-ray, and sputum culture.

■ ***TREATMENT.*** Extended antibiotic therapy is needed to rid the individual of the infection.

■ ***PREVENTION.*** TB is preventable with skin testing in high-risk populations or for individuals who might have been exposed, such as health care workers.

ADULT RESPIRATORY DISTRESS SYNDROME (ARDS)

■ ***DESCRIPTION.*** ARDS is also called shock lung. It is a sudden, life-threatening lung failure, a syndrome, not a specific disease, that usually develops within 24 to 48 hours of a major injury or illness.

■ ***ETIOLOGY.*** Approximately 30% of ARDS cases are caused by sepsis, a serious infection of the blood. Other conditions that can cause the syndrome include severe chest trauma, inhalation of smoke or toxic fumes, near-drowning, fat emboli, aspiration pneumonia, major burns, massive blood transfusion, and acute pancreatitis. In most cases, these conditions do not lead to the development of ARDS. It is unclear why some people develop the syndrome but others do not.

Following the trauma, the individual might be progressing smoothly when a sudden, life-threatening attack of ARDs occurs. ARDS is characterized by fluid escaping the vascular system and filling the alveoli, leading to acute respiratory failure.

■ ***SYMPTOMS.*** Symptoms develop suddenly and include extreme dyspnea, severe hypoxemia, tachypnea, cyanosis, and pulmonary hypertension (high blood pressure in the pulmonary arteries).

■ ***DIAGNOSIS.*** History and physical examination along with a chest X-ray and ABGs aid in diagnosis.

■ ***TREATMENT.*** Individuals suffer extreme dyspnea and need mechanical ventilation. Even with prompt and proper treatment, ARDs has a high mortality rate. Approximately one third of the affected individuals die within days, another third die within weeks, usually due to pneumonia and heart failure. Approximately one third recover, but many of these individuals have permanent respiratory damage and are more prone to respiratory-related illnesses thereafter.

■ ***PREVENTION.*** ARDS is prevented by avoiding diseases and conditions that damage the lung, for instance, preventing aspiration, treating with as low a level of oxygen as possible, and treating infection promptly.

SUDDEN ACUTE RESPIRATORY SYNDROME (SARS)

■ ***DESCRIPTION.*** SARS is the first severe, easily transmissible new disease to emerge in the twenty-first century. SARS is a respiratory illness that was first reported in Asia but spread to people in Europe, South America, and North America in February 2003. Public health officials worked quickly to halt the spread of the disease and actually contained it by July 2003. According to WHO, 8,098 people worldwide became sick with SARS, and 774 died in the 2003 outbreak. In the United States, only 8 people were infected, and all of these had traveled outside the United States to areas with SARS infection (WHO, 2008).

■ ***ETIOLOGY.*** World experts have determined that SARS is caused by a previously unknown type of coronavirus, a family of viruses that usually causes only mild to moderate illness such as the common cold. This new virus has been named the SARS coronavirus.

The SARS virus appears to be spread by respiratory droplets. Persons who have close person-to-person contact with an infected individual are most at risk. Close contact is defined as having cared for or lived with someone with SARS or having direct contact with the respiratory secretions of a person with SARS. Examples of close contact include sharing drinking and eating utensils, kissing, hugging, touching, or talking to someone within 3 feet. Close contact does not include walking past an infected individual or briefly sitting across from the person in a waiting room.

The SARS virus is thought to be easily spread when an infected individual coughs or sneezes and spreads the infected respiratory droplets into the air as far as 3 feet. Infection can occur when these droplets fall on or are inhaled onto the mucous membranes of the mouth, nose, and eyes of persons nearby. The virus also can spread when a person touches an infected surface or object and then touches his or her mouth, nose, or eyes.

■ ***SYMPTOMS.*** SARS usually begins with a high fever. Other symptoms include malaise, chills, headache, myalgia, dizziness, rigors, cough, sore throat, and runny nose. Incubation of the SARS virus appears to be approximately 7–10 days. In many cases, patients present with headache, dizziness, and myalgia. Temperature rises and becomes excessive as the disease progresses. In more acute cases, there is rapid deterioration with low oxygen saturation and acute respiratory distress requiring ventilatory support. ARDS has been observed in a number of patients in end-stage disease.

■ ***DIAGNOSIS.*** Diagnosis is suspected in any person who exhibits symptoms and has a history of travel to a foreign country where SARS has been identified. Positive chest X-rays showing small, patchy shadows that progress to generalized interstitial infiltrates are indicative of SARS. Several diagnostic test kits have been produced, but none have proved effective; thus, there is no rapid screening test for SARS.

■ ***TREATMENT.*** Antibiotics are ineffective against SARS because it is a viral disease. Treatment of symptoms includes antipyretic medications, oxygen administration, and ventilator support if needed. Steroids and antiviral medications have been tried but have not helped, and some research has suggested that these actually cause harm.

■ ***PREVENTION.*** Prevention includes avoiding contact with infected individuals and use of isolation procedures if contact is necessary. Respiratory isolation—including the use of gown, gloves, goggles, and an approved respiratory mask—are essential.

LUNG CANCER

■ ***DESCRIPTION.*** Lung cancer is a disease of uncontrolled cell growth in the tissues of the lung. The majority of primary lung cancers are derived from epithelial cells—cells lining the air passages. There are two types of primary tumors, called small-cell and non-small-cell.

GLIMPSE OF THE FUTURE

Changing Recommendations for Skin Testing for TB

The Centers for Disease Control and Prevention (CDC) recommend using the QuantiFERON-TB (QFT) test in the TB guidelines. This blood test is used like the PPD skin test for detecting latent TB infections but also has some advantages over the commonly used PPD test. The QFT is not as affected by Bacille-Calmette-Guerin vaccination as the PPD test. Also, since it is a blood test run by qualified laboratories, it reduces the errors found in the PPD testing from various personnel administering and reading the test. The test is recommended for targeted screening of persons who are at increased risk such as health care workers, immigrants, drug users, military personnel and residents and employees in jails. At this time, the test is not as widely used as the PPD test but, based on the CDC guidelines, it would be the test of choice for detecting TB in the future.

Source: Hudson (2006).

Small-cell tumors, also called oat cell, occur less frequently (16%) but grow rapidly and are often metastatic by the time they are discovered. They usually respond better to chemotherapy and radiation but still carry a much worse prognosis than non-small-cell tumors.

Non-small-cell tumors are more frequent (80%) and are usually treated surgically. This type of lung cancer is strongly associated with smoking.

Metastatic lung cancer is common and often due to metastasis from tumors in other parts of the body. Primary lung cancers also commonly metastasize to other areas, including the brain, bone, and liver.

Lung cancer is the leading cause of cancer deaths in the United States in both men and women. Most lung cancer can be prevented because approximately 90% is due to smoking. Lung cancer claims more lives than colon, prostate, lymph, and breast cancers combined.

■ ***ETIOLOGY.*** Lung cancer is rare among those under 40 and, in most cases, is caused by cigarette smoking. Ninety percent of lung cancer victims are smokers. Men are affected more commonly than women, although the increase in female smokers has increased the number of female lung cancer victims.

■ ***SYMPTOMS.*** Lung cancer is often asymptomatic until metastasis has occurred. Often, the first symptoms are those related to other organs affected by metastasis. Discovery by metastasis makes for a very poor prognosis; approximately 10% of lung cancer victims survive 5 years. Symptoms related to the lung tumor are dyspnea, coughing, and hemoptysis.

■ ***DIAGNOSIS.*** Diagnosis is made by X-ray and tissue biopsy.

■ ***TREATMENT.*** Treatment includes chemotherapy, surgery, and radiation. If the tumor is discovered early, surgical removal might confer cure, but this is rarely the case.

■ ***PREVENTION.*** To never smoke or to quit smoking is the best preventive action.

Diseases of the Pleura and Chest

Diseases of the pleura and chest can be caused by infection, trauma, or other diseases. Pain and shortness of breath are the common symptoms. The severity of such disorders can range from mild to severe, depending on the cause, the individual's age, medical history, and other complicating factors.

PLEURISY (PLEURITIS)

■ ***DESCRIPTION.*** Pleurisy is inflammation of the membranes covering the lung (visceral pleura) and lining the chest cavity (parietal pleura).

■ ***ETIOLOGY.*** Pleurisy can be due to bacterial infection of the pleura. Secondary pleurisy often follows trauma, pneumonia, TB, and neoplasm.

■ ***SYMPTOMS.*** The main symptom of pleurisy is a sharp, chest-area pain that increases with inspiration and coughing. Pain can be so severe that it limits movement in the affected area.

■ ***DIAGNOSIS.*** A distinctive pain with breathing is a classic symptom of pleurisy. This symptom, combined with auscultation of a characteristic friction rub or squeaky, rubbing sound with inspiration, confirm the diagnosis. Identifying the cause of the pleurisy might be more difficult. Identification efforts can include chest X-ray, CT scan, analysis of fluid in the pleural space, and biopsy.

■ ***TREATMENT.*** Treatment is aimed at the cause and includes symptomatic treatment with analgesics, heat application, and taping the chest to restrict movement and, thus, decreasing pain.

■ ***PREVENTION.*** Preventing or treating the various causes, maintaining a healthy lifestyle, and avoiding respiratory allergens are helpful.

PNEUMOTHORAX

■ ***DESCRIPTION.*** Pneumothorax is a collection of air in the pleural cavity, often resulting in partial or complete collapse of the lung on the affected side (Figure 9–13). Spontaneous pneumothorax occurs when air is leaked into the pleural space from the inside or from the lung.

■ ***ETIOLOGY.*** Common causes include pulmonary disease, tumor, or pulmonary tissue tear. Traumatic pneumothorax occurs when air enters the pleural cavity from outside the chest. Causes include gunshot wound, stabbing, or crushing of the chest. A rib fracture often causes a traumatic pneumothorax.

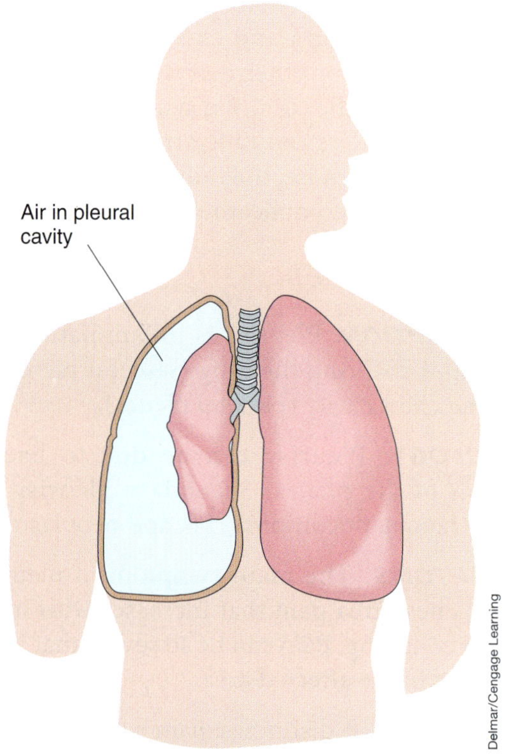

FIGURE 9–13 Pneumothorax.

■ ***SYMPTOMS.*** No matter the cause of the pneumothorax, symptoms are related to the degree of lung collapse. Complete lung collapse causes a sudden, severe chest pain, followed by severe dyspnea and symptoms of shock. Respirations are weak and shallow. Sucking breath sounds might be heard at the site of a traumatic wound. Increased air pressure on the affected side can cause a shift of the mediastinum toward the unaffected side. The condition of mediastinal shift is a medical emergency. Emergency treatment includes placing an occlusive dressing, clean hand, or plastic material over the sucking chest wound to prevent additional air from entering the chest.

■ ***DIAGNOSIS.*** Auscultation of the chest reveals decreased or absent breath sounds. Diagnosis is confirmed by chest X-ray.

■ ***TREATMENT.*** Further treatment can include performing a **thoracentesis** (THOR-rah-sen-TEE-sis; thora = chest, centesis = puncture) to insert a chest tube to withdraw air and assist in reexpanding the lung. Oxygen therapy and analgesics might also be prescribed.

■ ***PREVENTION.*** Preventative measures for noninjury related pneumothorax include not smoking and having respiratory problems treated promptly.

HEMOTHORAX

Hemothorax is the collection of blood in the chest cavity. Cause, symptoms, diagnosis, and treatments are the same as for a pneumothorax. Blood pressure and blood loss are monitored and treated as necessary.

PLEURAL EFFUSION (HYDROTHORAX)

■ ***DESCRIPTION.*** Pleural effusion, or hydrothorax, is a collection of fluid in the chest cavity.

■ ***ETIOLOGY.*** Causes of hydrothorax can include congestive heart failure, TB, or pneumonia.

■ ***SYMPTOMS.*** The affected individual might be asymptomatic or can exhibit signs of dyspnea and chest or pleuritic pain.

HEALTHY HIGHLIGHT

The Harmful Effects of Smoking

The 1982 U.S. Surgeon General's Report stated that, "Cigarette smoking is the major single cause of cancer mortality in the United States." This statement is as true today as it was in 1982 (American Cancer Society, 2008).

Smoking is responsible for nearly one in five deaths in the United States. Because cigarette smoking and tobacco use are acquired behaviors—activities that people choose to do—smoking is the most preventable cause of premature death in our society (American Cancer Society, 2008).

Smoking kills more people than alcohol, AIDS, car crashes, illegal drugs, murders, and suicides combined (Smoke Free Society, 2008).

The preceding facts stress how detrimental cigarette smoking is to the individual and to society. Some other harmful effects of smoking include:

- Its link to cancer, particularly cancer of the lung, larynx, esophagus, pancreas, bladder, kidney, and mouth.
- Heart and cardiovascular disease, especially stroke.
- Increased heart rate.
- Chronic bronchitis and emphysema.
- Decreased rate of lung tissue growth.
- Impaired level of lung function.
- Shortness of breath, especially with exercise, and increased phlegm production.
- Heartburn and peptic ulcers.
- Premature birth and low birth weight if used during pregnancy.
- Shortened life span with increased risk of morbidity.
- Addiction to nicotine.

■ ***DIAGNOSIS.*** Diagnosis is confirmed by X-ray.

■ ***TREATMENT.*** Treatment can include thoracentesis to remove the excess fluid.

■ ***PREVENTION.*** Correction of the condition causing hydrothorax is needed to prevent reoccurrence.

EMPYEMA

■ ***DESCRIPTION.*** Empyema is the collection of pus (py = pus) in the chest cavity.

■ ***ETIOLOGY.*** Empyema can be the result of a ruptured lung abscess or an ulcerated tumor. Empyema is not as common as it was prior to the development of antibiotics.

■ ***SYMPTOMS.*** Symptoms include coughing, dyspnea, and chest pain on the affected side.

■ ***DIAGNOSIS.*** Diagnosis is by X-ray and thoracentesis.

■ ***TREATMENT.*** Microbiologic cultures can be performed on the fluid to identify the infective organism. Antibiotic therapy is a common treatment for bacterial infections.

■ ***PREVENTION.*** Rapid and appropriate treatment of cause prevents this condition.

Diseases of the Cardiovascular and Respiratory Systems

The cardiovascular and respiratory systems are so closely related that many diseases affect both systems. The degree to which each system is affected also is often so similar that it becomes difficult to classify the disease by one system over the other. For this reason, these diseases need further consideration.

PULMONARY EMBOLISM (PE)

■ ***DESCRIPTION.*** PE is a sudden blockage of an artery in the pulmonary system by an embolism (Figure 9–14).

■ ***ETIOLOGY.*** Chapter 8, "Cardiovascular System Diseases and Disorders," discussed the pathology of an embolism. Remember that the floating material can be a blood clot, fat globule, or piece of tissue. Commonly, a blood clot or thrombus develops in the veins of the lower legs, thighs, or pelvis. This clot then breaks loose, floats in the vascular system, and sticks in a pulmonary artery, resulting in a pulmonary embolism.

■ ***SYMPTOMS.*** Symptoms of a PE vary greatly, depending on the size of the clot and the size of the area affected. Dyspnea, cough, chest pain, and apprehension are common symptoms. If the PE is severe, cyanosis, shock, and death can result.

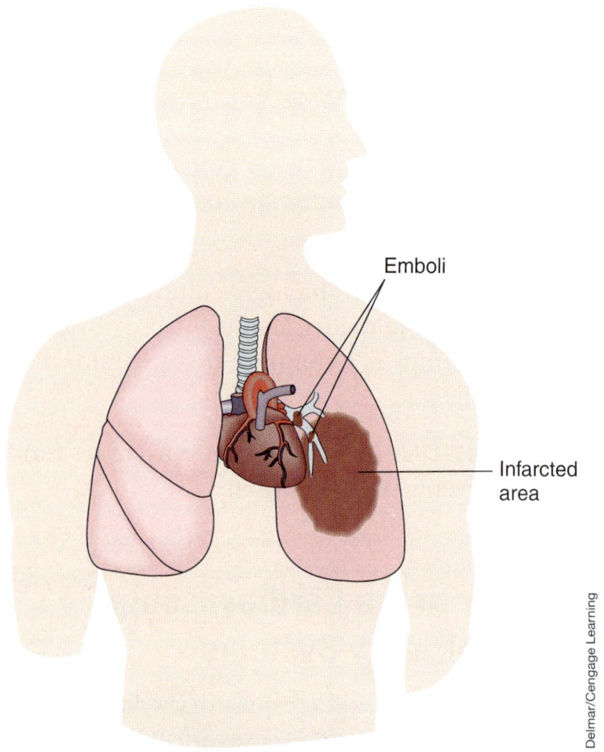

FIGURE 9–14 Pulmonary emboli.

Factors that contribute to the development of an embolism are prolonged bed rest, obesity, and trauma or fractures of the legs or pelvis.

■ ***DIAGNOSIS.*** Diagnosis is confirmed by X-ray examination and lung scans.

■ ***TREATMENT.*** Treatment is aimed at maintaining cardiopulmonary function by administering oxygen and anticoagulation medications.

■ ***PREVENTION.*** Prevention includes ambulation, antiembolic stockings, and leg exercises to improve blood flow and prevent clotting.

PULMONARY EDEMA

■ ***DESCRIPTION.*** Pulmonary edema, if severe, can be a life-threatening medical emergency. It affects the tissue and air spaces of the lungs by filling them with fluid. This fluid leaks out of the vascular system due to increased vascular pressure.

■ ***ETIOLOGY.*** Cardiovascular disease is the common cause of pulmonary edema. It is commonly seen as a result of congestive heart failure and resulting fluid buildup, but any disease that affects blood pressure, heart function, and blood fluid levels can lead to pulmonary edema. These diseases include hypertension, pulmonary embolism, and renal failure.

■ ***SYMPTOMS.*** Pulmonary edema is characterized by dyspnea, orthopnea (ortho = straight, pnea = breath), or difficulty breathing when lying down, and a blood-tinged frothy sputum.

■ ***DIAGNOSIS.*** Diagnosis is determined by ABGs and chest X-ray. ABGs will show an increased carbon dioxide level, and chest X-rays will exhibit increased opacity (whiteness).

■ ***TREATMENT.*** Treatment is aimed at reducing pressure and blood volume. Diuretics to increase urine output, cardiogenics to increase the contraction of the heart, and morphine to bring about venous dilatation might be prescribed. Mechanical respiratory ventilation might also be needed (Figure 9–15).

■ ***PREVENTION.*** Pulmonary edema might not be preventable. Reducing the risk of cardiovascular disease is helpful and includes not smoking, controlling blood pressure, limiting cholesterol, limiting salt intake, exercising daily, eating a heart-healthy diet, and managing stress.

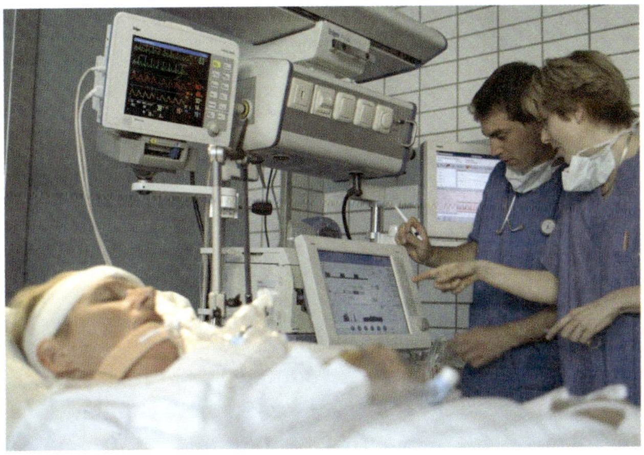

FIGURE 9–15 Respiratory ventilator.

COR PULMONALE

Cor pulmonale was discussed in Chapter 8. Remember that it is a right-sided heart failure related to acute or chronic pulmonary disease. Increased pulmonary blood pressure causes enlargement of the right ventricle and decreased pumping ability. Polycythemia (poly = many, cyt = cell- red cell, emia = blood) develops as the body tries to compensate for hypoxemia (hypo = not enough, ox = oxygen, emia = blood), leading to a thickening of the blood and further increasing workload on the heart.

TRAUMA

Pneumothorax and Hemothorax

Pneumothorax and hemothorax often occur due to some type of trauma. Examples of trauma that often cause these conditions are fractured ribs, gunshot wounds, stabbings, and crushing chest injuries. Collapse of the lung, shock, and death are potential outcomes.

Suffocation

Suffocation is the condition of not breathing to the point of unconsciousness and, eventually, death due to the lack of oxygen and the high level of carbon dioxide in the body tissues. The brain and heart are immediately affected.

Accidental suffocation often occurs with infants and small children playing with plastic bags. Criminal suffocation of homicide victims might be a common finding in forensic pathology. Suffocation can also be caused in a variety of other ways.

- **Aspiration** Aspiration of food that occludes or blocks the airway is common. This type of suffocation leads to the death of approximately one person a day in the United States! Treatment of food aspiration i s immediate attention and can include the performance of an abdominal thrust, previously known as the Heimlich maneuver (see pages 196).
- **Strangulation** Accidental, suicidal, or criminal strangulation can occur by hanging or squeezing the neck with the hands, rope, wire, or a variety of other objects.
- **Drowning** Drowning is a common cause of accidental death, especially in children and adolescent males. Drownings may be classified as wet or dry. Wet drownings are the most common (approximately 90%) and are characterized by water entering the airways and lungs, preventing the entry of oxygen into the system. Dry drownings are less common and are characterized by a reflex laryngospasm that closes the glottis and does not allow water or air to enter. Treatment of either type of drowning is immediate resuscitation and transport to an emergency department.

RARE DISEASES

Pneumoconioses

Pneumoconioses (new-mo-cone-ee-OH-sees) refers to a group of environmentally induced diseases that cause progressive, chronic inflammation and infection. This condition is caused by frequently inhaling the small dust particles of the offending agent for extended periods of time. Pneumoconiosis can occur within a few years, or it might take 20 or 30 years to develop. Types of pneumoconiosis, cause, and related occupations include:

- **Asbestosis**, the most frequently occurring form of the disease, related to insulating and fireproofing.
- **Anthracosis** from inhaling carbon and coal, often called coal miner's disease and black lung.
- **Silicosis** from inhaling silicone affects glass cutters, sand blasters, and stonemasons.

HEALTHY HIGHLIGHT

Abdominal Thrust

The abdominal thrust, previously known as the Heimlich maneuver, is a technique used to remove foreign material—usually food—from the respiratory tract of a choking victim. Choking is a medical emergency. First call 911 emergency medical services and then start the procedure. If the victim is able to talk or has wheezing breath sounds, this maneuver should not be performed; the abdominal thrust is performed only on individuals who are unable to breathe. Treatment for a choking person who cannot speak, turns blue, or stops breathing is based on age. The procedure described here is for an adult. The procedure can be performed with the victim in a standing, or sitting position.

To perform the abdominal thrust on a victim in a sitting or standing position, the rescuer assumes a position behind the victim. The rescuer wraps his or her arms around the victim's waist, allowing the victim's head, arms, and upper body to fall forward. The rescuer makes a fist with one hand and holds it in place with the other hand. The fist should be placed against the victim's abdomen at a point slightly above the umbilicus and below the rib cage. The maneuver calls for the rescuer to perform an upward thrust forcefully to this area. This maneuver can be repeated until the airway is cleared.

If the victim is or becomes unconscious, the rescuer should begin the steps for CPR.

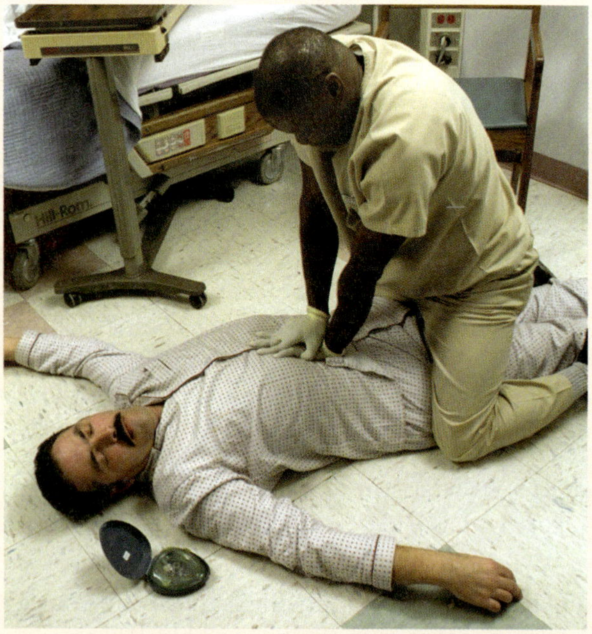

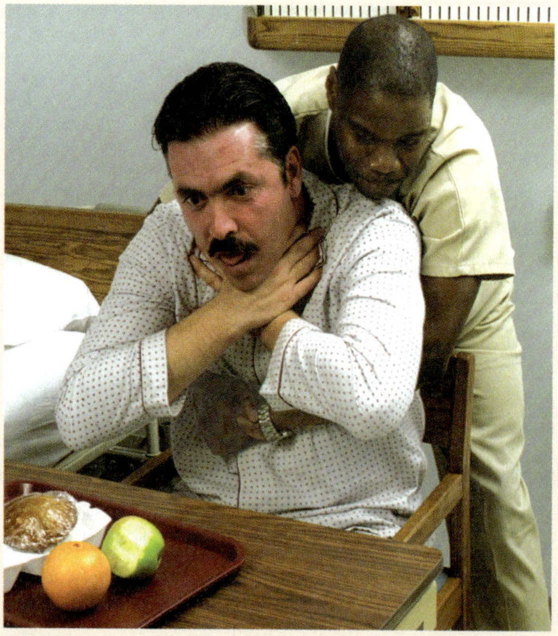

Abdominal thrust or Heimlich maneuver

HEALTHY HIGHLIGHT

If the victim is pregnant or obese, a chest thrust can be performed. The rescuer places both hands under the victim's armpits with the thumb side of the fist on the middle of the breastbone. The fist is covered with the other hand and thrust backward until the object is coughed out. If the victim becomes unconscious, the chest thrust is administered like the abdominal thrust noted previously but on the breastbone rather than below the ribs as in the abdominal thrust.

Fungal Diseases

Fungal diseases affecting the lungs are caused by inhaling an airborne fungus. The lung lesions caused by fungal diseases form granulomatous inflammations like TB, but they do not cavitate (cause cavities in the lung tissue). The fungus can spread through the lung tissue and cause acute illness with symptoms of dyspnea and fever. Treatment consists of rest and antifungal medications. Two forms include:

1. Histoplasmosis, which occurs primarily in the midwestern United States. This fungus is harbored in bird droppings such as those found in chicken houses, bat caves, and pigeon roosts.
2. Coccidioidomycosis (cox-sid-ee-OYD-o-my-co-sis), which occurs primarily in the southwestern United States. This fungus grows in hot, dry areas and produces spores that become windborne. Also known as desert fever and valley fever.

Legionnaires' Disease

Legionnaires' disease is a bacterial pulmonary infection so named as the result of an outbreak in 1976 at a convention of the American Legion held in Philadelphia. The causative bacterium is *Legionella pneumophilia*. This bacteria lives in water storage tanks and cooling systems. Legionnaires' disease can also be called Legionnaires' pneumonia because it produces typical pneumonia symptoms. It differs from other types of pneumonia in that it does not respond to the usual treatment, and it might cause permanent lung damage. Legionnaires' disease is not limited to the pulmonary system like typical pneumonia is; it can cause complications such as liver damage and renal dysfunction. Severe cases might need mechanical ventilation and can have a fatal outcome.

EFFECTS OF AGING ON THE SYSTEM

The effects of aging on the respiratory system increase the risk for the older adult to develop respiratory disease. Over time, the respiratory system loses some of its elasticity, becomes less efficient, and has less reserve. Weakened respiratory muscles contribute to the ineffectiveness of the system. It can also be adversely affected by changes in posture occurring with aging, by the long-term effects of chronic diseases such as COPD, and by the changes occurring in other systems. The older adult usually has a lower tolerance for exercise due to the increased need for oxygen during exercise and the inability of the body to meet that demand.

Changes in the immune responses that occur with aging put the older adult at increased risk for acute respiratory infections. Influenza and pneumonia are common but very serious diseases affecting older adults. Pneumonia is the leading cause of death due to infections in the older population. Another respiratory disease that older people are at increased risk of developing is TB. Their reduced immunity contributes to the high incidence of TB among older adults.

Chronic respiratory diseases are particularly difficult for older people. The nature of the disease, symptoms, effects, and treatments can all contribute to the increased respiratory dysfunction, and thus, the debilitation of the individual. Many older individuals have been heavy smokers for years. The effects of smoking might have already severely damaged respiratory function and will continue to inhibit effective breathing if the individual continues to smoke. Smoking is the major cause of the high incidence of cancer of the lung in older people. Cancer of the lung is the second leading cause of death in the older adult.

SUMMARY

The respiratory system is responsible for the intake of oxygen for the body and the removal of carbon dioxide. Decreased respiratory function greatly limits the ability of other systems because oxygen is necessary at the cellular level for all activities to occur. Diagnostic tests for respiratory diseases include physical examination, chest X-rays, ABGs, and PFTs. Respiratory diseases are a major cause of disability and death in the United States. Acute respiratory diseases such as the common cold, pneumonia, and influenza occur in all age groups. An increased incidence of influenza and other communicable respiratory diseases are causing concern among public health officials. Most chronic respiratory diseases are found in the older adult. Smoking is the greatest contributor to chronic respiratory disease, especially to cancer of the lung.

*Study*WARE™ Connection

View an animation on flail chest on your StudyWARE™ CD-ROM.

REVIEW QUESTIONS

Short Answer

1. What are the functions of the respiratory system?
2. Which signs and symptoms are associated with common respiratory system disorders?
3. Which diagnostic tests are most commonly used to determine the type and cause of respiratory system disorders?
4. What is the most effective preventive technique against the common cold?
5. What behavior puts an individual at highest risk for pulmonary disease?

Matching

6. Match the term on the left with the correct descriptive clause on the right.

_____ asthma	a. Inflammation of the mucous membranes of the sinuses
_____ pneumothorax	b. High-risk behavior for developing respiratory disease
_____ COPD	c. Best preventive behavior against respiratory infections
_____ hemothorax	d. Hypersensitivity reaction, causing constriction of the bronchi
_____ TB	e. Bacterial infection causing a primary lesion in the lung
_____ sinusitis	f. Collapse of part of the lung with blood in the space
_____ cor pulmonale	g. Group of chronic pulmonary diseases
_____ hand washing	h. Right-sided heart failure
_____ smoking	i. Collection of air in the pleural cavity

CASE STUDIES

■ Jake Cooper, a 37-year-old sales executive, recently returned from a business trip in Eastern Asia. He had read about avian flu while visiting clients in Hong Kong and now has some concerns for his own health. He has to return to the same area in 2 weeks and wonders whether he should cancel the trip. What can you tell him about avian (bird) flu? Might he be infected? What symptoms should he watch for? Could he infect his family or friends here? Should he see his family physician? Is there much of a threat to his health from his visit? Would you recommend that he cancel the next trip?

■ Mr. Loftin is a 78-year-old man who has been diagnosed with severe emphysema. He has been a heavy smoker since age 12 and continues to smoke. He complains about his shortness of breath, stating he cannot do much more than walk across the room without gasping for air. He has been cautioned about the effects of his continued smoking, but he responds with statements such as, "What difference does it make if I quit now? I've smoked all my life, and you can't go back and change that." How would you respond to this statement? Is it too late for him to quit and receive some benefit of that behavioral change? Is any of the damage from smoking reversible? How can you explain this to Mr. Loftin?

Workbook Practice

Go to your Workbook and complete the practice questions.

*Study*WARE™ Connection

To help you learn the content in this chapter, take a practice quiz or play an interactive game on your StudyWARE™ CD-ROM.

BIBLIOGRAPHY

American Cancer Society. (2008). Cigarette smoking. American Cancer Society. *www.cancer.org* (accessed May 2008).

American Lung Association. (2006). Tuberculosis skin test fact sheet. American Lung Association. *www.lungusa.org* (accessed May 2008).

American Lung Association. (2007). Chronic obstructive pulmonary disease fact sheet. American Lung Association. *www.lungusa.org* (accessed June 2008).

Banning, M. (2006). Chronic obstructive pulmonary disease: Clinical signs and infections. *British Journal of Nursing 15*(16), 874–880.

Bream-Rouwenhorst, H., Beltz, E., Ross, M., & Moores, K. (2008). Recent developments in the management of acute respiratory distress syndrome in adults. *American Journal of Health-System Pharmacy 65*(1), 29–36.

Centers for Disease Control and Prevention (CDC). (2008). MMWR recommendations and reports. CDC. *www.cdc.org* (accessed May 2008).

Chandler, T. (2007). Reducing re-admission for asthma: Impact of a nurse-led service. *Paediatric Nursing 19*(10), 19–21.

Ciutto, L., & Ashby, M. (2007). The importance of a community-based asthma helpline. *Journal of Asthma 44*(9), 705–710.

Dennison, C. (2008). Transfusion-related acute lung injury: A clinical challenge. *Dimensions of Critical Care Nursing 27*(1), 1–7.

Downs, C., & Appel, S. (2007). Chronic obstructive pulmonary disease and management. *Journal of the American Academy of Nurse Practitioners 19*(3), 126–132.

Eastwood, G., Gardner, A., & O'Connell, B. (2007). Low-flow oxygen therapy: Selecting the right device. *Australian Nursing Journal 15*(4), 27–30.

El Soh, A., Alhajhasan, A., Ramadan, F., & Pineda, L. (2007). A comparative study of community and nursing home acquired empyema thoracis. *Journal of the American Geriatrics Society 55*(11), 1847–1852.

Epstein, L. (2007). Beliefs about asthma differ. *American Journal of Nursing 107*(9), 20.

Fatigue in palliative care. (2007). *Nursing Standard 22*(1), 59.

Hagar, R., Michlitsch, J., Gardner, G., Vichinsky, E., & Morris, C. (2007). *British Journal of Haematology 140*(1). 104–112.

Henderson, Y. (2007). Recognizing dysfunctional breathing in asthma consultations. *Nursing Standard 22*(3), 40–41.

History of flu pandemics. (2007). *Nursing Standard 21*(38), 13.

Hudson, K. (2006). New treatment options push patient care forward. *Nursing Management 37*(8), 49–51.

Jenkins, P. (2007). The relationship between dyspnea and blood pressure in chronic obstructive pulmonary disease. *Journal of Cardiovascular Nursing 22*(5), 351–358.

Langmeier, J. (2007). Tuberculosis of the genitourinary system. *Nursing 27*(4), 279–321.

Linden, A., Berg, G., & Wadhwa, S. (2007). Evaluation of a Medicaid asthma disease management program. *Disease Management 10*(5), 266–272.

Pruitt, B. (2007). Taking an evidence-based approach to treating acute lung injury. *Nursing 37*(Supplement), 14–18.

Rebmann, T. (2005). Severe acute respiratory syndrome. *Journal of Perinatal & Neonatal Nursing 19*(4), 332–345.

Rootmensen, G., van Keimpema, A., Looysen, E., van der Schaaf L., de Haan, R., & Jansen, H. (2008). The effects of additional care by a pulmonary nurse for asthma and COPD patients at a respiratory outpatient clinic: Results from a double blind, randomized clinical trial. *Patient Education & Counseling 70*(2), 179–186.

Sims, J. (2007). An overview of pulmonary embolism. *Dimensions of Critical Care 26*(5), 182–186.

Smoke Free Society. (2008). Tobacco and You. *www.smokefreesociety.org* (accessed May 2008).

Stallard, L. (2007). Chronic obstructive pulmonary disease: A non-pharmacological approach. *Nursing Older People 19*(6), 32–36.

Tesfaigzi, Y., Meek, P., & Lareau, S. (2006). Exacerbations of chronic obstructive pulmonary disease and chronic mucus hypersecretion. *Clinical & Applied Immunology Reviews 6*(1), 21–36.

Tuberculosis diagnosis and management. (2007). *Thorax 62*(Supplement), A80–A83.

Triple inhaled therapy best for COPD. (2008). *Pulse 68*(1), 8.

Vally, H. (2008). Allergic and asthmatic reactions to alcoholic drinks: A significant problem in the community. *Clinical & Experimental Allergy 38*(1), 1–3.

Wagner, J., Jiang, Q., Harkema, J., Ames. B., Illek, B., Roubey, R., & Peden, D. (2008). Y-tocopherol prevents airway esinophilia and mucus cell hyperplasia in experimentally induced allergic rhinitis and asthma. *Clinical & Experimental Allergy 38*(3), 501–511.

Walke, L., Byers, A., Tinetti, M., Dubin, J., McCorkle, R., & Fried, T. (2007). Range and severity of symptoms over time among older adults with chronic obstructive pulmonary disease and heart failure. *Archives of Internal Medicine 167*(22), 2503–2508.

World Health Organization (WHO). (March 2006). Tuberculosis fact sheet: Global and regional incidence. WHO. *www.who.int* (accessed May 2008).

World Health Organization (WHO). (2008). Sudden Acute Respiratory Syndrome (SARS). WHO. *www.who.int* (accessed May 2008).

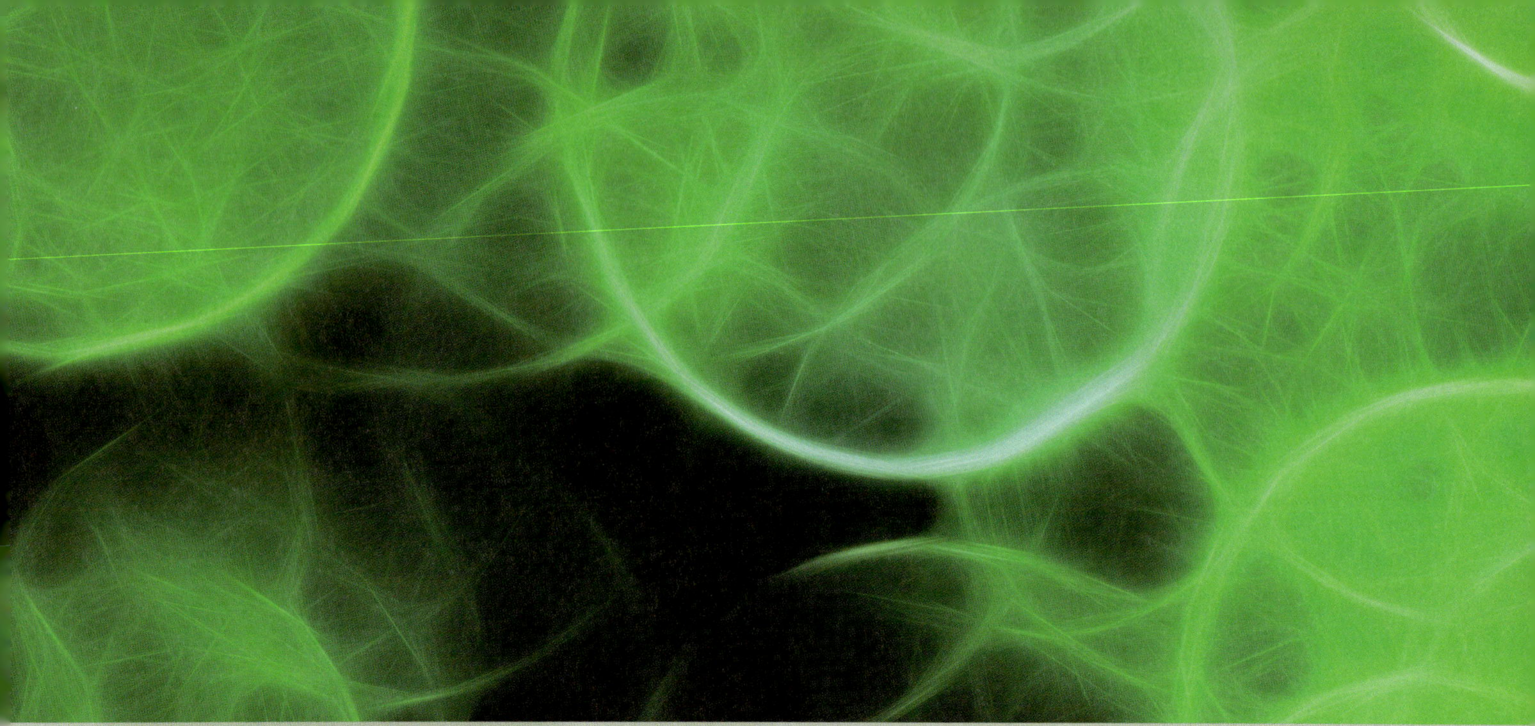

OUTLINE

- Anatomy and Physiology
- Common Signs and Symptoms
- Diagnostic Tests
- Common Diseases of the Lymphatic System
  Lymphadenitis
  Lymphangitis
  Lymphedema
  Lymphoma
  Mononucleosis
- Rare Diseases
  Kawasaki Disease
- Effects of Aging on the System
- Summary
- Review Questions
- Case Studies
- Bibliography

KEY TERMS

Lymph (p. 204)
Lymphadenopathy (p. 205)
Lymphangiography (p. 205)
Lymphangiopathy (p. 205)
Lymphocytes (p. 205)
Lymphocytopenia (p. 205)
Lymphocytosis (p. 205)

10

Lymphatic System Diseases and Disorders

LEARNING OBJECTIVES

Upon completion of the chapter, the learner should be able to:

1. Define the terminology common to the lymphatic system and the disorders of the system.
2. Discuss the basic anatomy and physiology of the lymphatic system.
3. Identify the important signs and symptoms associated with common lymphatic system disorders.
4. Describe the common diagnostics used to determine the type and cause of lymphatic system disorders.
5. Identify common disorders of the lymphatic system.
6. Describe the typical course and management of the common lymphatic system disorders.
7. Describe the effects of aging on the lymphatic system and the common disorders associated with aging of the system.

OVERVIEW

The lymphatic system is the infection-fighting system of the body. It works with the immune system to play an important role in preventing infection and maintaining one's immunity. The lymphatic system includes the lymph nodes, lymph vessels, and fluid lymph. It is a special vascular system that picks up excess tissue fluid and returns it to the blood. Disorders of the system include inflammatory conditions and neoplasms. The lymphatic system is so closely related to the immune system, the blood and blood-forming organs, and the cardiovascular system that many of the concepts and diseases of the system have already been discussed. Refer to these chapters for additional information on the lymphatic system. ■

ANATOMY AND PHYSIOLOGY

The lymphatic system includes lymph vessels, ducts, and nodes (Figure 10–1). It is important in protecting the body from infection and filters bacterial and nonbacterial products resulting from the inflammatory process. The goal of the system is to prevent these waste products from entering the general circulation, but this activity can cause some inflammation of the node filtering the waste products, causing swelling and redness of the involved node.

The lymphatic system depends, to some extent, on the vascular system because the lymphatic system returns its fluids and other materials to the vascular system. There is diffusion of fluid between the lymphatic vessels, the interstitial spaces, and the blood capillaries.

The fluid in the lymphatic system is called **lymph**, a clear liquid similar to plasma that contains many white cells. The conducting vessels of the lymphatic system include the capillaries, the smallest vessels, and the larger lymph vessels, which have valves much like the veins in the cardiovascular system. In the lymph vessels, the direction of flow is toward the thoracic cavity. The vessels meet in the right lymphatic duct or the left lymphatic duct, which drain into the venous system. The right lymphatic duct drains the lymph from the right half of the head, upper torso, and right arm. The rest of the lymph vessels in the body drain into the left lymphatic duct, also called the thoracic duct.

The lymph vessels have other functions besides the transportation of lymph. They also return important nutrients such as proteins and large particulate matter that have leaked out into the capillaries to the blood vessels (Figure 10–2). In the course of a day, approximately 3 liters of extra fluid is leaked into the tissue and not picked up by the venous system. The lymphatic system picks up this extra fluid and returns it to the blood. In addition, the lymph vessels transport toxic substances to the nodes for filtration.

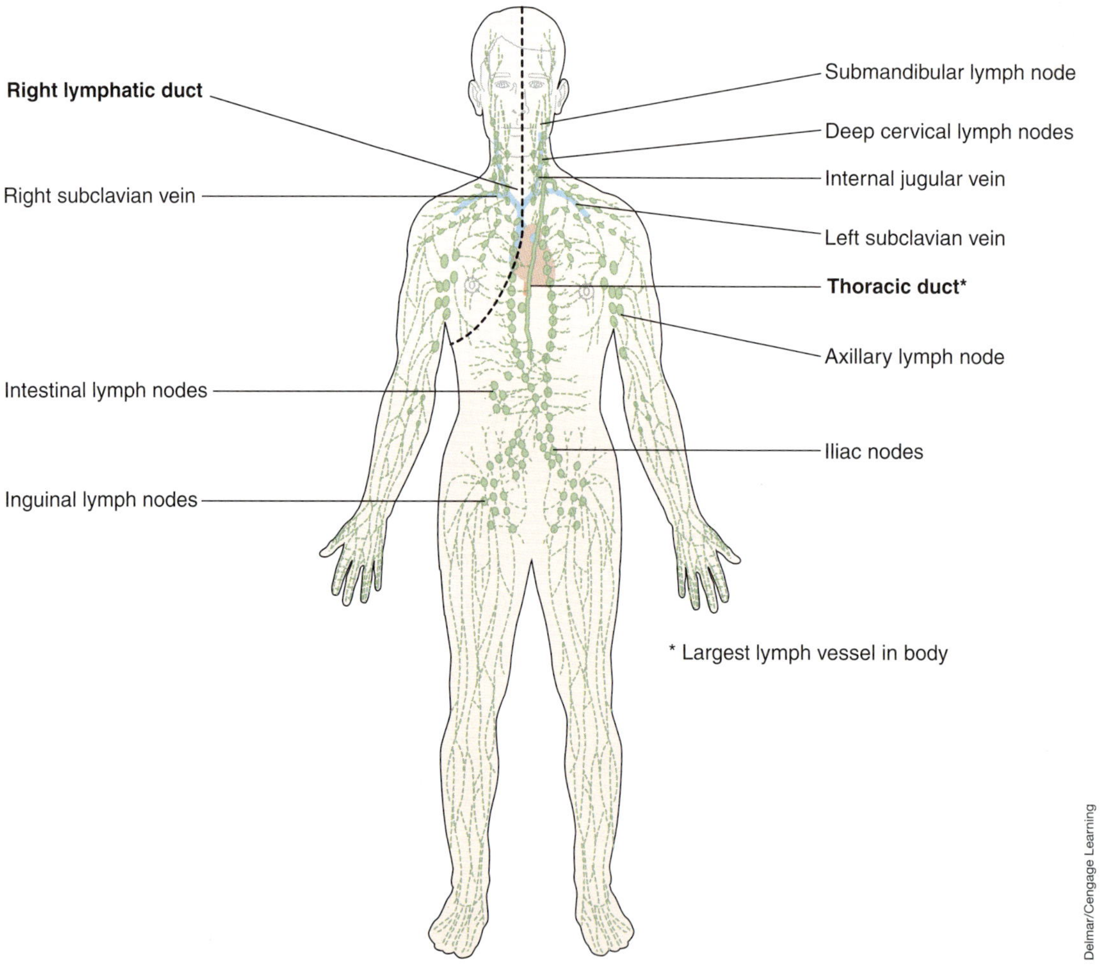

FIGURE 10–1 The lymphatic system.

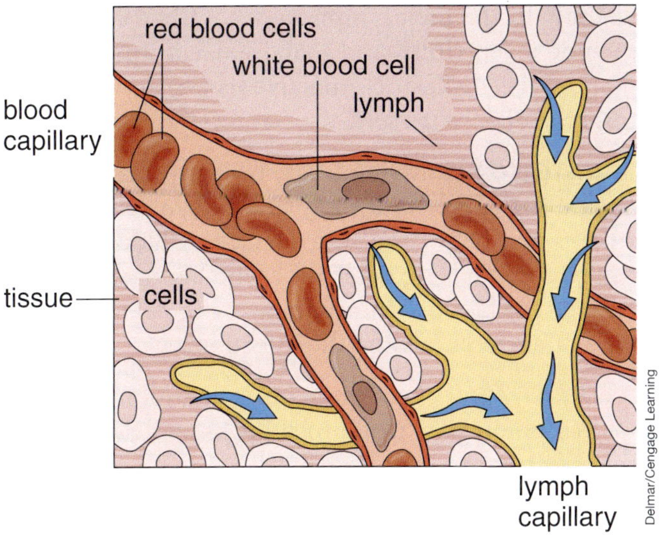

FIGURE 10–2 Exchange of fluids between the lymph and blood vessels.

In the digestive process, the vessels are important in the absorption of fats. The nodes are important in the filtering process, but they also produce lymphocytes and protect the body by developing immunity to some diseases.

Organs related to the lymph system are the tonsils, thymus gland, and spleen. These organs also play a part in the body's immunity and protection system. See Chapter 5, "Immune System Diseases and Disorders," for a discussion on immunity.

StudyWARE™ Connection

View an animation on the lymphatic system on your StudyWARE™ CD-ROM.

COMMON SIGNS AND SYMPTOMS

Enlargement of the lymph glands or nodes is common and is usually due to infection somewhere in the body. Infection stimulates activity of the nodes and glands to produce more **lymphocytes** (white cells created in the lymphatic system). Fever, fatigue, and weight loss are common with lymphatic diseases.

Most disorders of the lymphatic system are related to diseases of other systems. **Lymphocytosis** (lympho = lymph, cyto = cell, osis = increase or an abnormal increase in lymphocytes) and **lymphocytopenia** (lymphocyte = lymph cell, penia = decrease or an abnormal decrease in lymphocytes) in blood and tissue can accompany diseases of the immune system as well as of the lymphatic system.

DIAGNOSTIC TESTS

A complete blood count with white cell differential can assist in determination of inflammation or infectious diseases of the lymphatic system.

Lymphangiography (lim-FAN-jee-OG-rah-fee; lymph = lymph, angio = vessel, graphy = procedure) consists of injecting a contrast dye and taking X-rays. This procedure can be helpful in diagnosing vessel conditions. Magnetic resonance imaging (MRI) and computerized tomography (CT) can also be used.

Biopsy of lymph glands and nodes can assist in determination of lymphoma. A special connective tissue cell called a Reed–Sternberg cell confirms a diagnosis of Hodgkin's disease.

COMMON DISEASES OF THE LYMPHATIC SYSTEM

Diseases of the lymphatic system commonly include inflammatory conditions. Often, diseases of this system are the result of disease in another system. Disease of lymph glands collectively can be called **lymphadenopathy** (lim-FAD-eh-NOP-ah-thee; lymph = lymph, adeno = gland, opathy = disease). **Lymphangiopathy** (lim-FAN-jee-OP-ah-thee; lymph = lymph, angio = vessel, opathy = disease) is a general term to describe any disease of the lymph vessels.

Lymphadenitis

■ ***DESCRIPTION.*** Lymphadenitis (lim-FAD-eh-NIGH-tis; lymph = lymph, adeno = gland, itis = inflammation) is characterized by swelling of the lymph gland, nodes, or both.

■ ***ETIOLOGY.*** Lymphadenitis is usually caused by infection somewhere in the body. Drainage of bacteria or toxic substances can cause the swelling. The location of the affected nodes can assist in determination of cause.

■ ***SYMPTOMS.*** Swelling, pain, and tenderness of the gland or node are common.

■ ***DIAGNOSIS.*** A physical examination revealing swollen lymph nodes is indicative of lymphadenitis. A blood culture can be performed to determine spread of infection to the bloodstream. A biospy confirms the diagnosis.

■ ***TREATMENT.*** Antibiotic treatment is helpful with bacterial infections.

■ ***PREVENTION.*** Maintaining good general health is helpful in preventing any infection.

Lymphangitis

■ ***DESCRIPTION.*** Lymphangitis (lymph = lymph, angi = vessel, itis = inflammation) is a condition of swelling of the lymph vessel due to inflammation.

■ ***ETIOLOGY.*** This inflammation is commonly caused by infection with streptococcal bacteria following a trauma.

■ ***SYMPTOMS.*** Lymphangitis is often characterized by a red streak at the site of bacterial entry that extends to the area lymph nodes. Other symptoms include fever, chills, and malaise. Cellulitis (inflammation of cellular or connective tissue) and leukocytosis can also be present.

■ ***DIAGNOSIS.*** Diagnosis is immediate based on the high fever and the primary symptom of red streaks just below the skin surface. A blood culture can be completed to determine whether bacteria have entered the bloodstream. A biopsy can determine the type of bacteria causing the infection.

■ ***TREATMENT.*** Lymphangitis is commonly treated with antibiotics. Warm, moist packs and elevation of the affected area are also helpful.

■ ***PREVENTION.*** Good hygiene and maintaining good general health are preventive activities.

Lymphedema

■ ***DESCRIPTION.*** Lymphedema (lymph = lymph, edema = swelling) is an abnormal collection of lymph fluid, usually observed in the extremities (Figure 10–3).

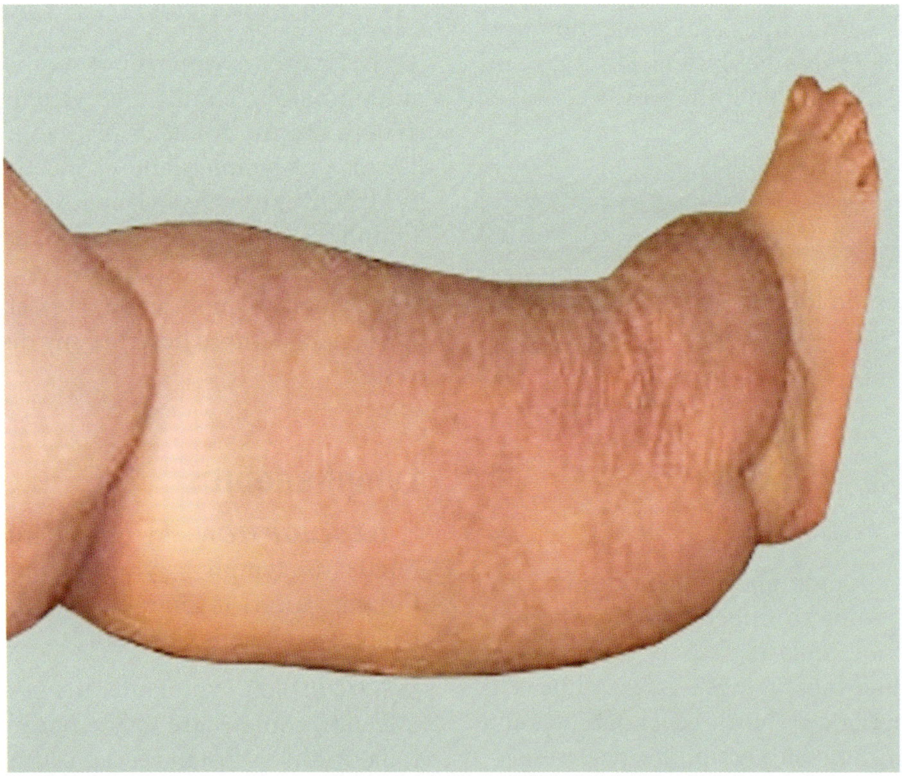

FIGURE 10–3 Lymphedema.

GLIMPSE OF THE FUTURE

Weight Reduction Programs Might Help Reduce Lymphedema

Clinical trials are testing the effects of weight reduction as a treatment for lymphedema in women who have had a mastectomy for breast cancer. Lymphedema in the upper extremities is a common side effect of this surgery. This trial studied women who had post-mastectomy-related lymphedema and were put on a weight reduction plan. The results showed that weight loss could significantly relieve the lymphedema in these subjects. Further study is needed, but in the future, weight reduction programs may be part of the standard treatment for individuals with lymphedema due to breast cancer surgery.

Source: Shaw, et al. (2007).

ETIOLOGY. The most common causes are:

- Surgery or radiation treatments for cancer, especially breast and testicular surgeries.

  Breast cancer surgery (mastectomy) and radiation can lead to a chronic lymphedema of the arm on the affected side. About 30% of all post-mastectomy patients are affected by lymphedema.
- Surgery on blood vessels of the arms or legs.
- Other surgical procedures, such as liposuction.
- Other causes such as pregnancy, burns, and trauma.

SYMPTOMS. Symptoms occur in the arms and legs and include swelling and heaviness. Swelling can also extend into the fingers and toes, causing tight-fitting rings and shoes.

DIAGNOSIS. History and physical examination of the affected area along with CT and MRI scans confirm the diagnosis.

TREATMENT. Treatment is dependent on the cause. Antibiotics might be needed to treat infections that worsen with lymphedema. Placing the affected arm or leg above heart level, while resting, and exercise to increase lymph flow can decrease the edema. Procedures such as obtaining blood pressure and drawing blood samples should not be performed on the affected side because affected tissue is more prone to infection.

Pregnancy and constrictive clothing often cause an increase in venous pressure, resulting in an accumulation of fluid in the ankles and feet. Decreasing venous pressure in these cases will relieve lymphedema. To reduce venous pressure in the pregnant female, lying on the left side helps improve venous

COMPLEMENTARY AND ALTERNATIVE THERAPY

Alternative Treatment for Lymphedema: Low-Level Laser Therapy

The Food and Drug Administration (FDA) in October 2006 approved the use of a new alternative treatment for post–breast cancer lymphedema. The FDA-approved device is the Riancorp LTU-904 Laser Therapy Unit. This is the only laser device approved by the FDA for lymphedema treatment, and it is approved only for post-mastectomy lymphedema. The laser therapy unit uses infrared lasers to penetrate tissue where the edema is located. There has been some success with this treatment, but the effects are not permanent. Most individuals have to be treated three times per week for 6 weeks. Long-term results are still being evaluated.

Source: Tassis (2006); RianCorp (2006).

flow because the inferior vena cava is to the right of midline. Constrictive clothing should be removed or loosened when lymphedema is observed.

Compression therapy might be needed temporarily or life long, depending on the cause of the condition. Compression aids in pushing the excessive fluid back into the venous or lymphatic system. Compression also aids in venous return or return flow of both the lymphatic and venous system. Compression gloves, arm wraps, and leg stockings are available for this purpose.

Surgery might be needed to remove excess tissue if the affected limb becomes so large and heavy that it interferes with the ability to move and walk.

■ ***PREVENTION.*** Activities to reduce the risk of lymphedema include protecting the affected extremity (arm or leg), elevating the area while at rest, avoiding heat directly on the area, avoiding tight clothing, and keeping the extremity clean to prevent infection.

Lymphoma

Lymphoma refers to several types of neoplasms that affect lymphoid tissue (lymph nodes, tonsils, spleen, and lymph fluid). There are many types of lymphoma, but all affect normal lymphocyte production, leading to an impaired immunity. Lymphoma is the most common type of blood cancer in the United States. Lymphoma is discussed in more detail in Chapter 7, "Blood and Blood-Forming Organs Diseases and Disorders," under the heading, "Disorders of White Blood Cells."

Mononucleosis

Mononucleosis is a viral infection that affects primarily children and young adults. It is somewhat contagious and is commonly called the kissing disease. This disease is discussed in more detail in Chapter 7 under the heading "Disorders of White Blood Cells."

RARE DISEASES

Kawasaki Disease

This disorder is also called mucocutaneous lymph node syndrome. It is an acute febrile disease found mostly in children and causes cervical lymphadenopathy. It resembles scarlet fever because the individual develops a rash and some edema of the hands and feet. Other symptoms include lethargy, congestion, irritability, fever, dry skin and reddened lips, tongue, and mucous membranes. Treatment is supportive because the disease does not respond to antibiotic therapy. This disease is rarely fatal in the acute stage, but children can die quite suddenly some years later due to coronary artery disease.

EFFECTS OF AGING ON THE SYSTEM

As the individual ages, there is decreased ability to produce antibodies, leading to decreases in the normal immune response, which interferes with the normal ability to ward off infections. If other chronic diseases are also present, the individual can be at an even higher risk for poor healing and development of infections. In addition, as the immune response becomes less effective, the individual is more susceptible to autoimmune disorders. Many diseases of the older adult have some direct relationship to the decreased immune response. Because the lymphatic system depends, for some of its functions, on the vascular system, additional problems arise in the older person who has impaired circulation or other vascular system diseases.

SUMMARY

The lymphatic system plays an important role in the body's ability to fight infection and maintain immunity. The system is composed of lymph, lymph nodes, and vessels to transport the lymph. The lymphatic system also transports fluid that has leaked into the interstitial areas between the blood vessels. Diseases of the system are usually caused by infections or neoplasms and can range from mild to severe. Treatment varies with the particular type of disease. Common symptoms include fever, fatigue, weight loss, and enlarged lymph nodes.

REVIEW QUESTIONS

Short Answer

1. What are the three main functions of the lymphatic system?

2. Name the four signs and symptoms associated with common lymphatic system disorders.

3. Which diagnostic tests are most commonly used to determine the type and cause of lymphatic system disorders?

True or False

4. T F Diseases of the lymphatic system commonly include inflammatory conditions.
5. T F Lymphangiography is a biopsy of a lymph node or several nodes.
6. T F Lymphadenitis is characterized by a swelling of the lymph nodes.
7. T F Lymphangitis is a condition of swelling of lymph vessels due to inflammation.
8. T F Lymphedema is always caused by obstruction of a lymphatic vessel.
9. T F Mononucleosis is a bacterial infection that usually affects children and young adults.
10. T F Lymphoma affects lymphocyte production and impairs immunity.

CASE STUDIES

■ Mrs. Talik is 78 years old and has been hospitalized frequently for repeated respiratory infections. Until the past 2 years, she has been relatively healthy. She has not been diagnosed with any serious chronic diseases but does have some osteoporosis. Based on your knowledge of the aging process and the lymphatic system changes, what might be contributing to the development of these repeated respiratory infections? What can she do to decrease her risk and improve her immunity to infections?

■ Mrs. Smithson is a 55-year-old woman who has had a mastectomy for breast cancer. She has severe lymphedema in her right arm. She had talked to her physician about treatments for this, and he recommended using compression wraps and keeping the arm elevated. Are there any other recommendations you could make to her? How would you explain the cause of her lymphedema to her? She states that she heard laser therapy would cure her condition. What should you tell her about that?

*Study***WARE**™ Connection

To help you learn the content in this chapter, take a practice quiz or play an interactive game on your StudyWARE™ CD-ROM.

Workbook Practice

Go to your Workbook and complete the practice questions.

BIBLIOGRAPHY

Appollo, K. (2007). Lower-extremity lymphedema in a patient with gynecologic cancer. *Oncology Nursing Forum 34*(5), 937–939.

Beesley V., Janda, M, Eakin, E., Obermair, A., & Battistutta, D. (2007). Lymphedema after gynecological treatment. *Cancer 109*(12), 2607–2614.

Carboon, I. (2008). Rethinking the evidence imperative: Why patients choose complementary and alternative medicine. *Leukemia & Lymphoma 49*(2), 181–182.

Eashall, A. (2007). Compression hosiery: Donning aids and garment removal. *British Journal of Community Nursing 12*(10), S10–S16.

FDA approvals: LYU-904, Ortho T, Cruzi, Paragon Z CRT. (2007). Medscape Medical News. *www.medscape.com* (accessed May 2008).

Gary, D. (2007). Lymphedema diagnosis and management. *Journal of the American Academy of Nurse Practitioners 19*(2), 72–78.

Honor, A. (2006). The staging of lymphedema and accompanying symptoms. *British Journal of Community Nursing 11*(10), S6–S8.

Horning, K. (2007). Lymphedema: An under-treated problem. *MEDSURG Nursing 16*(4), 221–227.

Ji, R. (2007). Lymphatic endothelial cells, inflammatory lymphangiogenesis, and prospective players. *Current Medicinal Chemistry 14*(22), 2359–2368.

Lacovara, J., & Yoder, L. (2006). Secondary lymphedema in the cancer patient. *MEDSURG Nursing 15*(5), 302–306.

Linnitt, N., & Davies, R. (2007). Fundamentals of compression in the management of lymphedema. *British Journal of Nursing 16*(10), 588–592.

Low level laser therapy (2007). Lymphatic Research Foundation. *www.lymphnotes.com/article* (accessed February 13, 2008).

Lymphedema. (2008) National Cancer Institute. *www.cancer.org* (accessed May 2008).

Marrs, J. (2007). Lymphedema and implications for oncology nursing practice. *Clinical Journal of Oncology Nursing 11*(1), 19–21.

RianCorp Pty Ltd. (2006). FDA clears laser-based lymphedema therapy. RianCorp Pty Ltd. *www.riancorp.com* (accessed February 13, 2008).

Shaw, C., Mortimer, P., & Judd, P. (2007). A randomized controlled trial of weight reduction as a treatment for breast-related lymphedema. *Cancer 110*(8), 1868–1874.

Stacker, S., Hughes, R., Williams, R., & Achen, M. (2006). Current strategies modulating lymphangiogenesis signaling pathways in human diseases. *Current Medicinal Chemistry 13*(7), 783–792.

Tassis, J. (2007). FDA approves LTU-940 low level laser for lymphedema treatment. Circle of Hope Lymphedema

Foundation, Inc. *www.lymphedemacircleofhope.org* (accessed February 13, 2008).

Tester, M., & Lakasing, E. (2007). Glandular fever: A practical lesson in acute inflammation. *Primary Health Care 17*(9), 40–42.

Williams, R. (2007). Fit for purpose. *Nursing Standard 21*(25), 55–57.

Zakaria, S., Johnson, R., Pockaj, B., & Degnim, A. (2007). Breast cancer presenting as unilateral arm edema. *Journal of General Internal Medicine 22*(5), 675–676.

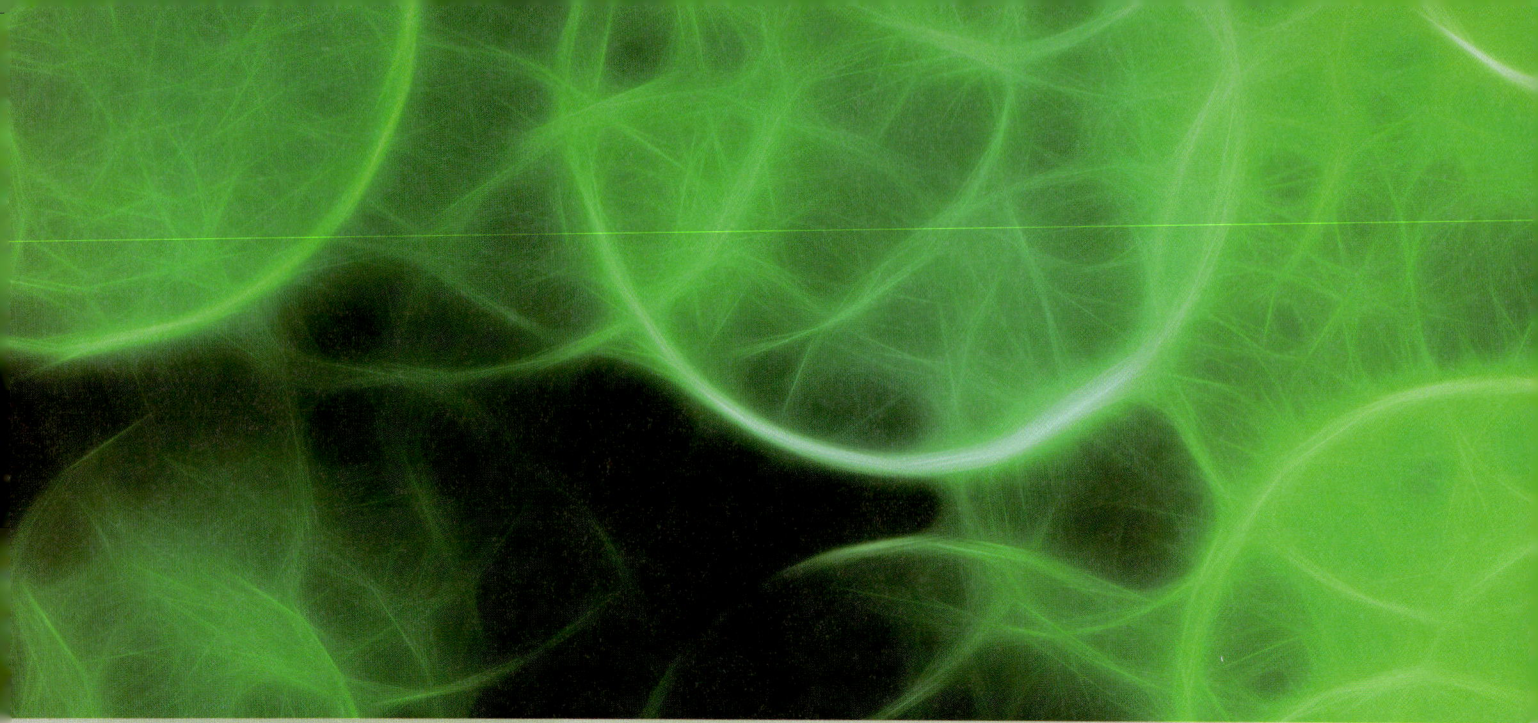

OUTLINE

- Anatomy and Physiology
- Common Signs and Symptoms
- Diagnostic Tests
- Common Diseases of the Digestive System
  Diseases of the Mouth
  Diseases of the Throat and Esophagus
  Diseases of the Stomach
  Diseases of the Small Intestine
  Diseases of the Colon
  Diseases of the Rectum
- Trauma
  Trauma to the Mouth
  Trauma to the Stomach and Intestines
- Rare Diseases
  Achalasia
  Gluten-Induced Enteropathy
  Intestinal Polyps
- Effects of Aging on the System
- Summary
- Review Questions
- Case Studies
- Bibliography

KEY TERMS

Achlorhydria (p. 222)
Adhesions (p. 227)
Asymptomatic (p. 221)
Colorectal (p. 232)
Defecate (p. 216)
Dental plaque (p. 218)
Enterotoxin (p. 229)
Exacerbation (p. 224)
Feces (p. 215)
Gingivitis (p. 218)
Hematemesis (p. 215)
Hematochezia (p. 215)
Ileus (p. 227)
Intrinsic factor (p. 215)
Intussusception (p. 227)
Malaise (p. 225)
Melena (p. 215)
Motility (p. 215)
Occult blood (p. 218)
Ova and Parasite (O&P) (p. 218)
Paralytic obstruction (p. 228)
Perforation (p. 215)
Peristalsis (p. 214)
Peritonitis (p. 215)
Polyp (p. 232)
Remission (p. 224)
Salmonella (p. 229)
Septicemia (p. 216)
Stool (p. 215)
Strep throat (p. 220)
Vermiform (p. 227)
Virulent (p. 220)
Volvulus (p. 227)

11

Digestive System Diseases and Disorders

LEARNING OBJECTIVES

Upon completion of the chapter, the learner should be able to:

1. Define the terminology common to the upper and lower digestive system and the disorders of the system.
2. Discuss the basic anatomy and physiology of the digestive system.
3. Identify the important signs and symptoms associated with common digestive system disorders.
4. Describe the common diagnostics used to determine type and cause of digestive system disorders.
5. Identify the common disorders of the digestive system.
6. Describe the typical course and management of the common digestive system disorders.
7. Describe the effects of aging on the digestive system and the common disorders associated with aging of the system.

OVERVIEW

The digestive system provides nutrients for the body through the processes of ingestion, digestion, and absorption and eliminates waste products from the system. Diseases or disorders of the digestive system are some of the most common medical problems. Because there are many differences in eating patterns, lifestyle behaviors, and inherited traits, digestive system problems vary considerably among individuals. Some digestive system problems are caused by poor nutritional habits, whereas others might be due to structural problems or a particular disease process. ■

ANATOMY AND PHYSIOLOGY

The digestive system has been described as a long tube running through the body. It has two main purposes: (1) to change the food we eat into simpler substances so they can be absorbed into the blood and carried to all cells of the body and (2) to eliminate waste products from the body. The two major parts of the digestive system are the alimentary canal and the accessory organs, including the tongue, teeth, salivary glands, gallbladder, pancreas, and liver.

The alimentary canal (Figure 11–1) is a continuous tube running from the mouth to the anus. The term *gastrointestinal (GI) tract* technically refers only to the stomach and intestines but is often used as a synonym for the alimentary canal. The alimentary canal is approximately 30 feet, or 9 meters, in length, but most of it is coiled up in the abdomen and surrounded by the peritoneum. The peritoneum is a large, serous membrane covering the organs in the abdomen and lining the walls of the abdominal cavity. It secretes fluid to prevent friction between organs in the abdomen as they move during the process of digestion. The alimentary canal starts at the mouth, where ingested food begins to be broken down to supply the body with needed nourishment. The teeth begin the process by breaking the food into smaller parts. The tongue, the organ of taste, assists the process by helping move the food in the mouth. The salivary glands, located outside the mouth with ducts leading from the glands to the mouth, secrete about 1,500 milliliters of saliva per day. The saliva continues the process of breaking down food and moistening it to make it easier to swallow. At the back of the mouth lies the pharynx, the channel for food to pass from the mouth to the esophagus.

The esophagus is a tube (about 9 inches in length) that extends from the pharynx to the stomach. The walls of the esophagus are very muscular. Movement of these muscles is called peristaltic contraction. These contractions, the process called **peristalsis**, move the food from the pharynx to the stomach.

The stomach is a sac-type receptacle that lies just under the diaphragm in the upper abdomen. The esophagus connects to the stomach at the cardiac

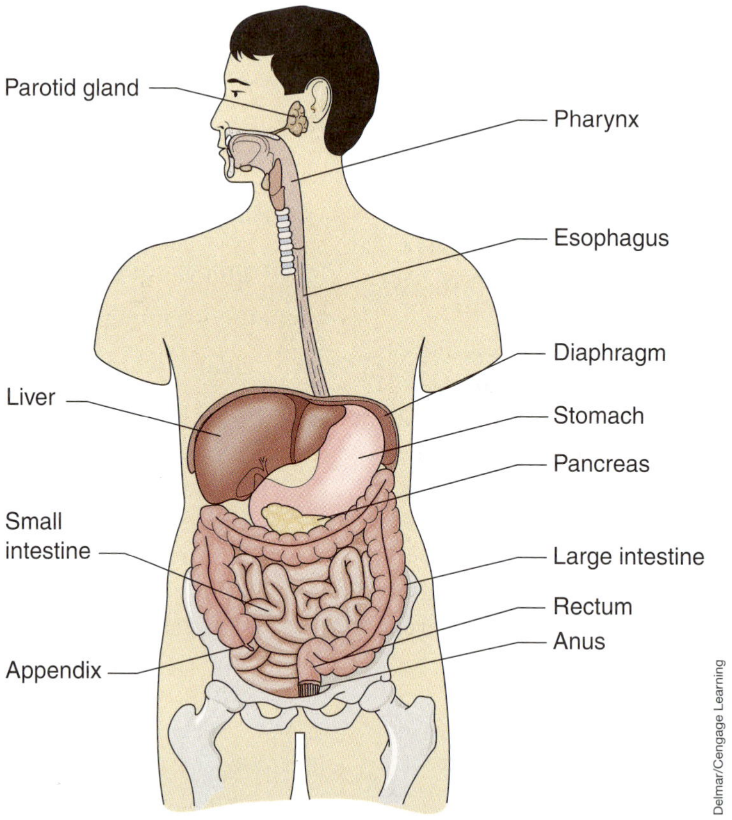

FIGURE 11–1 The digestive system.

orifice (opening). A thick ring of smooth muscle called the cardiac, or gastroesophageal, sphincter surrounds this opening. The upper portion of the stomach, at the cardiac orifice end, is called the fundus, and the middle portion of the stomach is called the body. Food is broken down in the stomach by a process of chemical changes from the action of pepsin—an enzyme—and hydrochloric acid secreted by cells in the stomach. Food is mixed with these chemicals by the contractions of the stomach. The lining of the stomach also secretes a substance called the **intrinsic factor**, which is necessary for the absorption of vitamin B_{12}. At the lower portion of the stomach, called the pyloric region, the stomach is connected to the first part of the small intestine, called the duodenum. The opening at this end of the stomach is the pyloric orifice, which is surrounded by the pyloric sphincter. Sphincter muscles control the cardiac and pyloric openings.

The small intestine extends from the pyloric orifice to the ileocecal valve at the beginning of the large intestine It is divided into three sections. The first section, the duodenum, is about 10 inches, or 25 centimeters, in length, the shortest of the three sections. The duodenum receives bile from the liver and pancreatic juices from the pancreas, which aid in the digestive process. The duodenum connects the stomach to the jejunum (jay-JUNE-um), the second section of the small intestine, on the left side of the upper abdomen. The jejunum extends from the duodenum to the ileum. It is about 7.5 feet, or 2 meters, in length and is coiled throughout the abdomen. The ileum is the third section of the small intestine, attaching to the jejunum at its beginning and ending at the ileocecal (il-ee-oh-SEE-cal) valve, the beginning of the large intestine.

The major function of the small intestine is digestion and absorption of food and fluids. Material is moved through the small intestine by muscular action (peristalsis). Most of digestion takes place in the small intestine. Finger-like projections called villi, containing lymph vessels and blood capillaries, are located on the inside surface of the intestine. Additional extensions called microvilli cover the villi, forming a velvety surface that greatly increases the surface area of the small intestine. As a result of this increased surface area, nutrient absorption is greatly increased. Nutrients pass into the vascular capillaries for delivery to the body cells.

The large intestine connects to the small intestine at the ileocecal valve in the lower-right portion of the abdomen. The first section of the colon is called the cecum. The appendix is attached to the cecum near the ileocecal valve. The large intestine, also called the colon, is about 5 feet, or 1.5 meters, long. Each section of the colon is named according to its anatomical position. The colon begins in the lower-right quadrant of the abdomen (cecum), rises to the mid-level (ascending colon), crosses the abdomen at the umbilicus level (transverse colon), and descends on the left side (descending colon) into the pelvic cavity, where it is called the sigmoid colon. The sigmoid colon forms an S-shaped tube that extends into the lower pelvic region, ending at the rectum and anus. The process of digestion and absorption continues in the large intestine, but the most important function of the large intestine is the absorption of water and electrolytes and the elimination of **feces**, the material not absorbed by the intestines.

> ***Study*WARE™ Connection**
>
> View an animation on digestion on your StudyWARE™ CD-ROM.

COMMON SIGNS AND SYMPTOMS

Diseases of this system usually result in signs and symptoms related to hemorrhage, **perforation**, and altered **motility** (movement) in the system. Hemorrhage can be mild or severe and can originate at any site along the system. Terms identifying bleeding are **hematemesis** (HEM-ah-TEM-eh-sis; hemat = blood, emesis = vomiting), **hematochezia** (HEM-at-toe-KEE-zee-ah, bright red blood in the feces), and **melena** (meh-LEE-nah, dark, tarry **stool**) due to the presence of blood.

Perforation in any area of the tract can be life-threatening due to the contaminating contents of the tract and the ease of spread in the abdominal cavity. Perforation in the stomach or intestines allows spillage of contents into the abdominal cavity, causing **peritonitis** (PER-ih-toe-NIGH-tis; an inflammation of the peritoneum), of which pain is a common symptom. Spilled gastric contents are high in gastric acid and are corrosive to abdominal organs, and intestinal contents have a normally high bacterial count. Spilling intestinal contents into the

HEALTHY HIGHLIGHT

Good Elimination Habits

To avoid constipation, defecation should be allowed to occur when reflexes are the strongest, usually early morning following breakfast, although elimination habits differ from individual to individual. Some people might have bowel movements after every meal; others will have a bowel movement daily or every 2 or 3 days. Other good elimination habits include a diet high in fiber (fruits, vegetables, grains, and cereals), daily exercise, and adequate intake of fluids. Laxatives and enemas should be avoided because these artificially stimulate the bowel and can alter its normal elimination pattern. Regular use of laxatives produces dependence on them for bowel elimination.

abdominal cavity causes infection, which can lead to **septicemia** (SEP-tih-SEE-me-ah; septic = dirty, emia = blood or bacteria in the bloodstream). Causes of perforation can include peptic ulcer, injury from gunshot or stab wounds, and untreated appendicitis.

Alteration in motility, or movement of food along the tract, commonly leads to a variety of signs and symptoms, including nausea, vomiting, diarrhea, or constipation. Diarrhea is a disorder characterized by frequent, watery stools. Irritability of the intestinal lining causes hyperactivity of muscle contractions (peristalsis), causing a rushing of the watery contents in the small intestine through the large intestine. This rushing denies the large intestine the time needed to reabsorb the water. The primary concern with diarrhea, especially in young children and older people, is loss of fluids, leading to dehydration. Causes of diarrhea include a sudden increase in stress or nervous condition, bacterial or viral infection, or food poisoning.

Constipation is the opposite of diarrhea. The stool in the colon remains for an extended period of time, too much water is reabsorbed, and the stool becomes hard, dry, and difficult to pass. Constipation is commonly caused by poor dietary and elimination habits. Avoiding the urge to **defecate** (have a bowel movement) increases the amount of time the stool remains in the colon and, thus, increases constipation.

DIAGNOSTIC TESTS

Diagnostic tests for the digestive system commonly include radiologic (X-ray) examinations and endoscopic (looking into the cavity with a lighted scope) examinations. An upper GI series, also called a barium swallow, allows visualization of the esophagus, stomach, and upper portion of the small intestine. In preparation for such an examination, the individual must be N.P.O. (*non per os*—nothing by mouth) for a minimum of 8 hours. Prior to the examination, the individual drinks a barium solution, which coats the inside of the upper tract, allowing visualization by X-ray. The physician can view a series, or several X-rays, to detect problems of the upper tract (Figure 11–2).

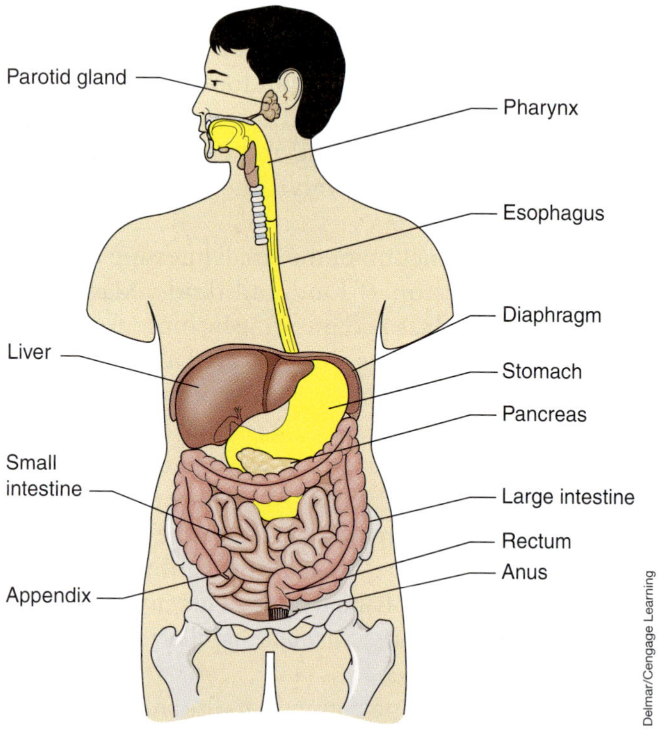

FIGURE 11–2 Upper GI; yellow area is visualized.

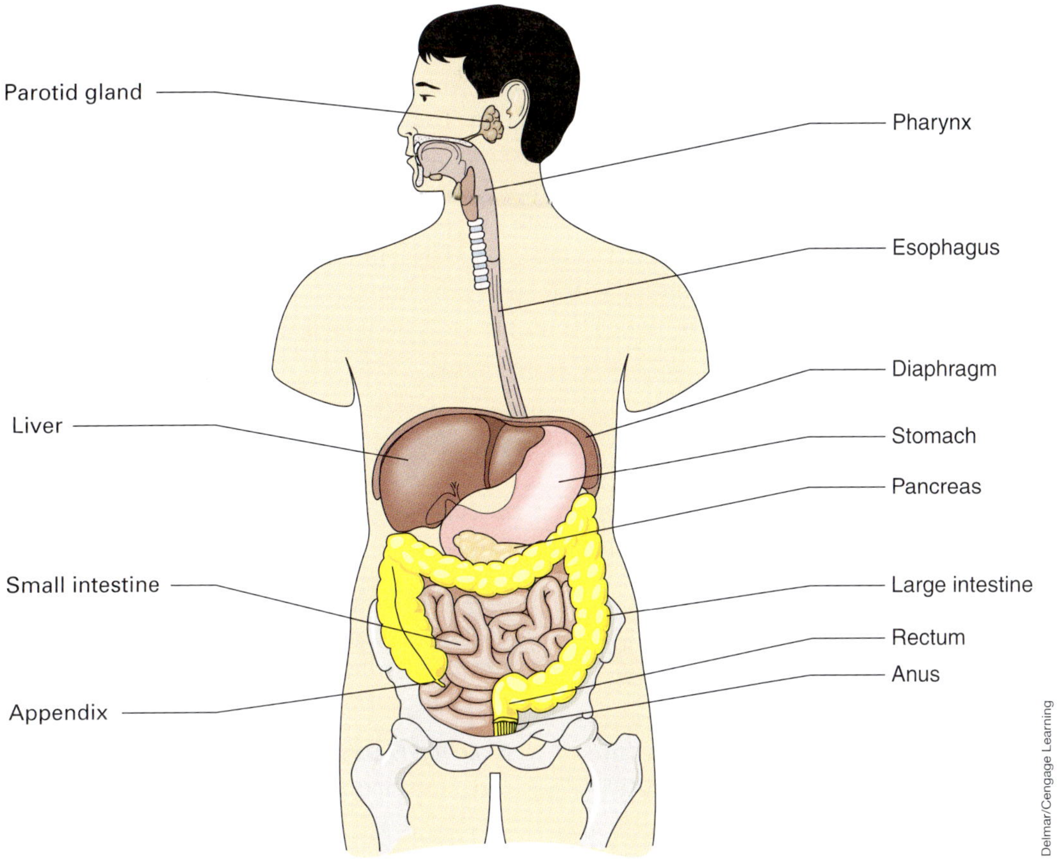

FIGURE 11–3 Lower GI; yellow area is visualized.

A lower GI series, also called a barium enema, provides visualization of the large intestine. In preparation for this radiologic examination, the individual is given an enema or laxatives the day before the examination to rid the colon of fecal material, and the diet is restricted to clear liquids. The day of the examination, an enema of barium solution is administered to coat the lower tract and allow X-ray visualization of the large intestine (Figure 11–3).

Endoscopic examination allows the physician to look directly into the digestive organs through a lighted scope (Figure 11–4). The name of each procedure is identified by naming the organ being scoped: stomach (gastroscopy), colon (colonoscopy), sigmoid colon (sigmoidoscopy), and entire upper GI area (esophagogastroduodenoscopy, EGD). During an endoscopic examination, a physician might obtain a biopsy (small piece of tissue for examination) to determine the presence of a neoplasm or other disease processes.

Video capsule endoscopy has recently been added as a diagnostic test. In this test, a capsule containing a miniature video camera is swallowed and travels through the small intestine. As it travels along, it sends video images of the lining to a receiver worn on a belt at the waist. The images can then be downloaded and

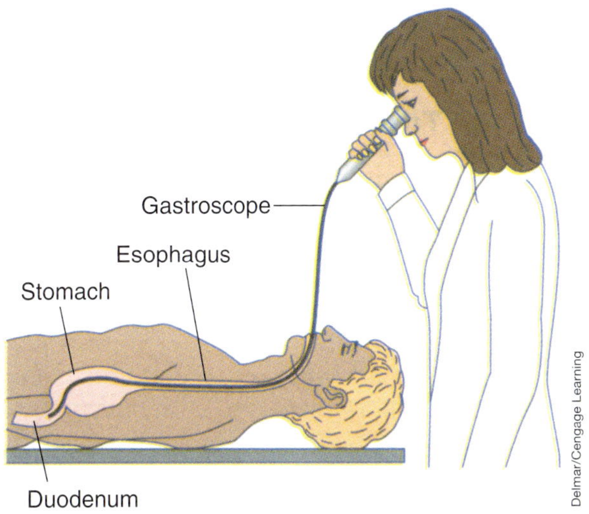

FIGURE 11–4 Esophagogastroduodenoscopy.

GLIMPSE OF THE FUTURE

A physician at the Mayo Clinic research center has developed a unique test that examines the stomach without the tubes (gastroscope or EGD) that are usually used for this visualization. The technique lets the physician see the stomach wall and measure its motor activity as well as its volume in less time and without the preparation and trauma to the patient that traditional gastroscopy causes. The test uses a computer to create a three-dimensional picture of the stomach and to analyze its activity. It can be used to diagnose conditions such as dyspepsia and other problems of the stomach. In the future, this test may replace the traditional endoscopic technique that is presently used to visualize the stomach.

Source: Mayo Foundation for Medical Research and Education (2008).

viewed on computer. The value of this test is the ease of viewing even very small or mild abnormalities. A disadvantage of this camera is that it cannot be used in patients with obstruction in the intestine because it might get stuck in the obstruction.

Several laboratory tests can be performed to assist in diagnosis of digestive system diseases. One of these is the Hemoccult®, which tests stool for **occult** (hidden) **blood**. A positive Hemoccult® can be indicative of colon cancer.

Another laboratory test is an **Ova and Parasite (O&P)**, an examination of a stool specimen for the presence of adult parasites or their eggs (ova). Parasites identified by an O&P might include roundworms, tapeworms, pinworms, or hookworms and protozoa such as *Giardia lamblia*. Stool or fecal cultures can be used to determine bacterial infections in the colon.

COMMON DISEASES OF THE DIGESTIVE SYSTEM

Diseases of the Mouth

The primary function of the mouth is to begin the breakdown of food into smaller particles. Diseases of the mouth include those related to inflammation and tumors.

DENTAL CARIES

■ ***DESCRIPTION.*** Dental caries is an infectious disease that damages the teeth; it primarily affects children and young adults.

■ ***ETIOLOGY.*** Microorganisms in the mouth attack the teeth, producing dental cavities. The cause of caries is twofold, requiring bacteria along with a diet high in carbohydrates (sugars). Left untreated, the disase can lead to infection, pain, and tooth loss.

■ ***SYMPTOMS.*** The bacteria stick to the tooth surface in a tough, sticky material called **dental plaque**. Acids produced by the bacteria erode the tooth surface.

■ ***DIAGNOSIS.*** Diagnosis involves inspecting the teeth for plaque, followed by X-rays revealing cavities.

■ ***TREATMENT.*** Treatment can range from simple dental fillings to oral surgery, depending on the extent of the caries.

■ ***PREVENTION.*** Prevention is based on frequently removing dental plaque by brushing and flossing the teeth. A decrease in carbohydrate (sugar) intake is also helpful. The use of fluoride in drinking water and toothpaste also reduces the incidence of caries.

PERIODONTAL DISEASE

■ ***DESCRIPTION.*** Periodontal disease affects the supporting structures of the teeth such as the gums. It is a disease that affects adults and incidence increases with aging. Most adults have some degree of periodontal disease, the main reason for tooth loss in an adult.

■ ***ETIOLOGY.*** Dental plaque, poor oral hygiene, and inadequate diet are common factors leading to this disease.

■ ***SYMPTOMS.*** Dental plaque sticks on the tooth at the gum line, often leading to **gingivitis** (inflammation of the gums with painful bleeding) (Figure 11–5).

■ ***DIAGNOSIS.*** A dentist can make a diagnosis by inspecting the gums and measuring the pocket depth of the teeth. Redness, puffiness, and bleeding along with a pocket depth of 3 millimeters indicates disease.

GLIMPSE OF THE FUTURE

An Alternative Herbal Therapy to Prevent Periodontal Disease

Myracrodruon urundeuva, also known as urundeúva, or Mu, is found in timber trees in South America. Mu and *Lippia sidoides* (Ls), which is from plants in Brazil, have been used for years as antimicrobial and anti-inflammatory agents. They have recently been combined into a topical gel and tested to treat periodontal disease. The results of the study showed significant benefits of the Mu/Ls gel in preventing bone loss associated with periodontal disease. The experimental study was done on rats but in the future, further research might be done using the same or similar combinations of these extracts to prevent periodontal disease in humans.

Source: Botelho, et al. (2007).

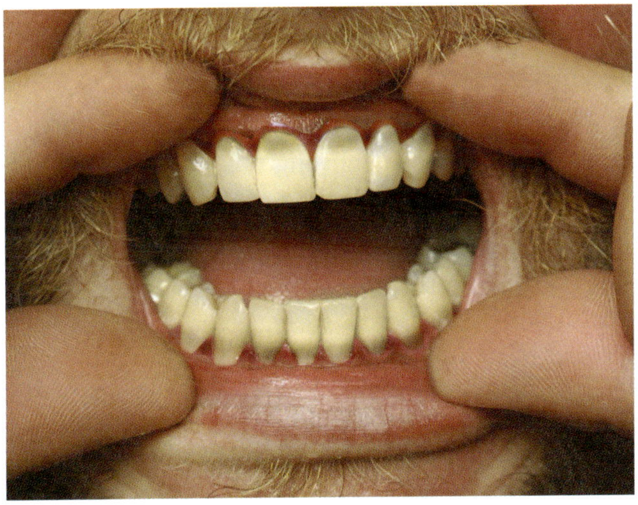

Courtesy of Mark L. Kuss.

FIGURE 11–5 Gingivitis (inflamed gingiva).

■ ***TREATMENT.*** Treatment involves removing the plaque and treating the inflammation.

■ ***PREVENTION.*** Prevention is based on frequent brushing and flossing of the teeth with special attention given to the gum line, regular dental care to remove plaque, and an adequate diet.

CANCER OF THE MOUTH

■ ***DESCRIPTION.*** Tumors of the mouth can occur on the lip, cheek, gum, palate, or tongue. A common oral cancer is squamous cell carcinoma of the lip.

■ ***ETIOLOGY.*** This tumor usually occurs on the lower lip of men and is related to exposure to sunlight, chewing tobacco, and smoking pipes or cigars (Figure 11–6).

■ ***SYMPTOMS.*** Symptoms usually include a small lump on the tongue, lip, or other mouth area and is often pale in color and painless.

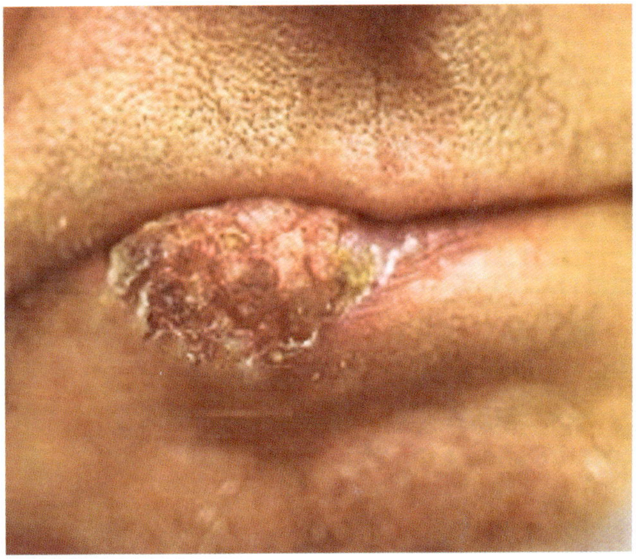

Courtesy of Mark L. Kuss.

FIGURE 11–6 Cancer of the lip.

■ ***DIAGNOSIS.*** A tissue biopsy of the lump is the most definitive diagnostic test.

■ ***TREATMENT.*** Treatment is usually quite effective and includes radiation therapy and surgical excision.

■ ***PREVENTION.*** Prevention is aimed at decreasing exposure to sunlight by using SPF sunscreen, wearing hats to shade the face, and eliminating the use of tobacco products.

Diseases of the Throat and Esophagus

There are many diseases of the throat and esophagus, ranging from mild to severe and acute to chronic. Infections and inflammatory conditions are some of the most common. Pharyngitis is often categorized as a respiratory problem because the pharynx can be considered part of the respiratory system as well as part of the digestive system.

PHARYNGITIS

■ ***DESCRIPTION.*** Pharyngitis is commonly called a sore throat.

■ ***ETIOLOGY.*** Pharyngitis can be caused by viral or bacterial microorganisms.

■ ***SYMPTOMS.*** The most frequent and earliest symptom of pharyngitis is a sore throat. Visual examination reveals redness in the area. A common type of pharyngitis is an inflammation of the tonsils called tonsillitis, in which the tonsils form crypts of pus, which give the tonsils a whitish appearance.

An acute type of pharyngitis is called **strep throat**, caused by **virulent** (VIR-u-lent; infectious, difficult to kill) bacteria, streptococcus. This bacteria can spread into the bloodstream and produce other diseases such as scarlet fever, rheumatic fever, glomerulonephritis, and endocarditis.

■ ***DIAGNOSIS.*** Diagnosis is made by examination and throat culture.

■ ***TREATMENT.*** Treatment of strep throat includes identification of the organism through laboratory cultures, followed by antibiotic treatment and follow-up culture to check effectiveness of antibiotic treatment. Antibiotic treatment is quite effective if taken as prescribed.

■ ***PREVENTION.*** Frequent and thorough hand washing is one of the best preventive methods, along with avoiding contact with people who are sick. Using a new toothbrush after an infection prevents reinfection.

REFLUX ESOPHAGITIS

■ ***DESCRIPTION.*** Reflux esophagitis, more recently called gastroesophageal reflux disease (GERD), is an inflammation of tissue at the lower end of the esophagus.

■ ***ETIOLOGY.*** GERD is caused by a reflux (backflow) of stomach acids through the cardiac sphincter upward into the esophagus.

■ ***SYMPTOMS.*** The most common symptom of reflux esophagitis is heartburn, a burning sensation in the mid-chest or epigastric (epi = above, gastric = stomach) area. Long-term reflux can lead to bleeding, ulceration, and scarring of the esophagus, which can cause stricture and difficulty swallowing.

HEALTHY HIGHLIGHT

Tips About Strep Throat

Sore throats need to be cultured routinely to diagnose the streptococcus infection, commonly called strep throat. An accurate diagnosis depends on obtaining a throat culture. Practitioners cannot determine this condition by simply viewing the throat. Even though culturing is more costly, this determination is extremely important because strep throat can lead to rheumatic heart disease and possibly heart valve deformity. Parents of children who have recurrent attacks of strep throat should also have throat cultures because they might be carriers of the strep infection. Strep throat is usually treated effectively with antibiotics.

Antibiotics should be taken as prescribed. They should always be taken until all tablets or capsules are gone. Even if the affected individual begins to feel better, the medication should be continued until completed because discontinuing the antibiotic or saving some medicine for later can lead to bacterial resistance. If an individual does not take the prescribed number of tablets, it is possible for many bacteria to survive the short dosage time and actually build up a resistance to that antibiotic. These bacteria can then cause another attack of strep throat that cannot be treated or cured with the previously prescribed antibiotic. Taking all antibiotics as prescribed should destroy all the bacteria and eliminate the risk of bacterial resistance.

■ ***DIAGNOSIS.*** Diagnosis is usually made by barium swallow X-ray (upper GI). If further diagnostic testing is needed, an EGD with biopsy can be performed.

■ ***TREATMENT.*** Treatment is directed at reducing reflux and can include recommendations to avoid large meals, spicy foods, caffeine, and tight clothing. Medications such as stool softeners, laxatives, and antacids might be helpful. Several drugs specifically for reflux problems are also available, some over the counter and others requiring a prescription. Activities that increase abdominal pressure might be restricted. Sleeping with the head of the bed elevated is often helpful. Surgery on the incompetent sphincter is usually not recommended and considered only in extreme cases.

■ ***PREVENTION.*** Preventive measures include controlling weight and avoiding smoking, caffeine, carbonated beverages, chocolate, and high-fat foods as well as late-night meals.

HIATAL HERNIA

■ ***DESCRIPTION.*** Hiatal hernia is a sliding of part of the stomach into the chest cavity.

■ ***ETIOLOGY.*** The stomach slides upward through the natural hole in the diaphragm where the esophagus passes through to the stomach (Figure 11–7). This herniation can increase in frequency with age and weakening of the cardiac sphincter.

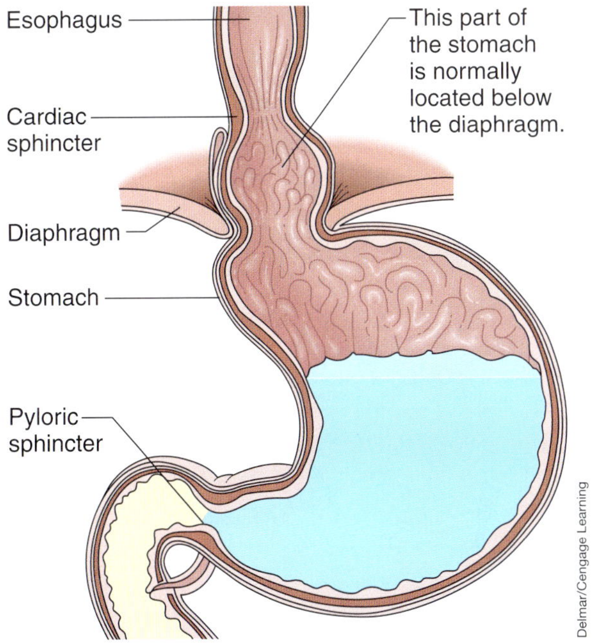

FIGURE 11–7 Hiatal hernia.

■ ***SYMPTOMS.*** Many hiatal hernias are **asymptomatic** (a = without, symptomatic = symptoms), but those that do cause discomfort are usually related to esophageal reflux.

■ ***DIAGNOSIS.*** Hiatal hernias are diagnosed by an upper GI X-ray.

■ ***TREATMENT.*** Treatment is often the same as for reflux esophagitis.

■ ***PREVENTION.*** Although it is difficult to prevent hiatal hernias totally, risk can be reduced by maintaining a healthy weight, avoiding heavy lifting, and not smoking.

ESOPHAGEAL VARICES

■ ***DESCRIPTION.*** Esophageal varices are extremely dilated varicose veins located in the esophagus.

■ ***ETIOLOGY.*** Unusually high pressure in the veins of the esophagus causes them to enlarge and become tortuous, resulting in esophageal varices. This increased venous pressure is due to blockage or reduced flow of blood into the liver, causing poor venous return from the esophagus. (For more information on liver disease, see Chapter 12, "Liver, Gallbladder, and Pancreas Diseases and Disorders.") Any condition that leads to venous congestion in the liver can lead to esophageal varices. Esophageal varices are usually related to cirrhosis of the liver. The most common cause of cirrhosis is excessive alcohol consumption. Hemorrhage of the varices can be a life-threatening condition.

■ ***SYMPTOMS.*** Symptoms include vomiting blood, black stools, and, on endoscopic examination, dilated esophageal blood vessels.

■ ***DIAGNOSIS.*** Physical examination can reveal low blood pressure, bloody stools, and signs of chronic liver disease. Diagnosis is confirmed with an EGD.

■ ***TREATMENT.*** The goal of treatment is to decrease venous pressure by methods such as portal vein bypass surgery and medication to lower blood pressure. Other treatments include limiting the diet to soft, nonirritating foods and the use of stool softeners to prevent straining, which increases esophageal venous pressure. Chronic bleeding of the vessels can be treated with a sclerosing agent that hardens or destroys the vessel. Treatment for acute bleeding includes instillation of cold saline washings, the application of pressure to the site through a nasogastric tube, or both.

■ ***PREVENTION.*** Treating or preventing liver disese can prevent this disease.

Diseases of the Stomach

Diseases of the stomach are common problems in the digestive system. Complaints of stomach pain, especially after eating, are frequently voiced to the physician. This problem increases with age due to the age-related changes in the system that are also complicated by other chronic diseases. Disorders of the stomach range from mild acute gastritis to more serious diseases such as cancer of the stomach.

GASTRITIS

■ ***DESCRIPTION.*** Gastritis is not a specific disease but a condition that results from several problems that all cause inflammation of the stomach.

■ ***ETIOLOGY.*** Commom causes are use of anti-inflammatory medications, or NSAIDS, such as aspirin or ibuprophen, smoking, alcohol consumption, and infection of a bacteria such as *Helicobacter pylori* (*H. pylori*).

H. pylori infection is common, with 20% of Americans under the age of 40 and more than 50% of those over 60 years of age suffering from it (NIDDK, 2008). The presence of the bacteria does not cause symptoms in the majority of people. Those persons affected might experience chronic gastritis. *H. pylori* weakens the protective mucous lining of the stomach, allowing acid to contact the sensitive tissues underneath. The bacteria, along with stomach acid, irritate the stomach lining, leading to pain and, often, ulceration. *H. pylori* gastritis is now thought to be a major factor in gastric ulcer formation.

Gastritis also increases with age. As people age, the number of acid-producing cells decreases, thus leading to atrophic gastritis, or **achlorhydria** (AH-klor-HIGH-dree-ah; no hydrochloric acid), because there is not enough hydrochloric acid to kill off ingested bacteria. Achlorhydria also leads to loss of intrinsic factor (a protein produced by the gastric mucosa), leading to pernicious anemia. (See Chapter 7, "Blood and Blood-Forming Organs Diseases and Disorders," for more information on anemia.)

■ ***SYMPTOMS.*** The most common symptom is abdominal pain. Other symptoms include nausea, belching, and vomiting.

■ ***DIAGNOSIS.*** Diagnosis is determined by blood test to check for anemia, stool test to look for presence of blood in the stool and *H. pylori* bacteria, and an upper GI endoscopy or EGD for visual confirmation.

■ ***TREATMENT.*** Medications to reduce stomach acid help relieve symptoms and promote healing. Treatment for *H. pylori* involves treatment with antibiotics. Avoiding irritating foods, medications, smoking, and alcohol is also helpful. Treating and resolving the underlying cause usually leads to resolution of gastritis.

■ ***PREVENTION.*** Avoiding irritating factors and promptly treating *H. pylori* when symptomatic aids in prevention of gastritis.

PEPTIC ULCER

■ ***DESCRIPTION.*** An ulcer is an area of tissue that has eroded, leaving a crater-like appearance (Figure 11–8). Peptic ulcers are those ulcers found in the stomach and duodenum that are caused, in part, by the action of pepsin. Peptic ulcers found in the stomach are called gastric ulcers, and those located in the duodenum are called duodenal ulcers.

■ ***ETIOLOGY.*** As many as 80% of these ulcers are associated with *H. pylori* (CDC, 2007). Other contributing factors include severe stress, heavy intake of drugs (such as aspirin, steroids, and alcohol), and smoking.

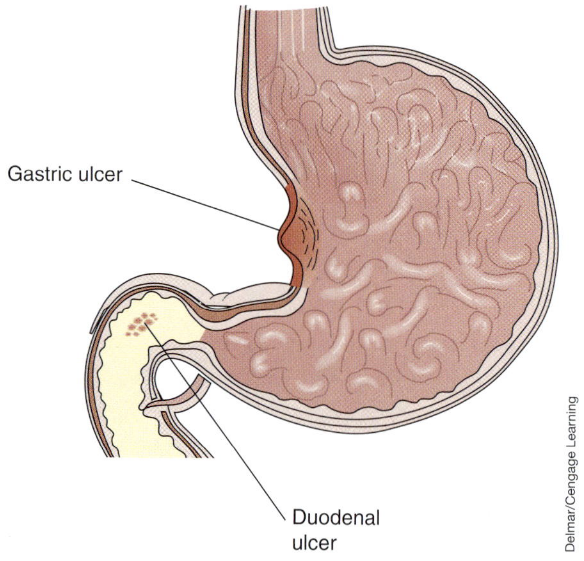

FIGURE 11–8 Peptic ulcers.

COMPLEMENTARY AND ALTERNATIVE THERAPY

Apricot Juice to Treat Stomach Disorders

The juice of the Japanese apricot (*Prunus mume*) has been used to treat dyspepsia for centuries. It has also been studied as a treatment for *H. pylori* bacteria, which causes stomach ulcers. The preparation used is called Bainiku ekisu, which is a concentrated juice made from the Japanese apricot. Research has shown positive effects of the juice on the bacteria, but it does not seem to completely eliminate it. More research is needed to determine the therapeutic effects of this herbal preparation.

Source: Nakajima, et al. (2006).

The stomach lining is normally protected by a thick mucous membrane lining. Pepsin is an enzyme secreted in the stomach that breaks down protein, but this same enzyme, to some degree, breaks down the stomach's lining, causing ulcers.

■ ***SYMPTOMS.*** Ulcer pain is caused by the hydrochloric acid in the stomach irritating the raw ulcerated area. Complications of peptic ulcers are massive bleeding, perforation, and obstruction.

■ ***DIAGNOSIS.*** Diagnosis is based on symptoms and the results of a gastroscopy or visual examination of the inside of the stomach

■ ***TREATMENT.*** Treatment is aimed at reducing the gastric acidity and healing the stomach lining. Antibiotics are also used to treat ulcers caused by *Helicobacter* bacteria. Other treatments include reduction or elimination of contributory factors. Antacids to neutralize gastric acids and other gastric medications might be helpful. Surgery is warranted in severe cases that might lead to hemorrhage, perforation, obstruction, or extreme pain.

■ ***PREVENTION.*** Infection with *H. pylori* is thought to be through water, food, or kissing someone who has the bacteria. At this time, routes of infection are unproven and the fact that many people with *H. pylori* do not develop peptic ulcers makes this cause unpreventable. Quick treatment of *H. pylori*, when discovered as an irritant, along with avoiding other irritants, is beneficial.

CANCER OF THE STOMACH

■ ***DESCRIPTION.*** Cancer of the stomach often spreads through the stomach tissue to nearby organs such as the pancreas, intestine, and esophagus. These cancer cells can also spread through the blood and lymphatic system to the liver, lungs, and lymph nodes all over the body. Often, this cancer goes undiagnosed until after it spreads outside the stomach and into other organs.

■ ***ETIOLOGY.*** The cause of stomach cancer is unknown, although research has proven certain causative factors. These include some correlation to food additives and foods that are smoked, salted, and pickled. Cigarette smoking is another risk factor along with gender, in that men are more affected than women.

■ ***SYMPTOMS.*** Symptoms are often vague and include loss of appetite, general stomach distress, and heartburn. Prognosis is good if the cancer is discovered early.

■ ***DIAGNOSIS.*** Diagnostic testing includes upper GI studies, endoscopy, and biopsy. Biopsy is the most definitive diagnostic test.

■ ***TREATMENT.*** Treatment can include surgical resection, chemotherapy, and radiation.

■ ***PREVENTION.*** Preventing causative factors might help in prevention.

Diseases of the Small Intestine

The small intestine, consisting of the duodenum, jejunum, and ileum, secretes enzymes and absorbs nutrients for cellular functions. Disorders of the small intestine frequently manifest themselves by pain that radiates across the abdomen, although this symptom alone is not enough to diagnose the specific disease process. Additional evaluation is needed, such as

COMPLEMENTARY AND ALTERNATIVE THERAPY

Herbs for Obesity

The leaves of a southeast Asian tree (*Lagerstroemia speciosa*), known as banaba, have been used historically for the treatment of a variety of illnesses such as diabetes and urinary problems. The effects of the banaba leaves in preventing diabetes have been confirmed in some studies. Recent research has tested the effects of a preparation of banaba leaves to treat or prevent obesity. This particular formula of the extract of the leaves shows some potential for preventing adipose tissue (fat) from developing.

Source: Klein, et al. (2007).

X-ray or computerized tomography (CT) scan. The disorders of the small intestine can range from mild intestinal upset to more severe chronic problems such as ulcers or regional enteritis.

DUODENAL ULCER

A duodenal ulcer, also called a peptic ulcer of the duodenum, was discussed previously under "Peptic Ulcer."

MALABSORPTION SYNDROME

■ ***DESCRIPTION.*** The primary purpose of the small intestine is to absorb nutrients. Malabsorption syndrome occurs when this process is altered and nutrients are not adequately absorbed into the blood.

■ ***ETIOLOGY.*** Persons with malabsorption syndrome can be unable to absorb nutrients (especially fat) and minerals. Other diseases such as diabetes mellitus, cystic fibrosis, pancreatic deficiencies, lactose intolerance, and gluten enteropathy can also lead to malabsorption syndrome. Malabsorption syndrome can range from mild intestinal upset to more severe chronic problems such as ulcers or regional enteritis.

■ ***SYMPTOMS.*** Symptoms include anemia, diarrhea, edema, muscle cramping, and weight loss. Heart arrhythmias can result from potassium deficiency, and blood clotting disorders can also occur. Children who are affected might exhibit signs of failure to grow.

■ ***DIAGNOSIS.*** Diagnosis is often very difficult and requires extensive testing. Basic testing will include a thorough medical and physical examination followed by a variety of blood tests, X-rays, stool samples, endoscopies, ultrasound, and CT and magnetic resonance imaging (MRI) scanning. All these test aid in measuring abnormalities of the GI tract.

■ ***TREATMENT.*** Most treatments include diet therapy for control. One of the complications of the disorder is a bleeding tendency due to the lack of vitamin K absorption.

■ ***PREVENTION.*** Many of the malabsorption syndromes are hereditary, so there are no preventive solutions. Genetic screening followed by early detection through routine physical exams and testing is of benefit. Prevention, in some cases, is as easy as avoiding the foods or substances that cause problems.

REGIONAL ENTERITIS (CROHN'S DISEASE)

■ ***DESCRIPTION.*** Regional enteritis is a chronic inflammatory disease most commonly affecting the small intestine, but it can also affect the large intestine. It is characterized by bouts of **remission** (slowing or stopping of symptoms) and **exacerbation** (x-AS-er-BAY-shun; flaring up of symptoms) (Figure 11–9) and is commonly classified as inflammatory bowel disease (IBD) until complete diagnosis is made. As regional enteritis progresses, the intestinal wall becomes thickened, resulting in a narrowing of the lumen.

■ ***ETIOLOGY.*** The cause of the disease has not yet been determined, although genetic, immunologic, infectious, and psychologic factors have been considered.

■ ***SYMPTOMS.*** Symptoms include anorexia, flatulence, abdominal pain, diarrhea, and constipation. Individuals with regional enteritis tend to experience relapse or exacerbations of the condition during periods of stress or emotional upset, factors that support the psychogenic theory. Young females are most often affected by regional enteritis.

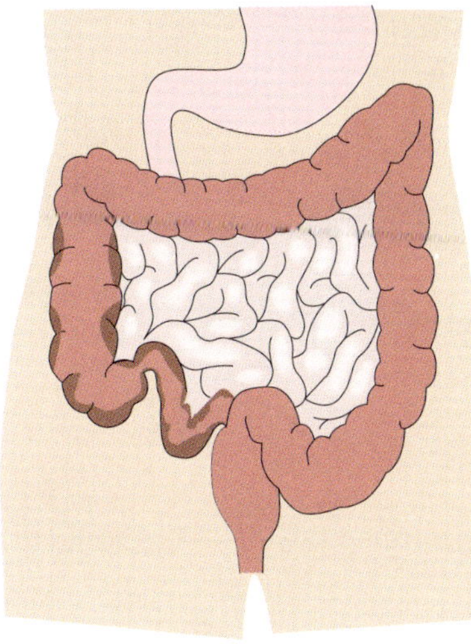

FIGURE 11–9 Regional enteritis.

■ ***DIAGNOSIS.*** Symptoms, along with blood test, upper GI series, CT scanning, and colonoscopy help determine the diagnosis. Recently, video capsule endoscopy has been added to diagnostic testing.

■ ***TREATMENT.*** Treatment is supportive but not likely to be curative. Approaches can involve a low-residue diet and medications to control diarrhea, inflammation, infection, and depression. Surgical resection is not curative and is performed to treat complications such as perforation and obstruction.

■ ***PREVENTION.*** Because Crohn's is thought to have some inherited tendency, there are no known preventive measures. To prevent flare-ups, maintaining a healthy diet and reducing stress are helpful.

GASTROENTERITIS

■ ***DESCRIPTION.*** Gastroenteritis (gastro = stomach, entero = intestines, itis = inflammation), as its name suggests, is inflammation of both the stomach and intestines (Figure 11–10).

■ ***ETIOLOGY.*** Causes can include bacterial, viral, or parasitic invasion; ingestion of tainted food; lactose intolerance; allergic reaction to food or drugs; and stress.

■ ***SYMPTOMS.*** Gastroenteritis can have an acute and violent onset with nausea, vomiting, abdominal cramping, and diarrhea, leading to rapid fluid and electrolyte loss. Or symptoms may be less violent, with stomach rumbling, **malaise** (ma-LAZ; general ill feeling), nausea, and mild diarrhea.

■ ***DIAGNOSIS.*** The symptoms usually help identify this illness. Identifying the cause might require stool samples to examine for viruses, bacteria, and parasites.

■ ***TREATMENT.*** Treatment focuses on symptoms and can include antinausea medication, antidiarrhea medication, antibiotics, fluids, and nutritional support and stress management. Prognosis is generally good.

■ ***PREVENTION.*** If the gastroenteritis is caused by a virus, it probably cannot be prevented. With bacterial gastroenteritis, the best preventive measures include hand washing and properly preparing and storing food because bacteria easily grow and multiply in poultry, egg, and cream products. Keeping foods such as potato and chicken salad refrigerated, especially during warm weather, is helpful. Avoiding contaminated food and water, especially in underdeveloped countries also prevents gastroenteritis.

If stress is the cause of the upset, then controling this with stress reduction, healthy diet, and regular exercise will help with prevention.

INGUINAL HERNIA

■ ***DESCRIPTION.*** An inguinal hernia is a common problem that affects the digestive system.

■ ***ETIOLOGY.*** An pouching of the small intestine and the peritoneum (abdominal cavity lining) into the groin area (Figure 11–11) causes this condition. Inguinal hernias are more common in males, perhaps due to a congenital defect that developed as the testes descended from the abdomen into the scrotum, thus pulling part of the peritoneum into the inguinal area. Inguinal hernias also develop in both sexes due to a weakness in the abdominal wall.

The portion of the intestine that herniates can become caught and twisted, thus cutting off blood supply to the organ. If this occurs, it is called a strangulated hernia, which can be life-threatening and needs immediate surgical intervention.

■ ***SYMPTOMS.*** Symptoms include a bulge in the groin or scrotum and groin pain that increases with bending or lifting and is relieved by lying down. If there is sudden pain, nausea, and vomiting, chances are the hernia has become strangulated.

■ ***DIAGNOSIS.*** Diagnosis depends on a thorough history and physical exam of the groin area. Ultrasound and CT scans can be used to finalize the diagnosis.

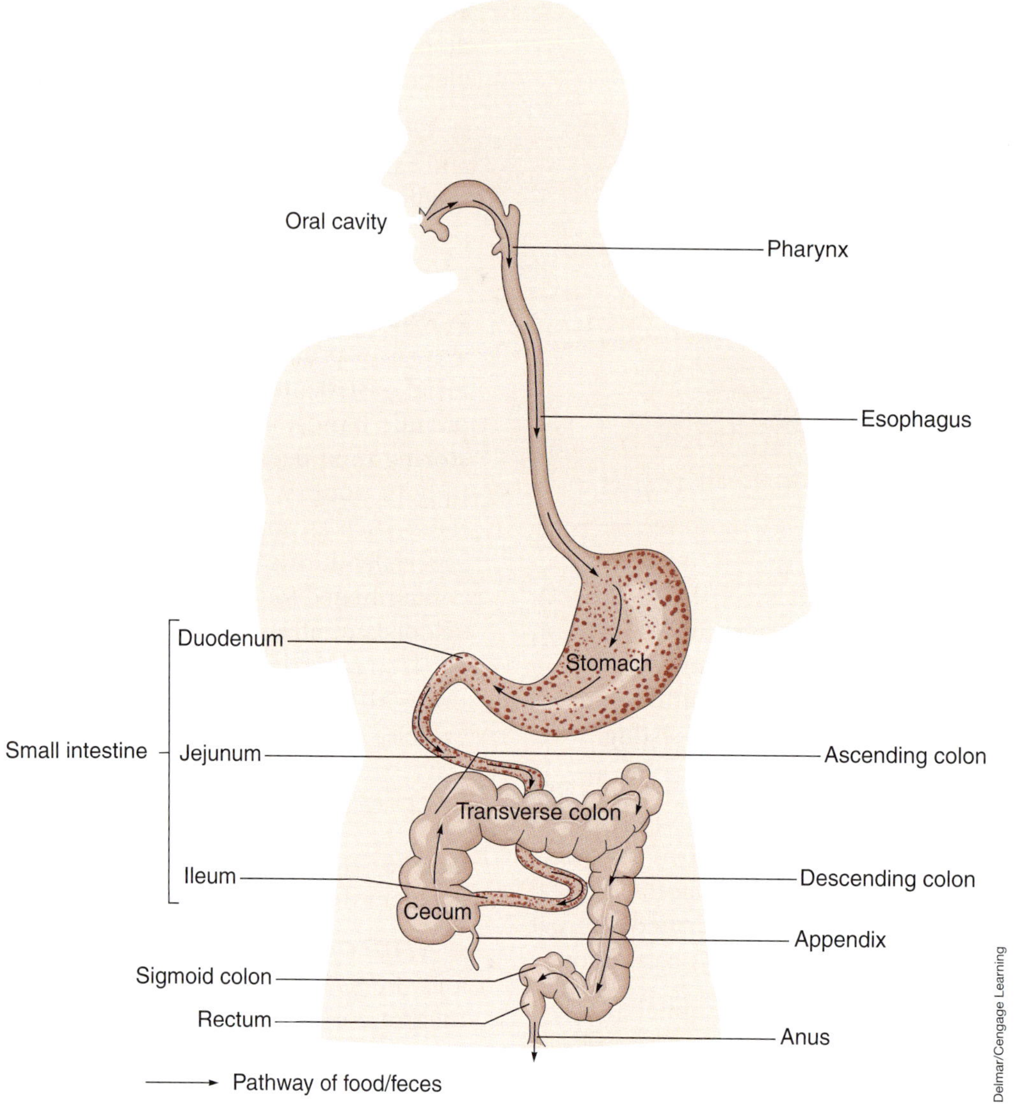

FIGURE 11–10 Gastroenteritis.

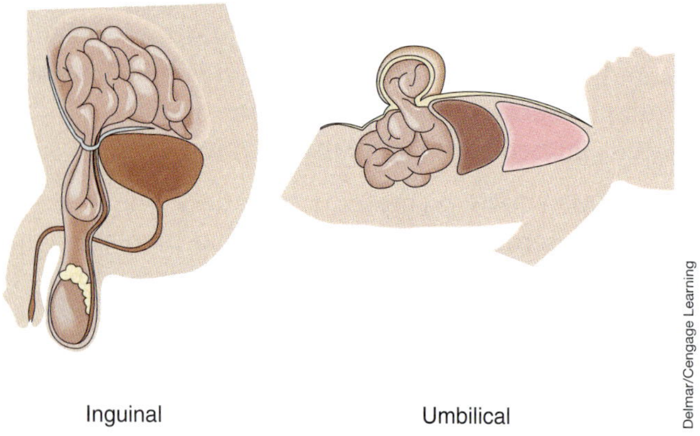

FIGURE 11–11 Hernias: inguinal and umbilical.

■ ***TREATMENT.*** Fortunately, inguinal hernias can be repaired surgically to prevent this potentially life-threatening situation.

Portions of the small intestine can also herniate through other openings in the body such as the femoral canal or the umbilicus. The femoral hernia, like the inguinal hernia, is more common in males. The umbilical hernia is most common in infants. Like the inguinal hernia, both are corrected surgically to prevent complications.

■ ***PREVENTION.*** Preventive measures include maintaining proper body weight, stopping smoking, using proper body mechanics during lifting, and avoiding constipation because straining to have a bowel movement increases abdominal pressure and can lead to a hernia.

Diseases of the Colon

Diseases of the colon or large intestine are common to all ages but are found most frequently in the middle-aged and older adult with the exception of appendicitis. Common problems such as ulcerative colitis and cancer of the colon are two of the more serious conditions of the colon.

APPENDICITIS

DESCRIPTION. The appendix is located near the junction of the small and large intestines, and although it is primarily composed of lymphoid tissues, the exact function is yet unknown.

ETIOLOGY. Appendicitis is the inflammation of the **vermiform** (VER-my-form; worm-like) appendix. Infection or obstruction usually causes appendicitis. The position of the appendix near the colon allows bacteria-laden fecal contents to drop into the appendix, causing obstruction and infection. The inflamed appendix swells (see Figure 11–12), decreasing circulation and potentially leading to gangrene.

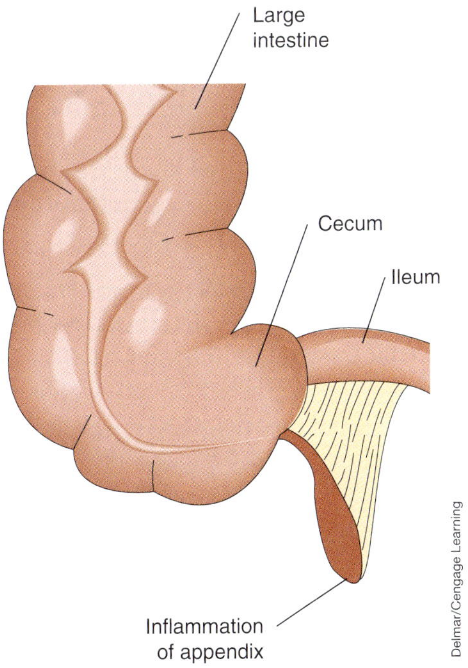

FIGURE 11–12 Appendicitis.

SYMPTOMS. The pain of appendicitis usually begins with generalized abdominal pain that shifts to the lower right quadrant. Other signs and symptoms include nausea, vomiting, fever, and leukocytosis. This combination of signs and symptoms also mimics other abdominal diseases such as kidney stones, pelvic inflammatory disease, and pancreatitis, which can lead to an incorrect diagnosis.

As appendicitis progresses, the wall of the appendix thins and can rupture. Rupture of the appendix usually relieves the pain for a short time but leads to the more severe complication of peritonitis. Before the development of antibiotics, peritonitis was usually fatal.

DIAGNOSIS. A physical examination revealing increased pain when gentle pressure is applied in the area of the appendix and then released, called rebound tenderness, is helpful in diagnosis. Blood tests revealing an elevated white blood cell count, along with a urinalysis to rule out bladder infection is helpful. Ultrasound and CT are used to confirm the diagnosis.

TREATMENT. Treatment for appendicitis requires surgical removal of the appendix, preferably before rupture occurs.

PREVENTION. There is no proven way to prevent appendicitis, but eating a healthy diet including fruits and vegetables might aid in prevention.

INTESTINAL OBSTRUCTION

DESCRIPTION. Intestinal obstruction may be classified as a symptom of a disease process or as a disease itself.

ETIOLOGY. Regardless of the classification, it is identified as an inability to move intestinal contents through the bowel. An obstruction can be due to a blockage of the intestine or to a disease or **ileus** (ILL-ee-us; absence of peristalsis).

Blockage can occur due to tumors, hernias, or **adhesions** (ad-HE-zhuns) (Figure 11–13). Adhesions are areas within the colon that abnormally link together, resulting from a previous abdominal surgery or from inflammation. Blockage also can occur if the colon becomes twisted (**volvulus**; VOL-view-lus) (Figure 11–14). If the colon telescopes on itself, the condition can lead to a blockage called **intussusception** (IN-tus-sus-SEP-shun).

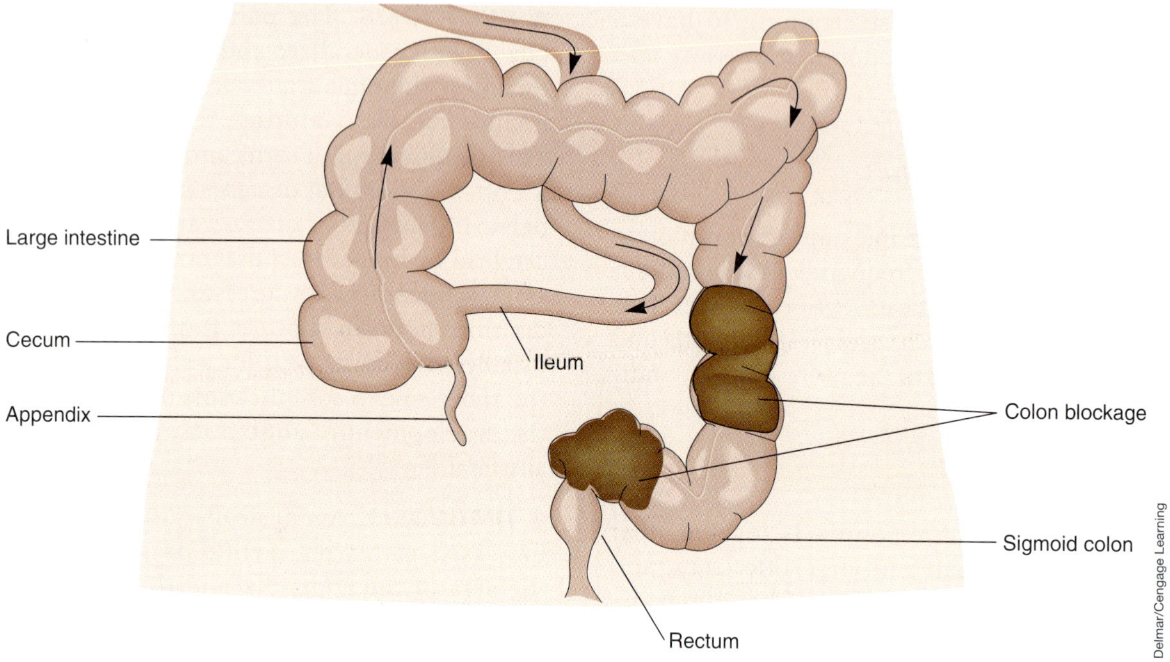

FIGURE 11–13 Colon blockage.

A decrease or absence of peristalsis that causes intestinal obstruction is classified as a **paralytic obstruction**—colon action is paralyzed (unable to move). This type of obstruction can be a postoperative complication or a result of peritonitis.

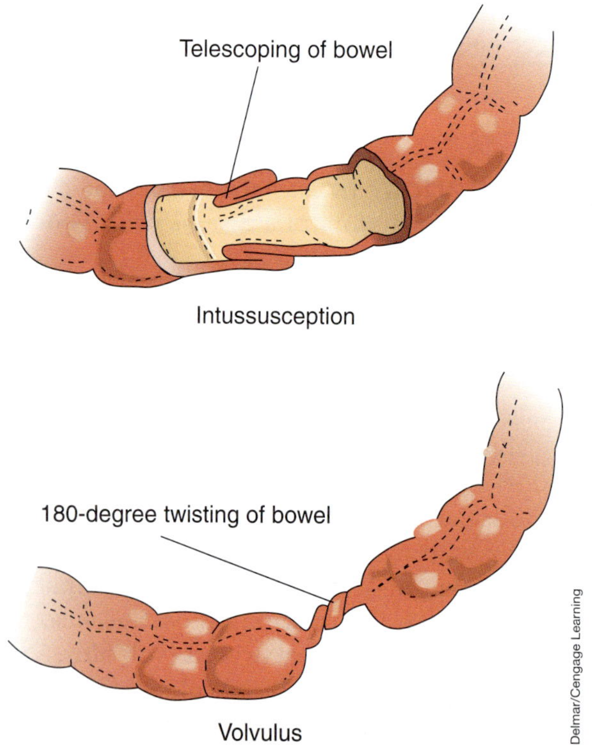

FIGURE 11–14 Volvulus and intussusception.

■ ***SYMPTOMS.*** Symptoms depend on the type and severity of the obstruction. The individual might experience mild to severe abdominal pain and distention, nausea, and vomiting.

■ ***DIAGNOSIS.*** Barium enema, abdominal CT scan, upper GI, and abdominal films all aid in the diagnosis.

■ ***TREATMENT.*** Intestinal obstruction can be relieved by nasogastric suctioning, but more commonly, surgery is required.

■ ***PREVENTION.*** Prevention depends on the cause. If the condition is related to adhesions, intussusception, or volvulus, intestinal obstruction might not be preventable. Treatment of other causes, such as tumors and hernias, is helpful in prevention of intestinal obstruction.

ULCERATIVE COLITIS

■ ***DESCRIPTION.*** Ulcerative colitis is a chronic inflammation of the colon (Figure 11–15) that causes inflammation and ulcers in the lining of the rectum and colon. Like regional enteritis, it is commonly called inflammatory bowel disease until diagnosis is confirmed.

HEALTHY HIGHLIGHT

Food Poisoning

Microorganisms that we ingest (eat) can cause GI upset in a variety of ways. Most microorganisms that we ingest are easily incapacitated and destroyed by the acid in the stomach. Some microorganisms will cause illness only if we ingest great numbers of them at a time. Ingestion of these great numbers allows a large number of microorganisms to escape the acid environment, invade the small intestine, and cause illness. An example of this type of microorganism is **Salmonella** (SAL-moh-NEL-ah). For salmonella to make us ill, we must eat food that has been tainted with it. The bacteria reproduce in the food product before we eat it, thus providing the circumstances for ingestion of a large number of bacteria at one time. Salmonella bacteria invade the lining of the small intestine and bring about symptoms, usually 24 to 48 hours after ingestion of the food. Salmonella food poisoning can be prevented by refrigerating foods and by cooking foods thoroughly. Salmonella food poisoning is determined by a stool culture.

Other types of microorganisms also are very virulent and are thus able to withstand the stomach's acid environment. Ingestion of even small numbers of these will allow passage into the small intestine and cause illness. These organisms include viruses, amoebae, and *Shigella*, which are frequently spread by a fecal–oral route.

Another way that microorganisms make us ill is by producing a toxin (poisoning). The bacteria itself does not cause the harm, but the **enterotoxin** (intestine poison) they produce does the damage. Staphylococcal food poisoning is of this type. Staphylococcal organisms contaminate nonrefrigerated food and release enterotoxins. When these enterotoxins are ingested, they quickly invade the lining of the stomach and small intestine, leading to symptoms within 1 to 4 hours. Staphylococcal food poisoning can be prevented by proper refrigeration of food products. This type of food poisoning is determined by a food culture. Prognosis is good, and symptoms usually resolve within 24 hours.

Observing the following measures can prevent most GI upset caused by contaminated food:

- Always wash your hands before and after preparing food.
- Wash your hands before and after a meal.
- Keep eating utensils and plates clean and stored until ready for use.
- Cover and refrigerate food properly.
- Cook foods thoroughly, especially meats and seafood.

■ ***ETIOLOGY.*** The cause of ulcerative colitis is unknown. Exacerbations of the disease often occur during stressful times, leading to the belief that a psychogenic factor is involved. Other causative theories include hereditary, autoimmune, and dietary factors. Patients with ulcerative colitis are at high risk for developing colon cancer.

■ ***SYMPTOMS.*** The colon and rectum have multiple ulcerations that lead to lower abdominal pain, blood in the stools, anemia, and diarrhea.

■ ***DIAGNOSIS.*** Diagnostic tests include blood tests to check for anemia, stool sample, CT scan, and colonoscopy. A colonoscopy is the best test to confirm the diagnosis.

■ ***TREATMENT.*** Treatment can include dietary limitations, stress reduction, mild sedatives, and anti-inflammatory medications. Surgery is usually considered only if conservative treatment fails. Surgical intervention often results in a colostomy (opening in the colon), either temporary or permanent

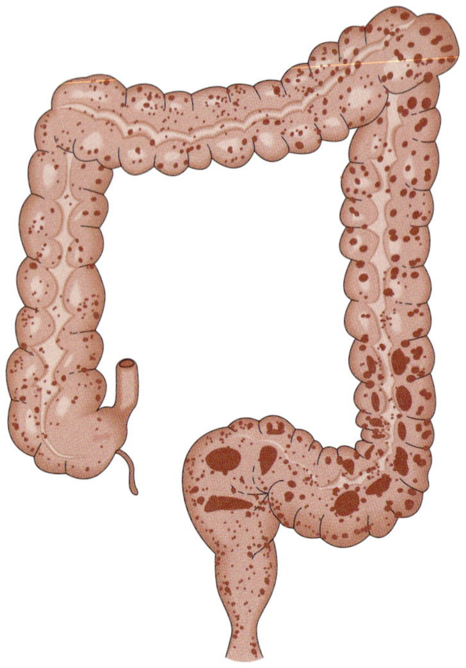

FIGURE 11–15 Ulcerative colitis.

(Figure 11–16). If the colostomy is permanent, a portion of the colon might be removed.

■ ***PREVENTION.*** Because the cause is unknown, prevention is not possible. Taking steps to reduce stress is helpful in reducing the severity of the symptoms.

INFLAMMATORY BOWEL DISEASE (IBD)

IBD refers to both regional enteritis (Crohn's disease) and ulcerative colitis. Both diseases (as previously discussed) are chronic in nature with undetermined etiology. However, a general diagnosis of IBD can be used until a definite diagnosis of another bowel disorder is made.

IRRITABLE BOWEL SYNDROME (SPASTIC COLON)

■ ***DESCRIPTION.*** Irritable bowel syndrome (IBS) is the most common intestinal disorder and commonly can be confused with IBD, but they are not the same. IBD is an inflammation of the bowel with chronic lesions. There are neither inflammation nor lesions in IBS.

■ ***ETIOLOGY.*** The cause of IBS is unknown, but a strong psychogenic factor has been considered. IBS is chronic, and onset usually occurs in the young adult. Frequent recurrence over the years is very frustrating to the affected individual and the physician.

■ ***SYMPTOMS.*** IBS is a functional disorder of motility and can cause a group of symptoms, including abdominal pain and altered motility. Typically, an individual suffering from IBS has bouts of diarrhea, constipation, or both.

Spicy foods, caffeine, alcohol, and seasonings can irritate the colon and bring about symptoms of IBS. Stress also has an adverse effect and often causes alterations in intestinal motility.

■ ***DIAGNOSIS.*** Tests to assist in diagnosis include stool sampling, blood test, X-rays, and endoscopy. Colonoscopy is the most helpful in confirming the diagnosis.

■ ***TREATMENT.*** Avoidance of causative factors and stress reduction techniques often allow the colon to return to its normal functional state.

■ ***PREVENTION.*** IBS cannot be prevented, but symptoms can be reduced. Avoiding causative agents along with stress reduction techniques will help prevent symptoms. Stress reduction techniques include counseling, biofeedback, regular exercise, yoga, meditation, deep breathing, and hypnosis.

DYSENTERY

■ ***DESCRIPTION.*** Dysentery is a general term for a group of GI disorders characterized by acute inflammation. Dysentery commonly affects those in underdeveloped countries and those who travel to these countries. According to the Centers for Disease Control and Prevention (CDC), most cases in the United States occur in immigrants, in those who live in inner-city housing, in frequent travelers, in children in day care, and in people in nursing homes.

■ ***ETIOLOGY.*** Invasion of microorganisms into the lining of the colon causes dysentery, usually as a result of ingestion of contaminated food, water, or both due to poor sanitary conditions.

■ ***SYMPTOMS.*** The main symptom is massive bloody or watery diarrhea along with severe abdominal pain and cramping. Dysentery is the disease and should not be confused with diarrhea, the symptom.

■ ***DIAGNOSIS.*** Diagnosis is based on stool samples showing the presence of causative microorganisms.

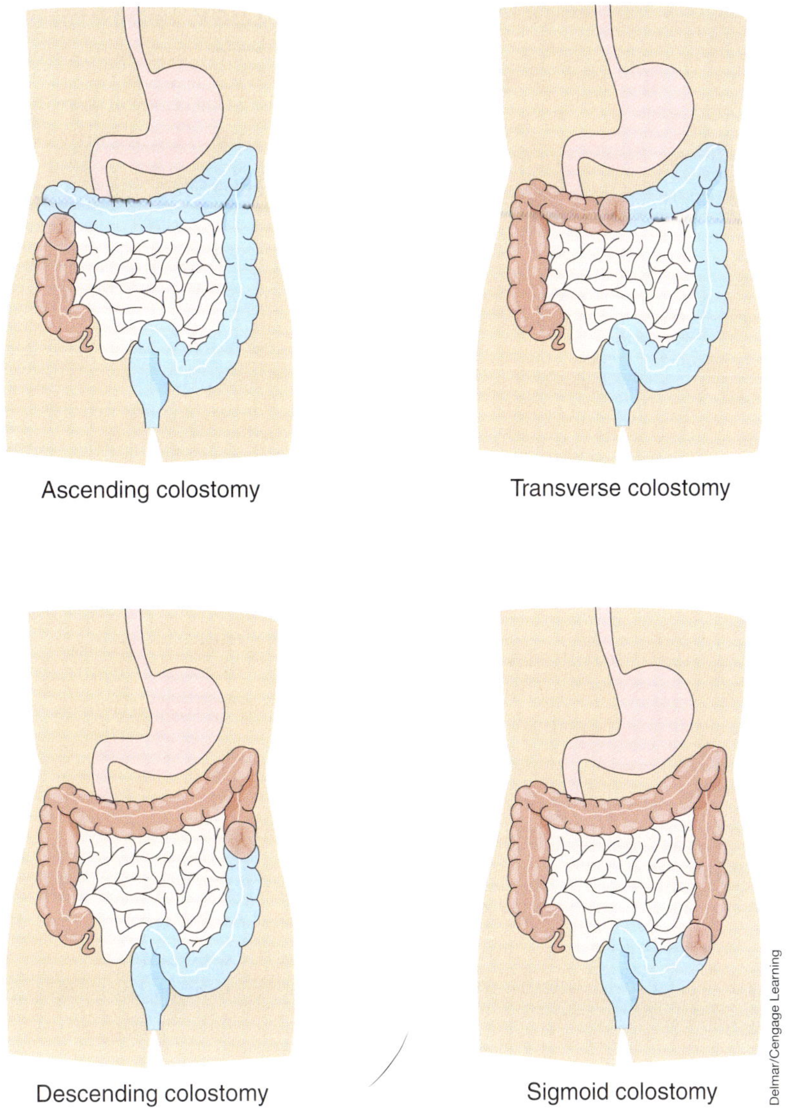

FIGURE 11–16 Colostomy locations *(blue section may be surgically removed if colostomy is permanent).*

■ ***TREATMENT.*** Treatment depends on the cause of the disease. Antibiotics are usually effective for dysentery caused by a bacterial infection.

■ ***PREVENTION.*** Dysentery is spread by poor hygiene. Preventive steps include hand washing and not sharing eating utensils and straws. If traveling to an underdeveloped country, do not drink the water, use ice cubes, or eat salad or any fresh fruit or vegetables.

DIVERTICULOSIS/DIVERTICULITIS

■ ***DESCRIPTION.*** Diverticulosis is a condition of having diverticula, or little pouches, in the colon (Figure 11–17), especially in the sigmoid colon. It can be asymptomatic (without symptoms) until the pouches become packed with fecal material and become irritated and inflamed. Once inflamed, the condition is called diverticulitis.

■ ***ETIOLOGY.*** Diverticulitis increases in incidence with age and has been associated with poor dietary habits, lack of physical activity, and poor bowel habits.

■ ***SYMPTOMS.*** Low abdominal pain and cramping are indicative of diverticulitis. Because this inflammatory disease progresses, it can lead to hemorrhage, perforation, or narrowing of the lumen of the colon and, thus, obstruction.

■ ***DIAGNOSIS.*** Diagnosis is easily made by performing a colonoscopy and visualizing the pouches.

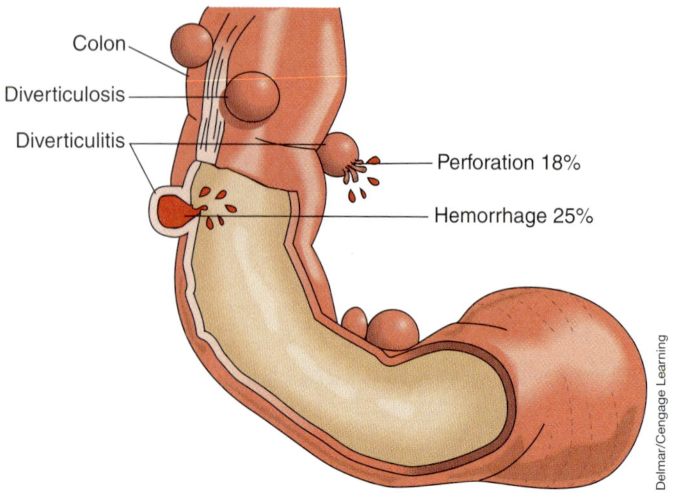

FIGURE 11–17 Diverticulosis/Diverticulitis.

■ ***TREATMENT.*** Increasing the amount of fiber in the diet is usually effective in relieving symptoms and preventing complications. Foods high in fiber include fruits, vegetables, beans, potatoes, rice, and cereals. Fiber keeps the stool soft, allowing it to move more easily through the colon. Antibiotics might be needed if acute diverticulitis develops.

■ ***PREVENTION.*** A high-fiber diet can aid in prevention of diverticulosis. Some believe that avoiding any foods with seeds and nuts is helpful, although this concept has not been proven.

COLON POLYPS

■ ***DESCRIPTION.*** A **polyp** (PAH-lip) is an inward projection of the mucosal lining of the colon (Figure 11–18).

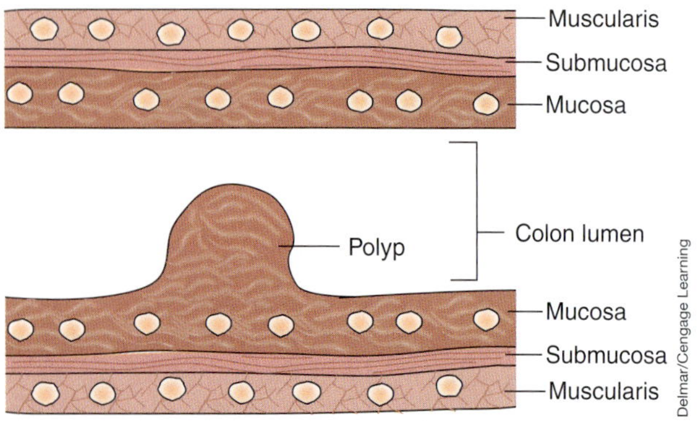

FIGURE 11–18 Colon polyp.

■ ***ETIOLOGY.*** Polyps can be due to an inflammatory reaction or caused by a benign or malignant neoplasm.

■ ***SYMPTOMS.*** Colon polyps can cause rectal bleeding, but most commonly, they are asymptomatic.

■ ***DIAGNOSIS.*** These growths are often diagnosed during a routine colonoscopy (colon = colon, oscopy =procedure to look into) or sigmoidoscopy (sigmoid = sigmoid portion of the colon).

■ ***TREATMENT.*** Suspicious polyps can be excisionally biopsied during these procedures. Cancerous polyps are removed by excisional biopsy or surgical resection, depending on the number and type of polyps present.

■ ***PREVENTION.*** Colon polyps might not be preventable, but making healthy lifestyle changes and lowering certain risk factors is helpful. Preventive activities include eating healthy, limiting fat intake, limiting alcohol consumption, stopping smoking, maintaining a healthy body weight, and exercising.

CARCINOMA OF THE COLON AND RECTUM

■ ***DESCRIPTION.*** Commonly called **colorectal** cancer, this classification covers a variety of carcinomas that arise in the colon and rectum. These tumors are usually adenocarcinomas that arise from the mucosal lining. Colorectal cancer commonly affects both sexes.

■ ***ETIOLOGY.*** The cause of colorectal cancer is unknown. Some identified predisposing factors include ulcerative colitis, familial polyposis (many colon polyps), and a diet high in red meat and low in fiber.

■ ***SYMPTOMS.*** Signs and symptoms of colorectal cancer depend on the site of the malignancy. Common symptoms can include a change in bowel habits (diarrhea or constipation), pencil-sized stools, blood in the stools, anemia (due to tumor bleeding), abdominal discomfort, and obstruction.

Adenocarcinomas (the most common type found in colorectal cancer) tend to grow slowly. Eventually, the tumor can grow large enough to obstruct the lumen and spread through the colon wall. After it has spread through the colon wall, it can gain access to the lymphatic and vascular systems and spread throughout the body. The most common site of metastasis is the liver. Prognosis is good if the carcinoma is detected before metastasis; after metastasis, prognosis is poor.

■ ***DIAGNOSIS.*** Diagnosis of colorectal cancer can be made by stool examinations for occult blood, colonoscopy, and barium enema. Some rectal tumors also can be palpated by digital examination.

■ ***TREATMENT.*** Colorectal carcinoma is one of the leading causes of death from cancer in the United States. If detected early, it is potentially curable by surgical resection.

Resection is a major surgery and involves removing part (partial or hemicolectomy) or all of the colon (colectomy). If only part of the colon is removed, connecting the two healthy bowel ends back together is possible and is called an anastomosis; however, if a large amount of the colon is removed, an anastomosis might not be possible. In this case, a permanent or temporary opening called a colostomy might be required (see Figure 11–16).

A colostomy is developed by bringing the end of the colon through an opening in the abdominal wall. The new opening is called a stoma (Greek word for mouth), so named because it is pink in color like the inside of the mouth. This stoma will have bowel material passing through, so it is covered by a special colostomy bag which is emptied several times a day.

Some colostomies are temporary and are developed to allow the bowel to heal after surgery. In this case, the colon is reconnected in a second surgery, usually several weeks or months later.

Other treatments for colon cancer include chemotherapy and radiation. These can be used in conjunction with surgery or used separately, depending on the treatment plan and prognosis.

■ ***PREVENTION.*** Prevention of colorectal cancer focuses on dietary changes, which include decreasing red meat and increasing fiber consumption. It is also recommended that stool examination be performed on individuals annually, beginning at age 50.

Diseases of the Rectum

The rectum is the terminal or end part of the digestive system. The most common rectal problem is hemorrhoids. Rectal fissures and other minor problems can also occur, but cancer of the rectum is one of the most serious diseases of the rectum. Cancer of the rectum is more commonly diagnosed in the older adult than at any other age.

HEMORRHOIDS

■ ***DESCRIPTION.*** Hemorrhoids are varicose veins, either internal or external, in the rectum (Figure 11–19). Internal hemorrhoids can be examined by a physician using a proctoscope (procto = rectum, scope = instrument used to view). Internal hemorrhoids are located on the rectal wall; external hemorrhoids are located in the lower anal canal.

HEALTHY HIGHLIGHT

Colon Cancer Prevention

Colon cancer commonly occurs after age 50. It is, therefore, recommended that everyone age 50 and older should have an annual clinical exam, including a stool examination for occult blood. This relatively easy examination can assist with early detection of colon cancer. If the individual is at risk, if something is found at the clinical exam, or if the occult blood test is positive, a colonoscopy is recommended. If nothing is found during the colononoscopy, another one is not necessary for 10 years if the yearly exam and occult blood test continue to be negative. If any abnormality is found during the colonoscopy, another one should be done in 3 years. Prognosis for colon cancer is good if it is discovered in its early stages.

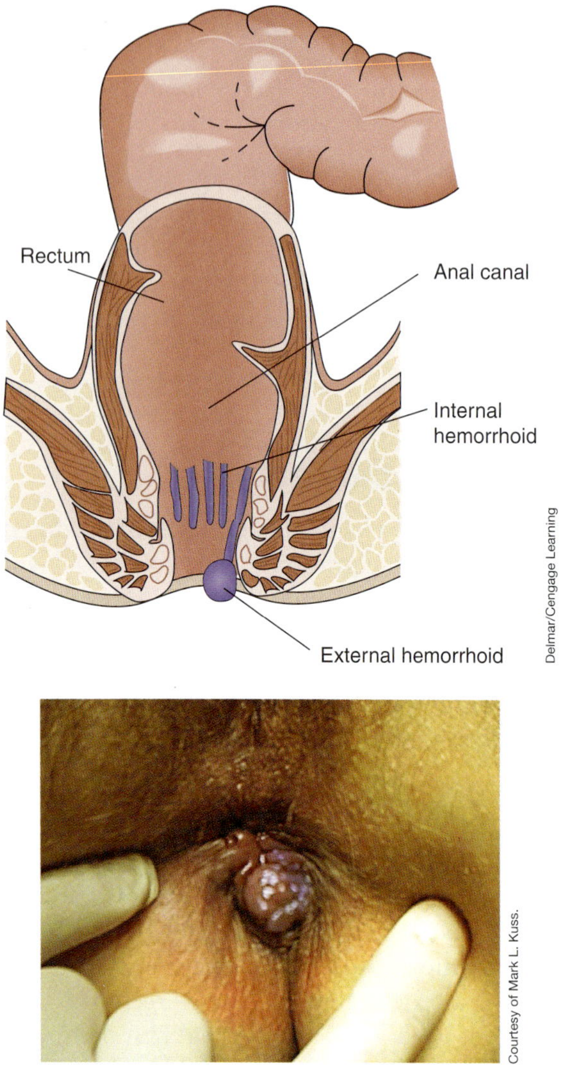

FIGURE 11–19 Hemorrhoids: internal and external.

External hemorrhoids are developed when internal hemorrhoids are pushed or prolapsed through the anal opening. External hemorrhoids are the ones commonly known as hemorrhoids and can be viewed around the anal opening. External hemorrhoids are bluish in color and might bleed with straining during bowel movements.

■ ***ETIOLOGY.*** Factors that increase the risk of developing hemorrhoids include any activity that increases pressure in the anal area such as straining to have a bowel movement, frequent bouts of constipation, prolonged standing, prolonged sitting, pregnancy, and childbirth. Other causes can be related to heredity and loss of muscle tone.

■ ***SYMPTOMS.*** The most common symptoms are itching, bleeding with bowel movements, and rectal pain.

■ ***DIAGNOSIS.*** External hemorrhoids are easily diagnosed by physical examination including a digital rectal exam. During this exam, the physician uses a gloved, lubricated finger to feel for abnormalities. Internal hemorrhoids might need visual inspection with an anoscope (lighted tube to examine the anus) or proctoscope (lighted tube to examine the rectum).

■ ***TREATMENT.*** Treatment of hemorrhoids can include medications and warm sitz baths to ease the pain. Manual reduction, cryosurgery, and hemorrhoidectomy can be optional treatments, depending on the severity of the disease.

■ ***PREVENTION.*** Preventive measures are focused on softening the stool (which decreases constipation and straining with bowel movements). These measures include good bowel habits (defecating when reflexes are strong), adequate fluid intake, increased fiber intake, exercise, and avoiding laxative use.

CARCINOMA OF THE RECTUM

See "Carcinoma of the Colon and Rectum."

TRAUMA

Trauma to the Mouth

Trauma to the mouth can be due to motor vehicle accidents, falls, abuse, burns, or any other blunt or perforating injury. The result can be broken teeth or jawbones or lesions and lacerations. Depending on the severity of the injury and the treatment needed, the individual might have difficulty eating. If the jaw is broken, the individual might need to have the jaw wired closed for a period of time, requiring a special liquid nutrition program to maintain adequate intake of fluids, vitamins, and minerals. Burns and lacerations also interfere with the normal oral intake of fluid and food. The individual might need alternate feeding methods such as parenteral (intravenous) or enteral (tube feeding) nutrition.

Trauma to the Stomach and Intestines

Trauma to the digestive system other than to the mouth is usually due to perforation (a hole through the organ), which can be the result of a stabbing, gunshot wound, or piercing by some other kind of object. This is a medical emergency because the contents of the stomach or intestines can spill out into the abdominal cavity, causing peritonitis. Commonly, the wound is surgically repaired and the individual is given antibiotics for the infection.

RARE DISEASES

Achalasia

Achalasia (eh-cha-LAY-see-ah) is a disorder of the esophagus that causes pain with swallowing. The peristaltic movement of the lower portion of the esophagus does not function properly. The cause of the disorder is unknown. Treatment might involve surgery, drug therapy, or both.

Gluten-Induced Enteropathy

This disease is also called celiac sprue disease (nontropical sprue disease), an immune problem that sensitizes the individual to gluten proteins. This protein is found mainly in wheat and rye products but also in oat and barley foods. Individuals with gluten-induced enteropathy have impaired absorption of some vitamins and proteins, fats, and carbohydrates. Gluten-induced enteropathy is treated by a dietary measure, restricting all gluten-containing foods.

Intestinal Polyps

Intestinal polyps are benign (noncancerous) tumors found along the lining of the intestine. Although they usually do not cause any symptoms for the individual, they are often surgically removed as a preventive treatment because polyps can increase the risk of cancer.

EFFECTS OF AGING ON THE SYSTEM

Disorders of the digestive system are common in the aging population, so the incidence of problems increases with age. Some of the problems occurring with age in the system are caused by changes in the cardiovascular or neurologic system, which causes disruptions in the functioning of the digestive system. In the upper digestive system, the most common problem with aging is related to loss of teeth. Preventive dentistry has lessened teeth and gum problems in recent years, but it is still a significant factor in the older adult. Further, the sense of taste becomes less sensitive, and the motility in the esophagus decreases and can cause some distress, but it is generally asymptomatic.

Changes in the lining of the stomach and decreased secretion of hydrochloric acid increase the likelihood of digestive disorders in the older adult. Decreased circulation to the stomach increases the incidence of ulcer disease.

Lower digestive disorders are common in the older adult. The lower intestinal lining is affected much like the stomach lining. Absorption of some nutrients such as vitamin B_{12} and fats can decrease. Decreased circulation to the intestines can cause ischemia and pain in the abdomen, and decreased motility can contribute to constipation problems. The development of inflammatory disease and hemorrhoids is common to the aging process but also can be caused by earlier problems or other predisposing factors.

SUMMARY

The digestive system is a long, hollow tube that extends from the mouth to the anus. Its purpose is the ingestion, digestion, and absorption of fluids and nutrients and elimination of wastes. Accessory organs of the digestive system include the liver, pancreas, and gallbladder. The most common diseases of the system are infections, ulcers, and cancer. Physiologic and lifestyle changes in older adults put them at higher risk for diseases of the digestive system.

REVIEW QUESTIONS

Short Answer

1. What are the functions of the digestive system?

2. Which signs and symptoms are associated with common digestive system disorders?

3. Which diagnostic tests are most commonly used to determine type and cause of the digestive system disorders?

Matching

4. Match the disorders listed in the left column with the correct region of the digestive system in the right column:

_____ Pharyngitis	a. disease of the small intestine
_____ Gastritis	b. disease of the mouth
_____ Hemorrhoids	c. disease of the colon
_____ Periodontal disease	d. disease of the throat or esophagus
_____ Regional enteritis	e. disease of the rectum
_____ IBS	f. disease of the stomach

Multiple Choice

5. Which of the following behaviors might contribute to digestive system problems?
   a. Eating four to six small meals per day
   b. Improperly cooking food
   c. Failure to wash hands after toileting
   d. Poor dietary habits
   e. Straining with bowel movements
   f. Drinking plenty of fluids daily
   g. Frequent use of laxatives and enemas

True or False

6. T F The alimentary canal is a continuous tube from the mouth to the anus.
7. T F Strep throat should always be treated because it can lead to rheumatic heart disease.
8. T F The main function of the large intestine (colon) is the digestion of food.
9. T F The *Helicobacter* bacteria are contributing factors in the development of peptic ulcers.
10. T F The effects of aging put the older adult at an increased risk for digestive system problems.

CASE STUDIES

■ Stacey Erin is a 32-year-old accountant who has just been diagnosed with peptic ulcer disease. She would like some information about her disorder and to find out what to expect in the future and how to cope with it. What would you tell her about peptic ulcer disease? How can she prevent continued problems with her ulcer?

■ Mr. Montgomery was recently diagnosed with colon cancer. He is 67 years old and was recently widowed. He has no family members nearby to assist him during the ordeal of coping with the diagnosis, surgical treatment, and postoperative care. He asks you to explain the treatment and the care that he will need after surgery. He was told that his cancer has not metastasized, so the surgeon will just do a resection of the colon. What would you tell him? How can you help Mr. Montgomery with his questions and fear for his future? What resources can you give him for more information and support?

StudyWARE™ Connection

To help you learn the content in this chapter, take a practice quiz or play an interactive game on your StudyWARE™ CD-ROM.

Workbook Practice

Go to your Workbook and complete the practice questions.

BIBLIOGRAPHY

Ando, T., Nobata, K., Watanabe, O., Kusugami, K., Maedam O., Ishiguro, K., Ohmiya, N., Niwa, Y., & Goto, H. (2007). Abnormalities in the upper gastrointestinal tract in inflammatory bowel disease. *Inflammopharmacology 15*(3), 101–104.

Barakzai, M., Gregory, J., & Fraser, D. (2007).The effect of culture on symptom reporting: Hispanics and irritable bowel syndrome. *Journal of the American Academy of Nurse Practitioners 19*(5), 261–267.

Beers, Mark H., MD, & Berkow, Robert, MD, eds. (2004). Malabsorption syndromes.. In *The Merck manual of diagnosis and therapy* (section 3, chapter 30). Whitehouse Station, NJ: Merck Research Laboratories.

Botelho, M., Roa, V., Carvalho, C., Bezerra-Fiho, J., Fonseca, S., Vale, M., Montenegro, D., Cunha, F., Ribeiro, R., & Brito, G. (2007). *Lippia sidoides* and *Myracrodruon urundeuva* prevent alveolar bone resorption in experimental periodontitis in rats. *Journal of Ethnopharmacology 113*(3),471-478.

Brown-Guttovz, H. (2007). Intussusception. *Nursing 37* (2), 80.

Brown-Guttovz, H. (2008). About irritable bowel syndrome. *Nursing 38*(2), 28.

Castledine, G., Grainger, M., Wood, N., & Dilley, C. (2007). Researching the management of constipation in long-term care. Part 1. *British Journal of Nursing 16*(18), 1128–1131.

Centers for Disease Control and Prevention, National Center for Infectious Diseases. Travelers' health. New medication approved for treatment of giardiasis and amebiasis. *www.cdc.gov/travel* (accessed May 2008).

Centers for Disease Control and Prevention. (July 1998) Helicobacter pylori and Peptic Ulcer Disease. Fact Sheet for Healthcare Providers. *www.cdc.gov/ncidod/hpylori.htm* (accessed April 2009).

Cotterill, N., Norton, C., Avery, K., Abrams, P., & Donavan, J. (2008). A patient-centered approach to developing a comprehensive symptom and quality of life assessment of anal incontinence. *Diseases of the Colon & Rectum 51*(1), 82–87.

Digestive Diseases Research Centers. (2008). National Institutes of Health and the United States Department of Health and Human Diseases. *www2.niddk.nih.gov* (accessed May 2008).

Diggle, L. (2007). Rotavirus diarrhea and future prospects for prevention. *British Journal of Nursing 16*(16), 970–974.

Freeman, L. (2007). Responding to small bowel obstruction. *Nursing 37*(5), 65–66.

Grainger, M., Castledine, G., Wood, N., & Dilley, C. (2007). Researching the management of constipation in long-term care. Part 2. *British Journal of Nursing 16*(19), 1212–1217.

Greenway, F., Liu, Z., Martin, C., Kai-Yuan, W., Nofziger, J., Rood, J., Yu, Y., & Amen, R. (2006). Safety and efficacy of NT, an herbal supplement in treating human obesity. *International Journal of Obesity 30*(12), 1737–1441.

Hamer, H., Jonkers, D., Venema, K., Vanhoutvin, S., Troost, F., & Brummer, R. (2008). Review article: The role of butyrate on colonic function. *Alimentary Pharmacology & Therapeutics 27*(2), 104–119.

Harrison, S. (2007). Helping patients to cope with fecal incontinence. *Nursing Older People 19*(7), 26.

Hertig, V. (2007). Daily stress and gastrointestinal symptoms in women with irritable bowel syndrome. *Nursing Research 56*(6), 399–406.

Klein, G., Jaekyung, K., Himmeldirk, K., Yanyan, C., & Xiaozhuo, C. (2007). Antidiabetes and anti-obesity activity of lagerstroemia speciosa. *Evidence-Based Complementary and Alternative Medicine 4*(4), 401–407.

Koslap-Petraco, M. (2006). Homecare issues in rotavirus gastroenteritis. *Journal of the American Academy of Nurse Practitioners 18*(9), 422–428.

Krouse, R., Grant, M., Ferrell, B., Dean, G., Nelson, R., & Chu, D. (2007). Quality of life outcomes in 599 cancer and non-cancer patients with colostomies. *Journal of Surgical Research 138*(1), 79–87.

Lee, J., Chae, K., Ha, J., Park, B., Hee, S., Jeong, S., Kim, M., & Yoon, M. (2008). Regulation of obesity and lipid disorders by herbal extracts from *Morus alba*, *Melissa officinalis* and *Artemisia* capillaries in high-fat diet-induced obese mice. *Journal of Ethnopharmacology 115*(2), 263–270.

Mayo Foundation for Medical Education and Research. (2008) Virtual reality: Examination without the tubes. *Discovery's Edge*, Mayo Clinic's Online Research Magazine. *www.discoverysedge.mayo.edu* (accessed February 25, 2008).

National institute of Diabetes and Digestive and Kidney Diseases (NIDDK). (2008). *H. pylori* and peptic ulcer. *www.digestive.niddk.nih.gov/ddiseases* (accessed May 2008).

Nakajima, S., Fujita, K., Inoue, Y., Nishio, M., & Seto, Y. (2006). Effect of the folk remedy, Bainiku-ekisu, a concentrate of *Prunus mume* juice, on *Helicobacter pylori* infection in humans. *Helicobacter 11*(6), 589–591.

National Program of Cancer Registries. (2008). Centers for Disease Control and Prevention. *www.cdc.gov* (accessed May 2008).

Reavis, C. (2005). Rural health alert: *Helicobacter pylori* in well water. *Journal of the American Academy of Nurse Practitioners 17*(7), 283–289.

Tod, A., Stringer, E., Levery, C., Dean, J., & Brown, J. (2007). Rectal irrigation in the management of functional bowel disorders: A review. *British Journal of Nursing 16*(14), 858–864.

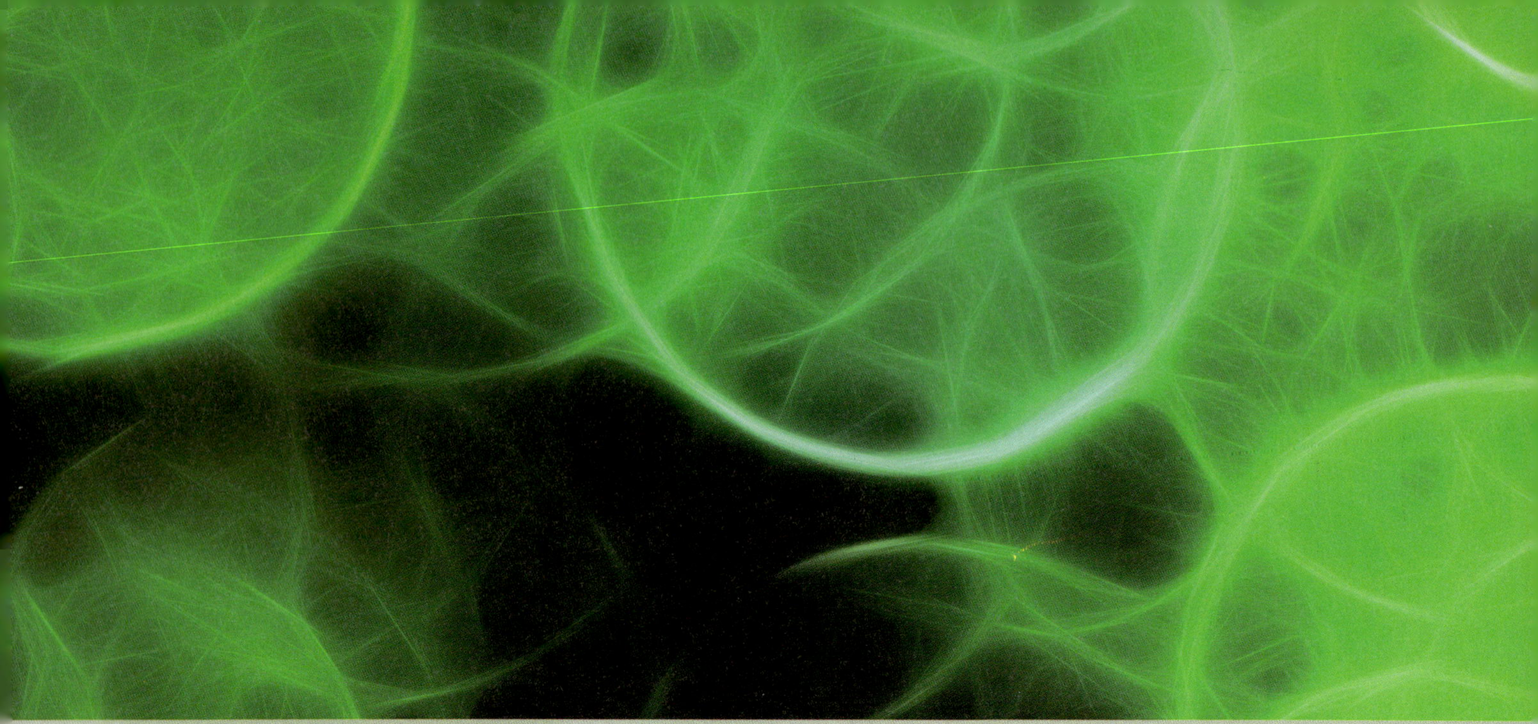

OUTLINE

- Anatomy and Physiology
- Common Signs and Symptoms
- Diagnostic Tests
- Common Diseases of the Accessory Organs of Digestion
  - *Liver Diseases*
  - *Gallbladder Diseases*
  - *Pancreatic Diseases*
- Rare Diseases
  - *Primary Biliary Cirrhosis*
  - *Gilbert's Syndrome*
  - *Hemochromatosis*
- Effects of Aging on the System
- Summary
- Review Questions
- Case Studies
- Bibliography

KEY TERMS

Abdominocentesis (p. 248)
Albumin (p. 248)
Amylase (p. 251)
Ascites (p. 248)
Autodigestion (p. 251)
Caput medusae (p. 247)
Cholecystectomy (p. 249)
Delirium tremens (p. 248)
Esophageal varices (p. 247)
Fulminant (p. 245)
Gynecomastia (p. 248)
Hematemesis (p. 248)
Hepatomegaly (p. 244)
Jaundice (p. 243)
Palmar erythema (p. 248)
Portal hypertension (p. 247)
Spider angiomas (p. 248)
Splenomegaly (p. 247)

12

Liver, Gallbladder, and Pancreatic Diseases and Disorders

LEARNING OBJECTIVES

Upon completion of the chapter, the learner should be able to:

1. Define the terminology common to the liver, gallbladder, and pancreas and the disorders of the organs.
2. Discuss the basic anatomy and physiology of the liver, gallbladder, and pancreas.
3. Identify the important signs and symptoms associated with common liver, gallbladder, and pancreas disorders.
4. Describe the common diagnostics used to determine the type and cause of liver, gallbladder, or pancreas disorders.
5. Identify common disorders of the liver, gallbladder, and pancreas.
6. Describe the typical course and management of the common liver, gallbladder, and pancreas disorders.
7. Describe the effects of aging on the liver, gallbladder, and pancreas and the common disorders associated with aging of the organs.

OVERVIEW

The liver, gallbladder, and pancreas are the accessory organs of digestion. Although these organs are not considered part of the digestive system, they have important roles in the digestive process as well as in many other functions in the body. Disorders of the liver, gallbladder, or pancreas can cause serious digestive problems and many other systemic disorders. ■

ANATOMY AND PHYSIOLOGY

The liver is the largest solid organ of the body, taking second place only to the skin as the largest organ overall (Figure 12–1). The liver has many functions, most of which are related to its chemical actions. It plays a role in digestion, absorption, metabolism, blood clotting, the manufacture of important chemicals, and storage of nutrients. The liver is composed of two lobes, weighs about 3.5 pounds, and lies in the right upper quadrant of the abdomen. Some of the most important functions of the liver include:

- Production and secretion of bile used for fat digestion.
- Production of cholesterol.
- Oxidation of fatty acids and glycerol used for body energy.
- Metabolism of carbohydrates, fats, and protein.
- Conversion of glucose to glycogen for storage and the reverse process for energy.
- Synthesis of amino acids.
- Detoxification of many drugs and other toxins.
- Storage of vitamins and other minerals.
- Production of fibrinogen and prothrombin for blood clotting.

The liver receives blood from the portal system through the portal vein and the hepatic artery. About 1,450 ml of blood flows through the liver every minute. The blood returns to the circulatory system through the hepatic vein to the inferior vena cava.

Bile to emulsify, or break down, lipids in the intestine is continually produced in the liver and conducted through the hepatic duct to the duodenum. When bile is not needed in the digestive process, excess bile is stored in the gallbladder until needed by the intestine in the digestive process.

The gallbladder is a small, pear-shaped organ lying just under the liver (see Figure 12–1). Bile travels from the gallbladder to the duodenum via the cystic duct and the common bile duct.

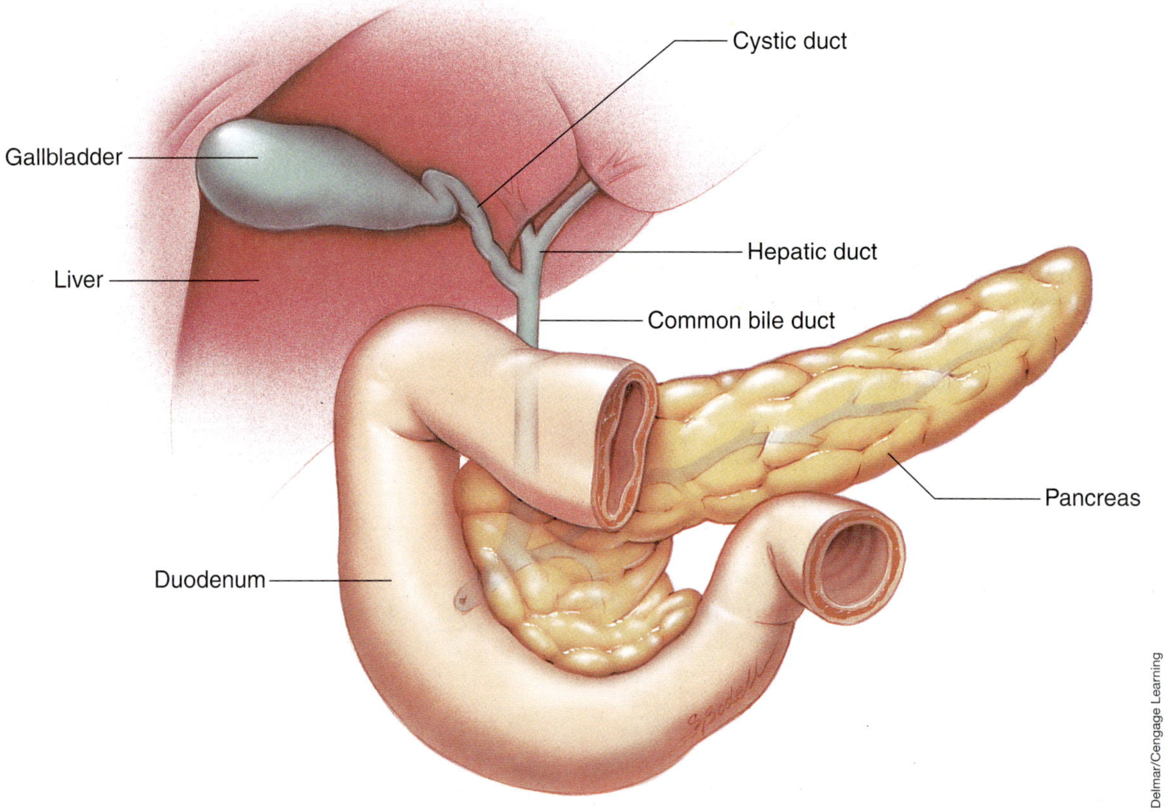

FIGURE 12–1 The liver, gallbladder, and pancreas.

The pancreas lies in the abdomen behind the stomach between the duodenum and the spleen (see Figure 12–1); it is both an endocrine gland (the islet cells secrete hormones) and an exocrine gland, producing and secreting most of the digestive enzymes. The pancreas secretes intestinal juices consisting of chymotrypsin and trypsin, which break down proteins; amylase, which breaks down starch; and lipase, which breaks down fats. The pancreatic juices exit the gland by way of the pancreatic duct to the duodenum.

StudyWARE™ Connection

View an animation on the pancreas on your StudyWARE™ CD-ROM.

COMMON SIGNS AND SYMPTOMS

Jaundice (JAWN-dis, a yellowish discoloration of the skin) is an obvious symptom of liver disease and can be secondary to gallbladder disease as well. If a bile duct is blocked, for instance, the bile backs up into the liver and leads to jaundice.

Jaundice is caused by high levels of bilirubin in the blood. Bilirubin is a by-product of the breakdown of heme, the main component of hemoglobin in red blood cells. The liver filters bilirubin out of the blood and excretes it in bile. If the liver is unable to filter bilirubin and excrete it, hyperbilirubinemia (hyper = too much, bilirubin, emia = blood), or excessive bilirubin in the blood, occurs. This excess leaks into the tissues, and the individual's skin, mucosa, and sclera (white part of the eye) become yellowish in color.

Bilirubin can be broken down in the skin by exposure to sunlight or direct lighting, which explains the use of bili lights to clear bilirubin in a jaundiced newborn infant. Excessive bilirubin is also filtered out of the blood by the kidneys, causing dark brown urine.

Pain is a common symptom of gallbladder disease, pancreatitis, and end-stage pancreatic cancer. With gallbladder disease, right-sided abdominal pain commonly occurs following a meal containing fat. Acute abdominal pain occurs with pancreatitis and pancreatic cancer.

DIAGNOSTIC TESTS

Liver function tests are blood tests to measure levels of bilirubin, albumin (blood protein), and alkaline phosphatase (enzyme). Impaired liver function will lead to elevated bilirubin and alkaline phosphatase levels and low albumin levels.

Ultrasound is used to evaluate the liver, gallbladder, and pancreas for size, shape, and position. X-ray examinations of the gallbladder and the vessels of the gallbladder (cholecystogram and cholangiogram, respectively) use radiopaque dye to show the presence of gallstones, tumors, and function of the gallbladder. Ultrasonography is used more often than the previously mentioned radiologic examinations.

Computer axial tomography (CAT or CT) scans can be performed to visualize the liver, gallbladder, and pancreas. Visualization of these organs aids in diagnosis of hepatic and pancreatic cancer. A liver biopsy can be performed by needle biopsy or during laparoscopic surgery. Biopsy is the most reliable test for determination of chronic hepatitis, cirrhosis, and cancer.

Blood tests to measure pancreatic function commonly include serum amylase and lipase. Amylase and lipase are digestive enzymes produced by the pancreas that break down carbohydrates and fats, respectively.

COMMON DISEASES OF THE ACCESSORY ORGANS OF DIGESTION

Diseases of the accessory organs of digestion can seriously affect the digestion and metabolism of nutrients. Symptoms of these disorders reflect an interference with the particular organ's function. Over 25 million individuals—1 in 10—in the United States have been diagnosed with liver or gallbladder diseases (American Liver Foundation, 2006).

Liver Diseases

Liver diseases can range from mild inflammation to those that destroy the liver and result in liver failure. Any disease of the liver can have serious consequences by interfering with the many functions of the liver.

HEPATITIS

■ ***DESCRIPTION.*** Hepatitis is inflammation of the liver that can lead to abnormal function and other diseases or conditions.

■ ***ETIOLOGY.*** Hepatitis might be caused by the chemical action of drugs or toxic substances. Chronic alcoholism often leads to hepatitis prior to the functional changes seen with cirrhosis, but the most common cause of hepatitis is a group of viruses. This form of hepatitis is often called viral hepatitis and is the form most commonly thought of when one considers hepatitis.

Viral hepatitis is the most prevalent liver disease in the world and is often asymptomatic. When symptoms do occur, they can be so vague that the disease is misdiagnosed, which explains why approximately 40% of Americans have antibodies to hepatitis A and 10% have antibodies to hepatitis B, yet these individuals do not recall ever having hepatitis.

Viral hepatitis occurs in five basic types. A different virus causes each type. The types of hepatitis are A, B, C, D, and E.

Hepatitis A (HAV). The most benign or harmless form of hepatitis. Total recovery occurs 98% of the time. This virus is spread by fecal–oral route and commonly affects children and young adults, especially in areas where there is poor sanitation and overcrowding. Symptoms are usually very vague and similar to flu, often leading to misdiagnosis. The virus is shed in the feces, and the affected individual does not become a carrier of the disease. HAV never leads to chronic hepatitis or cirrhosis. A vaccine is available and is recommended for those traveling or living in a high-risk area.

Hepatitis B (HBV). A serious form of hepatitis formerly called serum hepatitis. It was once thought that HBV was spread only by contact with blood, as occurs with blood transfusions and contaminated needles. However, it is now known that saliva, urine, feces, and semen can spread the virus, which also qualifies it as a sexually transmitted disease. HBV is 100 times more infectious than HIV, the virus that causes AIDS (Hepatitis Foundation, 2008). HBV also can be spread transplacentally (across the placenta from mother to unborn infant). This virus is a major health problem because individuals can become carriers of the virus and carry it for years or even a lifetime. Approximately 46,000 new infections occur every year in the United States (CDC, 2008). Carriers are not only a threat to others but also are at high risk for developing chronic hepatitis and cirrhosis. About 1 out of every 250 persons is a carrier of HBV. Those at high risk for HBV are drug addicts, homosexuals, blood recipients, and health care workers. A vaccine is available and is 95% effective in prevention of the disease.

Hepatitis C (HCV). Similar to HBV because it also is spread by blood or sexual contact but differs from B in that it attacks the RNA of a cell, whereas hepatitis B attacks the DNA. After HCV was distinguished from HBV, it was found to be the cause of most cases of hepatitis following blood transfusion (posttransfusion hepatitis). HCV is more likely to become chronic hepatitis than form B is, with approximately 50% of those affected with HCV developing chronic hepatitis and cirrhosis. Approximately 3% of the world's population, or some 170 million individuals, are infected with HCV (Hepatitis Foundation, 2008).

Hepatitis D (HDV). Also called the delta virus. It requires the presence of HBV to replicate. Infection with both B and D can cause more prominent symptoms and a greater risk of developing chronic and fulminant hepatitis.

Hepatitis E (HEV). Similar to HAV in that it is spread through the fecal–oral route. It is commonly due to water contamination. Chronic hepatitis does not develop with HEV, but this virus in pregnant women can be fatal.

■ ***SYMPTOMS.*** Jaundice is often the first symptom that signals a liver problem, although not all individuals become yellow. Interestingly, those who become more jaundiced are more likely to have a good recovery than those who are less jaundiced. Individuals with mild jaundice are more likely to develop chronic hepatitis. Other symptoms include malaise, anorexia, myalgia (myo = muscle, algia = pain), fever, and abdominal pain. Physical examination might reveal **hepatomegaly** (HEP-ah-toh-MEG-ah-lee; hepato = liver, megaly = enlargement). Dark-colored urine and clay- or light-colored stools are related to the inability of the liver to form normal bile.

■ ***DIAGNOSIS.*** A blood test showing hepatitis virus antibodies is adequate for diagnosis.

■ ***TREATMENT.*** Treatment for viral hepatitis is symptomatic. Adequate rest and good nutrition are essential.

Approximately 85% of affected individuals recover in 6 weeks. The most serious complications with hepatitis are development of chronic hepatitis and **fulminant** (FULL-ma-nant; to occur suddenly and with great intensity) hepatitis. Chronic hepatitis develops in one out of four cases and often leads to cirrhosis of the liver. Fulminant hepatitis is an acute hepatitis that causes extensive necrosis of liver tissue. Symptoms include a high fever, hemorrhages from the skin and mucous membranes, confusion, and stupor. Coma often develops and leads to death. Even with prompt and supportive care, fulminant hepatitis is 90% fatal.

PREVENTION. Prevention of hepatitis involves good hygiene and special care when handling needles and body secretions.

- Other activities that aid in prevention include:
- Avoiding excessive alcohol consumption.
- Avoiding use of illegal drugs or snorting cocaine.
- Avoiding unprotected sex, especially with multiple partners.
- Receiving the hepatitis vaccines, especially for those in a high-risk group.

GLIMPSE OF THE FUTURE

Improving Treatments for Hepatitis B

Chronic hepatitis B viral (HBV) infection is a major cause of cirrhosis and even cancer of the liver. Interferon is one of the treatment strategies used at this time, along with antiviral medications, to treat the infection. New and, hopefully, more effective treatments with fewer side effects are now being studied. One treatment, called RNA interference (RNAi), uses small interfering RNA (siRNA) to treat the HBV infection. There is still research to be completed on this method before being assured that it is effective and marketable. RNAi may be useful in the future as a treatment for HBV if researchers find it to be successful and if the side effects are minimal.

Source: Guofeng & Ram (2008).

COMPLEMENTARY AND ALTERNATIVE THERAPY

Herbal Medicines Mixed with Statins Might Cause Harm to the Liver

A variety of herbal medicines is used by postmenopausal women since the use of hormone replacement therapy has declined. Black cohosh (*Cimicifuga racemosa*) is an herbal preparation that is often used to reduce hot flashes. Recent research has shown some adverse interactions between this preparation and atorvastatin (one of the statins from a class of hypolipidemic drugs used to lower cholesterol levels). Elevated liver enzymes have been seen in patients who are taking these two drugs. It is recommended that patients who are taking both herbal preparations to avoid postmenopausal symptoms and cholesterol-lowering medications check with a physician or pharmacist about possible side effects that could be harmful to the liver or other organs.

Source: Patel & Derkits (2007).

OTHER DISEASES OF THE LIVER

CIRRHOSIS

DESCRIPTION. Cirrhosis (sir-ROH-sis) of the liver is a chronic, irreversible, degenerative disease also known as end-stage liver disease. It is characterized by the replacement of normal liver cells with nonfunctioning, fibrous scar tissue, giving the surface of the liver a nodular appearance known as hobnail liver. This change in structure and function of the liver cells leads to impaired blood flow and altered function of the liver.

ETIOLOGY. The most common cause of cirrhosis is chronic alcoholism. Cirrhosis is more common in males than females. It also can be idiopathic or the end result of other diseases such as chronic hepatitis and congestive heart failure. The development of the disease often takes years. Symptoms usually do not appear until serious structural and functional changes in the liver tissue have occurred. If symptoms occur, they are usually mild and nonspecific and might include loss of appetite, nausea, indigestion, weakness, and weight loss.

As the disease progresses, the abnormal scar tissue alters blood flow through the liver and leads to a variety of complications such as blood backing up in the hepatic portal vein. The relationship of the liver, hepatic portal system, and digestive system is as follows:

- The purpose of the hepatic portal system is to carry venous blood from the spleen and digestive organs (esophagus, stomach, and intestines) to the liver (Figure 12–2). The liver plays a major role in the digestive system by detoxifying and metabolizing nutrients before releasing them into the systemic blood in the inferior vena cava.

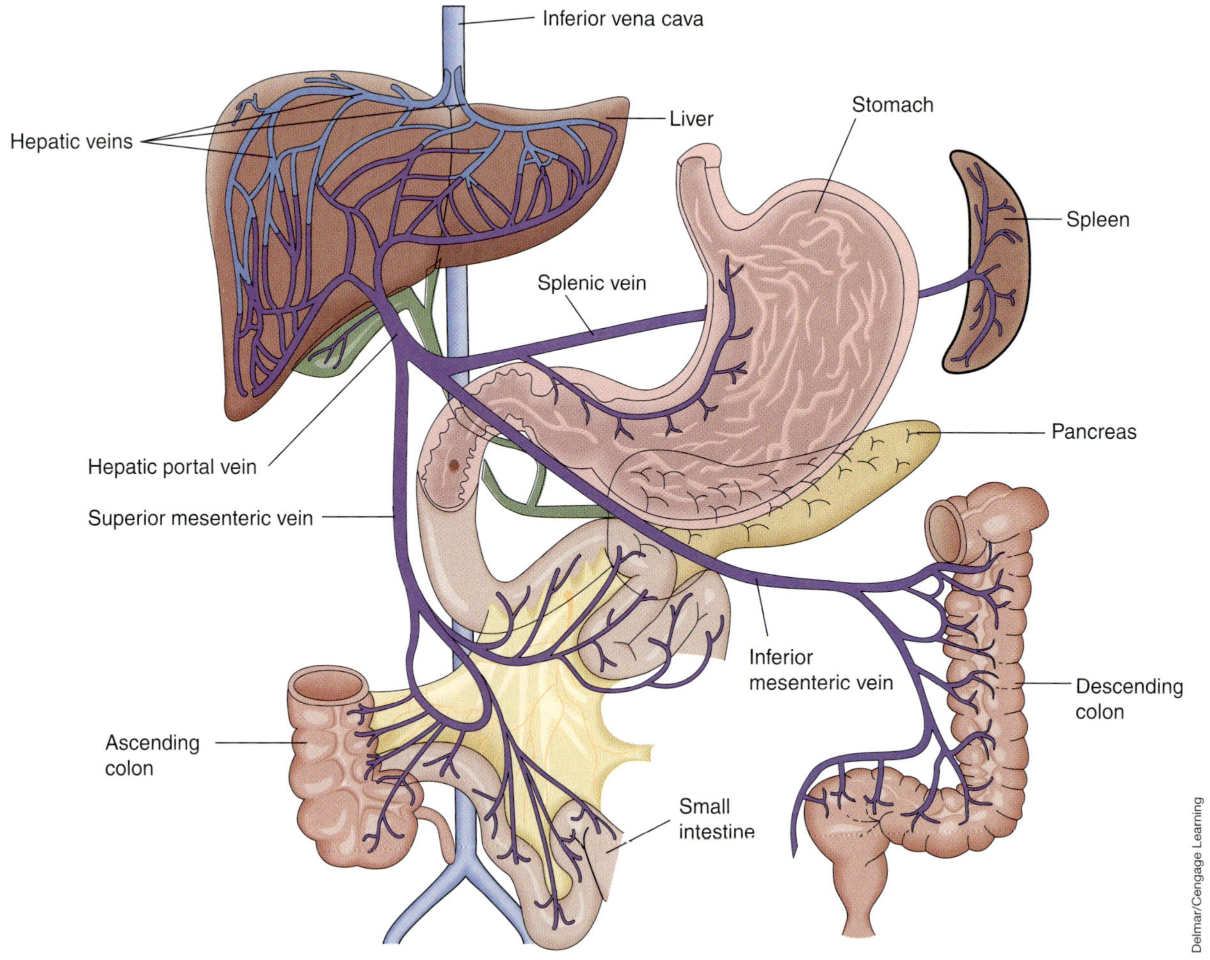

FIGURE 12–2 Hepatic portal system.

For example, if an individual consumes a meal with an alcoholic beverage, these nutrients are absorbed into venous blood in the small intestine and transported to the liver to be filtered, detoxified, and stored. The liver's responsibility, in part, is to keep blood glucose levels from soaring when an individual eats a high-carbohydrate meal. Nutrients are filtered, metabolized, stored, and released as needed into the systemic circulation by the liver. Toxins such as alcohol are detoxified. If alcohol consumption is too great or outpaces the liver's ability to detoxify the blood, the blood alcohol level will rise.

- If the liver is obstructed for any reason, blood will back up in this portal system. As blood backs up, pressure increases in the portal vein and is called **portal hypertension**.

SYMPTOMS. Complications of severe cirrhosis can include:

1. **Varicosities** Portal hypertension causes varicosities (varicose veins) of the veins of the digestive system organs. Varicosities are commonly located in the esophagus (**esophageal varices**) (Figure 12–3). Esophageal varices (VAIR-ah-SEEZ) are prone to rupture, leading to massive hemorrhage, shock, and death. Other sites of varicosities include the rectum (hemorrhoids) and anterior abdominal wall. Varicosities across the front of the abdomen are often quite tortuous and unsightly, a condition called **caput medusae** (Medusa's head) because the physician who named the condition was reminded of Medusa's head when observing the varicosities. Medusa, in Greek mythology, was a woman who had snakes on her head in place of hair.
2. **Splenomegaly** Portal hypertension also causes increased pressure on the organs that are connected to or drained by the portal system. Often, this passive congestion in the spleen leads to **splenomegaly** (SPLEE-no-MEG-ah-lee; spleno = spleen, megaly = enlarged). Splenomegaly often causes increased blood cell destruction, leading to anemia, leukopenia, and thrombocytopenia. Thrombocytopenia (thrombo = clot, cyto = cell, penia = decrease) increases the risk of bleeding.

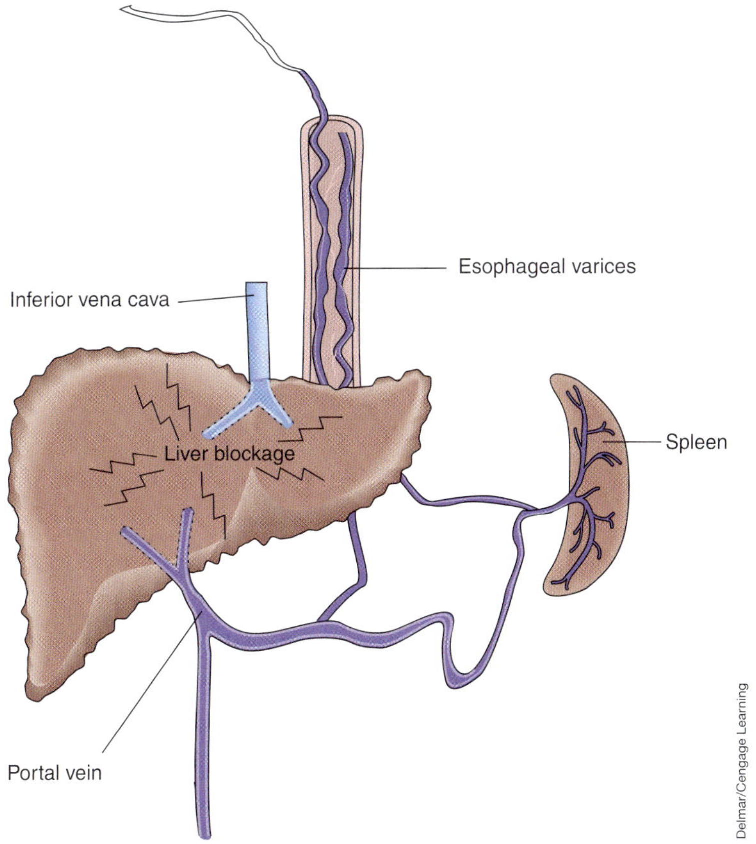

FIGURE 12–3 Esophageal varices.

3. **Gastrointestinal hemorrhage** This condition occurs due to thrombocytopenia and inability of the liver to secrete blood proteins essential for clotting. **Hematemesis** (HEM-ah-TEM-eh-sis; hemat = blood, emesis = vomiting) is often the first symptom of severe cirrhosis.
4. **Ascites** (ah-SIGH-teez) This is an accumulation of fluid in the abdominal cavity that develops as a result of liver failure and portal hypertension. The increased pressure on the veins of the portal system causes leaking of serum into the abdomen. Often, this fluid enlarges the abdomen to the point of causing difficult breathing. Excessive abdominal fluid can be drained by piercing the abdominal wall with a large-bore needle a procedure called **abdominocentesis** (ab-DOM-ih-no-sen-TEE-sis; abdomino = abdomen, centesis = puncture). The malnutrition of cirrhosis leads to spindly arms and legs despite the bloated abdomen.
5. **Edema** This often develops in the ankles and feet as a result of liver failure. The normal liver produces a blood protein called **albumin** (AL-byou-men), which is responsible for the osmotic pressure of blood, the movement of fluid from the blood through the capillaries to the tissues and back into the blood. Without osmotic pressure, blood fluid tends to leak into the tissues and remain there. A decrease in albumin allows this to occur, leading to edema in the feet and ankles.
6. **Jaundice** This usually results from the obstruction of the bile ducts as normal tissue is replaced by fibrous scar tissue, a characteristic of cirrhosis.
7. **Altered sex hormone metabolism** The normal liver inactivates small amounts of estrogen secreted by the adrenal glands in both the male and female. The cirrhotic liver is not capable of inactivating estrogen; thus, the male develops characteristics related to excessive estrogen. Such characteristics include:
   - **Gynecomastia** (GUY-neh-koh-MAS-tee-ah) An enlargement of the breasts
   - **Palmar erythema** Palms of the hands become reddened in color
   - **Spider angiomas** Small dilated blood vessels on the face and chest
   - **Female hair distribution** Absent or reduced chest and pubic hair
   - **Testicular atrophy** Decrease in testicle size
8. **Hepatic encephalopathy** The liver is often unable to detoxify the blood of nitrogenous waste products such as ammonia. This waste product can circulate in the blood and can affect the brain, causing mental confusion, stupor, and a characteristic shaking or tremor. This shaking, combined with hallucinations, is called **delirium tremens** (dee-LIR-ee-um TREE-mens) or DTs. Further depression of the nervous system can lead to hepatic coma and, ultimately, death. The clinical features of cirrhosis of the liver in the male are shown in Figure 12–4.

■ ***DIAGNOSIS.*** An examination revealing the physical characteristics described in Figure 12–4, along with blood testing, including elevated liver enzymes, elevated bilirubin, low serum albumin, and enlarged liver seen on abdominal X-ray, are all indicative of liver cirrhosis. A liver biopsy will confirm the diagnosis.

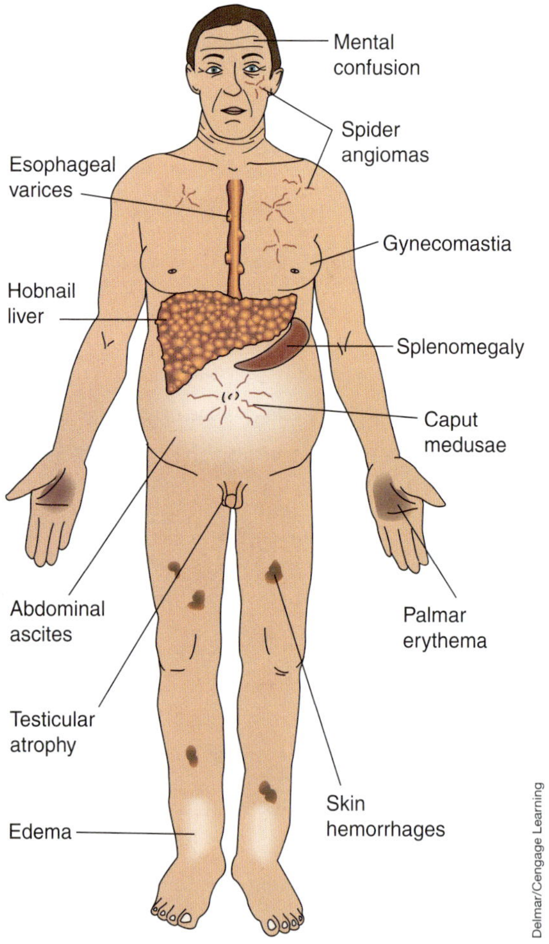

FIGURE 12–4 Clinical features of cirrhosis of the liver in the male.

■ ***TREATMENT.*** Treatment of cirrhosis is directed at the cause in an attempt to prevent further liver damage. Alcohol is strictly prohibited regardless of the cause of the cirrhosis. Adequate nutrition and rest are necessary. Vitamins, minerals, and diet supplements might be needed to prevent malnutrition. Diuretics might be necessary to reduce edema and ascites.

Cirrhosis has an unfavorable prognosis with most individuals surviving only 10 to 15 years after diagnosis. The appearance of ascites is a prognostic indicator because a majority of individuals with cirrhosis die within 5 years after the onset of ascites. Individuals usually die of massive bleeding from esophageal varices, hepatic encephalopathy, and other metabolic disorders.

■ ***PREVENTION.*** Although not all cases of cirrhosis are preventable, preventive measures include avoiding alcohol and exposure to all types of hepatitis and obtaining vaccinations for hepatitis A and B.

LIVER CANCER

■ ***DESCRIPTION.*** Primary and benign tumors (or those arising directly from liver tissue) are rare. When primary tumors do develop, they are more likely to occur in individuals with cirrhosis. Men are five times more likely to develop liver cancer than women. Secondary liver tumors (those that metastasize from other organs) are the most common and usually are the result of cancers in the breast, digestive system, and lungs.

■ ***ETIOLOGY.*** The cause of liver cancer, like most cancers, is not fully understood.

■ ***SYMPTOMS.*** Liver cancer is usually discovered late or at end stage because symptoms of anorexia, weight loss, and abdominal discomfort are so nonspecific.

■ ***DIAGNOSIS.*** Diagnosis is confirmed by biopsy.

■ ***TREATMENT.*** Treatment of liver cancer can involve surgery, chemotherapy, and radiation. Even with aggressive treatment, prognosis is very poor with only 10% of affected individuals living 5 years after diagnosis.

■ ***PREVENTION.*** In many cases, avoiding the spread of cancer from other organs is not possible. The best prevention is to avoid hepatitis, cirrhosis, and other liver diseases by reducing risks for these diseases.

Gallbladder Diseases

Gallbladder disorders usually cause symptoms related to indigestion when eating fatty foods. Nausea, pain, and excessive gas are the most common symptoms. Nutritional changes and a variety of surgical procedures can be used to treat the disease.

CHOLECYSTITIS

■ ***DESCRIPTION.*** Cholecystitis (KOH-lee-sis-TYE-tis; chole = bile or gall, cyst = bladder, itis = inflammation) is inflammation of the gallbladder.

■ ***ETIOLOGY.*** Cholecystitis is usually caused by obstruction of bile flow due to a gallstone. When bile flow is obstructed, bile in the gallbladder becomes overly concentrated and irritates the lining of the gallbladder, leading to inflammation. When a fatty meal is eaten, fat in the duodenum stimulates the gallbladder to contract and release bile.

■ ***SYMPTOMS.*** This contraction of the inflamed gallbladder causes mild to severe pain in the upper right quadrant of the abdomen. This pain, combined with a history of nausea and vomiting after meals, is indicative of cholecystitis.

■ ***DIAGNOSIS.*** Ultrasound and cholecystogram confirm the diagnosis of cholecystitis. Cholecystogram involves swallowing a dye that is absorbed by the liver and excreted into the bile. Radiographic pictures can confirm the presence of stones.

Complications of cholecystitis include rupture of the gallbladder, leading to peritonitis. Chronic cholecystitis can cause bile to back up into the liver, leading to liver damage and cirrhosis.

■ ***TREATMENT.*** Treatment for cholecystitis is aimed at the cause. Gallstones often obstruct the gallbladder or one of its ducts. Treatment of choice for cholecystitis caused by stones is surgical removal by a procedure called **cholecystectomy** (KOH-lee-sis-TECK-toh-me; chole = bile or gall, cyst = bladder, ectomy = removal).

Cholecystectomy can be performed using an abdominal incision or by using a laparoscope (laparo = abdomen, scope = scope). Removal of the gallbladder using a laparoscope is called laparoscopic cholecystectomy (LAP-ah-row-SKOP-ic KOH-leh-sis-TECK-toh-me). Laparoscopic cholecystectomy is performed by passing a small, thin tubular scope through a small cut made just below the umbilicus (navel), allowing the surgeon to view the gallbladder during surgery. Three other small incisions are made in the abdomen to insert surgical tools. The gallbladder is also removed through one of these incisions. This type of procedure drastically reduces pain, hospital stay, length of recovery, and missed workdays compared to surgery with a larger abdominal incision.

After a cholecystectomy, the bile continues to be excreted by the liver into the common bile duct and simply drips into the duodenum as it is produced. As long as the individual does not take in an excessive amount of fatty foods, the amount of bile will be sufficient to break down the consumed fat, and normal digestion will occur.

■ **PREVENTION.** Preventive measures include maintaining a healthy body weight and eating a diet high in fiber, including vegetables and fruit.

CHOLELITHIASIS

■ **DESCRIPTION.** Cholelithiasis (KOH-lee-lih-THIGH-ah-sis; chole = bile or gall, lith = stone, iasis = condition) is the presence of gallstones in the gallbladder or bile ducts (Figure 12–5). Gallstones affect 1 in 5 women and 1 in 10 men—approximately 20 million people. In the United States, there are approximately one million new cases per year with 600,000 undergoing surgery for removal of the stones (American Liver Foundation, 2007).

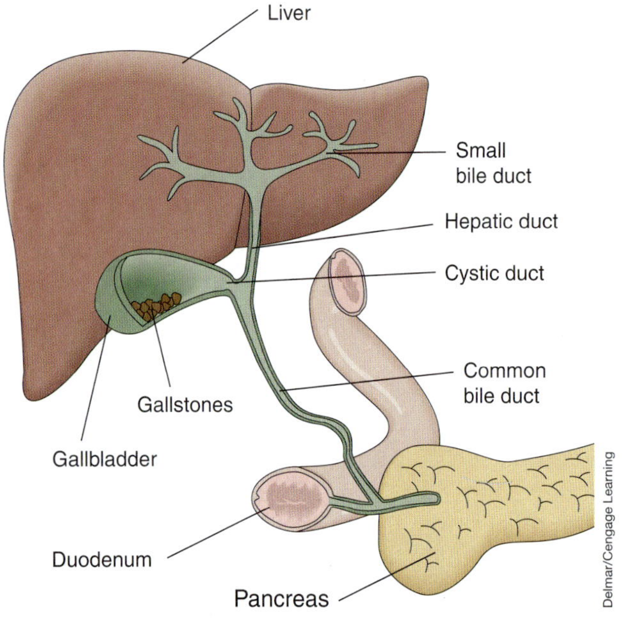

FIGURE 12–5 Cholelithiasis.

■ **ETIOLOGY.** Gallstones form from bile salts and cholesterol and can vary in size, shape, number, color, and composition. Cholesterol stones are by far the most common and are formed when a change in the composition of bile occurs. When bile becomes highly saturated with cholesterol, it crystallizes and forms a stone.

The three most important risk factors for developing gallstones include excessive body weight, increasing age, and being female. In general, individuals developing cholelithiasis have several factors in common, called the five Fs of cholelithiasis: (1) Female (2) Fair complexion (3) Fat or obese (4) Fertile or has had children (5) Forty years of age or older.

■ **SYMPTOMS.** Gallstones are often asymptomatic. If symptoms do occur, they are usually related to blocking the outflow of the gallbladder or of its ducts. Symptoms can include nausea, vomiting, and upper-right quadrant pain following meals containing fat. Complications of cholelithiasis include cholecystitis and jaundice.

■ **DIAGNOSIS.** A cholecystogram and ultrasound, along with a positive history, will confirm the diagnosis.

■ **TREATMENT.** Extracorporeal shockwave lithotripsy (litho = stone, tripsy = destruction) (ESWL) can be performed to break up the stones so they can be passed. If this procedure is not effective or is not recommended, cholecystectomy is performed.

■ **PREVENTION.** Decreasing fat intake in the diet will not aid in disolving stones, but may be helpful in prevention.

Pancreatic Diseases

Diseases of the pancreas are often quite advanced by the time symptoms appear. Some pancreatic disorders are associated with alcoholism. Replacement or supplements of pancreatic enzymes and insulin might be necessary when the pancreas is not functioning properly or is surgically removed.

PANCREATITIS

■ **DESCRIPTION.** Pancreatitis is an inflammation of the pancreas that can range from mild to fatal. With pancreatitis, the pancreas becomes inflamed, edematous, hemorrhagic, and necrotic.

Pancreatitis differs from inflammation of other organs because of the powerful digestive enzymes the pancreas produces. As this organ becomes diseased, these enzymes often escape the pancreatic cells and ducts, causing digestion of the pancreas (**autodigestion**) and the surrounding tissues. If this destruction extends into blood vessels, hemorrhage occurs, leading to severe pain and shock. Acute hemorrhagic pancreatitis usually follows an alcohol-drinking spree and is often fatal in spite of emergency medical attention.

■ ***ETIOLOGY.*** This disease is similar to cirrhosis of the liver in that most cases of severe pancreatitis are due to alcoholism.

Pancreatitis can also be caused by blockage of pancreatic ducts by gallstones. Many cases of pancreatitis are idiopathic (of unknown cause).

■ ***SYMPTOMS.*** An acute attack of pancreatitis causes sudden, severe abdominal pain that often radiates to the back. The individual may find some relief by drawing the knees up toward the abdomen. Other symptoms exhibited during an acute attack are nausea, vomiting, diaphoresis (sweating), and tachycardia.

Individuals with chronic pancreatitis might complain of constant back pain and frequent bouts of mild symptoms similar to those of an acute attack. As the disease progresses, the pancreatic tissue is replaced with fibrous tissue, and function is lost. As endocrine function is lost, the individual exhibits symptoms of diabetes mellitus. Digestive disorders, including malabsorption, occur when exocrine function is impaired.

■ ***DIAGNOSIS.*** Diagnosis of pancreatitis is often made based on the individual's history and is confirmed by blood testing. A high blood **amylase** (pancreatic enzyme) is indicative of pancreatitis.

■ ***TREATMENT.*** Treatment and prognosis of pancreatitis depends on the cause. If it is caused by gallstones, it is treated successfully by removing the gallbladder and the involved stones. Treatment for idiopathic and alcohol-related pancreatitis is palliative because there is no cure. Individuals must stop drinking alcohol and are treated with analgesics and nutritional support. Prognosis for these types of pancreatitis is poor.

■ ***PREVENTION.*** In some cases, pancreatitis might not be preventable. Actions that reduce risk include:

- Limiting alcohol intake. If any symptoms of pancreatitis develop, alcohol should be avoided completely.
- Stopping smoking. Tobacco use increases the risk of pancreatitis.
- Eating a healthy, low-fat diet. Increased consumption of fat increases the risk of gallstones and, thus, increases the risk of pancreatitis.

PANCREATIC CANCER

■ ***DESCRIPTION.*** Pancreatic cancer is usually an adenocarcinoma that occurs in the head of the pancreas. This cancer spreads very rapidly and its poor prognosis makes it a leading cause of cancer death.

■ ***ETIOLOGY.*** The cause of this tumor is unknown, but known carcinogens include cigarette smoking, high coffee consumption, chemical exposure, and consumption of a high-fat diet.

■ ***SYMPTOMS.*** Symptoms usually do not occur until late in the disease process, after metastasis has already occurred. As pancreatic tissue is destroyed, the individual can experience abdominal pain, back pain, nausea, vomiting, loss of appetite, weakness, jaundice, and fatigue.

■ ***DIAGNOSIS.*** Ultrasound and CT and magnetic resonance imaging (MRI) imaging can be helpful in making a diagnosis. A biopsy is the definitive test.

■ ***TREATMENT.*** Treatment can include surgical resection, chemotherapy, and radiation. This tumor usually responds poorly to all therapies, and prognosis is very poor. Supportive care can be provided, including pain management and nutritional support.

■ ***PREVENTION.*** There is no proven prevention. Activities to reduce risk include not smoking, maintaining a healthy weight, eating a healthy diet, and exercising regularly.

RARE DISEASES

Primary Biliary Cirrhosis

Primary biliary cirrhosis is a chronic liver disease that gradually destroys the bile ducts in the liver. The cause is unknown, but it might be related to immune system dysfunction. Destruction of bile ducts decreases bile excretion from the liver and causes a chronic inflammation, resulting in cirrhosis. The disease is much more common in middle-aged females than in males.

Signs and symptoms of the disease include jaundice, edema, itching, and abnormal liver function studies. Treatment is directed at relieving the symptoms. A liver transplant might be necessary.

Gilbert's Syndrome

Gilbert's syndrome is a congenital liver disorder that usually has its onset in the teenage or young adult years and is more common in males. Symptoms include increased serum bilirubin and jaundice, but it is usually left untreated because it does not seem to affect liver function adversely.

Hemochromatosis

Hemochromatosis is a disorder in which the body absorbs and stores excessive amounts of iron. It is the most common inherited disease, affecting approximately one million people in the United States (American Liver Foundation, 2003). Eventually, damage to the liver can occur. It is diagnosed by blood tests for iron levels, and treatment requires blood (about 1 to 2 units) to be removed weekly until iron levels return to normal. This regimen must be continued every 4 months for life to keep the iron levels within normal limits.

EFFECTS OF AGING ON THE SYSTEM

The older adult who develops hepatitis usually undergoes a more severe infection than a younger person does with the same disease. The mortality rate for hepatitis increases with age. Older people can be at an increased risk for developing hepatitis if any of the following factors are present:

- A depressed immune system
- Increased contact with a variety of caregivers
- Poor nutrition
- Increased intake of medications
- Poor hygiene
- Multiple blood transfusions

Cirrhosis in an older person can be of unknown etiology or due to chronic alcohol intake. It is usually progressive and severe, and the prognosis is poor. Bile stones are also seen more frequently in the older adult. Surgery is usually the treatment of choice but might not be an option due to the age of the individual and other complicating disorders. Pancreatic disease is also common in the older adult population, so replacement of pancreatic enzymes might be needed if the pancreas is not producing adequate amounts.

SUMMARY

Diseases of the liver, gallbladder, and pancreas have serious effects on digestion and metabolism. The liver has many functions in the body, so when it is diseased, a variety of other disorders can result. If the liver fails completely, a transplant is necessary. Hepatitis is the most common liver disorder and is usually viral in nature. Cirrhosis of the liver is a chronic, progressive disease most commonly related to alcohol ingestion.

Gallbladder disease, most commonly caused by gallstones, affects thousands of individuals annually. Pancreatic disorders are often not diagnosed until late in the disease process because early symptoms are often not apparent. If the pancreas is not functioning properly, pancreatic enzymes and hormones might need to be supplemented. The older adult is at increased risk for developing disorders of the liver, gallbladder, and pancreas.

REVIEW QUESTIONS

Short Answer

1. What are the functions of the liver, gallbladder, and pancreas?

2. Which signs and symptoms are associated with common liver, gallbladder, and pancreatic disorders?

3. Which diagnostic tests are most commonly used to determine the type and cause of liver, gallbladder, or pancreatic disorders?

Multiple Choice

4. Which of the following is the cause of jaundice?
   - a. Increased levels of amylase in the blood
   - b. Decreased levels of pancreatase in the blood
   - c. Increased levels of bilirubin in the blood
   - d. Decreased levels of lipase in the blood

5. Impaired liver function reveals an elevation in which of the following tests?
   - a. Bilirubin and alkaline phosphatase
   - b. Albumin and bilirubin
   - c. Alkaline phosphatase and amylase
   - d. Amylase and albumin

6. Diseases of the liver, gallbladder, or pancreas generally have an adverse effect on which of the following?
   - a. The immune system
   - b. Digestion and metabolism
   - c. The inflammatory process
   - d. The endocrine system

7. Which of the following types of hepatitis is the most common?
   - a. Hepatitis A
   - b. Hepatitis B
   - c. Hepatitis C
   - d. Hepatitis D

8. Individuals at high risk for developing HBV include which of the following?
   - a. Drug addicts
   - b. Blood recipients
   - c. Health care workers
   - d. All of the above

9. Which of the following is the best definition of cirrhosis?
   - a. A chronic, degenerative disease of the pancreas
   - b. An acute irreversible disease of the liver
   - c. An abnormality of the liver caused by alcoholism
   - d. A chronic, degenerative, irreversible disease of the liver

10. Ascites is an accumulation of fluid in the abdominal cavity, usually due to which of the following conditions?
   a. Pancreatic cancer
   b. Liver failure and portal hypertension
   c. Cholelithiasis
   d. Cirrhosis

True or False

11. T F Gallbladder disorders usually cause symptoms related to indigestion when eating high-fat foods.
12. T F A cholecystogram is a radiographic exam used to diagnose cholecystitis.
13. T F Gallstones are most commonly found in obese, middle-aged men.
14. T F A high serum amylase is usually diagnostic for pancreatitis.
15. T F The older adult who develops hepatitis usually experiences a much milder episode of the disease than does a young person.

CASE STUDIES

- Ms. Fisher is a 68-year-old woman with the classic symptoms of gallbladder disease. She is diagnosed with gallstones and is scheduled for surgery in 2 weeks. She asks you about the cause of gallstones and why she would develop them. How would you respond to her? What typical factors put an individual at risk for developing gallstones?

- Mr. Swicky came to the clinic with complaints of abdominal pain, sweating, fever, and anorexia. His physician sent him to the hospital for an in-depth evaluation. He was diagnosed with viral hepatitis A. Mr. Swicky's wife is very concerned about his condition. What can you tell her about type A hepatitis? Should she be vaccinated for hepatitis A now? Are there other treatments? What precautions should the family practice to prevent transmitting hepatitis? Where can she find more information about hepatitis?

*Study*WARE™ Connection

To help you learn the content in this chapter, take a practice quiz or play an interactive game on your StudyWARE™ CD-ROM.

Workbook Practice

Go to your Workbook and complete the practice questions.

BIBLIOGRAPHY

American Association for the Study of Liver Diseases. (2008). *www.aasld.org* (accessed May 2008).

American Liver Foundation, 2003.

American Liver Foundation. (2006). *www.liverfoundation.org* (accessed May 2008).

American Liver Foundation. (2007). *www.liverfoundation.org* (accessed May 2008).

Centers for Disease Control. (2008). Viral hepatitis. Centers for Disease Control. *www.cdc.gov/Features/ViralHepatitis/* (accessed May 2008).

Connor, S., & Garden, O. (2006). Bile duct injury in the era of laparoscopic cholecystectomy. *British Journal of Surgery 93*(2), 158–168.

Demi, A. (2008). Commentary by Demi. *Western Journal of Nursing Research 30*(2), 228–229.

Guofeng, C., & Ram, M. (2008). RNAi for treating hepatitis B viral infection. *Pharmaceutical Research 25*(1), 72–86.

Hepatitis Foundation International. (2008). ABCs of Hepatitis. Hepatitis Foundation International. *www.hepfi.org/living* (accessed May 2008).

Kohnke, M. (2008). Approach to the genetics of alcoholism: A review based on pathophysiology. *Biochemical Pharmacology 75*(1), 160–177.

Logeswaran, R., & Eswaran, C. (2007). Stone detection in MCRP images using controlled region growing. *Computers in Biology & Medicine 37*(8), 1084–1091.

Mallette, C., Flynn, M., & Promrat, K. (2008). Outcome of screening for hepatitis C virus infection based on risk factors. *American Journal of Gastroenterology 103*(1), 131–137.

National Liver Foundation. (2008). *www.nlfindia.com* (accessed May 2008).

National Program of Cancer Registries. (2008). Centers for Disease Control and Prevention. *www.cdc.gov* (accessed May 2008).

Patel, N., & Derkits, R. (2007). Possible increase in liver enzymes secondary to atorvastin and black cohosh administration. *Journal of Pharmacy Practice 20*(4), 341–346.

Pearce, B., & Grant, I. (2008). Acute liver failure following therapeutic paracentamol administration in patients with muscular dystrophies. *Anaesthesia 63*(1), 89–91.

Peginterferons plus ribavirin comparable for hep C. (January 26, 2008). *Iphfarma Weekly* (1662), 16.

Research & Development. (January 5, 2008). *Inpharma Weekly* (1619), 8–11.

Reid, K., Ramos-De la Medina, A., & Donohue, J. (2007). Diagnosis and surgical management of gallbladder disease: A review. *Journal of Gastrointestinal Surgery 11*(5), 671–681.

Subinfection with hepatitis C after needlestick injury. (2007). *Nursing Standard 21*(23), 16–17.

Tan, A., Yeh, S., Chun-Jen, C., & Chen, P. (2008). Viral hepatocarcinogenesis: From infection to cancer. *Liver International 28*(2), 175–188.

Treatment of gallstone and gallbladder disease. (2007). *Journal of Gastrointestinal Surgery 11*(9), 1222–1224.

Wong, C., & Ng, I. (2008). Molecular pathogenesis of hepatocellular carcinoma. *Liver International 28*(2), 160–174.

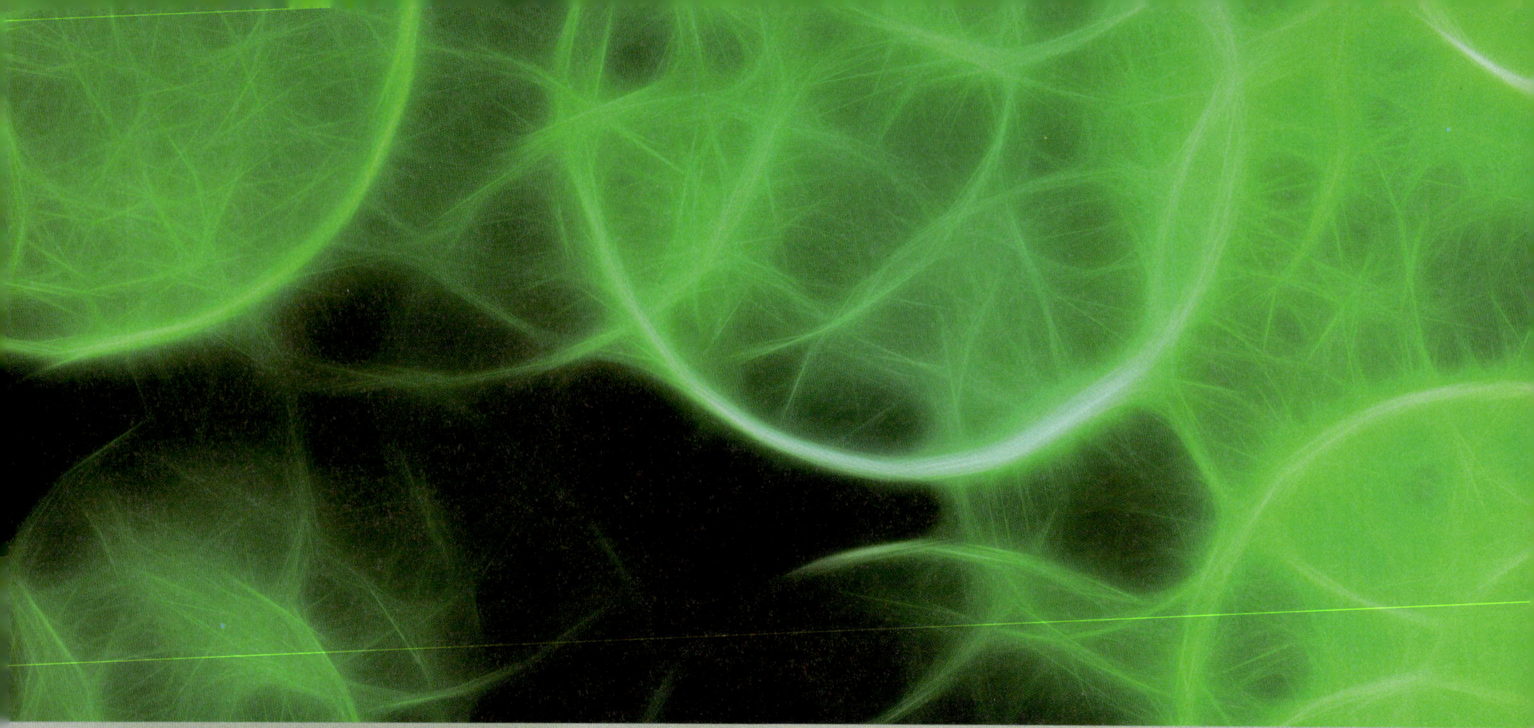

OUTLINE

- Anatomy and Physiology
- Common Signs and Symptoms
- Diagnostic Tests
- Common Diseases of the Urinary System
  - *Urinary Tract Infection (UTI)*
  - *Diseases of the Kidney*
  - *Diseases of the Bladder*
- Trauma
  - *Straddle Injuries*
  - *Neurogenic Bladder*
- Rare Diseases
  - *Goodpasture Syndrome*
  - *Interstitial Cystitis*
- Effects of Aging on the System
- Summary
- Review Questions
- Case Studies
- Bibliography

KEY TERMS

Albuminuria (p. 258)
Anuria (p. 258)
Blood urea nitrogen (BUN) (p. 259)
Catheterization (p. 260)
Clean catch (p. 259)
Creatinine (p. 259)
Creatinine clearance test (p. 259)
Cystogram (p. 259)
Cystoscopy (p. 260)
Dysuria (p. 258)
Frequency (p. 258)
Hematuria (p. 258)
In and out catheterization (p. 260)
Indwelling catheter (p. 260)
Intravenous pyelogram (IVP) (p. 259)
Kidneys-ureter-bladder (KUB) (p. 259)
Lithotripsy (p. 266)
Nephrectomy (p. 270)
Nocturia (p. 258)
Oliguria (p. 258)
Proteinuria (p. 258)
Pyuria (p. 258)
Radical cystectomy (p. 272)
Suprapubic catheter (p. 260)
Transurethral resection (TUR) (p. 272)
Urea (p. 259)
Uremia (p. 259)
Urgency (p. 258)
Urinalysis (p. 259)
Urine culture and sensitivity (C&S) (p. 259)

13

Urinary System Diseases and Disorders

LEARNING OBJECTIVES

Upon completion of the chapter, the learner should be able to:

1. Define the terminology common to the urinary system and the disorders of the system.
2. Discuss the basic anatomy and physiology of the urinary system.
3. Identify the important signs and symptoms associated with common urinary system disorders.
4. Describe the common diagnostics used to determine the type and cause of urinary system disorders.
5. Identify common disorders of the urinary system.
6. Describe the typical course and management of the common urinary system disorders.
7. Describe the effects of aging on the urinary system and the common disorders associated with aging of the system.

OVERVIEW

The urinary system maintains homeostasis in the body by excreting and reabsorbing important electrolytes, compounds, and water. It also excretes wastes from the body in the form of urine. Disturbances in other systems such as the circulatory or nervous systems can adversely affect the functioning of the urinary system. Urinary disorders range from mild infections to very serious diseases such as cancer of the bladder or kidneys. ■

ANATOMY AND PHYSIOLOGY

The urinary system includes the kidneys, ureters, bladder, and urethra (Figure 13–1). The kidneys are located behind the intestines at the mid-back level; each is about the size of a man's fist and weighs about 150 grams. The kidneys are responsible for removing waste products from the bloodstream. Every minute, about one fourth of the blood circulating in the body passes through the kidneys, where toxic wastes and unused nutrients are filtered and pass out of the body as urine. The kidneys also regulate fluid, electrolyte, and acid–base balances, assist in the metabolism of calcium, and help regulate blood pressure. The kidneys are composed of nephrons that act as filters, selectively filtering, excreting, or reabsorbing what is needed by the body to maintain homeostasis. They monitor the amount of salts and other chemicals needed for proper body functioning. The kidneys also produce an active form of vitamin D necessary for strong bones.

The ureters are tubules that run from the kidney to the bladder (see Figure 13–1) and transport the urine from the renal pelvis to the bladder, where it is stored until emptied, usually voluntarily by the individual. The bladder, the muscular organ that holds urine, can usually store about 350–500 ml. This amount varies from individual to individual and is affected by many other factors, especially bladder tone, neurologic disease, and urologic disorders. Micturition is the process of voiding, or emptying, the bladder. This usually occurs in response to stimuli to the pelvic nerves.

The urethra is a hollow tube, significantly longer in males than in females, running from the bladder to the external opening (the meatus) for excretion (see Figure 13–1). The urethra serves as the passageway for urine in the female and for both urine and semen ejaculation in the male.

Urine is normally clear, slightly yellow to gold in color, and free of sediments. Some drugs can change the color of urine. Urine has its own distinct odor but is not foul-smelling unless disease is present. Some foods, however, will change the odor of urine as their by-products are excreted, such as asparagus. Urine has a normal specific gravity of 1.005–1.030 and a pH of about 6. Changes in these values can indicate disease.

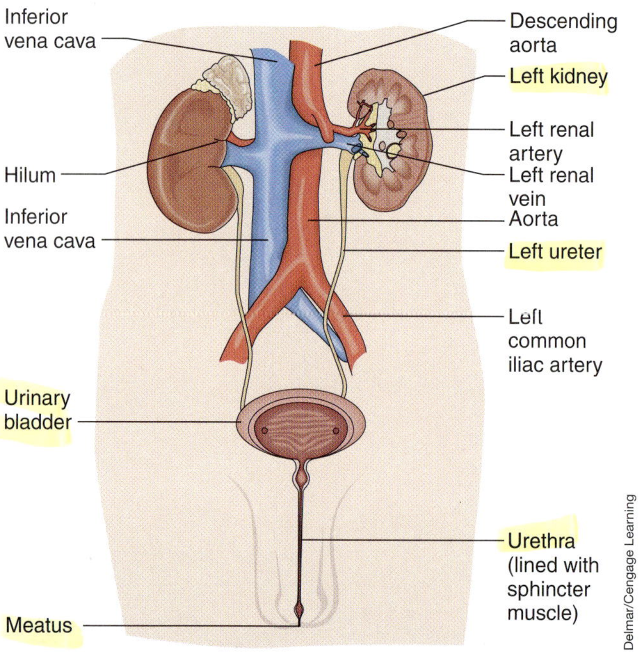

FIGURE 13–1 The urinary system.

StudyWARE™ Connection

View an animation on the formation of urine on your StudyWARE™ CD-ROM.

COMMON SIGNS AND SYMPTOMS

Common signs and symptoms of urinary tract diseases include any abnormality in urine or in the ability to urinate. Some of these include:

- **Hematuria** (hem-ah-TOO-ree-ah; hema = blood, uria = urine), blood in the urine.
- **Pyuria** (pye-YOU-ree-ah; py = pus, uria = urine), pus in the urine.
- **Proteinuria**, protein in the urine. A specific protein, albumin, can be identified, revealing **albuminuria**.
- **Dysuria** (dis-YOU-ree-ah; dys = difficult or painful, uria = urine), difficulty or pain with urination.
- **Nocturia** (nock-TOO-ree-ah; noc = night, uria = urine), increased voiding at night.
- **Oliguria** (OL-ih-GOO-ree-ah; olig = scanty or few, uria = urine), a decrease in urine output.
- **Anuria** (ah-NEW-ree-ah; an = without, uria = urine), no urine output.
- **Frequency**, urinating frequently.
- **Urgency**, the need to urinate immediately.

Varying degrees of pain in the low back or flank area also can indicate urinary disease; other symptoms include nausea, vomiting, malaise, and fatigue. Urinary system diseases also can affect the cardiovascular and respiratory systems, leading to hypertension, edema, and shortness of breath.

DIAGNOSTIC TESTS

A **urinalysis** (YOU-rih-NAL-ih-sis; urine analysis) is the most common test performed to diagnose urinary system diseases. This test is important because the results can confirm the presence of various urinary tract disorders. It tests a urine sample for pH; specific gravity; and presence of protein, glucose, sugar, and blood. Such a test also includes a microscopic examination to determine the presence of bacteria, crystals, and casts (tube-shaped particles made up of red cells, white cells, and kidney cells). The specific test, normal findings, abnormal findings, and pathologies are summarized in Table 13–1.

A **urine culture and sensitivity (C&S)** test can be performed in the laboratory if the urinalysis shows an abnormal number of white cells or bacteria in the urine. If the bacteria count is greater than 100,000 bacteria per ml or cc of urine, a diagnosis of urinary tract infection is confirmed. A smaller number can indicate a contaminated specimen or the presence of a mild infection. A culture helps determine the type of bacteria present and a sensitivity test will help determine the most effective antibiotic to prescribe for treatment.

A urine specimen collected for a culture can be obtained by the **clean catch** method or by sterile technique. The clean catch method involves cleaning the urethral meatus, voiding a moderate amount of urine to flush out the urethra, and then catching a urine specimen in a sterile container. Catching the specimen after urinating as described above is considered a mid-stream catch and is part of the proper technique of obtaining a clean catch specimen. A sterile technique involves placing a sterile urinary catheter into the bladder to obtain a sterile urine specimen.

Blood tests can be performed to determine whether waste products are being filtered out adequately by the glomerulus, thus checking kidney function. The two most common nitrogenous waste products normally filtered from the blood are **urea** and **creatinine**. A **blood urea nitrogen (BUN)** test will determine the levels of urea nitrogen or waste product in the blood. A **creatinine clearance** test is a blood test to determine the ability of the renal glomeruli to filter creatinine out of the blood after creatinine is ingested by the subject. High levels of waste products in the blood is called **uremia** (you-REE-me-ah; ur = urine, emia = blood), a toxic condition of the blood.

Radiologic examination of the urinary system includes **kidneys-ureter-bladder (KUB)**, **intravenous pyelogram (IVP)**, and **cystogram**. A KUB is a common X-ray of the structures of the urinary tract to determine abnormalities. An IVP is an X-ray taken after injecting dye into the individual's bloodstream. The dye accumulates in the urinary tract, improving the ability to visualize and identify obstructions, tumors, and deformities. A cystogram

TABLE 13–1 Urinalysis Values

Urinalysis	Normal Values	Abnormal Results
Color	Clear amber	Very light or very dark; cloudy
Odor	Pleasantly aromatic	Offensive, unpleasant
Albumin (protein)	Negative	Albuminuria
Acetone	Negative	Ketonuria
Red blood cells	2–3/HPF	Hematuria
White blood cells	4–5/HPF	White, cloudy urine
Bilirubin	Negative	Bilirubinuria
Glucose	Negative	Glycosuria
Specific gravity	1.005–1.030	Higher or lower than normal
Bacteria	Negative	Present
Casts	Rare	Present, several to many
pH	4.6–8.0	Higher or lower than normal

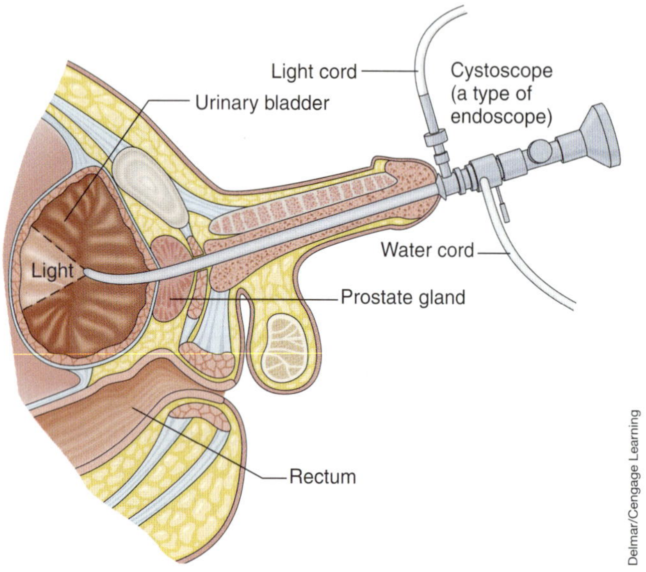

FIGURE 13–2 Cystoscopy

(cysto = bladder, gram = picture) is an X-ray taken of the bladder after a radiopaque dye is instilled into the bladder by using a urinary catheter; the procedure is called a cystography (cysto = bladder, ography = procedure to graph or take a picture). A cystogram helps determine shape and function of the bladder.

Cystoscopy (sis-TOS-koh-pee; cysto = bladder, scopy = procedure to look) is an invasive procedure to look into the urethra and bladder by using a lighted scope (Figure 13–2). Stones, tumors, and areas of infection and inflammation can be viewed with a cystoscope. Additional instruments might be used to allow the physician to obtain a tissue biopsy or to crush bladder stones.

Biopsies of the kidney and bladder are often performed to determine the presence of disease. Bladder biopsies are often obtained by using a cystoscope as previously mentioned; renal biopsies are often obtained by using X-ray technique to guide a fine needle through the flank area to remove a core of renal tissue.

Catheterization of the urinary bladder is a sterile procedure. Sterile technique must be maintained to prevent urinary tract infections. A soft catheter is passed through the urethra and into the bladder to instill fluids or medication into the bladder or to remove urine. Urinary catheterization to remove urine can be performed to relieve urinary retention, empty the bladder prior to a procedure, obtain a sterile urine specimen for testing, or as a treatment for incontinence.

If the catheter is removed as soon as the urine is drained, the catheterization is temporary and is called an **in and out catheterization**. If the catheter is placed for a longer period of time, as commonly occurs for urinary incontinence, a balloon on the end of the catheter is inflated after placement to hold the catheter in the bladder, and the catheterization is called an **indwelling catheter**. If the catheter is inserted surgically through the pelvic wall, as is often done after urinary tract surgeries, it is called a **suprapubic catheter** (Figure 13–3).

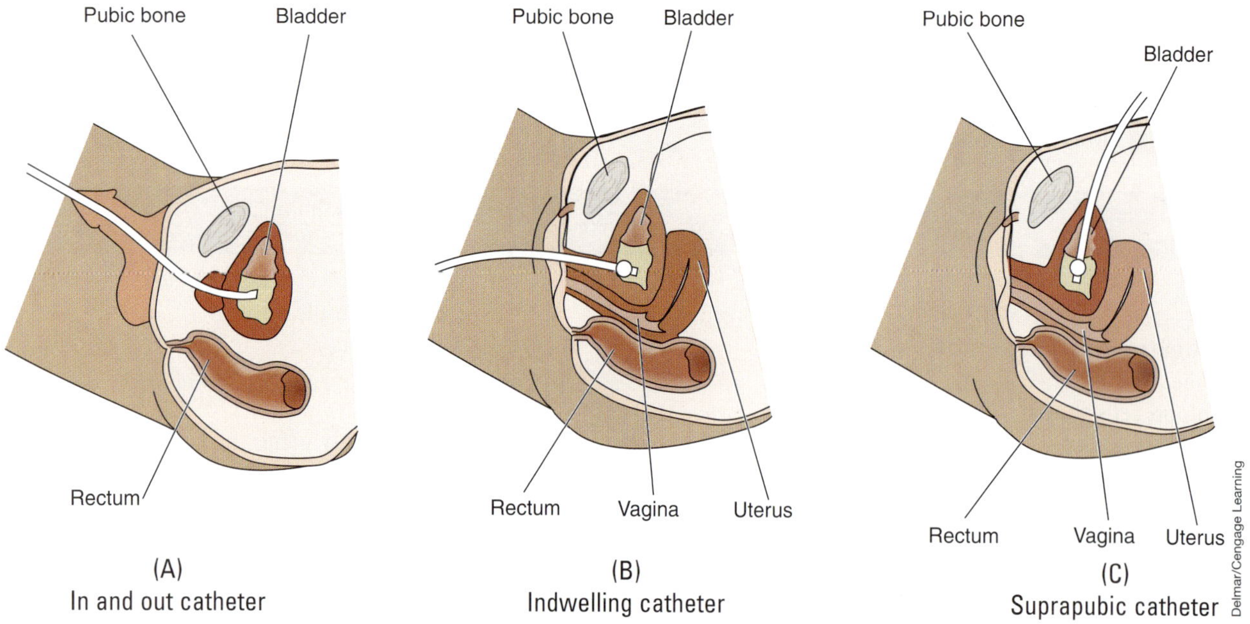

FIGURE 13–3 Types of urinary catheters.

COMMON DISEASES OF THE URINARY SYSTEM

Diseases of the urinary system can affect either gender at any age. Urinary tract infections are the most common disorders of the system. Many of the diseases of the urinary system, such as dysuria, oliguria, and frequency of urination, have similar symptoms in their early stages of development.

Urinary Tract Infection (UTI)

DESCRIPTION. UTI is a broad diagnosis covering any infection of the urinary tract, including the urethra, bladder, and kidneys (Figure 13–4a).

ETIOLOGY. UTIs can be caused by a virus or fungus, but by far, the most common infection is due to bacteria.

Bacteria can reach the urinary tract through the blood (hematogenous infection) or by entering the tract through the urethra (ascending infection). Hematogenous infection is less common and is usually the result of septicemia. In this case, the urinary tract is a site of secondary infection. Primary infection might begin in the respiratory or gastrointestinal tract and be carried to the urinary tract through the blood.

The most common route for infection of the urinary tract is the ascending route by which bacteria enter the urethra and climb, or ascend, upward toward the kidneys, infecting the various organs as they progress.

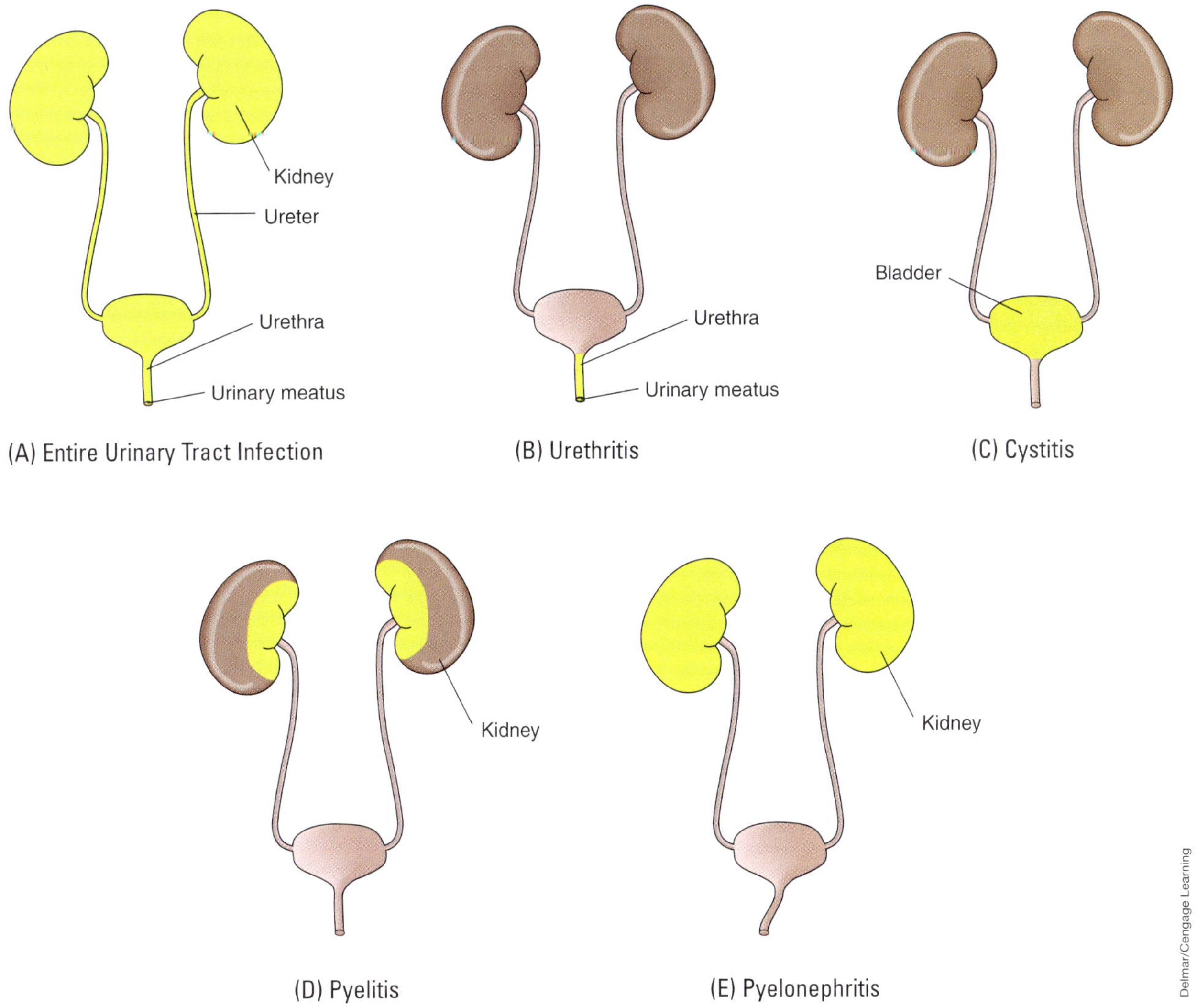

FIGURE 13–4 Yellow areas indicate sites of urinary tract infections.

Approximately 80% of the time, the bacteria causing ascending infection are *Escherichia coli* (*E. coli*). This bacterium is a normal flora of the intestine and is commonly found in large numbers around the anal and perineal area. Sexual intercourse, bladder catheterization, and surgical procedures increase the risk of ascending infection.

UTIs in males are quite rare and are usually related to obstruction of the tract by an enlarged prostate or a sexually transmitted disease. Ascending UTIs are far more common in females than in males for the following reasons:

- Anatomically, the female urethra is shorter than the male urethra, allowing bacteria to ascend more easily.
- Anatomically, the female urethral opening is closer to the rectal area than that of the male, allowing migration of bacteria from the rectal area to the urethra.
- Improper female toileting habits or wiping improperly from the back (rectal area) toward the front (vulva area) pulls rectal bacteria toward and into the urethral opening.
- Vaginal secretions can harbor bacteria and contaminate the urethral area.
- Sexual intercourse can cause trauma to the urethra and bladder, leading to inflammation and potential infection.
- Pregnant females are more susceptible to infection due to the pressure of the heavy uterus on the urinary tract and because pregnancy hormones tend to relax the organs of the urinary tract, allowing easier entry by bacteria.
- Male prostatic secretions have an antibacterial effect, reducing the risk of UTI.

SYMPTOMS. Signs and symptoms of UTI can include dysuria, flank pain, urinary frequency and urgency, hematuria, and low back pain.

DIAGNOSIS. UTIs are commonly diagnosed by urinalysis and culture of a urine specimen. Bacterial counts of 100,000 bacteria or greater per milliliter of urine confirms UTI.

TREATMENT. Antibiotic treatment is usually effective. A bacterial sensitivity test helps in the selection of the most effective antibiotic for treatment.

PREVENTION. There are several natural preventive measures against UTIs. The act of urination actually washes most bacteria out of the urethra. A low pH (acidity) and the presence of urea in the bladder have a bactericidal effect. Also, the ureters close off

HEALTHY HIGHLIGHT

Preventing Urinary Tract Infections

Females who suffer frequent UTIs might find the following measures helpful to prevent them.

- Drink six to eight glasses of water a day.
- Drink cranberry juice to lower the pH or acidify the urine.
- Follow correct female toileting habits—wiping front to back.
- Avoid tight-fitting jeans and body suits.
- Wear underwear and pantyhose with absorbent cotton perineal panels.
- Avoid perfumed soaps, bubble baths, douches, and feminine deodorants.
- Cleanse the genital area before and after sexual intercourse.
- Urinate before and after sexual intercourse.
- Use a water-soluble lubricant if needed during sexual intercourse.
- Remove a contraceptive diaphragm or sponge as soon as possible.

As previously discussed, UTI includes infection of any of the organs of the urinary tract. Types of urinary tract infection include urethritis, cystitis, pyelitis, and pyelonephritis. A brief discussion of each follows.

during urination to prevent urine from refluxing up the ureter to the kidney. Other preventive measures are discussed in the following Healthy Highlight.

URETHRITIS

Urethritis (YOU-reh-THRIGH-tis; urethri = urethra, itis = inflammation) is more common in males than in females as a symptom of gonorrhea (Figure 13–4b). In females, urethritis can also be the result of irritation from tight clothing, application of soaps or powders to the genital area, or sexual intercourse. Urethritis commonly occurs in conjunction with cystitis. In males and females, it can be a symptom of herpes genitalis or chlamydia. Symptoms of urethritis can include swelling of the urethra, dysuria, and a urethral discharge.

CYSTITIS

Cystitis (sis-TYE-tis; cyst = bladder, itis = inflammation) is commonly called a bladder infection (Figure 13–4c). Cystitis, occurring in females as they become sexually active, is called honeymoon cystitis. Antibiotic treatment is usually effective. Antispasmodic medications, such as Pyridium, might be prescribed in addition to antibiotics to decrease the discomfort of bladder spasms. Individuals taking Pyridium should be warned that this medication normally stains the urine a reddish orange, which will permanently stain clothing. After treatment is completed, a follow-up urinalysis and culture is important to ensure complete elimination of all bacteria because recurrent infections are common.

PYELITIS

Pyelitis (PYE-eh-LYE-tis; pyelo = pelvis of kidney, itis = inflammation) is a fairly common disease among young female children (Figure 13–4d). It is usually the result of an ascending infection from the bladder (cystitis) but also can be spread by blood (hematogenous infection). Rapid diagnosis and treatment must be initiated to prevent the spread of infection to adjacent tissue, which can cause pyelonephritis.

PYELONEPHRITIS

Pyelonephritis (PYE-eh-loh-neh-FRY-tis; pyelo = pelvis of kidney, nephr = kidney, itis = inflammation) can be due to an ascending or a hematogenous infection and can affect one or both kidneys (Figure 13–4e). Obstruction or urine flow blockage in the urinary tract caused by pregnancy, prostate enlargement, stones, or tumors increases the risk of pyelonephritis. Commonly, abscesses form in the kidney and rupture, filling the kidney pelvis with pus and leading to pyuria (pyo = pus, uria = urine). Other symptoms include a sudden onset of fever and chills with flank pain and hematuria. Pyelonephritis is usually treated effectively with antibiotics, but repeated bouts of acute pyelonephritis or chronic pyelonephritis leads to scarring of the kidney. Chronic pyelonephritis can eventually lead to uremia and kidney failure.

Diseases of the Kidney

Diseases of the kidney affect the filtering system of the body. This, in turn, affects the homeostatic balance of fluids and electrolytes and, if left untreated, kidney diseases can affect all other body systems and interrupt their functioning. Therefore, symptoms of kidney disease can first appear in an affected system rather than in the urinary system. An example of this is an elevated blood pressure caused by inappropriate reabsorption of sodium and water.

GLOMERULONEPHRITIS (ACUTE)

■ **DESCRIPTION.** Acute glomerulonephritis is an inflammation of the glomerulus, or filtering unit, of the kidney. It is the most common disease of the kidney.

■ **ETIOLOGY.** This disease usually affects children and young adults within 1 to 4 weeks following a strep throat infection. Other streptococcus infections such as scarlet fever and rheumatic fever also can cause this problem. Glomerulonephritis with this etiology also may be called acute poststreptococcal glomerulonephritis. In addition to streptococcus bacterial infections, virus, other bacteria, and parasites can lead to this disease.

Glomerulonephritis is nonsuppurative, or in other words, it is not associated with bacterial infection and pus formation. Inflammation in this case is the result of tissue destruction caused by the individual's immune system. Glomerulonephritis is a type of allergic or immune disease caused by an antigen–antibody reaction. The causative agent (bacteria, virus, or parasites) produces antigen that stimulates the individual's immune system to produce antibodies. These antibodies stick to the antigen, thus producing large antigen–antibody complexes that circulate in the bloodstream until they become trapped in the tiny capillaries of the glomerulus, thus blocking the glomerulus. This leads to increased pressure, irritation, and the inflammatory response.

The outpouring of neutrophils and serum as part of the inflammatory response increases pressure and decreases blood flow to the glomerulus. Ultimately, the glomerulus weakens and becomes permeable, allowing red blood cells and blood plasma proteins to leak into Bowman's capsule and appear in the urine.

■ ***SYMPTOMS.*** Signs and symptoms of glomerulonephritis are flank pain, fever, loss of appetite, and malaise (general ill feeling). The eyes and ankles might appear edematous (swollen). Oliguria and hematuria are frequent signs of glomerulonephritis. A urinalysis can show albuminuria (albumin = a blood protein, uria = urine) and casts (proteins that mold to the shape of the kidney tubules).

■ ***DIAGNOSIS.*** A routine urinalysis can show red blood cells, indicating possible damage to the glomeruli; white blood cells, indicative of infection; and increased protein, which might indicate nephron damage. Blood tests revealing increased levels of creatinine or urea are also positive indicators of the condition. An X-ray, ultrasound, and computerized tomography (CT) of the kidney can also be completed. A biopsy confirms the diagnosis.

■ ***TREATMENT.*** Treatment is usually supportive. Antipyretic (anti = against, pyretic = fever) and diuretic (to increase urine output) medications can be prescribed. Dietary management might include restrictions of salt, protein foods, and fluids. If a secondary bacterial infection occurs, antibiotics can be prescribed.

■ ***PREVENTION.*** Prevention is aimed at proper antibiotic treatment for streptococcal infections. Proper treatment of strep throat in children and young adults decreases the number of antigen–antibody complexes, thus reducing the risk of developing glomerulonephritis.

Prognosis for glomerulonephritis is generally good. Children usually recover at a slightly better rate than adults. Those who do not recover may progress into chronic glomerulonephritis.

GLOMERULONEPHRITIS (CHRONIC)

■ ***DESCRIPTION.*** Chronic glomerulonephritis occurs when there is a slow, progressive destruction of the kidney's glomeruli. This chronic condition is among the leading causes of chronic kidney failure and end-stage kidney disease and often leads to chronic hypertension.

■ ***ETIOLOGY.*** Repeated bouts of acute glomerulonephritis can lead to a chronic condition that might extend over several years with periods of remission and exacerbation. During this time, a number of the glomeruli are destroyed, leading to an inability of the kidney to produce urine. This decrease in urine output leads to edema, an increase in fluid volume in the blood, retention of salt, and, ultimately, hypertension.

Approximately 25% of people with this condition have no prior history of kidney disease. In most of these cases, the cause of the condition is unknown, but it is thought to be related to an unidentified abnormality of the immune system.

■ ***SYMPTOMS.*** Symptoms of chronic glomerulonephritis include those mentioned in the acute disease plus hypertension. Uremia (you-REE-me-ah; ur = urine, emia = blood or urine waste in the blood) and kidney failure can occur during late stages of the disease.

■ ***DIAGNOSIS.*** Diagnosis is based on testing and symptoms. An abnormal urinalysis, complete blood count (CBC), BUN, and creatinine along with symptoms of anemia and uremia may be indicative of the disease. A CT scan and kidney ultrasound might also be completed; biopsy confirms the diagnosis.

■ ***TREATMENT.*** The primary treatment goal is control of symptoms. High blood pressure can be difficult to control and is often the most important aspect of treatment. Various medications can be tried to control high blood pressure. Dietary restrictions of salt, protein, and fluids might be recommended to help control hypertension and prevent kidney failure. Steroids and immunosuppressive medications can treat some forms of glomerulonephritis. End-stage disease might require hemodialysis or kidney transplant to control symptoms and sustain life.

■ ***PREVENTION.*** There is no specific prevention for most cases of chronic glomerulonephritis, but prompt treatment of the acute form might be beneficial.

HYDRONEPHROSIS

■ ***DESCRIPTION.*** Hydronephrosis (HIGH-droh-neh-FROH-sis; hydro = water, nephro = kidney, osis = condition of) is a collection of urine in the renal pelvis, due to some type of obstruction. This accumulation of urine leads to dilation and distention of the kidney pelvis.

■ ***ETIOLOGY.*** Causes of obstruction include congenital defects in urinary tract structure, kidney stones, tumors, enlarged prostate, and urinary tract infections. If the obstruction is unrelieved, permanent damage can occur, and the kidney pelvis will become nonfunctioning.

■ ***SYMPTOMS.*** Symptoms of hydronephrosis depend on whether the obstruction is acute or chronic. One or both kidneys can be affected, depending on the position of the obstruction (Figure 13–5). If one kidney is affected, the disease can go undetected because the other kidney continues to function adequately. A symptom that occurs regardless of where the obstruction lies is loin or flank pain. An enlarged kidney might be palpable on physical examination. If both kidneys are involved, anuria and uremia can develop.

■ ***DIAGNOSIS.*** Blood tests can show elevated creatinine and electrolyte imbalance. Diagnosis is confirmed by pyelogram.

■ ***TREATMENT.*** Treatment involves immediate draining of the kidney pelvis by surgical intervention and immediate relief of the obstruction.

■ ***PREVENTION.*** The causes of hydronephrosis usually cannot be prevented. Prompt treatment of conditions that cause it, such as kidney failure, reduces the risk of complications.

RENAL CALCULI

■ ***DESCRIPTION.*** Renal calculi are commonly called kidney stones. These stones are often composed of calcium salts and other substances. Size, location, and number of stones can vary (Figure 13–6). Urinary stones are more common in males than in females and commonly occur between ages 30 and 50.

■ ***ETIOLOGY.*** Cause of stone formation is unknown in most cases, but some precipitating factors include dehydration, chronic urinary tract infection, and immobility or prolonged bed rest, leading to release of calcium from the bones. Less commonly, stones are the result of metabolic disorders such as hyperparathyroidism, severe bone disease, and gout.

Staghorn calculi are one of the more common types of stones. These form in the pelvis of the kidney and can become so large that they fill the entire kidney pelvis. Calculi commonly form in the kidney, but they also can form in the urinary bladder. Bladder stones cause difficulty with emptying the bladder, often leading to frequent or chronic bladder

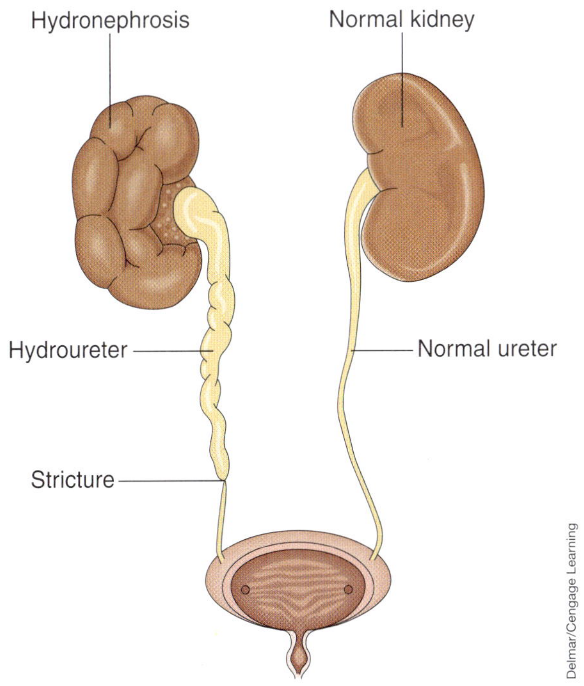

FIGURE 13–5 Hydronephrosis.

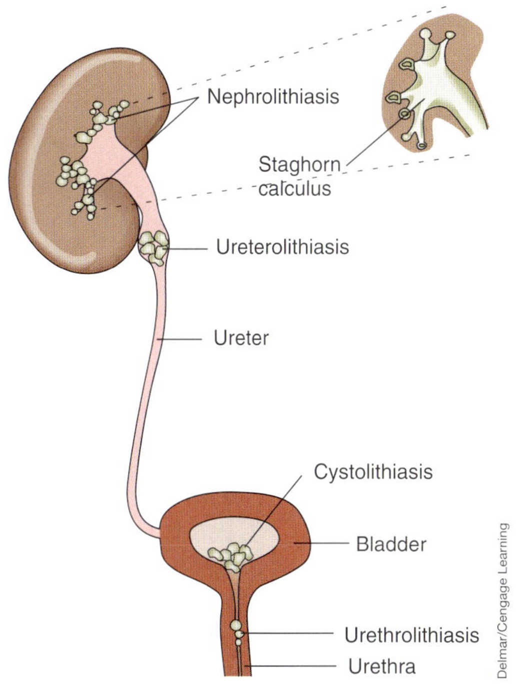

FIGURE 13–6 Types and location of renal calculi.

infections. Individuals can frequently form small kidney stones that easily pass through the urinary tract unnoticed, and stones can be present in the kidney yet cause no problems. It is only when stones become caught in the ureters or obstruct the urinary tract that problems and symptoms arise.

■ ***SYMPTOMS.*** Typical symptoms of kidney stones are hematuria and renal or urinary colic. Urinary colic is an extreme, spasmodic flank pain caused by the contraction of an obstructed ureter. This pain is often described as "the worst pain I've had in my entire life."

■ ***DIAGNOSIS.*** Diagnosis is commonly confirmed by using an IVP. A KUB and renal ultrasound also can be beneficial for diagnosis.

■ ***TREATMENT.*** Treatment during an acute attack of kidney stones includes administering pain medication and increasing fluid intake with the hope the stone will pass in the urine. Urine is often strained through a filtering device in an effort to catch the stone for identification. Even though stones feel like they should be quite large to the individual passing them, the ones that are voided and filtered are usually quite small, ranging in size from a grain of salt to a small piece of rice.

If the urinary tract is totally obstructed, emergency surgery must be performed to prevent hydronephrosis and kidney damage. Surgery called a stone basket procedure can be performed in which a retrieval instrument is passed through the urethra, bladder, and ureter to remove the stone. Another method is to break the stones into pieces for retrieval or in hopes that the pieces can be passed. This breaking of the stone is called **lithotripsy** (litho = stone, tripsy = breaking). During lithotripsy, the affected individual is placed in a tub of water and external shock waves are emitted into the water, shattering the hard stones (Figure 13–7).

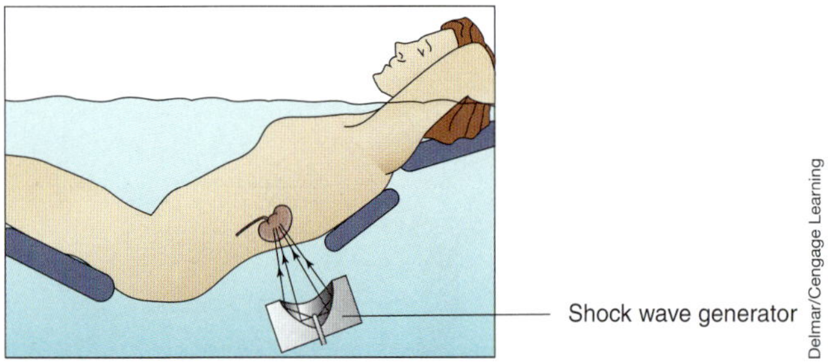

FIGURE 13–7 Lithotripsy.

■ ***PREVENTION.*** Prevention of further stone development can include medications, correcting any causative metabolic conditions, and increasing water intake.

POLYCYSTIC DISEASE

■ ***DESCRIPTION.*** Polycystic kidney disease (PKD) causes massive enlargement of both kidneys due to development of multiple grape-like cysts (Figure 13–8). These cysts can cause the kidneys to increase to a weight of 20 or 30 pounds. Polycystic disease is a slow, progressive disease that affects teenagers and young adults, usually leading to renal failure by age 30 or 40. There is no cure for the disease.

■ ***ETIOLOGY.*** PKD is an inherited disorder. Most commonly, it is autosomal-dominant, meaning if one parent has the disease, there is a 50% chance that the disease gene will pass to a child.

■ ***SYMPTOMS.*** As the disease progresses, kidney tissue is destroyed and function becomes increasingly impaired. Hypertension generally develops as the kidneys fail. Symptoms include lumbar pain, hematuria, and recurrent UTIs.

■ ***DIAGNOSIS.*** Diagnosis includes a family and clinical history. CT scan, especially when combined with dye infusion, is one of the most sensitive tests available and confirms the diagnosis.

■ ***TREATMENT.*** Treatment involves management of hypertension and UTIs. Dialysis and kidney transplant are often needed for end-stage treatment.

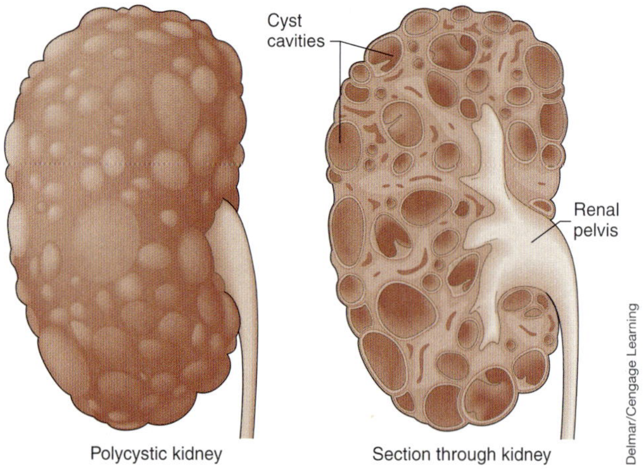

FIGURE 13–8 Polycystic kidney.

■ ***PREVENTION.*** PKD is an inherited disease and is not preventable.

RENAL FAILURE

■ ***DESCRIPTION.*** Renal failure is the failure of the kidneys to cleanse the blood of waste products. The primary method of cleansing the body of waste involves the formation of urea in the liver, which the kidneys filter out of the blood and excrete in urine. When the kidneys fail, the urea remains in the blood. A high urea level in the blood is called uremia, meaning, literally, urine in the blood. Urea is eventually converted to ammonia, leading to toxicity and related symptoms in all systems of the body (Figure 13–9).

■ ***ETIOLOGY.*** Acute renal failure is usually related to decreased blood flow to the kidneys due to conditions such as hemorrhagic or surgical shock, embolism, congestive heart failure, and dehydration. Blockage of urine flow, caused by tumors, stones, or enlarged prostate, also can lead to acute failure. Reversal of acute renal failure, which involves treating the cause of the failure, is usually quite successful. Dialysis might be needed temporarily to remove toxic wastes from the individual's blood until kidney function is restored. Individuals in acute renal failure are placed on a limited diet to allow the kidneys to rest and regenerate function.

Chronic renal failure occurs slowly and is usually the result of chronic kidney disease such as glomerulonephritis, pyelonephritis, renal hypertension, and PKD. Long-term substance abuse, alcoholism, and diabetes also can cause chronic renal failure.

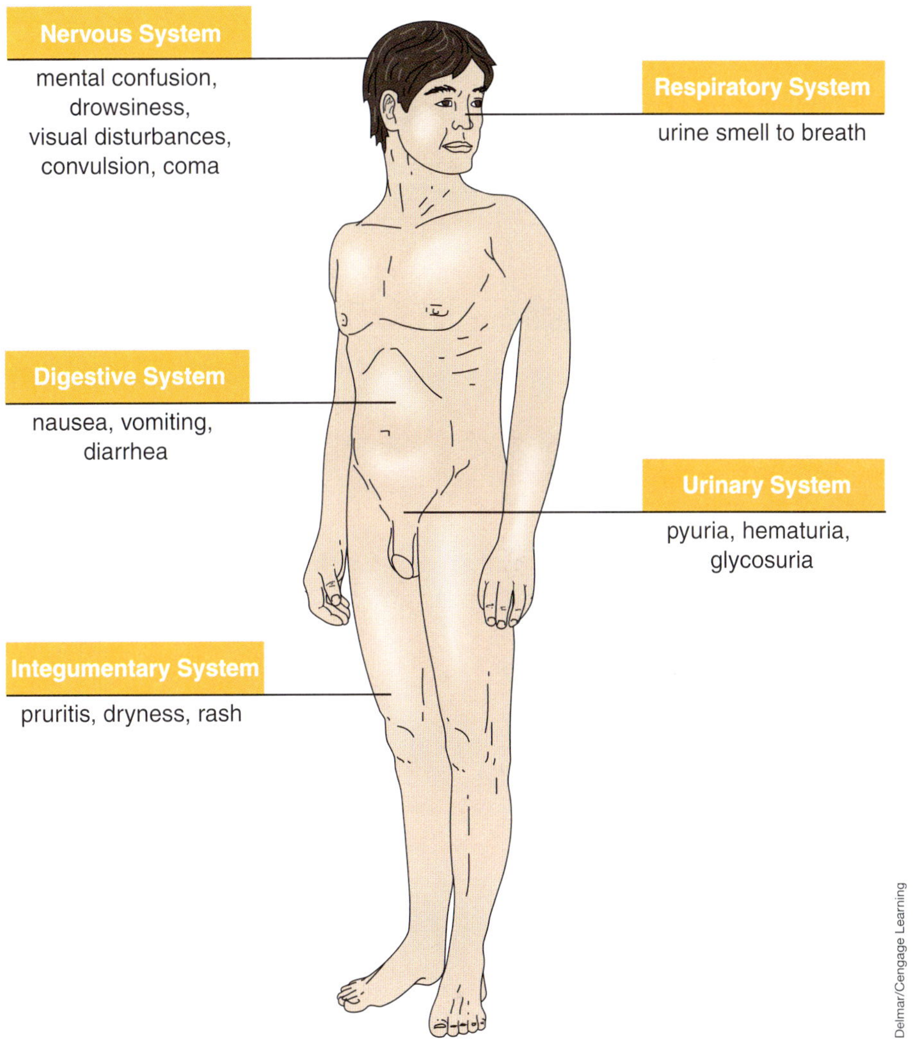

FIGURE 13–9 Areas of the body affected by toxic levels of circulating ammonia.

■ ***SYMPTOMS.*** Symptoms of renal failure are not significant until approximately 75% of kidney function has been destroyed. Symptoms can include those of acute failure and problems of infertility; impotence; and bone weakness, leading to pain and fractures.

■ ***DIAGNOSIS.*** History and physical exam along with blood testing assist in diagnosis. Elevated blood creatinine levels along with an elevated BUN are indicative of kidney failure.

■ ***TREATMENT.*** Treatment includes management of the related cause of the failure, limiting protein and sodium in the diet, and monitoring fluid intake and urine output. Medications can include antihypertensives, diuretics, and antibiotics as needed. Dialysis and kidney transplantation might be options for long-term treatment.

Dialysis is a procedure that cleanses the blood of waste products when the kidneys have failed or are failing to perform this function. There are two types of dialysis; both require the same components: the patient's blood, a semipermeable membrane, and a washing or dialyzing solution. In both types of dialysis, the waste products in the individual's blood pass through the semipermeable membrane by diffusion to enter the dialyzing solution, thus cleansing the blood.

The most common type of dialysis is hemodialysis (Figure 13–10). During hemodialysis, the individual's blood is routed out of an artery (usually the brachial or radial artery) and through an artificial kidney machine, or hemodialyzer, which mechanically cleans the blood. This machine is filled with a semipermeable, cellophane-like material and dialyzing solution. As blood passes through the machine, the waste products diffuse through the membrane into the dialyzing solution to cleanse the blood. The clean blood reenters the patient through a venous access.

One common problem with hemodialysis is maintaining vascular access. Usually, an arteriovenous (AV) shunt is created by placing catheters in the needed artery and vein (Figure 13–11), which are then connected (shunted) with silicone rubber tubing. Complications of AV shunts include infection and clotting.

The other type of dialysis is peritoneal dialysis. This procedure involves performing a paracentesis to instill dialyzing solution into the peritoneal cavity. This type of dialysis uses the membrane that lines the peritoneal cavity to act as the semipermeable membrane. The dialyzing solution is allowed to stay in the abdomen for varying amounts of time (dwell time), during which waste products diffuse out of the peritoneal capillaries and into the dialyzing solution. Solution is then drained and disposed of. Peritoneal

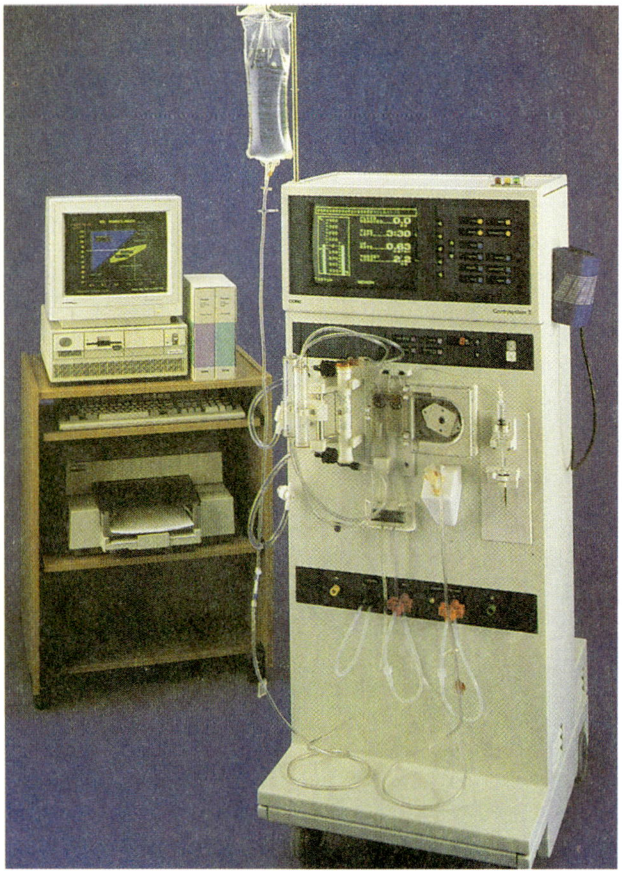

Delmar/Cengage Learning

FIGURE 13–10 Hemodialysis unit.

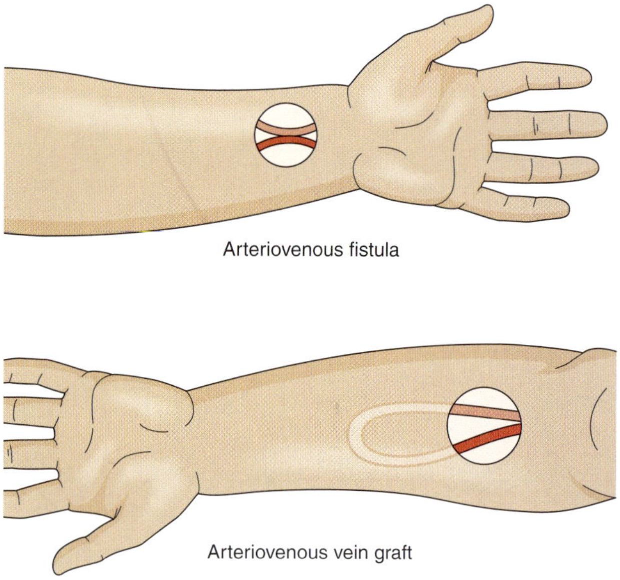

Delmar/Cengage Learning

FIGURE 13–11 Hemodialysis sites: AV Shunts.

dialysis can be performed by several methods such as the following:

- **Continuous ambulatory peritoneal dialysis (CAPD)** is a self-dialysis that does not use a machine. Solution drains by gravity into and out of the peritoneal cavity by way of a permanently connected catheter into a bag worn around the individual's waist. CAPD is performed several times a day and usually once at night (Figure 13–12).

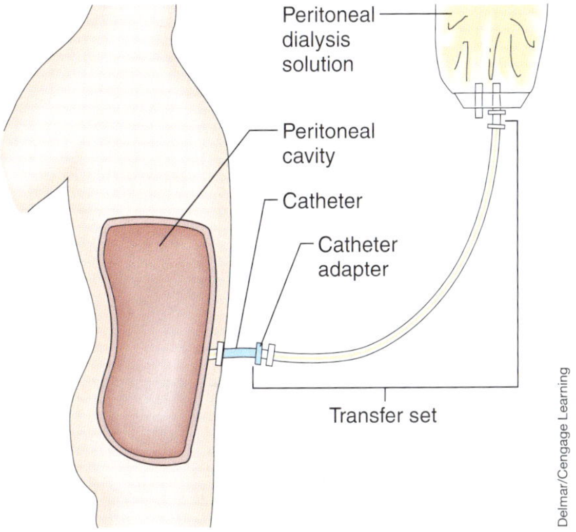

(A) infusion of solution.

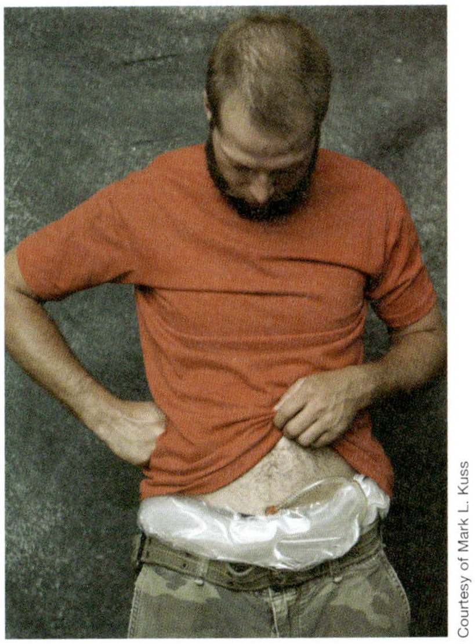

(B) Empty solution container is rolled up and hidden under clothing.

FIGURE 13–12 Continuous ambulatory peritoneal dialysis.

- **Continuous cycling peritoneal dialysis (CCPD)** uses a cycling machine and proceeds while the individual sleeps.
- **Intermittent peritoneal dialysis (IPD)** is performed several times a week, usually in a medical clinic.

Hemodialysis is a much faster and more efficient process than peritoneal dialysis, but it is also much more expensive and more time-consuming. Also, access to an artificial kidney machine might be limited to large metropolitan areas.

Renal transplantation is a procedure to transplant a kidney of a donor into a recipient. This is a relatively simple surgical procedure performed on individuals with chronic renal failure commonly due to diabetes, hypertension, and glomerulonephritis.

Best results from kidney transplants are obtained when the donor and recipient are close human leukocyte antigen (HLA) matches or are histocompatible. An identical twin provides the greatest probability of match, with a fraternal twin, sibling, parent, and biological child the next best matches, in that descending order. The greatest problems with renal transplant are obtaining a kidney that is histocompatible with the recipient, dealing with postoperative organ rejection and complications with lifelong administration of immunosuppressant medications.

PREVENTION. Some causes of kidney failure might not be preventable. Controlling risk factors and conditions that cause kidney failure is the best preventive method. Because kidney disease is often caused by hypertension and diabetes, keeping these under control is important. Other preventive activities include not smoking, maintaining a healthy weight, eating healthy, and exercising regularly.

ADENOCARCINOMA OF THE KIDNEY

DESCRIPTION. Cancer of the kidney is relatively uncommon. When it does occur, the most common type is renal cell carcinoma or renal cell adenocarcinoma. These tumors are more common in men than in women and usually affect men 55 years of age or older.

ETIOLOGY. The cause of this tumor is unknown, although cigarette smoking is considered to be a risk factor. Adenocarcinoma of the kidney frequently metastasizes to the liver, brain, and bone before symptoms appear.

COMPLEMENTARY AND ALTERNATIVE THERAPY

An Herbal Medicine Linked to Bladder Cancer

Reports about a case of a gentleman who developed bladder cancer, kidney problems, and, eventually, renal failure after taking an herbal medicine might be a warning to others. The man was taking *Longdan Xieganwan* for liver enhancement. This is a Chinese herbal supplement that has been used to treat irritability and headaches associated with stress. It is also used to treat gall stones, gallbladder diseases, hepatitis, herpes, shingles, cystitis, hyperthyroidism, and jaundice. The herbal preparation contains aristolochic acid, which has been associated with bladder cancer and kidney damage. Recent research has shown that aristolochic acid is a urological carcinogen. In this reported case, the man stopped taking the drug after 5 years but still developed bladder tumors and kidney failure. He had to be put on dialysis. This herbal medicine has been banned in many countries but can be obtained via the Internet.

Source: Herbal Medicines (2006).

■ ***SYMPTOMS.*** The most common initial symptom is painless hematuria. Later, as the tumor increases in size, the individual experiences flank pain and fever.

■ ***DIAGNOSIS.*** A KUB, IVP, CT scan, and biopsy of the kidney can confirm the diagnosis.

■ ***TREATMENT.*** Treatment, whether metastasis has occurred or not, is **nephrectomy** (neh-FRECK-toh-me; nephr = kidney, ectomy = excision or removal). If metastasis has occurred, chemotherapy and radiation also might be employed, but prognosis varies with the extent of spread. Cure might be possible if no metastasis has occurred, but with metastasis, prognosis is poor.

■ ***PREVENTION.*** Kidney cancer might not be preventable, but controlling risk factors by living a healthy lifestyle, including not smoking, eating more fruits and vegetables, staying active, maintaining normal body weight, and controlling blood pressure all might be helpful in prevention.

Diseases of the Bladder

With the exception of incontinence, diseases of the bladder are relatively uncommon compared to the many other disorders of the urinary system. However, incontinence is very common, especially in the older adult. It can cause many physical and psychological problems for an individual.

URINARY INCONTINENCE

■ ***DESCRIPTION.*** Urinary incontinence is the loss of control of urine flow. It is estimated that more than 15 million people have this disorder, and 85% of them are female. Forty percent of females age 60 and older suffer with urinary incontinence.

■ ***ETIOLOGY.*** Pregnancy, childbirth, hysterectomy, and menopause can all affect female continence. Males are also affected by incontinence but not nearly as often as females. As males age, the prostate is often enlarged, leading to urinary dribbling, the inability to control flow. Prostate surgery also can affect continence.

■ ***SYMPTOMS.*** Incontinence affects all areas of an individual's life by disrupting sleep, physical activity, travel plans, and sexual activity. Often, the fear of urinary accidents drives affected individuals away from social activity and into a life of seclusion.

There are several types of incontinence. Stress incontinence is the inability to hold urine when the bladder is stressed by coughing, sneezing, or laughing. Urge incontinence occurs with a sudden uncontrollable urge to empty the bladder. Overflow incontinence is caused by the bladder not properly emptying and leaking when overfilled.

■ ***DIAGNOSIS.*** A complete medical history and physical exam, including a voiding diary, is helpful in diagnosis. Diagnostic testing can include urinalysis and CBC to determine any underlying infections.

Specialized urodynamic testing uses cystometry to measure anatomic and functional status of the bladder and urethra. Post-void residual volumes of the bladder use a urinary catheter placed into the bladder to measure any urine remaining in the bladder after voiding. Cystoscopy might help identify the presence of bladder tumors, cysts, or foreign bodies.

■ ***TREATMENT.*** Incontinence can be managed by wearing sanitary napkins, incontinence pads, adult diapers, or waterproof briefs. Males also might use external appliances to catch the urine.

Stress incontinence can be improved by different treatments, depending on the cause of the incontinence. A common noninvasive treatment employs frequently emptying the bladder and exercising the pelvic muscles and external sphincter to strengthen these structures. Exercises of these muscles are called Kegel exercises. These exercises are performed by tightening or contracting the pelvic muscles as one would do to hold or stop urine flow. Performing repetitions of 20 to 40 Kegel exercises several times a day can be quite effective in controlling some types of stress incontinence (Figure 13–13).

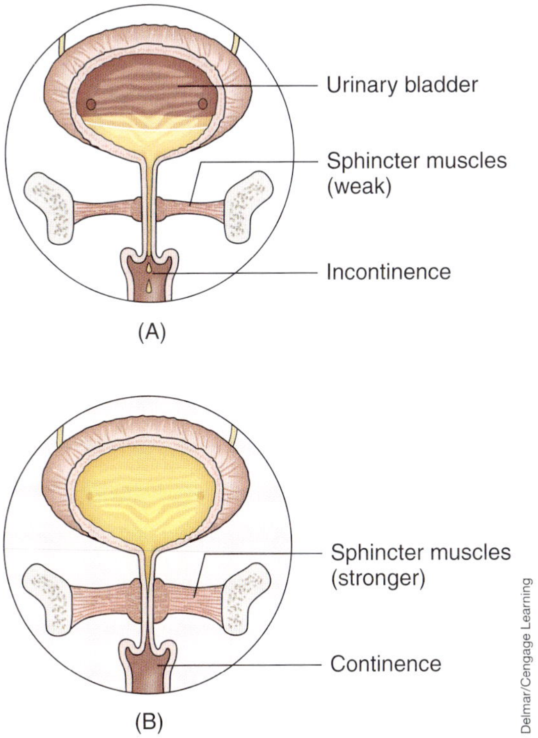

FIGURE 13–13 Kegel exercises: (A) Before exercises, pelvic muscles are thin, the sphincter is weak, and the urethra cannot close; (B) After exercises (3 months), the muscles are thicker and stronger, closing the sphincter.

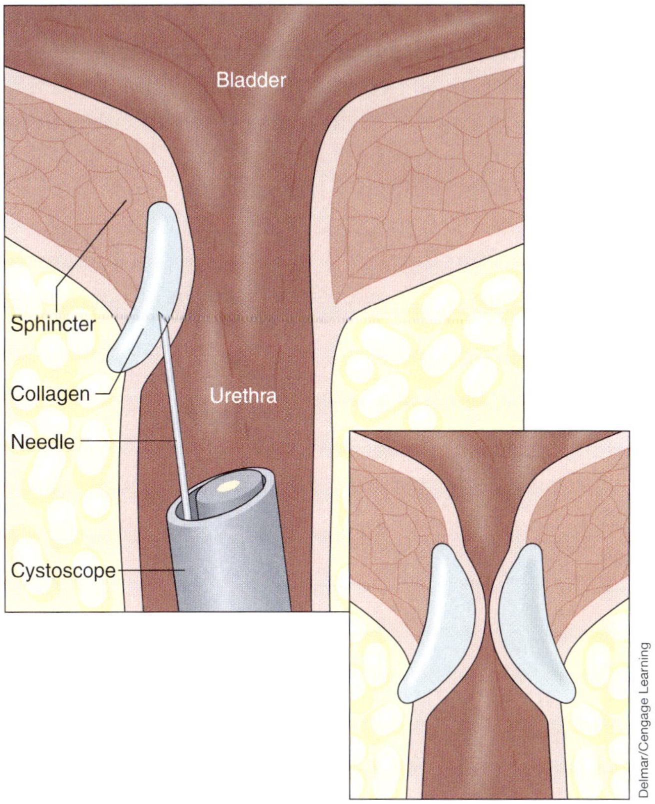

FIGURE 13–14 Collagen injection for incontinence.

Another treatment for stress incontinence involves collagen injections near the external sphincter to narrow the urethra (Figure 13–14). Laparoscopic bladder suspension also might be a treatment of choice. Another surgical procedure performed to suspend the bladder neck and urethra to correct urinary incontinence is called Marshall-Marchetti-Krantz (MMK). Female stress incontinence can be improved with estrogen therapy because low estrogen levels weaken the urethral sphincter.

Overflow incontinence can be controlled with medications, self-catheterization, or both. If the bladder has herniated through the pelvic floor or if there is vaginal prolapse, surgery might be necessary.

Urge incontinence can be improved by bladder training. Bladder training consists of emptying the bladder every hour for 7 to 10 days and then gradually increasing the length of time until one is toileting every 3 hours. Kegel exercises also might help. Surgery is usually a last alternative because it is quite expensive.

In males, urinary incontinence is common following prostate surgery. To control this incontinence, exercise is necessary. If exercise does not control the incontinence, collagen injections might be needed. Another treatment option is surgical insertion of an artificial sphincter. This artificial device has a valve that an individual can activate to control urine flow.

Urinary incontinence in both sexes can be related to other diseases such as stroke and UTI. Sleeping pills, antihistamines, muscle relaxants, and medications to control hypertension also might cause urinary incontinence.

■ ***PREVENTION.*** Incontinence is not always preventable. Decreasing risk involves maintaining a healthy weight, not smoking, performing Kegel exercises, avoiding bladder irritants such as coffee, eating more fiber, and remaining physically active.

TRANSITIONAL CELL CARCINOMA OF THE BLADDER

■ ***DESCRIPTION.*** Bladder cancer is the most common neoplasm of the urinary tract. It usually occurs in males after age 60 and is three times more common in males than in females. Transitional cell carcinoma arises from the lining of the bladder. Bladder cancer commonly metastasizes before symptoms appear, making it highly malignant.

■ ***ETIOLOGY.*** The cause of these tumors is unknown, but the most important risk factor is cigarette smoking, which increases the chance of cancer proportionate to the number of cigarettes smoked during the life of the affected individual. Other predisposing factors include exposure to industrial chemicals and chronic cystitis.

■ ***SYMPTOMS.*** Symptoms include hematuria, dysuria, and nocturia, but these symptoms do not usually appear until late in the course of the disease.

■ ***DIAGNOSIS.*** Diagnosis can be confirmed by cystoscopy and biopsy.

■ ***TREATMENT.*** Treatment depends on the stage of the tumor. **Transurethral resection (TUR)** (trans = through, urethral = urethra; resection = partial excision) can be performed to remove the tumor, or, more frequently, a **radical** (radical = a treatment that seeks to cure; aggressive, not palliative or conservative) **cystectomy** (sis-TECT-toh-me, cyst = bladder, ectomy = excision or removal) is performed. If metastasis has occurred, radiation and chemotherapy also might be used. Prognosis depends on the stage of the tumor when discovered. Usually, discovery is late in the course of the disease, and prognosis is poor.

■ ***PREVENTION.*** Prevention consists of not smoking, avoiding exposure to industrial chemicals, and promptly treating cystitis.

TRAUMA

Straddle Injuries

Straddle injuries commonly cause injury to the urethra. This type of injury occurs when an individual accidentally falls in a straddling position. These injuries are more common in males. Instances when straddle injuries can occur include walking a fence or roof beam or, in some cases, riding a horse or motorcycle. Treatment varies, depending on the severity of the injury.

GLIMPSE OF THE FUTURE

Probiotics for Bladder Cancer

Probiotic bacteria are presently being used to treat a variety of conditions from diarrhea to allergies. Probiotics are dietary supplements of bacteria or yeast that supplement normal gastrointestinal flora. Research has shown they are effective in the treatment of traveler's diarrhea, colitis, and some UTI. In addition, they have been shown to prevent some cases of respiratory infections, dental disease, irritable bowel syndrome, and inflammatory bowel disease. The probiotics most commonly used are strains of *Lactobacillus* and *Bifidobacterium*. In the future, there might be many more uses for probiotic bacteria. Studies using probiotics for bladder cancers and colon cancers are on the horizon.

Source: Goldin & Gorbach (2008).

Neurogenic Bladder

DESCRIPTION. Neurogenic bladder is dysfunction of the bladder due to some type of injury to the nervous system supplying the urinary tract or bladder.

ETIOLOGY. A common trauma that causes neurogenic bladder is a spinal cord injury such as those sustained in motor vehicle accidents or diving accidents. Other traumatic causes include cerebrovascular accidents, strokes, tumors, and herniated lumbar disks. Diabetes, dementia, and Parkinson's disease are metabolic disorders that often lead to neurogenic bladder.

SYMPTOMS. Symptoms of neurogenic bladder vary, depending on the nerves involved. Individuals might have no feeling of the need to void, or they might feel like they need to void all the time. Other symptoms are mild to severe urinary incontinence, difficulty or inability to empty the bladder, and bladder spasms.

DIAGNOSIS. Neurogenic bladder is difficult to diagnose. A detailed history, physical and neurologic examinations, and a series of urologic studies might be needed to confirm a diagnosis.

TREATMENT. Treatment goals are aimed at prevention of UTIs and controlling incontinence. Indwelling urinary catheters can control incontinence. Intermittent self-catheterization can be taught to individuals unable to empty the bladder to prevent hydronephrosis and possible renal failure.

The prognosis of neurogenic bladder depends on the possibility of reversing the nerve damage. Herniated lumbar disks that cause neurogenic bladder are commonly repaired and rapidly restore bladder function. If nerve damage is permanent, neurogenic bladder will also be permanent.

PREVENTION. Neurogenic bladder, in many cases, is not preventable. In other cases, prevention is aimed at rapid diagnosis and treatment of the cause.

RARE DISEASES

Goodpasture Syndrome

Goodpasture syndrome is an autoimmune disorder characterized by glomerulonephritis and pulmonary hemorrhage. For some unknown reason, the body's own antibodies attack the membranes of the kidneys and lungs, leading to symptoms of hemoptysis (he-MOP-tih-sis; hemo = blood, ptysis = saliva), or coughing or spitting up blood; dyspnea (dys = difficulty, pnea = breathing); chest pain; and anemia. Goodpasture syndrome usually results in renal failure and, ultimately, death.

Interstitial Cystitis

Interstitial cystitis is a chronic nonbacterial cystitis due to inflammation of the inner lining of the bladder. Typically, this disease affects young women and is thought to be autoimmune in nature.

The inflammation and swelling of the inner lining of the bladder decreases the capacity of the bladder, leading to the need to urinate frequently. Often, the lining is ulcerated, leading to hematuria. Other symptoms include pain above the pubic area and lower abdomen, bladder fullness, and urgency.

Treatment includes instillation of liquid medications into the bladder to distend the bladder and treat the disorder. Treatment can be needed for up to 12 weeks, but response to treatment is generally good.

EFFECTS OF AGING ON THE SYSTEM

The most common problem of the urinary system in the older adult is urinary incontinence. It is frequently due to changes in other body systems in the aging process rather than to the urinary system. Because the urinary elimination process is primarily controlled by the nervous system, changes with aging or diseases of this system can affect the individual's ability to control urine flow. Individuals with Alzheimer's disease, brain tumor, or other disorders of the nervous system might not be aware of the urge to urinate or be able to communicate the need to urinate.

In older males, benign prostatic hypertrophy is a common disorder that often causes urinary frequency, dribbling, pain or burning with urination, and difficulty starting the urine flow. In older females, the changes in estrogen levels can cause a decrease in vaginal muscle tone and, along with the changes in structure, cause increased frequency and some urine incontinence. Changes in lower abdomen muscle tone, usually the result of multiple pregnancies or obesity, also contribute to some urinary incontinence in the older adult female.

(See Chapter 17, "Reproductive System Diseases and Disorders," for more information on changes in the female and male reproductive systems.)

Older individuals with other common system disorders such as stroke or severe circulatory impairment might not feel the urge to urinate and, thus, have urinary incontinence. Chronic UTIs also can affect bladder function so that the result over time is urinary incontinence.

Urinary problems in the older adult might not be due to the aging process at all, however, but to many other events occurring in the individual's life. For instance, fecal impactions that are common in the institutionalized older individual also can cause urinary incontinence.

Some medications can cause changes in the ability of the bladder to empty thoroughly, causing overflow incontinence. Many older adults take medications such as antidepressants, narcotic pain relievers, or cardiac drugs that can cause some urinary retention, eventually resulting in incontinence.

Older adults who have mobility problems frequently have urinary incontinence. Individuals who have some difficulty rising from a chair or bed, or who walk slowly, often have periods of incontinence simply because they cannot get to the restroom in time. Lack of mobility causes the individual to be dependent on others for toileting, and this frequently leads to urinary incontinence problems. This is a common problem for the institutionalized older adult.

SUMMARY

The urinary system includes the kidneys, ureters, bladder, and urethra. This system maintains homeostasis in the body by excreting and reabsorbing important electrolytes, compounds, and water. Urinary disorders range from mild infections to very serious diseases such as cancer. The most common signs and symptoms of urinary dysfunction include an abnormality in the urine or in the individual's ability to urinate. The most common disorders of the urinary system include infections and incontinence.

Some diseases are diagnosed by urinalysis or urine culture and sensitivity, but radiologic examinations are also used. A cystoscopy can be performed for diagnostic or treatment purposes. In the older adult, urinary incontinence is the most frequent problem of the system. Urinary disorders can be the result of urinary system pathology or of disease or malfunction of other body systems.

REVIEW QUESTIONS

Short Answer

1. What are the functions of the urinary system?

2. Which signs and symptoms are associated with common urinary system disorders?

3. Which diagnostic tests are most commonly used to determine the type and cause of urinary system disorders?

4. What is the most common urinary problem in the older adult population?

Matching

5. Match the disorders listed in the left column with the correct definition in the right column.

_____ Urethritis	a. most commonly used diagnostic test for urinary system disorders
_____ Pyuria	b. pus in the urine
_____ Oliguria	c. an inflammation of the filtering components of the kidney
_____ Anuria	d. difficulty urinating
_____ Nocturia	e. excision of the kidney
_____ Cystectomy	f. inflammation of the urethra
_____ Dysuria	g. frequent urination at night
_____ Nephrectomy	h. surgical removal of the bladder
_____ Urinalysis	i. scanty urine output
_____ Pyelonephritis	j. absence of urine output
_____ Glomerulonephritis	k. inflammation of the kidney pelvis

CASE STUDIES

■ Ms. Hayden, age 55, has been noticing a small amount of urine leakage at intervals when she participates in her low-impact aerobics class. She has noticed this problem for about a year, now, but thinks it is nothing to worry about. She tells you that this occurs every time she does aerobics and asks what you think the cause might be. She is also embarrassed to ask her physician about it. How would you respond to Ms. Hayden? Do you think this is a problem for concern? Should she seek medical advice?

■ Jeremy is a 30-year-old truck driver who has had several episodes of kidney stones. Although he states the episodes are extremely painful, he has been able to pass the stones each time he has been afflicted and has not had to have surgery or lithotripsy treatment. He asks you how he might be able to prevent kidney stones from developing in the future. Are there some lifestyle interventions he can institute to prevent the recurrence of kidney stones? What would you tell him? Where could he find additional information about this?

StudyWARE™ Connection

To help you learn the content in this chapter, take a practice quiz or play an interactive game on your StudyWARE™ CD-ROM.

Workbook Practice

Go to your Workbook and complete the practice questions.

BIBLIOGRAPHY

Allen, P. (2007). Basic research may improve approach to UTI, CPPS. *Urology Times 35*(6), 11.

American Kidney Fund. (2008). *www.kidneyfund.org* (accessed June 2008).

Brandau, S., & Suttmann, H. (2007). Thirty years of BCG immunotherapy for non-muscle invasive bladder cancer: A success story with room for improvement. *Biomedicine & Pharmacotherapy 61*(6), 299–305.

Campbell, B. (2006). Bladder cancer. *Nursing 36*(4), 54–57.

Commissioning care. (2008). *Nursing Management-UK 14*(9), 4.

Evans, C., Debruyne, F., Payne, H., Solsona, E., Teillac, P., & Tubaro, A. (2007). Bladder cancer: Management and future directions. *European Urology Supplements 6*(3), 365–373.

Flagg, L. (2007). Dietary and holistic treatment of recurrent calcium oxalate kidney stones: Review of literature to guide patient education. *Urologic Nursing 27*(2), 113–143.

Goldin, B., & Gorbach, S. (2008). Clinical indications for probiotics: An overview. *Clinical Infectious Diseases S2*(46), S96–S100.

Herbal medicines. (July 29, 2006). *Reactions Weekly 1112*, 15.

History of gonorrhea in men is linked to bladder carcinogenesis. (2007). *Nursing Standard 21*(24), 14–15.

In the public eye. (2006). *Urology Times 34*(8), 57.

Kohmann, K. (2007). The future of SWL: A global perspective. *AIP Conference Proceedings 900*(1), 340–350.

National Center for Complementary and Alternative Medicine. (2008). National Institutes of Health (NIH). *www.nccam.nih.gov* (accessed June 2008).

National Kidney Foundation (2008). *www.kidney.org* (accessed June 2008).

Nguyen, C., & Jones, J. (2008). Defining the role of NMP22 in bladder cancer surveillance. *World Journal of Urology 26*(1), 51–58.

Pei, Z. (2007). Innovations in lithotripsy technology. *AIP Conference Proceedings 900*(1), 317–325.

Ponholzer, A., & Madersbacher, S. (2007). Lower urinary tract symptoms and erectile dysfunction: Links for diagnosis, management and treatment. *International Journal of Impotence Research 19*(6), 544–550.

Powles, T., Murray, I., Brock, C., Oliver, T., & Avril, N. (2007). Molecular positron emission tomography and PET/CT imaging in urological malignancies. *European Urology 51*(6), 1511–1521.

Rittenmeyer, H. (2008). Sacral nerve neuromodulation (InterStim) Part I: Case studies. *Urologic Nursing 28*(1), 15–20.

Rittenmeyer, H. (2008). Sacral nerve neuromodulation (InterStim) Part III: Review of the InterStim system. *Urologic Nursing 28*(1), 26–28.

Rodhe, N., Englund, L., Molstad, S., & Samuelsson, E. (2008). Bacteriuria is associated with urge urinary incontinence in older women. *Scandinavian Journal of Primary Health Care 26*(1), 35–39.

Simon Foundation (2008). *www.simonfoundation.org* (accessed June 2008).

Suttmann, H., KIamradt, J., Lehman, J., & Stockle, M. (2007). Improving the prognosis of patients after radical cystectomy: The role of perioperative chemotherapy. *BJU International 100*(6), 1225–1228.

Tasty treatment for kidney stones. (2006). *Nursing 36*(8), 35.

United States Cancer Statistics. (2008) Centers for Disease Control and Prevention. *www.cdc.gov*

Wagg, A., Potter, J., Peel, P., Irwin, P., Lowe, D., & Pearson, M. (2008). National audit of continence care for older people: Management of urinary incontinence. *Age & Ageing 37*(1), 39–44.

Washburn, D. (2007). Intravesical antineoplastic therapy following transurethral resection of bladder tumors: Nursing implications from the operating room to discharge. *Nursing 11*(4), 553–559.

Wendt-Nordahl, G., Krombach, P., Hannak, D., Michel, M., Alken, P., & Knoll, T. (2007). Prospective evaluation of acute endocrine pancreatic injury as collateral damage of shock-wave lithotripsy for upper urinary tract stones. *BJU International 100*(6), 1339–1343.

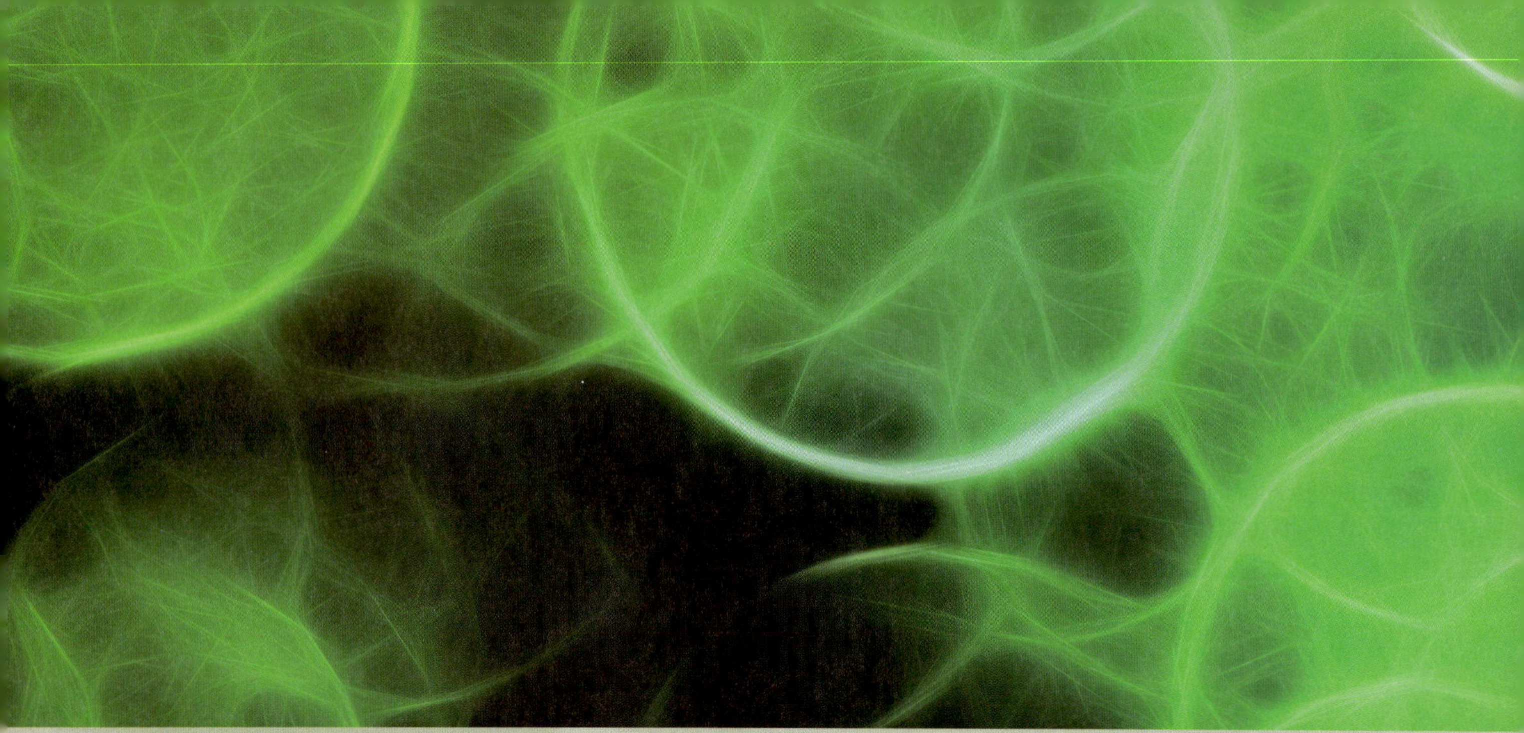

OUTLINE

- Anatomy and Physiology
- Common Signs and Symptoms
- Diagnostic Tests
- Common Diseases of the Endocrine System
  - *Pituitary Gland Diseases*
  - *Thyroid Gland Diseases*
  - *Parathyroid Gland Diseases*
  - *Adrenal Gland Diseases*
  - *Pancreatic Islets of Langerhans Diseases*
  - *Reproductive Gland Diseases*
- Trauma
- Rare Diseases
- Effects of Aging on the System
- Summary
- Review Questions
- Case Studies
- Bibliography

KEY TERMS

Acromegaly (p. 283)
Adenoma (p. 285)
Aldosterone (p. 289)
Amenorrhea (p. 291)
Androgens (p. 282)
Cortisol (p. 282)
Cortisone (p. 289)
Cretinism (p. 287)
Diabetic retinopathy (p. 294)
Dwarfism (p. 284)
Estrogen (p. 282)
Exophthalmos (p. 286)
Giantism (p. 283)
Glucagon (p. 282)
Glucocorticoids (p. 282)
Glycogen (p. 293)
Glycosuria (p. 293)
Goiter (p. 286)
Goitrogenic (p. 287)
Gonad (p. 296)
Gynecomastia (p. 291)
Hirsutism (p. 291)
Hydrocortisone (p. 289)
Hyperglycemia (p. 293)
Hypoglycemia (p. 291)
Insulin (p. 282)
Islets of Langerhans (p. 291)
Ketoacidosis (p. 293)
Ketones (p. 000)
Lipids (p. 294)
Mineralocorticoids (p. 282)
Myxedema (p. 287)
Panhypopituitarism (p. 284)
Polydipsia (p. 285)
Polyuria (p. 285)
Precocious (p. 291)
Progesterone (p. 282)
Striae (p. 290)
Tetany (p. 289)
Thyroid storm (p. 286)
Vasopressin (p. 282)
Virilism (p. 291)

14

Endocrine System Diseases and Disorders

LEARNING OBJECTIVES

Upon completion of the chapter, the learner should be able to:

1. Define the terminology common to the endocrine system and the disorders of the system.
2. Discuss the basic anatomy and physiology of the endocrine system.
3. Identify the important signs and symptoms associated with common endocrine system disorders.
4. Describe the common diagnostics used to determine the type and cause of endocrine system disorders.
5. Identify common disorders of the endocrine system.
6. Describe the typical course and management of the common endocrine system disorders.
7. Describe the effects of aging on the endocrine system and the common disorders associated with aging of the system.

OVERVIEW

The endocrine system is a highly complex system of glands that secrete important hormones for a variety of body functions. The glands of the system work in harmony, discharging the hormones into the bloodstream as needed. The disorders of the system can be caused by problems in the primary gland or in another gland whose secretions control the primary gland. Disorders of the endocrine system can be related to oversecretion or undersecretion of the gland's hormones. ■

ANATOMY AND PHYSIOLOGY

The endocrine system consists of many glands located throughout the body (Figure 14–1). It includes the following glands:

1. hypothalamus—located beneath the thalamus in the area of the third ventricle of the brain
2. pituitary or hypophysis—located at the base of the brain
3. pineal—located behind the midbrain
4. thymus—located in the mediastinal cavity under the sternum, near the heart
5. thyroid—located in the neck on each side of the trachea
6. parathyroids—usually four glands, embedded in the posterior part of the thyroid
7. adrenals—two glands, one on top of each kidney
8. pancreatic islets—embedded in the pancreas
9. ovaries (female) and testes (male)—one ovary on each side of the uterus and one testis in each side of the scrotal sac

Each of these glands has a unique function and delivers its secretion as needed into the bloodstream. Table 14–1 lists the glands, their hormones, and the functions of each hormone. The mechanism known as negative feedback controls the amount of hormones secreted into the bloodstream. Although the hypothalamus monitors the hormone secretions, negative feedback regulates the amount secreted. In the negative feedback system, levels of the particular hormone in the bloodstream trigger the release of the hormone as needed. If the concentration of the hormone in the blood is low, the sequence of events stimulates the gland to secrete more hormones. In like manner, if the concentration of the hormone in the blood is higher than normal, the feedback mechanism triggers the gland to suppress the release of more hormones.

The hypothalamus, located in the third ventricle area of the brain, contains neurosecretory cells that secrete hypothalamic hormones. These hormones regulate the function of the anterior pituitary gland. The hypothalamus also produces the two hormones stored in the neurohypophysis or posterior pituitary gland.

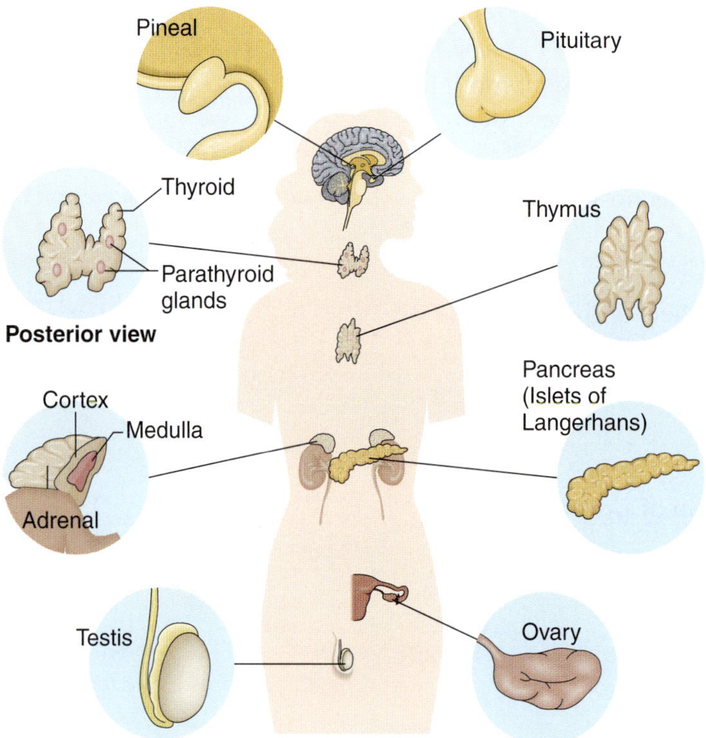

FIGURE 14–1 The endocrine system.

TABLE 14–1 The Endocrine Glands: Their Hormones and Hormone Functions

Endocrine Gland	Hormone	Hormone Function
Hypothalamus (Pituitary)	Inhibiting hormones and releasing hormones	Inhibits or releases hormones from the anterior pituitary
Hypophysis Adenohypophysis (Anterior Pituitary)	Adenocorticotropin hormone (ACTH) Thyrotropin hormone (TSH) Somatotropin hormone (STH) Melanocyte stimulating hormone (MSH) Lactogenic hormone (prolactin) Follicle-stimulating hormone (FSH) Luteinizing hormone (LH; also called interstitial cell-stimulating hormone, ICSH)	Stimulates release of adrenal cortex hormones Stimulates release of thyroid gland hormones Stimulates growth Stimulates melanin production Stimulates mammary glands and lactation Induces ovulation in females and testosterone secretion in males
Neurohypophysis	Antidiuretic hormone (ADH)	Increases reabsorption of water in the distal tubules of the kidneys
(Posterior Pituitary)	Oxytocin	Stimulates uterine contraction and the initiation of breast milk flow in females and increases the ejection of sperm into the seminal fluid in males
Pineal	Melatonin	Affects circadian rhythms
Thymus	Thymopoietin	Causes immune response development in the newborn and maintains it in the adult
Thyroid	Triiodothyronine (T_3) Thyroxine (T_4) Calcitonin	Stimulates growth and development regulates metabolism Increases calcium deposits into the bones
Parathyroid	Parathormone (PTH)	Regulates calcium and phosphate levels and increases reabsorption of calcium from the bones
Adrenals		Affects stress reactions; promotes protein and fat use to raise blood sugar
Adrenal Cortex	Glucocorticoids Mineralocorticoids Sex hormones	Affects sodium and water reabsorption Promotes sodium and water reabsorption Develops secondary sex characteristics
Adrenal Medulla	Epinephrine	Fight or flight response Increases blood pressure and metabolism
	Norepinephrine	Causes vasoconstriction and increases blood pressure
Pancreas Islets		
Alpha Cells	Glucagon	Increases blood glucose levels and is counterregulatory to insulin
Beta Cells	Insulin	Regulates protein, carbohydrate, and fat metabolism
Delta Cells	Somatostatin	Counterregulatory to insulin, glucagon, and somatotropin (STH)
Ovaries	Estrogen Progesterone	Regulates development, maturation, secondary sex characteristics and the reproductive cycle in females
Testes	Testosterone	Regulates growth and development, maturation, secondary sex characteristics and the reproductive system in males

The pituitary gland, also known as the hypophysis gland, is divided into two distinct parts. The adenohypophysis, or anterior part of the gland, produces several hormones that affect other endocrine glands. These include adenocorticotropin hormone (ACTH), thyrotropin hormone (TSH), somatotropin hormone (STH), melanocyte-stimulating hormone (MSH), lactogenic hormone (prolactin), follicle-stimulating hormone (FSH), and luteinizing hormone (LH; also called interstitial cell–stimulating hormone, ICSH).

The posterior pituitary, also called the neurohypophysis, stores two hormones that are secreted by the hypothalamus. Oxytocin (pitocin) helps the progress of labor in the pregnant female and causes uterine contractions after childbirth. It also affects the cells in the breasts, causing a release of milk during lactation. The antidiuretic hormone ADH, also known as **vasopressin**, is also released from the neurohypophysis. It affects the reabsorption of water from the renal tubules.

The pineal gland, located behind the midbrain, secretes melatonin. It might also secrete other hormones that interact with the hypothalamus and the pituitary gland to cause the secretion of hormones from other glands.

The thymus gland, located just below the clavicle behind the sternum, secretes thymopoietin, a hormone that stimulates the development of lymphocytes. Lymphocytes are important for immunity development and prevention of infections.

The thyroid gland, located in the neck on either side of the trachea, secretes thyroxine (T_4), triiodothyronine (T_3), and calcitonin. These hormones are released as needed in response to the thyroid-stimulating hormone secreted by the pituitary gland. T_4 and T_3 increase metabolic activity. Calcitonin affects the regulation of calcium and works in opposition to the hormone secreted by the parathyroid gland.

Embedded in the posterior part of the thyroid gland are the parathyroid glands. There are usually four of these, but there can be more. The parathyroid glands secrete parathormone, important in the regulation of calcium and phosphorus in the body.

The adrenal glands, located on top of each kidney, have two distinct parts. The cortex, the outer part, secretes **mineralocorticoids**, **glucocorticoids**, and **androgens**. The mineralocorticoids promote sodium retention. The glucocorticoids affect the metabolism of protein, glucose, and fats. **Cortisol** is the main glucocorticoid and is important for metabolism of carbohydrates. The androgens enhance masculinization. The most common androgen hormone is testosterone. The adrenal medulla or middle section secretes epinephrine and norepinephrine.

The beta cells located in the pancreas secrete **insulin**, another important hormone. Insulin is most important in the metabolism of glucose, but it also promotes fatty acid synthesis and amino acid entry into cells. Insulin secretion is regulated by the feedback mechanism and by counterregulatory hormones such as **glucagon**, cortisol, epinephrine, and the growth hormone.

The ovaries and testes secrete the sex hormones, as they are commonly known. The ovaries secrete **estrogen** and **progesterone**, important for development and maturation and maintaining the functions of the reproductive system. The testes secrete testosterone, important for growth and development, secondary sex characteristics, and maintaining the reproductive system functions. See Chapter 17, "Reproductive System Diseases and Disorders," for more information about the reproductive system.

StudyWARE™ Connection

View an animation on the endocrine system on your StudyWARE™ CD-ROM.

COMMON SIGNS AND SYMPTOMS

Most endocrine disorders are due to hypo- or hypersecretion by a gland; diagnosis depends on matching the signs and symptoms with the hormone dysfunction. The difficulty in diagnosing endocrine disorders is related to tracking the problem to the correct source. For instance, a pituitary dysfunction can easily lead to signs and symptoms of multiple gland disorders; a decreased secretion of thyroid-stimulating hormone from the pituitary might initially lead one to believe that the thyroid gland itself is dysfunctional. Some common signs and symptoms of endocrine system disorders include mental abnormalities, lethargy or fatigue, and tissue atrophy.

DIAGNOSTIC TESTS

The only endocrine glands that can be physically examined are the thyroid glands and testes; enlargement or atrophy of these glands can be felt, and severe enlargement can be seen. Assessment of proper function of the endocrine organs can be accomplished with blood or urine testing for the hormones they produce. Blood glucose and HbA1C are used to diagnose diabetes mellitus and to monitor the progression of the disease. Computerized tomography (CT) and magnetic resonance imaging (MRI) can be used to check for presence of tumors or alteration in organ size.

COMMON DISEASES OF THE ENDOCRINE SYSTEM

Endocrine diseases are the result of abnormally high or low hormone secretion by endocrine glands. Abnormal secretion might be due to the size of the gland: abnormally large or hypertrophied glands tend to produce abnormally high hormone levels, whereas abnormally small or atrophied glands tend to produce abnormally low levels. Abnormal gland size can be the result of injury to the gland by surgery, trauma, infection, or radiation. Abnormal function of endocrine glands leads to many physical and mental abnormalities. Abnormalities vary with the amount of hormone secreted (hypersecretion or hyposecretion) and the age of the individual involved.

Pituitary Gland Diseases

The anterior pituitary gland produces tropic (going toward or changing) hormones. These hormones stimulate target organs to grow or produce specific hormones. Growth hormone (GH or somatotropin) promotes growth and development of all body tissues. Other target organs are the thyroid, adrenal gland, testes, and ovaries.

HYPERPITUITARISM

DESCRIPTION. Hyperpituitarism is an abnormal increase in the activity of the pituitary gland. This oversecretion especially affects GH production, leading to excessive growth of bones and tissues.

ETIOLOGY. The most common cause is benign pituitary tumors, which lead to excessive secretion of the adenohypophyseal trophic hormones. Carcinoid tumors can also cause hyperpituitarism. This condition often affects other areas controlled by the pituitary such as thyroid and prolactin hormones.

SYMPTOMS. If hyperpituitarism occurs before puberty, **giantism** occurs (Figure 14–2). Children affected with hyperpituitarism can grow as much as 6 inches in a year. Sexual development is usually slowed; mental development might be normal or slowed.

If hyperpituitarism occurs in an adult, **acromegaly** (ACK-roh-MEG-ah-lee; acro = extremity, megaly = enlargement) occurs: the long bones are unable to grow in length, but the small bones of the hands, feet, and face enlarge. Common symptoms include large, doughy hands and large feet. Abnormal facial features include enlarged jaw with widely spaced teeth, tongue enlargement leading to slurred speech, large forehead, and oily, tough skin with skin pigmentation changes—darker or lighter. Females can also have excessive hair growth.

Acromegaly is a chronic, disfiguring disease that usually shortens life expectancy and often leads to congestive heart failure and respiratory and cerebrovascular diseases.

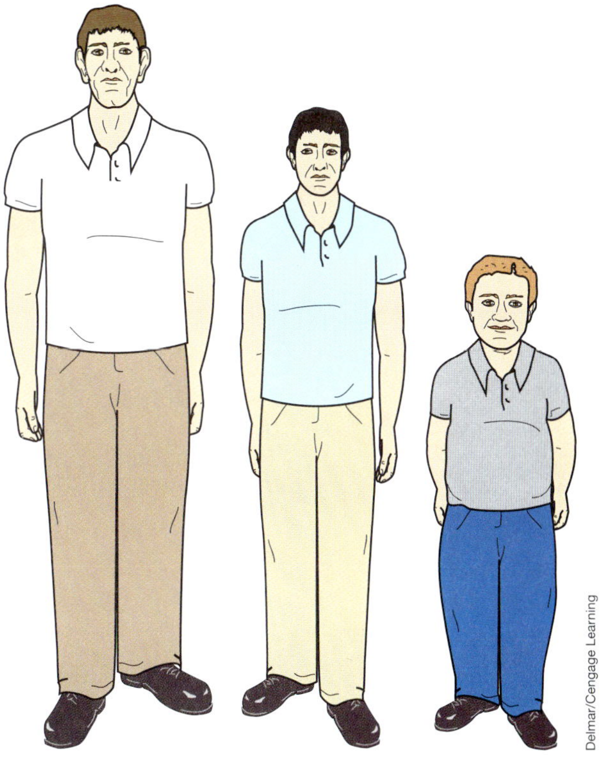

FIGURE 14–2 Giantism and dwarfism. (Right) A dwarf. (Left) A giant. A normal sized individual is in the center.

■ ***DIAGNOSIS.*** Diagnosis is made through examination of physical characteristics of abnormal or excessive growth in children and acromegaly in adults. Blood testing reveals high levels of GH, thyroid, and prolactin. MRI often reveals a pituitary tumor.

■ ***TREATMENT.*** In children, microsurgical removal, radiation, and drug therapy can decrease the secretion of GH and slow the growing process. Prognosis for giantism is usually good. In adults, surgical removal of pituitary tumors often leads to hypopituitarism, and these tumors tend to recur.

■ ***PREVENTION.*** There is no known prevention for hyperpituitarism except to prevent injury or trauma to the gland.

HYPOPITUITARISM

■ ***DESCRIPTION.*** Hypopituitarism is an abnormal decrease in the activity of the pituitary gland, leading to a deficiency or absence of any or all of the tropic hormones.

■ ***ETIOLOGY.*** A common cause is a tumor on the pituitary gland. As the tumor increases in size, damage to the gland interferes with hormone production. Other diseases and traumas can also damage the pituitary, including radiation treatments, head injuries, stroke, brain surgery, brain turmors, and infection.

■ ***SYMPTOMS.*** Because the pituitary gland is the master gland, hypopituitarism can lead to a variety of problems involving the function of all target organs (Figure 14–3). GH and gonadotropin are the most common deficiencies in hypopituitarism. The degree of hypopituitarism can range from mild to severe.

A decrease in growth hormone leads to impaired growth of all body tissues with the most severe decreases causing **dwarfism** (see Figure 14–2). Children affected with dwarfism are proportionately small and underdeveloped sexually and might or might not suffer from mental challenges. Gonadotropin deficiency can lead to abnormal development or absence of secondary sexual characteristics.

In adult women, this deficiency can cause amenorrhea and infertility. Adult men might have a lowered testosterone level, decreased libido (la-BE-doe; sex drive), and abnormal loss of facial and body hair. A decrease in ACTH and TSH can lead to metabolic disorders.

If the pituitary gland is destroyed or nonfunctional, a condition called **panhypopituitarism** (pan = all) exists and can lead to all the preceding disorders and result in fatal complications.

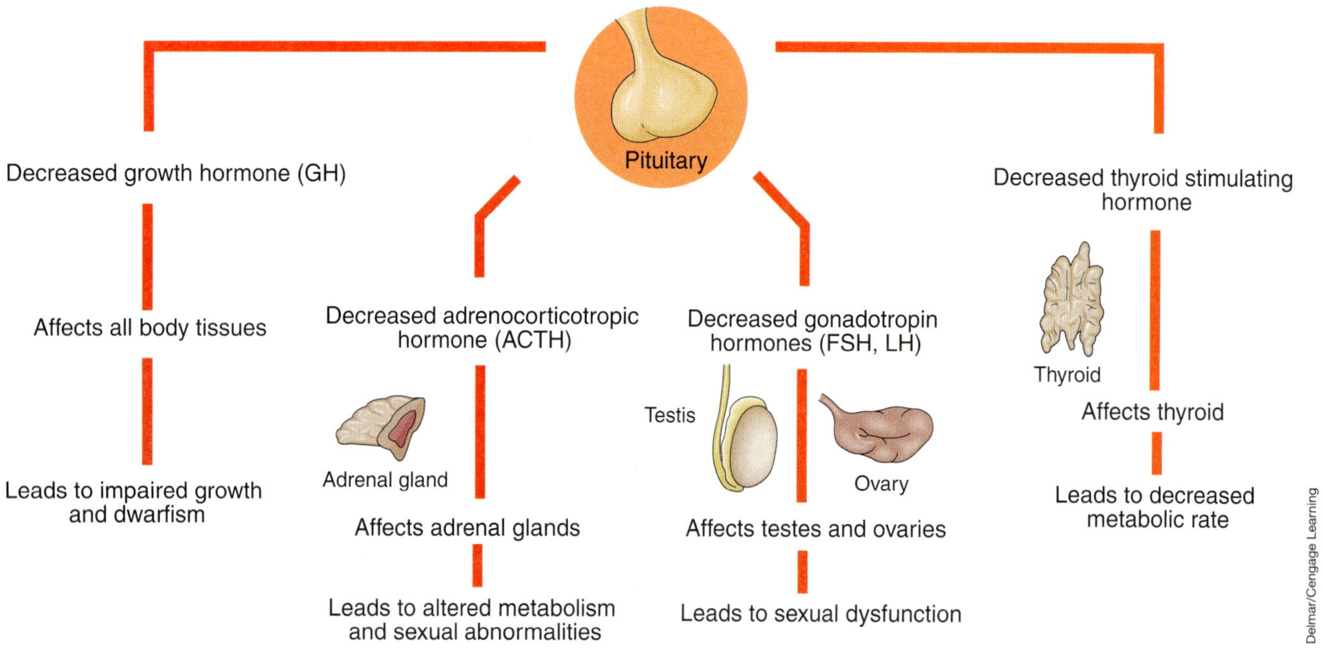

FIGURE 14–3 Effects of hypopituitarism.

■ ***DIAGNOSIS.*** Diagnosis and area of dysfunction can be confirmed by clinical history and blood testing. The dysfunction could involve the pituitary, the individual target organ, or both. Specific blood hormone tests to determine pituitary function can include each tropic hormone (GH, TSH, FSH, LH, ACTH). Target organ function can be assessed by testing blood levels of each individual organ hormone (T_3, T_4, estrogen, progesterone, testosterone, cortisol).

■ ***TREATMENT.*** Treatment of hypopituitarism involves hormone replacement of needed hormones. Constant monitoring and adjusting of hormone levels is needed for optimum results.

■ ***PREVENTION.*** There is no known prevention for hypopituitarism except to prevent injury or trauma to the gland.

DIABETES INSIPIDUS (DI)

■ ***DESCRIPTION.*** *Diabetes* is a general term meaning "passing through," and describes a variety of disorders characterized by **polyuria** (POL-ee-YOU-ree-ah; poly = many, uria = urine), excessive urination. There are several types of diabetes, but diabetes mellitus, a disorder of the pancreas, is the disease most often thought of as diabetes. Diabetes mellitus and gestational diabetes will be discussed later in the chapter.

DI is a disorder characterized by severe thirst and polyuria. There are two types of insipidus, depending on the cause, central DI (pituitary related) and nephrogenic DI (kidney related).

■ ***ETIOLOGY.*** Central DI is caused by a decrease in the release of vasopressin, or ADH, by the posterior portion of the pituitary gland. The cause is damage to the pituitary gland by tumor, surgery, traumatic head injury, or infection.

Nephrogenic DI occurs when there is a defect in the kidney tubules leading to inability of the kidney to respond to ADH. The defect can be be an inherited (genetic) disorder or related to chronic kidney disease or kidney damage caused by certain medications. In many cases, the cause is unknown.

■ ***SYMPTOMS.*** Without antidiuretic (anti = against, di = run through, uri = urine) hormone, the individual has excessive polyuria and might urinate between 2 and 15 gallons of urine in 24 hours. The urine quality is colorless and dilute. The individual experiences excessive **polydipsia** (POL-ee-DIP-see-ah; poly = many, dipsia = thirst or drinking) in an effort to overcome dehydration. Other symptoms include hypotension, dizziness, and constipation.

■ ***DIAGNOSIS.*** Testing for DI includes a urinalysis and a water restriction test. The urinalysis of an affected individual will show colorless urine with a very low specific gravity. The water restriction test includes limiting the suspected individual's water intake for several hours while measuring the urine output, blood pressure, and urine concentration. After several hours, the individual is given vasopressin medication. If the medication decreases urine output and increases urine concentration, the diagnosis of DI is confirmed. MRI of the kidney and pituitary gland assist in locating the cause.

■ ***TREATMENT.*** Central DI can be controlled with vasopressin administered as either a nasal spray or as tablets. Nephrogenic DI is treated with fluid intake to match urine output and drugs that lower urine output. Prognosis is generally good.

■ ***PREVENTION.*** Many cases might not be preventable. Prompt treatment of infections, injuries, and tumors can reduce risk, however.

Thyroid Gland Diseases

The activity of the thyroid gland affects the entire body. The hormone released by the thyroid gland (T_4) regulates metabolism, the rate at which calories are used. In this way, T_4 also regulates body heat, ensuring that the body is kept warm even in a cold environment. T_4 also stimulates the gastrointestinal system by increasing gastric secretions and peristalsis. To make T_4, the thyroid gland requires iodine. Diseases of the thyroid gland are primarily those of hypersecretion and hyposecretion.

HYPERTHYROIDISM

■ ***DESCRIPTION.*** Hyperthyroidism occurs when the thyroid gland secretes excessive T_4. This condition is also known as thyrotoxicosis.

■ ***ETIOLOGY.*** The cause of hyperthyroidism can be idiopathic (unknown), but there are several known causes of hyperthyroidism, including tumors or **adenoma** (AD-eh-NO-ma; adeno = gland, oma = tumor), heredity, excessive dietary intake of iodine (found in seaweed and liver), and taking too much thyroid hormone medication.

The most common cause is an autoimmune condition called Graves' disease. In this condition, antibodies stimulate the thyroid, leading to glandular hypertrophy. Graves' disease commonly affects young women.

■ ***SYMPTOMS.*** No matter the cause, the thyroid gland becomes enlarged and produces a characteristic **goiter** (GOI-ter), a noticeable protrusion of the thyroid gland (Figure 14–4). Overproduction of T_4 increases metabolism, leading to symptoms of tachycardia, nervousness, hyperactivity, weakness, and excessive excitability. The individual has a tremendous appetite but loses weight to the point of extreme thinness. Diarrhea is common because T_4 speeds up peristalsis of the gastrointestinal tract. High metabolic rate causes high heat production, leading to excessive sweating and an intolerance to heat. The skin can be moist, and the individual might have extreme thirst due to this water loss.

One very distinguishing characteristic of hyperthyroidism is a stare in the eyes due to **exophthalmos** (ECK-sof-THAL-mos; abnormal protrusion of the eyeballs) (Figure 14–5) from edema in the tissues behind the eyes. It can be so severe that the eyelids will not close. Unfortunately, this condition might not totally resolve when the hyperthyroidism is corrected.

■ ***DIAGNOSIS.*** A diagnosis is made based on history and physical examination and is confirmed with blood tests. An elevated thyroid-stimulating hormone is usually all that is needed to confirm the diagnosis.

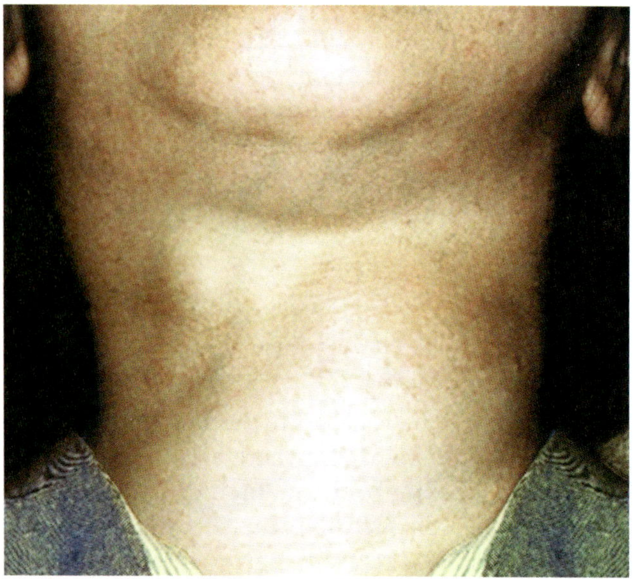

FIGURE 14–4 Goiter.

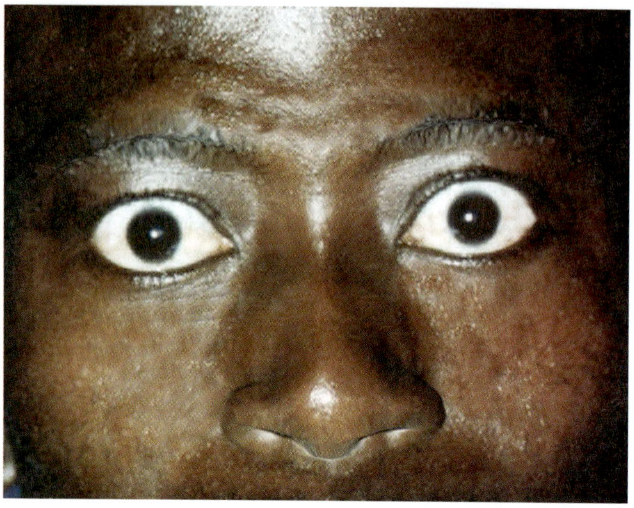

FIGURE 14–5 Exophthalmos in Graves' disease.

■ ***TREATMENT.*** Hyperthroidism can be treated with medication, radiation of the thyroid, or surgical removal of all or part of the gland. If the entire gland receives eradication radiation or is surgically removed, hormone replacement medication will be needed for the life of the individual.

A sudden, life-threatening exacerbation of all symptoms of hyperthyroidism is called thyroid storm. This condition can occur in an individual with severe hyperthyroidism or during the immediate postoperative period following a thyroidectomy (ectomy = excision or removal of). Symptoms of **thyroid storm** include severe tachycardia with heart rates reaching 200 beats per minute, tachypnea, and loss of temperature regulation characterized by a rapid and steady increase in body temperature. Emergency medical intervention must be initiated to save the individual's life.

■ ***PREVENTION.*** There are no general preventive measures for hyperthyroidism, but people who smoke are more likely to develop Graves' disease and ophthalmopathy than people who do not smoke (Shomon, 2008).

SIMPLE GOITER

■ ***DESCRIPTION.*** Simple goiter is an enlargement of the thyroid gland. It occurs as the thyroid attempts to produce adequate amounts of T_4.

■ ***ETIOLOGY.*** Causes of goiter include:

- A family history of goiter incidence.
- Eating large amounts of **goitrogenic** (goiter-producing) foods that inhibit production of thyroid hormone. These include soy, peanuts, peaches, spinach, turnips, cabbage, Brussels sprouts, seaweed, and millet.
- Regular use of medications that affect thyroid production, including lithium and propylthiourcil.
- Iodine deficiency is rare in the United States due to the use of iodized table salt, but some people in other parts of the world have iodine deficiency.

■ ***SYMPTOMS.*** This condition usually affects females and can be asymptomatic until the thyroid gland enlarges to the point of forming a noticeable mass at the front of the neck. If the gland is extremely enlarged, it can cause pressure on the trachea and esophagus and cause dyspnea and dysphagia (dys = difficulty, phagia = swallowing). The main symptom is a swollen thyroid gland. The size can range from a single small nodule to a large neck lump.

■ ***DIAGNOSIS.*** A physical examination including palpation (feeling the enlarged thyroid gland) along with blood tests, ultrasound, and fine-needle biopsy help confirm the diagnosis.

■ ***TREATMENT.*** Treatment includes administration of potassium iodide initially, followed by increasing iodine in the diet with iodized salt. If the cause is related to goitrogenic foods or drugs, avoidance of these often leads to cure. If the goiter is unresponsive to treatment, surgery might be needed to reduce the size of the gland. Treatment is aimed at stopping the enlargement of the gland, but it will not reduce the current size of the gland. Surgery also might be needed to improve physical appearance and decrease difficulty with breathing and swallowing.

■ ***PREVENTION.*** Monitoring dietary intake of goitrogenic foods and medications, along with ensuring adequate intake of iodine, helps prevent some types of goiter.

HYPOTHYROIDISM

■ ***DESCRIPTION.*** Hypothyroidism is the decrease in normal T_4 production.

Advanced hypothyroidism in an adult is called **myxedema** (MICK-seh-DEE-mah). Myxedema commonly occurs in middle-aged women.

Hypothyroidism in infants is rare in the United States. It is caused when any part of the fetus's thyroid fails to develop properly. Congenital hypothyroidism is called **cretinism**. It can be quite devastating, leading to mental and physical growth challenges in the infant and young child.

■ ***ETIOLOGY.*** There are two fairly common causes of hypothyroidism. The first and most common natural cause is an autoimmune disorder called Hashimoto's disease. This condition occurs most frequently in women. It is believed that lymphocytes react with thyroid tissue, leading to destruction of the thyroid gland tissue. This loss of tissue leaves the thyroid unable to produce adequate amounts of thyroid hormone.

The second cause is the result of medical treatments. Oftentimes, treatments to cure hyperthyroidism lead to destruction of part or all of the thyroid gland, leading to hypothyroidism.

In underdeveloped countries, congenital hypothyroidism is more common and is due to an iodine deficiency during the mother's pregnancy.

Symptoms, diagnosis, and treatment plan for hypothyroidism are quite similar regardless of the cause.

■ ***SYMPTOMS.*** Symptoms of hypothyroidism are the opposite of those for hyperthyroidism. The affected individual is fatigued, drowsy, and sensitive to cold temperature; has thin nails and brittle hair; and gains excessive weight. The individual becomes sluggish, mentally and physically.

> An individual with myxedema can exhibit all these symptoms as well as a characteristic swelling or bloating of the facial tissue, thickened tongue, and puffy eyelids.

Children with hypothyroidism, cretins, are dwarfed with a short, stocky body build and a protruding tongue and abdomen. The face is abnormal, with a broad nose, puffy eyelids, and small eyes. Sexual organs fail to develop (Figure 14–6). Muscle growth is slowed to the point that the child is unable to stand or walk. The earlier this condition is discovered, the better the prognosis. For this reason, many states mandate a thyroid blood test on newborns.

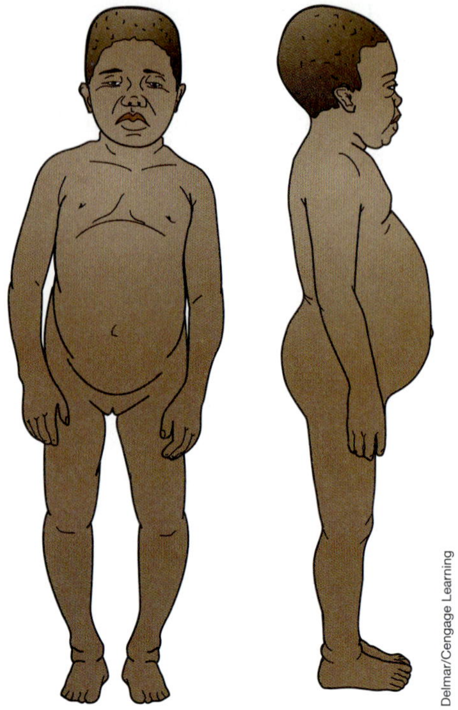

FIGURE 14–6 Cretinism.

DIAGNOSIS. Diagnosis is confirmed by review of symptoms along with thyroid hormone blood test, including T_4, T_3, and free T_4 index (FTI).

TREATMENT. This condition responds well to treatment with thyroxine hormone replacement. Symptoms usually disappear after a few months of treatment.

PREVENTION. Most cases of hypothyroidism in the United States are caused by Hashimoto's thyroiditis and cannot be prevented.

Parathyroid Gland Diseases

Parathyroid glands regulate blood calcium levels. Most of the body's calcium (approximately 99%) is stored in the bones, but the remaining 1% circulates in the blood. Blood calcium plays a vital role in blood clotting and muscle contraction, thus affecting heart function. If blood calcium levels drop, parathyroid hormone (parathormone, PTH) increases the level by increasing calcium absorption in the digestive tract, releasing calcium from bone stores, and saving calcium excretion in urine. When blood calcium levels are restored to normal, parathormone is no longer released. Like other endocrine glands, most endocrine diseases of the parathyroid are related to hypersecretion or hyposecretion.

HYPERPARATHYROIDISM

DESCRIPTION. Hyperparathyroidism is a condition of overproduction of parathormone by one or more of the four parathyroid glands.

ETIOLOGY. Oversecretion is usually due to a glandular tumor or idiopathic hyperplasia of the gland. Excessive parathormone production causes excessive blood calcium levels called hypercalcemia (hyper = excessive, calc = calcium, emia = blood).

SYMPTOMS. As previously discussed, this calcium is pulled from the bones, leading to bone weakness and spontaneous fractures. Hypercalcemia also leads to kidney stones because the urinary system—under the influence of parathormone—retains calcium, further increasing blood calcium levels. The digestive system increases absorption of calcium, leading to abdominal pain, vomiting, and constipation. Hypercalcemia also leads to hyperactivity of cardiac muscle, thus causing arrhythmias.

DIAGNOSIS. Blood tests for parathormone levels assist with diagnosis.

TREATMENT. Treatment of hyperparathyroidism is directed at the cause. Removal of a tumor or removal of the parathyroid glands might be necessary. Only half of one parathyroid gland is necessary to maintain normal parathormone levels. Other treatments include diuretics to increase urine output, thus forcing excretion of calcium, and limiting dietary intake of calcium. Prognosis is generally good with adequate treatment, although cardiac arrest can occur with severe hyperparathyroidism.

PREVENTION. There is no known way to prevent primary hyperparathyroidism.

HYPOPARATHYROIDISM

DESCRIPTION. Hypoparathyroidism is a decrease in the normal amount of parathormone secreted, which leads to abnormally low blood calcium levels.

ETIOLOGY. This condition is usually the result of surgical removal of all parathyroid glands in an effort to treat hyperparathyroidism or following a thyroidectomy.

■ ***SYMPTOMS.*** Low blood calcium levels (hypocalcemia) cause irritability to muscles, called **tetany**. Tetany should not be confused with the infectious disease tetanus (lockjaw). The tetany associated with hypoparathyroidism affects the face and hands primarily, causing uncontrolled contraction of these muscles. Testing for hypocalcemia and hypoparathyroidism involves checking for Chvostek's (VOHS-tecks) and Trousseau's (true-SOHs) signs (Figure 14–7).

■ ***DIAGNOSIS.*** Physical examination reviewing for symptoms, along with blood tests revealing low blood calcium level and low parathyroid hormone level, aid in diagnosis. X-rays for bone density might reveal weak bone structure related to abnormal calcium levels.

■ ***TREATMENT.*** Treatment with calcium and vitamin D, which controls absorption of calcium from the gastrointestinal tract, will cure the problem.

■ ***PREVENTION.*** There are no preventive measures for hypoparathyroidism.

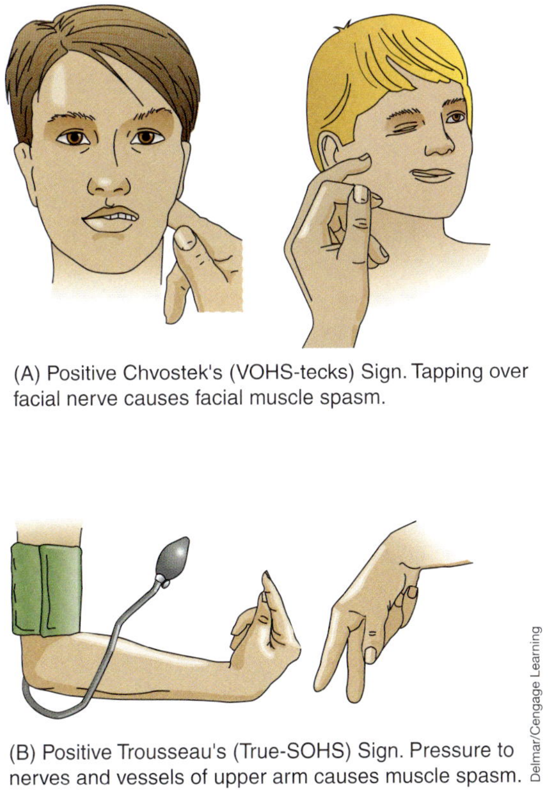

(A) Positive Chvostek's (VOHS-tecks) Sign. Tapping over facial nerve causes facial muscle spasm.

(B) Positive Trousseau's (True-SOHS) Sign. Pressure to nerves and vessels of upper arm causes muscle spasm.

Delmar/Cengage Learning

FIGURE 14–7 Tetany of the hand and face: (A) Chvostek's sign. (B) Trousseau's sign.

Adrenal Gland Diseases

The adrenal glands, also called the suprarenals because they sit atop the kidneys, have two distinct parts that function quite differently. The inner part, called the medulla, releases two hormones, epinephrine (adrenaline) and norepinephrine, when stimulated by the nervous system. These hormones have a direct effect on the vascular system and are known as fight-or-flight hormones. The cortex, or outer part of the adrenal gland, is controlled by the pituitary gland's release of ACTH. The adrenal cortex secretes several hormones.

- **Mineralocorticoids** The primary hormone is **aldosterone**, which regulates salt balance.
- **Glucocorticoids** The primary hormone is cortisol (**cortisone**), or **hydrocortisone**, which regulates carbohydrate metabolism.
- **Sex hormones** The primary ones are androgens and estrogens, which provide male and female characteristics, respectively. Males and females have both of these androgenic sex hormones.

Cortisone is a hormone frequently used to treat inflammatory diseases such as arthritis because it acts as an anti-inflammatory agent. Cortisone does not cure the inflammatory condition; it only relieves the inflammation and the associated pain. Prolonged use of cortisone is avoided whenever possible because it has some detrimental side effects including hypertension, ulcers, puffy face called moon face, and drowsiness. The anti-inflammatory properties of cortisone reduce the body's inflammatory response. This alteration in the immune system can mask the symptoms of an infection, allowing it to go unnoticed until it is in advanced stages. This side effect of prolonged cortisone use can be potentially life-threatening.

HYPERADRENALISM

Hyperadrenalism is the oversecretion of hormones by the adrenal cortex. The specific forms of hyperadrenalism depend on which hormones are secreted in excess. Three syndromes identified with hyperadrenalism are Conn's, Cushing's, and androgenital syndromes.

CONN'S SYNDROME

■ ***DESCRIPTION.*** Conn's, also called hyperaldosteronism, is due to an overproduction of aldosterone, a mineralocorticoid that plays an important role in maintaining blood volume pressure and electrolyte balance. It affects people between ages 30 and 50 and is more common in women than in men.

■ ***ETIOLOGY.*** This form of hyperadrenalism is most often due to an adrenal cortex tumor.

■ ***SYMPTOMS.*** Symptoms include hypokalemia (low potassium levels), alkalosis (increased blood pH), and hypertension.

■ ***DIAGNOSIS.*** Conn's should be suspected in those with hypertension that is resistant to standard treatment. Diagnosing Conn's is important because it represents a cause of hypertension that might be curable. Blood testing for the two hormones that play a role in stimulating aldosterone is helpful and includes aldosterone and rennin testing. Positive testing reveals high aldosterone and low rennin levels.

■ ***TREATMENT.*** Removal of the tumor usually leads to a good prognosis.

■ ***PREVENTION.*** There is no known prevention for most causes of hyperaldosteronism.

CUSHING'S SYNDROME

■ ***DESCRIPTION.*** Cushing's syndrome is due to an overproduction of the cortisol glucocorticoid.

■ ***ETIOLOGY.*** Cushing's might be caused by a tumor on the pituitary gland or on the adrenal cortex. Prolonged administration of large doses of glucocorticoid steroids (cortisone) will also cause this syndrome.

■ ***SYMPTOMS.*** Classic symptoms include a round, moon-shaped face and a buffalo hump on the upper back. Other symptoms include fatigue, weakness, poor wound healing, a rotund abdomen with pencil thin arms and legs, hypertension, and **striae** (stretch marks) on the skin (Figure 14–8).

■ ***DIAGNOSIS.*** Blood test to measure cortisol levels and MRI to view tumors aids in diagnosis.

■ ***TREATMENT.*** Surgical removal of the tumor or the adrenal cortex may correct the condition. Lifetime hormone therapy to replace this hormone is then needed. Cushing's syndrome may develop in individuals receiving long-term glucocorticoid steroids. These individuals need to be carefully monitored for symptoms of Cushing's syndrome.

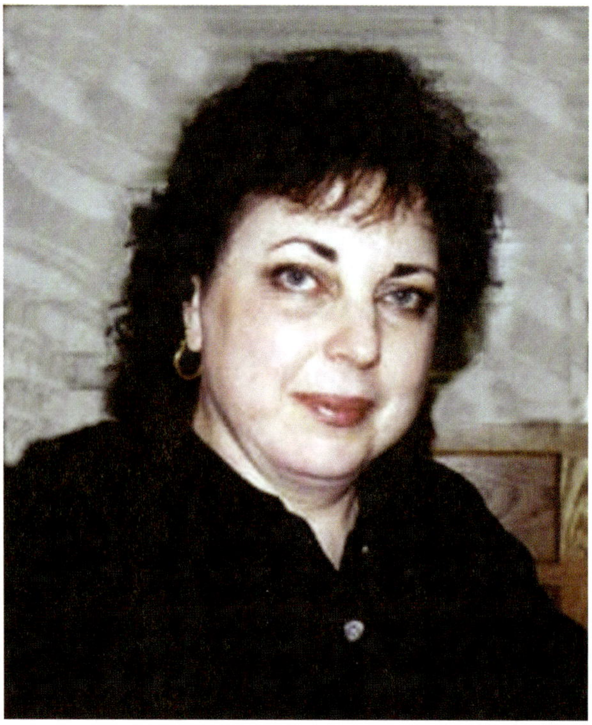

(A)

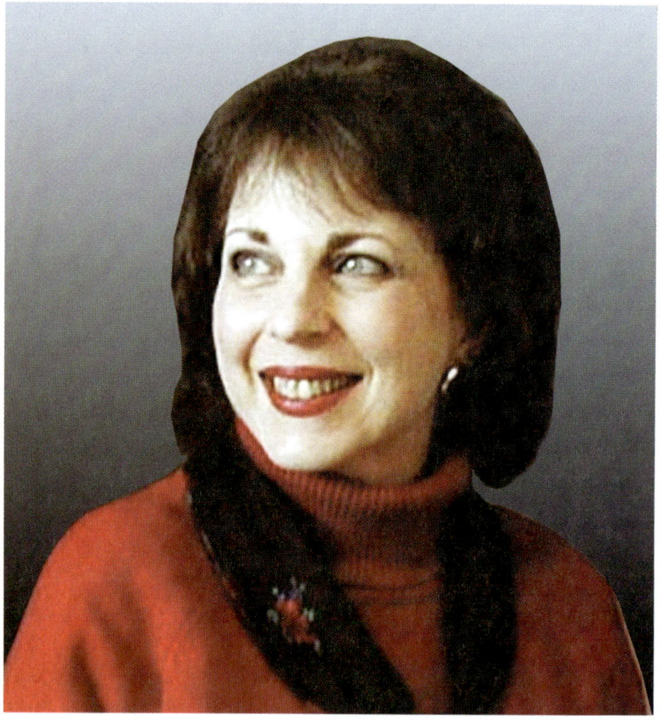

(B)

FIGURE 14–8 Cushing's syndrome. (A) Individual affected with Cushing's. (B) Same individual after treatment.

PREVENTABLE. Cushing's syndrome may be prevented by early detection and treatment of the associated symptomns.

ANDROGENITAL SYNDROME

DESCRIPTION. Androgenital syndrome is due to an overproduction of sex hormones by the adrenal cortex. It is also known as adrenal **virilism** (masculinization or feminization), depending on the excessive hormone.

ETIOLOGY. Androgenital syndrome is hereditary. Most of these conditions involve excessive, or hypersecretion of, androgen.

SYMPTOMS. Increased androgen leads to premature sexual development in male children, also called **precocious** (early development) puberty. In female children, overproduction of androgen leads to excessive hair growth on the legs, chest, and abdomen; an enlarged clitoris; a deepened voice; and **amenorrhea** (ah-MEN-oh-REE-ah; a = without, menorrhea = menses).

If adrenal feminization occurs due to excessive estrogen production, female children experience premature sexual development (precocious puberty). Male children with an overproduction of estrogen experience **gynecomastia** (GUY-neh-koh-MAS-tee-ah; excessive breast development), testicular atrophy, and decreased libido.

Virilism in the adult female leads to symptoms of **hirsutism** (HER-soot-izm), or abnormal hair on the face and body; decreased breast size; and amenorrhea.

DIAGNOSIS. Physical exam of symptoms along with blood testing for elevated ACTH aids in diagnosis.

TREATMENT. Treatment of adrenal cortex tumors usually involves surgical removal of the tumor.

PREVENTION. Because this is a hereditary disease, it is not preventable.

OTHER DISEASE OF THE ADRENAL GLANDS

HYPOADRENALISM

DESCRIPTION. Hypoadrenalism, Addison's disease, is an uncommon undersecretion of hormones by the adrenal cortex.

ETIOLOGY. Causes of Addison's disease include an autoimmune disorder, tumor of the pituitary gland, tuberculosis, and prolonged steroid hormone therapy. As much as 90% of the adrenal cortex can be destroyed before hyposecretion occurs.

SYMPTOMS. Symptoms of Addison's disease can be mild to life-threatening. Lack of mineralocorticoids allows depletion of sodium, leading to diarrhea and dehydration. Deficiency in glucocorticoids affects blood sugar levels, leading to **hypoglycemia** (HIGH-poh-gly-SEE-me-ah; hypo = decreased, glyc = glucose, emia = blood). Increased ACTH levels by the pituitary lead to a hyperpigmentation, or increased skin coloring, ranging from yellow to dark brown. This increased skin color affects the palms, elbows, scars, and skin folds and the areola of the nipples.

DIAGNOSIS. Diagnosis is based on medical history, symptoms, physical examination, and blood tests, including cortisol and ACTH.

TREATMENT. Treatment includes a combination of glucocorticoids and mineralocorticoids to replace the adrenal insufficiency.

PREVENTION. There are no guidelines for preventing Addison's disease.

Pancreatic Islets of Langerhans Diseases

The pancreas is both an exocrine and endocrine gland. As an exocrine gland, it secretes digestive juices through ducts into the digestive system. As an endocrine gland, it secretes two hormones—insulin and glucagon—directly into the blood. Both of these hormones are secreted by specialized tissue called **islets of Langerhans** that are scattered throughout the pancreas; however, insulin and glucagon have an antagonistic relationship. Insulin lowers blood sugar, whereas glucagon raises it. The overall effect of these hormones maintains a normal blood sugar level (80–120 mg/dl).

When blood sugar levels rise, for instance after a meal, insulin is secreted. Insulin assists in moving sugar out of the blood and into the tissues, thus decreasing the blood sugar level (Figure 14–9). Without adequate insulin, the blood sugar level rises, and the tissues are depleted of sugar.

HEALTHY HIGHLIGHT

Using Steroids Therapeutically

- Anabolic steroids are synthetic derivatives of testosterone that have anabolic (tissue-building) effects. These drugs were initially used by athletes to increase strength and endurance, but because of their potential for abuse, steroids have been placed in the Controlled Substance Act in category C-III. General uses include treatment for chronic infections, some types of anemia, extensive burns, and severe trauma.
- Use of steroids to enhance athletic performance is not recommended and has been banned in professional athletics. Serious irreversible side effects occur with long-term use of steroids and include kidney damage, increased risk of liver tumors, and increased risk of heart disease. Long-term steroid users exhibit increased irritability and aggressive behavior. In women, masculinization occurs as evidenced by hirsutism, menstrual difficulties, male patterned baldness, and a deepening of the voice. Males experience a decrease in testosterone production, leading to testicular atrophy; decrease in sperm production; and impotence. Individuals taking steroids need to follow the following recommended guidelines:
    - A well-balanced diet, including adequate proteins and carbohydrates, should be followed during steroid therapy.
    - Never share steroid medications with others.
    - Do not stop taking these medications abruptly. A scheduled weaning regimen should be determined and monitored by a qualified physician.

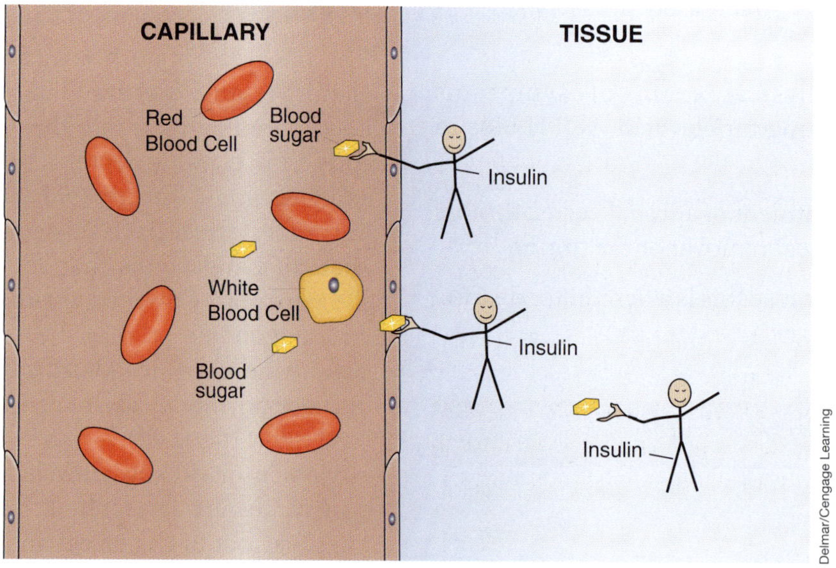

FIGURE 14–9 Effect of insulin on blood sugar. Insulin assists in moving sugar out of the blood and into the tissues, thus decreasing blood sugar levels. Think of insulin as "offering a hand" in pulling blood sugar levels down.

Sugar, or glucose, is the primary source of energy for all tissue cells. Without glucose, cells must burn fats and proteins for energy. When tissue cells burn fat and protein, they produce a waste product called **ketones**. Ketones are picked up by the blood to be filtered and excreted by the kidneys. Acetone, a part of this ketone waste, is excreted by the respiratory system, giving the affected individual a fruity or sweet-smelling breath. This condition of having ketones in the blood, breath, and urine is called ketosis. Chemically, a large part of ketones is acidic in nature, which leads to metabolic acidosis, or a low pH, in the body tissues. For this reason, ketosis is often called **ketoacidosis**.

When carbohydrates or sugars are eaten, the extra sugar, the amount not needed for immediate energy, is stored, primarily, in the liver as **glycogen**. If blood sugar levels drop, for instance during exercise, the pancreas secretes glucagon. Glucagon circulates in the blood and stimulates the liver to release glycogen in the form of glucose, thus raising the blood sugar to normal.

DIABETES MELLITUS (DM)

■ ***DESCRIPTION.*** DM, commonly known simply as diabetes, is the most common major disease of the endocrine pancreas.

■ ***ETIOLOGY.*** DM is a chronic disease affecting carbohydrate, or sugar, metabolism due to inadequate production of insulin by the pancreatic islets of Langerhans.

■ ***SYMPTOMS.*** Diabetes is characterized by symptoms of polyuria (excessive urination), polydipsia (excessive thirst), and polyphagia (excessive eating). **Glycosuria** (GLYE-koh-SOO-ree-ah; glyco = glycogen or sugar, uria = urine), or the spilling of sugar in the urine, is also a common symptom. The excessive sugar in the blood, known as **hyperglycemia** (hyper = excessive, glyc = glycogen or glucose, emia = blood), causes the kidney to filter out part of the excess, resulting in glycosuria. Hyperglycemia indicates that sugar is not being pulled into the tissues, and cells are using fat for energy, resulting in the formation of ketones (the waste product of fat metabolism). Ketones can be found in the blood and urine and smelled on the breath.

There are two types of DM:

Type 1 formerly known as insulin-dependent diabetes mellitus (IDDM) or juvenile-onset diabetes. This form of diabetes is the most serious and usually occurs quite suddenly. It affects children and young adults before age 25 and requires daily injections of insulin. Insulin must be injected because digestive juices would destroy oral forms. Type 1 is thought to be caused by an autoimmune disorder. The tendency for the disease also is thought to be genetically inherited. The immune system, when triggered by a virus or some other stressor, develops antibodies and begins warring against the islets of Langerhans, thereby destroying the insulin-secreting cells. Affected individuals generally do not secrete any insulin, making regulation of blood glucose levels quite difficult. Individuals with Type 1 must follow a strict diet, monitor blood sugar levels on a regular basis, and administer the needed amounts of insulin. Exercise and stress can alter insulin needs and must be considered as part of the treatment plan.

Type 2 formerly known as noninsulin-dependent diabetes mellitus (NIDDM) or adult onset-diabetes. This is the more common form of DM. Until recently, this type of diabetes was seen primarily in obese females over age 40, but due to the dramatic increase in childhood and adolescent obesity, the trend is changing. Obesity has led to a dramatic increase in the incidence of Type 2 diabetes among children and adolescents over the past two decades. The Centers for Disease Control and Prevention (2007) reports that, from the mid-1970s to mid-1990s, overweight children aged 2–5 increased from 5% to 13.9%; those overweight aged 6–11 increased from 6.5% to 18.8%; and those overweight aged 12–19 increased from 5% to 17.4%. These drastic increases raise concern about the future of Americans' health. It is well known that obesity increases the risk of many diseases, including Type 2 diabetes.

This form of diabetes is thought to be due to a wearing out of the pancreatic islets of Langerhans. It is believed that excessive carbohydrate consumption over the life of the individual places such a heavy demand on the pancreas to produce the needed insulin. This increased demand literally wears out the pancreatic cells, leading to Type 2 diabetes. Insulin injections are rarely needed because Type 2 is usually controlled with diet, exercise, and oral medications that stimulate insulin secretion.

Complications of DM may be classified as immediate or long term. Immediate and life-threatening complications of Type 1 diabetes include diabetic coma and insulin shock. Both of these complications occur as a result of improper insulin administration, either too much or not enough insulin. Diabetic coma can occur as a result of not administering enough insulin or taking in too many carbohydrates in the diet. Symptoms of diabetic coma are those related to hyperglycemia and include polyuria, polydipsia, dehydration, and ketoacidosis. Diabetic coma usually progresses rather slowly. The affected individual becomes lethargic and, if untreated, slips into a coma. The individual in a coma will have a slow deep-breathing pattern and fruity or sweet-smelling breath. They require emergency medical treatment with insulin and intravenous fluids.

Insulin shock occurs quite rapidly and is the result of taking too much insulin, not eating enough food, or participating in excessive exercise. The affected individual becomes hypoglycemic with symptoms of diaphoresis (sweating), light-headedness, and trembling. Without treatment, the affected individual progresses quite rapidly into a state of confusion followed by coma. Individuals in insulin shock need immediate emergency medical treatment with intravenous glucose to raise blood sugar levels (Table 14–2).

Long-term complications of diabetes usually appear gradually after many years. With improper carbohydrate metabolism, **lipids** or fats are pulled into the bloodstream for cellular energy. This increase in lipids in the vascular system leads to atherosclerosis.

Atherosclerosis leads to a variety of complications, including myocardial infarction, cerebrovascular accidents or strokes, and peripheral vascular disease. The poor circulation caused by peripheral vascular disease is the cause of diabetic gangrene in the feet and legs, which can lead to amputation, and poor wound healing.

Atherosclerosis also affects the vessels of the eyes and kidneys. The retinas of the eyes become damaged, causing **diabetic retinopathy** (retino = retina, opathy = disease) and leading to blindness. Damage to the kidney leads to kidney failure, a frequent cause of death in individuals affected with diabetes.

■ ***DIAGNOSIS.*** Diagnosis is confirmed by a positive history of symptoms along with blood glucose testing.

■ ***TREATMENT.*** Diabetes cannot be cured. Management of the disease is dependent on education and a lifetime commitment to following the treatment regimen of diet, medication, and exercise. Frequently monitoring blood glucose levels and controlling these is beneficial in avoiding long-term complications.

TABLE 14–2 Emergency Treatment of Diabetic Coma or Insulin Shock

Step 1: Determine a Need for Intervention
Unfortunately, it is usually difficult to determine whether an affected individual is suffering from diabetic coma or insulin shock, especially if found in a comatose state. The best rule to follow in this case is, "when in doubt—sugar." Raising an already elevated glucose level is not as life-threatening as allowing the blood sugar level to remain low or to drop even further.
Step 2: Administer Glucose
If the individual is still alert, drinking fruit juice with sugar added can be effective in raising blood sugar level. If juice is not available, candy of any type will help. If the individual is unconscious and emergency medical assistance is not available, turn the individual on his or her side and place table sugar or hard candy in the lower cheek of the mouth to help raise blood sugar. Emergency medical assistance should be sought immediately.
Additional Important Information
Diabetics should wear a diabetic alert tag and should carry some type of carbohydrate treat with them at all times for use during a hypoglycemic reaction. If an incident occurs, the tag alerts the medical responder or other individuals aiding the person that he or she is diabetic and, thus, could be having a hypoglycemic or hyperglycemic reaction. This saves time between assessing the victim for probable cause of the problem and treating the person. The diabetic alert tag also helps those who are assisting the individual to recognize the fruity breath of a hyperglycemic diabetic as ketone breath rather than mistaking it as alcohol breath. Allowing a hyperglycemic individual to sleep it off can be a fatal mistake.

The American Diabetes Association recognizes HbA1C testing as a standard in medical care of diabetes. This is a test that measures glycosylated hemoglobin in the blood and is a good indicator of diabetes management.

Glycosated hemoglobin is formed when the hemoglobin component of the blood is exposed to high glucose levels. Once the hemoglobin is glycosated it remains that way for the duration of the red blood cells' 2- to 3-month life. A high level of glycosated hemoglobin indicates that the blood glucose levels of the individual have been high during the previous 2 to 3 months.

The higher the HbA1C, the greater the risk of developing complications such as eye disease, kidney disease, nerve damage, heart disease, and stroke. This is especially true if the HbA1C level remains high for long periods of time.

The closer the HbA1C is to normal, the lower the risk for complications. A normal HbA1C is 5% or less. Results above 7% indicate that diabetes is poorly controlled. Managing blood glucose levels and bringing the HbA1C level down decreases the risk of long-term complications. Testing is recommended every 3 to 6 months.

■ ***PREVENTION.*** Type 1 diabetes has a hereditary etiology and cannot be prevented. Research has demonstrated that people at risk for type 2 diabetes can prevent or delay developing type 2 diabetes by losing weight and exercising.

GESTATIONAL DIABETES

■ ***DESCRIPTION.*** Gestational diabetes is a type of diabetes that occurs only during pregnancy. It is usually short-lived, with blood sugar levels returning to normal soon after delivery.

■ ***ETIOLOGY.*** During pregnancy, the placenta produces estrogen and progesterone to maintain pregnancy. These hormones make the body cells more resistant to insulin. The mother's pancreas usually produces more insulin to overcome this resistance. As the placenta grows, more hormones are produced, placing more demand on the pancreas. If the pancreas reaches a point at which it cannot produce enough insulin to meet the need, less glucose moves into the body cells, and blood glucose levels rise. The developing fetus is also affected by the hyperglycemia and is usually overweight at birth.

■ ***SYMPTOMS.*** The condition can present the same symptoms as DM or be asymptomatic.

■ ***DIAGNOSIS.*** This type of diabetes is usually discovered with routine urine testing during prenatal visits. It is important to discover this condition and treat it because, otherwise, it can lead to fetal or neonatal mortality.

■ ***TREATMENT.*** Gestational diabetes is treated, like DM, with exercise, dietary control of carbohydrate intake, and medications. Injectable insulin might be needed to control blood sugar levels. Oral hypoglycemic medications are contraindicated because these pass across the placenta and can lead to fetal birth defects or hypoglycemia. Gestational diabetes usually disappears after delivery. If this condition does not disappear after delivery, the affected individual will need to continue diabetic management. Women affected with gestational diabetes are often affected later in life by adult-onset diabetes.

■ ***PREVENTION.*** There is no absolute prevention, but those who observe a healthy lifestyle and a normal weight at conception are at less risk of developing the condition.

GLIMPSE OF THE FUTURE

Using Vitamin D to Prevent Diabetes Mellitus

A link has been found between vitamin D deficiency and the body's ability to metabolize glucose and insulin. Researchers have stated vitamin D may stimulate insulin secretion and may affect the action of insulin on glucose. Further research and clinical trials still need to be completed to confirm the biological effect of this association. Although the relationship of vitamin D to insulin and glucose metabolism is still being investigated, in the future, vitamin D may be given to persons who are deficient to help prevent DM.

Source: Tai, et al. (2008).

COMPLEMENTARY AND ALTERNATIVE THERAPY

Alternative Therapy for Type 2 Diabetes

Complementary and alternative therapies have been used in many populations for treatment of DM. *Clerodendrum capitatum* (CC) is a traditional African therapy for Type 2 diabetes. A recent study has looked at the glucose-lowering effects of an extract of the plant. In this study, rats were used to observe the effect of CC. The results revealed there was a glucose-lowering effect of the herbal preparation, but it did not affect the weight gain of the rats. The study also found that CC contained flavonoids (antioxidants), alkaloids, tannin, glycosides, and reducing sugars. The researchers reported there is some evidence that CC used in traditional folk medicine has a positive effect in the treatment of Type 2 diabetes.

Source: Adeneye, et al. (2008).

HYPOGLYCEMIA

■ **DESCRIPTION.** Hypoglycemia (HIGH-poh-gly-SEE-me-ah; hypo = decreased, glyc = glucose, emia = blood) is an abnormally low blood sugar. Hypoglycemia occurs whenever the blood glucose level drops below 60 mg/dl, although individuals can become symptomatic at different blood glucose levels. Some individuals tolerate unusually low blood glucose levels, whereas others do not.

■ **ETIOLOGY.** Some common causes of hypoglycemia are fasting, skipping meals, and excessive exercise. Hypoglycemia is also caused by administration of too much insulin, as previously discussed. Other causes of hypoglycemia include pancreatic adenoma, gastrointestinal disorders, and some hereditary disorders.

■ **SYMPTOMS.** Symptoms are the same as previously discussed for diabetes and include light-headedness, diaphoresis, and trembling. If untreated, symptoms can progress to include mental confusion and coma. Most individuals have had an episode of hypoglycemia at one time or another.

■ **DIAGNOSIS.** Physical examination to observe symptoms, along with blood glucose testing, aid in the diagnosis. A blood glucose level of less than 70 mg/dL at the time of symptoms and relief after eating confirm the diagnosis.

■ **TREATMENT.** Treatment of hypoglycemia is dependent on cause. Diabetics should carry glucose tablets or candy to take at the first sign of hypoglycemia. Acute hypoglycemia needs immediate emergency treatment with intravenous glucose administration.

■ **PREVENTION.** Preventive measures include eating a well-balanced diet, eating small meals often, keeping snacks available, avoiding sugary foods on an empty stomach, avoiding drinking alcohol on an empty stomach, keeping body weight at a healthy level, not smoking, and maintaining an exercise program.

Reproductive Gland Diseases

Sexual development can be affected by the release of androgens from the adrenal cortex, as previously discussed; by the pituitary; and by the sex organ (**gonad**). The male gonad is the testis, and the female gonad is the ovary. Gonads function as endocrine glands in the production of hormones, and the pituitary controls the function of the gonads by releasing gonadotropin. Gonadotropin stimulates the testes to produce the male hormone, testosterone, and the ovaries to produce the female hormone, estrogen. Dysfunction of the pituitary or the gonad can lead to endocrine disorders.

HYPERGONADISM

■ **DESCRIPTION.** Hypergonadism is the condition of increased hormone production before puberty, which produces precocious sexual development in both sexes.

■ ***ETIOLOGY.*** Causes of hypergonadism include unknown causes, testicular tumors, and pituitary tumors. Hypergonadism in females is primarily due to idiopathic causes. Uncommon causes include ovarian and adrenal tumors.

■ ***SYMPTOMS.*** In the male, onset of puberty usually occurs around age 13; with hypergonadism, this development occurs before age 10. Signs of precocious sexual development in the male include the growth of a beard and pubic hair and enlargement of the penis and testes. Spermatogenesis occurs, rendering the individual fertile. Rapid growth of muscle and bone leads to early uniting of the epiphyses and a premature stoppage of growth in the long bones.

In the female, onset of puberty usually occurs around age 10; with hypergonadism, this development occurs before age 8. Signs of precocious sexual development in the female include onset of menarche, appearance of pubic and underarm hair, and breast enlargement. Ovarian development renders the individual fertile, making pregnancy possible.

■ ***DIAGNOSIS.*** Diagnosis of hypergonadism is confirmed by positive clinical history and blood testing for evidence of elevated sex hormones.

■ ***TREATMENT.*** Treatment for both sexes involves removal or radiation of tumors and administration of hormones to suppress or counteract the sex hormone.

■ ***PREVENTION.*** There is no known prevention for hypergonadism.

HYPOGONADISM

■ ***DESCRIPTION.*** Hypogonadism is the condition of decreased sex hormone production by the age of normal puberty.

■ ***ETIOLOGY.*** In the male, causes of hypogonadism include dysfunctional testes, undescended testes, or loss of the testes due to castration. Testes also might fail to develop due to a pituitary disorder, resulting in the lack of gonadotropin. In the female, causes of hypogonadism include missing or dysfunctional ovaries.

■ ***SYMPTOMS.*** Loss of the male gonads before puberty causes eunuchism, or the lack of development of sex characteristics, because male characteristics are brought about by testosterone. Castration in the adult male will lead to a decrease in libido, but masculinity is maintained.

Without estrogen, female sex characteristics do not develop. Female children become abnormally tall because the long bones do not fuse normally without estrogen.

■ ***DIAGNOSIS.*** Hormone testing for males includes testosterone, thyroid level, and sperm count. For females, hormone testing of estrogen, FSH, LH, prolactin, thyroid, and anemia aid in diagnosis. If pituitary disease is suspected, an MRI or CT scan of the brain might be needed.

■ ***TREATMENT.*** Administration of testosterone is quite effective in treating hypogonadism in the male, and administration of estrogen is quite effective in treating hypogonadism in the female.

■ ***PREVENTION.*** Most cases cannot be prevented, but maintaining a healthy body weight and lifestyle might aid in prevention.

TRAUMA

Head injury can lead to multiple-organ dysfunction if the pituitary is involved. Hypersecretion and hyposecretion can occur with injury to any of the individual organs. Organ destruction and failure can be life-threatening when the pituitary, pancreas, and adrenal glands are all involved.

RARE DISEASES

Most previously discussed diseases of the endocrine system are relatively uncommon, with the exception of thyroid problems and DM. Other extremely rare endocrine disorders can be found in children or young adults, however. Cancer of most of the glands of the endocrine system is also somewhat rare, although the thyroid, ovaries, and testes are the most common sites for cancer development.

EFFECTS OF AGING ON THE SYSTEM

As the individual ages, changes occur in the endocrine glands. Decreases in the secretions from the glands alter the body's ability to respond to stressors, diseases, and other changes that occur from aging.

The older adult is at high risk for hypoglycemic reactions and excessive fluid loss due to reduced levels of glucocorticoids and aldosterone. Digestive and metabolism problems are common due to reduced secretions of pancreatic and thyroid hormones. The secretions from the gonads are reduced, resulting in changes in secondary sex characteristics. Because glucose tolerance lessens with age, the serum glucose levels tend to be higher in the older adult. DM is common in the older population but usually can be regulated by dietary adjustments. With all the other changes that occur during the aging process, diabetes becomes a very serious condition, adversely affecting many systems.

SUMMARY

The endocrine system is a complex system of many glands located throughout the body. Each of the glands has a unique function and delivers its hormones into the bloodstream. The hormones help the body's growth, regulation, and metabolism. Overproduction or underproduction of any one gland can cause dysfunction in other systems. If the gland malfunctions in childhood, the result is a different disorder than if the gland malfunctions in adulthood. The most common endocrine disorder overall is DM. Although, historically, Type 2 diabetes was most commonly found in middle-aged or older adults, it is now frequently diagnosed in younger populations and is related to the increasing rate of obesity in the population. The older adult with an endocrine disorder is at risk for other systemic problems. Secretions from the endocrine glands decrease slowly with age.

REVIEW QUESTIONS

Short answer

1. What are the functions of the endocrine system?

2. Which signs and symptoms are associated with common endocrine system disorders?

3. Which diagnostic tests are most commonly used to determine the type and cause of endocrine system disorders?

Multiple Choice

4. Which of the following is not an endocrine gland?
   a. Pituitary
   b. Adrenal
   c. Liver
   d. Ovaries

5. What function does the somatotropin hormone perform?
   a. Promotes absorption of calcium in the bones
   b. Stimulates the thyroid to produce its hormones
   c. Stimulates growth
   d. Promotes development of sex characteristics

6. Acromegaly is defined as which of the following?
   a. An overgrowth of the long bones of the body
   b. An abnormal decrease in the activity of the pituitary gland
   c. A tumor located in the anterior pituitary
   d. A chronic disorder characterized by large feet, hands, and facial bones

7. Cretinism is defined as which of the following?
   a. Congenital hypothyroidism
   b. Congenital hypopituitarism
   c. Severe chronic lack of growth hormone
   d. An impaired growth of all body parts

8. Hypoadrenalism is also known as which of the following disorders?
   a. Acromegaly
   b. Myxedema
   c. Cushing's syndrome
   d. Addison's disease

9. In Type 1 DM, the individual needs replacement of which of the following?
   a. Steroids
   b. Antidiuretic hormone
   c. Insulin
   d. Estrogen

10. The individual affected by Type 2 DM can usually control the disorder by:
    a. Insulin injections
    b. Diet and oral medications
    c. Replacement hormones
    d. Steroid therapy

Matching

11. Match the hormone in the left column with its gland in the right column. Some glands may be used more than once.

_____ ACTH	a. anterior pituitary
_____ T_3	b. posterior pituitary
_____ Oxytocin	c. pineal
_____ Mineralocorticoids	d. thyroid
_____ Melatonin	e. adrenals
_____ Estrogen	f. testes or ovaries
_____ Insulin	g. pancreatic islets
_____ Norepinephrine	
_____ ADH	
_____ Calcitonin	

CASE STUDIES

■ Ms. Jenson is a young woman who routinely uses a variety of herbal products to treat and prevent diseases. She knows there is a strong history of Type 2 diabetes in her family and has read on the Internet about using vitamin D to prevent diabetes. She asks you whether you think that would work for her. What should you tell her? Do you think it is a good option for her? What has the research shown about vitamin D as a preventive treatment for diabetes? Where could she find evidence-based information about this?

■ Mrs. Webb is 78 years old and has been hospitalized frequently for repeated respiratory infections. Until the past 2 years, she has been relatively healthy. She has not been diagnosed with any serious chronic diseases but does have some osteoporosis. Based on your knowledge of the aging process and the endocrine system changes, what might be contributing to the development of these repeated respiratory infections? What can she do to decrease her risk and improve her immunity to infections?

*Study*WARE™ Connection

To help you learn the content in this chapter, take a practice quiz or play an interactive game on your StudyWARE™ CD-ROM.

Workbook Practice

Go to your Workbook and complete the practice questions.

BIBLIOGRAPHY

Adeneye, A. A, Adeleke, T., & Adeneye, A. K. (2008). Hypoglycemic and hypolipidemic effects of the aqueous fresh leaves extract of *Clerodendrum capitatum* in Wistar rats. *Journal of Ethnopharmacology 116*(1), 7–10.

Aldiss, S. (2008), Research digest. *Paediatric Nursing 20*(1), 9.

Al-Hussein, F. (2008). A tale of two audits: Statistical process control for improving diabetes care in primary care settings. *Quality in Primary Care 16*(1), 53–60.

American Diabetes Association. (2007). Standards of medical care in diabetes: 2007. *Diabetes Care 30*(Suppl. 1): S4–S41.

American Diabetes Association. (2008). *www.diabetes.org* (accessed June 2008).

Aschenbrenner, D. (2008). Revisions to the labeling of erectile dysfunction and diabetes drugs. *American Journal of Nursing 108*(2), 79.

Canderelli, R., Lecesse, L., Miller, N., & Unruh, J. (2007). Benefits of hormone replacement therapy in postmenopausal women. *Journal of the American Academy of Nurse Practitioners 19*(12), 635–641.

Carey, J. (February 7, 2008). Surprising new diabetes data. *Business Week Online www.businessweek.com*, 10, (accessed June 2008)

Centers for Disease Control and Prevention. (2007). Overweight and obesity. Centers for Disease Control and Prevention. *www.cdc.gov* (accessed May 2008).

Chalmers, J., Joshi, R., & Patel, A. (2008). Advances in reducing the burden of vascular disease in type 2 diabetes. *Clinical & Experimental Pharmacology & Physiology 35*(4), 434–437.

Dominguez, L., Bevilacqua, M., DiBella, G., & Barbagallo, M. (2008). Diagnosing and managing thyroid disease in the nursing home. *Journal of the American Medical Directors Association 9*(1), 9–17.

Fraser, M., Cuerrier, A., Haddad, P., Arnason, J., Owen, P., & Johns, T. (2007). Medicinal plants of Cree communities (Quebec, Canada): Antioxidant activity of plants used to treat type 2 diabetes. *Canadian Journal of Physiology & Pharmacology 85*(11), 1200–1214.

Geerlings, S. (2008). Urinary tract infections with diabetes mellitus: Epidemiology, pathogenesis and treatment. *International Journal of Antimicrobial Agents 31*(Supplement 1), 54–57.

Goel, A., Kunnumakkara, A., & Aggarwal, B. (2008). Curcumin as "curecumin": From kitchen to clinic. *Biochemical Pharmacology 75*(4), 787–809.

Hatcher, E., & Whitmore, R. (2007). Hispanic adults' beliefs about type 2 diabetes: Clinical implications. *Journal of the American Academy of Nurse Practitioners 19*(10), 536–545.

Klein, G., Jaekyung, K., Himmeldirk, K., Yanyan, C., & Xiaozhuo, C. (2007). Antidiabetes and anti-obesity activity of *Langerstroemia speciosa. Evidence-Based Complimentary & Alternative Medicine 4*(4), 401–407.

Kuger, D., & Kulkarni, K. (2007). Insulin treatment of patients with diabetes and the problem of weight gain. *Internet Journal of Advanced Nursing Practice 9*(1), 2.

Levine, A., & Brennan, A. (2007). Rethinking sliding-scale insulin. *American Journal of Nursing 107*(10), 74–79.

Lifestyle interventions as effective as drug treatment in preventing onset of type 2 diabetes. (2007). *Journal of Cardiovascular Nursing 22*(6), 426.

Milar, B. (2006). A little learning. *Nursing Standard 20*(37), 20–22.

Moore, A. (2008). Taking control. *Nursing Standard 22*(23), 24–25.

Older drugs are as good as new. (2007). *Nursing 37*(10), 30.

Palmer, D., & Luther, B. (2007). Screening for metabolic syndrome. *Orthopaedic Nursing 26*(5), 293–295.

Quillen, T. (2006). About multiple endocrine neoplasia type 1. *Nursing 36*(5), 31.

Shomon, M. (2008). Smoking and thyroid disease. Thyroid-Info. *www.thyroid-info.com* (accessed June 2008).

Solan, J., & McKiernan, J. (2007). Thyroidectomy: The ambulatory nurse's role in preventing long-term sequelae. *Oncology Nursing Forum 34*(2), 515.

Standardizing HbA1C reporting. (2007). *Nursing 37*(12), 33.

Sternberg, S. (February 7, 2008). Blood sugar study in diabetes halted. *USA Today* News Section, 1.

Tai, K., Need, A., Horowitz, M., & Chapman, I. (2008). Vitamin D, glucose, insulin, and insulin sensitivity. *Nutrition 24*(3), 279–285.

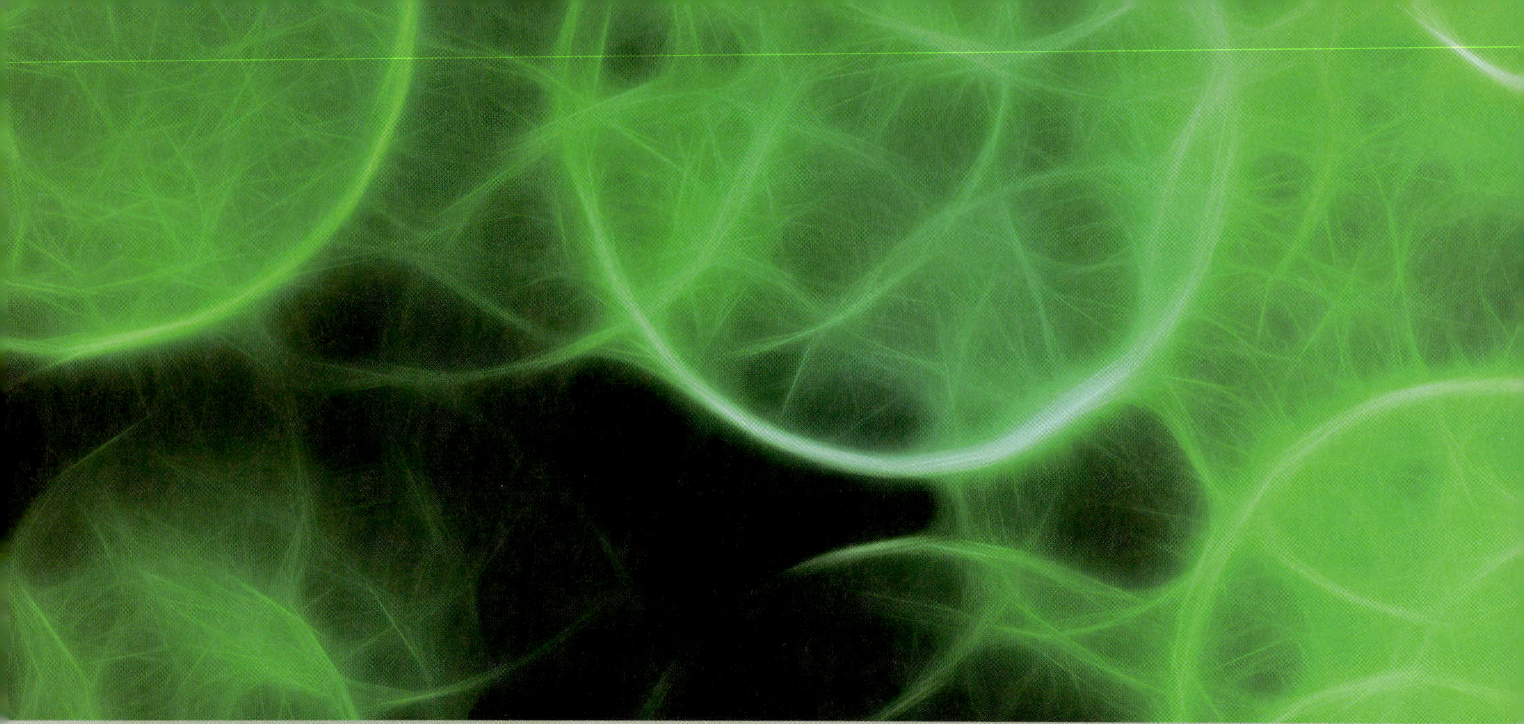

OUTLINE

- Anatomy and Physiology
  - *The Central Nervous System*
  - *The Peripheral Nervous System*
- Common Signs and Symptoms
- Diagnostic Tests
- Common Diseases of the Nervous Systm
  - *Infectious Diseases*
  - *Vascular Disorders*
  - *Functional Disorders*
  - *Dementias*
  - *Sleep Disorders*
  - *Tumors*
- Trauma
  - *Concussions and Contusions*
  - *Skull Fractures*
  - *Epidural and Subdural Hematomas*
  - *Spinal Cord Injury: Quadriplegia and Paraplegia*
- Rare Diseases
  - *Amyotrophic Lateral Sclerosis*
  - *Guillain-Barré Syndrome*
  - *Huntington's Chorea*
  - *Multiple Sclerosis*
- Effects of Aging on the System
- Summary
- Review Questions
- Case Studies
- Bibliography

KEY TERMS

Amnesia (p. 321)
Aura (p. 314)
Carotid endarterectomy (p. 312)
Cauterization (p. 323)
Cephalalgia (p. 313)
Chorea (p. 326)
Convulsion (p. 315)
Decompress (p. 324)
Dysphagia (p. 311)
Dysphasia (p. 311)
Epidural (p. 323)
Grand mal (p. 315)
Hemiparesis (p. 311)
Hydrophobia (p. 309)
Hypothermia (p. 324)
Intractable (p. 313)
Nuchal rigidity (p. 308)
Paraplegia (p. 324)
Paresthesia (p. 326)
Petit mal (p. 315)
Quadriplegia (p. 324)
Seizure (p. 315)
Spinal stenosis (p. 313)
Status epilepticus (p. 315)
Subdural (p. 323)

15

Nervous System Diseases and Disorders

LEARNING OBJECTIVES

Upon completion of the chapter, the learner should be able to:

1. Define the terminology common to the nervous system and the disorders of the system.
2. Discuss the basic anatomy and physiology of the nervous system.
3. Identify the important signs and symptoms associated with common nervous system disorders.
4. Describe the common diagnostics used to determine the type and cause of nervous system disorders.
5. Identify common disorders of the nervous system.
6. Describe the typical course and management of the common nervous system disorders.
7. Describe the effects of aging on the nervous system and the common disorders associated with aging of the system.

OVERVIEW

The nervous system is a complex network that provides communication from the brain to the rest of the body and from the body back to the brain. It facilitates the individual's ability to reason, interact with other individuals, understand complex ideas, and respond both intellectually and physically. Disorders of the system can affect any or all other normal functioning in the individual. Because brain and spinal cord injury often causes irreversible damage, the individual with a nervous system disorder can become a victim of severe, permanent, neurological deficits. ■

ANATOMY AND PHYSIOLOGY

The nervous system is composed of the brain, spinal cord, and nerves (Figure 15–1). It is divided into the central nervous system (CNS) and the peripheral nervous system (PNS). The CNS includes the brain and the spinal cord. The PNS includes the autonomic nervous system (ANS), the cranial nerves, and the spinal nerves. The CNS communicates with organs and other body systems through the PNS.

The Central Nervous System

The brain is a complex structure located within the protective covering of the skull. It is divided into the cerebrum, cerebellum, and brain stem. The cerebrum is divided into two hemispheres that can be further subdivided into lobes. Each of these lobes has a specialized function (Figure 15–2). The basal ganglia, called the gray matter, is located deep in the hemispheres. Another part of the cerebrum is called the diencephalon. This is where the hypothalamus and thalamus are located. They are active in controlling the body's sleep–wake pattern and are involved in the actions of the pituitary gland. (See Chapter 14, "Endocrine System Diseases and Disorders," for more information.)

The cerebellum, important in coordination and fine motor movements, is located in the lower back part of the brain.

The brainstem makes up the last part of the brain. It is subdivided into the midbrain, pons, and medulla; contains some nerves; and is responsible for

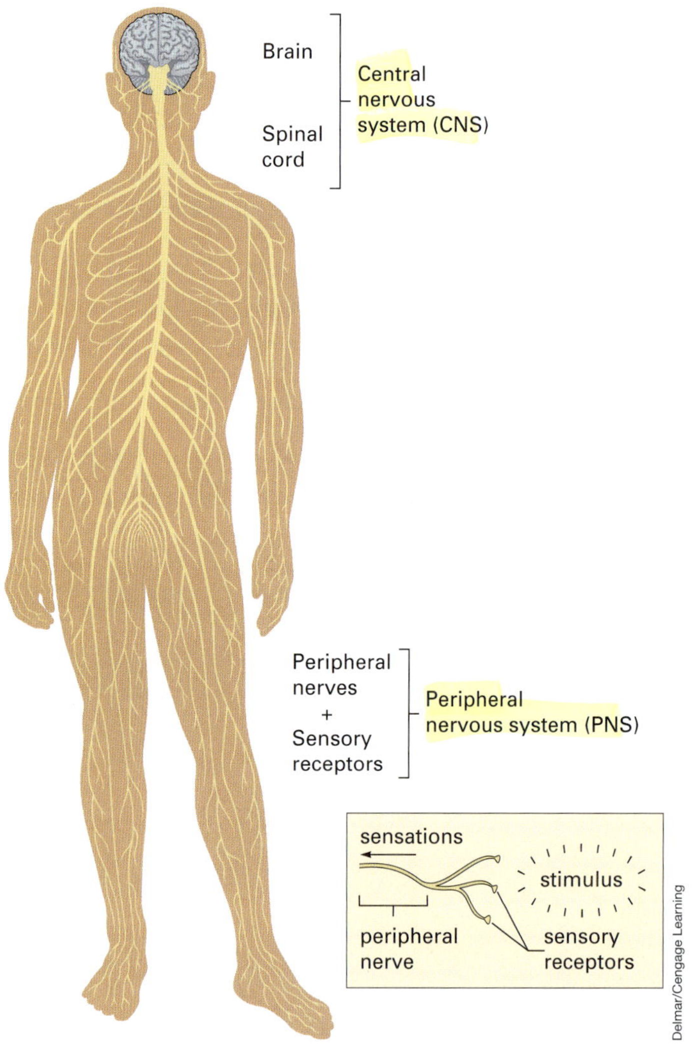

FIGURE 15–1 The nervous system.

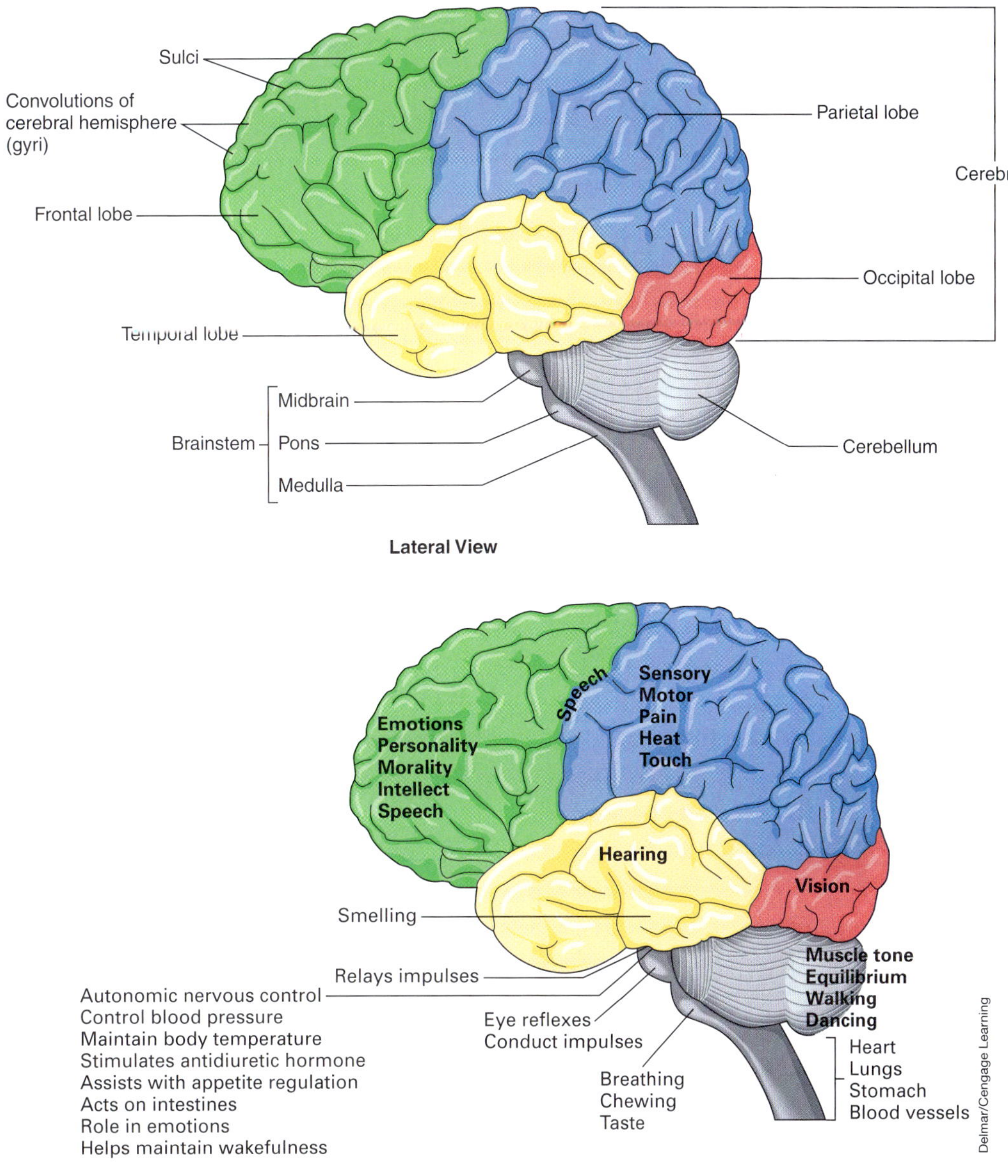

FIGURE 15–2 The cerebral lobes and their specialized functions.

transmitting impulses that control respiration, swallowing, wakefulness, and other activities.

The spinal cord is a continuous structure running through the vertebral column from the medulla to the tailbone. The spinal cord is composed of both white and gray matter. It has ascending and descending pathways that transmit impulses. Sensory impulses (pain, temperature, and touch) travel from the spinal cord to the brain. Motor impulses (for movement of muscles) travel from the brain to the spinal cord.

The meninges are membranes that cover the brain and spinal cord. The meninges are divided into three layers: the dura mater (outer cover), the arachnoid (middle layer), and the pia mater (inner layer). They provide both protection and support for the system.

The Peripheral Nervous System

The ANS controls the functions of the body's organs, and innervates smooth muscle and cardiac muscle. It is divided into the parasympathetic and sympathetic systems. The parasympathetic system controls the changes in the body needed to relax and restore function, such as returning blood pressure to normal after it has increased in response to some need. The sympathetic system controls the changes in the

TABLE 15–1 The Cranial Nerves

Cranial Nerve	Function
I. Olfactory	Smell
II. Optic	Sight
III. Oculomotor	Movement of the eyeball, pupil, and eyelid
IV. Trochlear	Movement of the eyeball
V. Trigeminal	Chewing; pain, temperature, and touch of face and mouth
VI. Abducens	Movement of the eyeball
VII. Facial	Movement of the face and secretion of saliva; taste
VIII. Auditory	Hearing and balance
IX. Glossopharyngeal	Swallowing and secretion of saliva; taste and sensation in the mouth and pharynx
X. Vagus	Sensation and movement in the pharynx, larynx, thorax, and gastrointestinal system
XI. Accessory	Movement of the head and shoulders
XII. Hypoglossal	Movement of the tongue

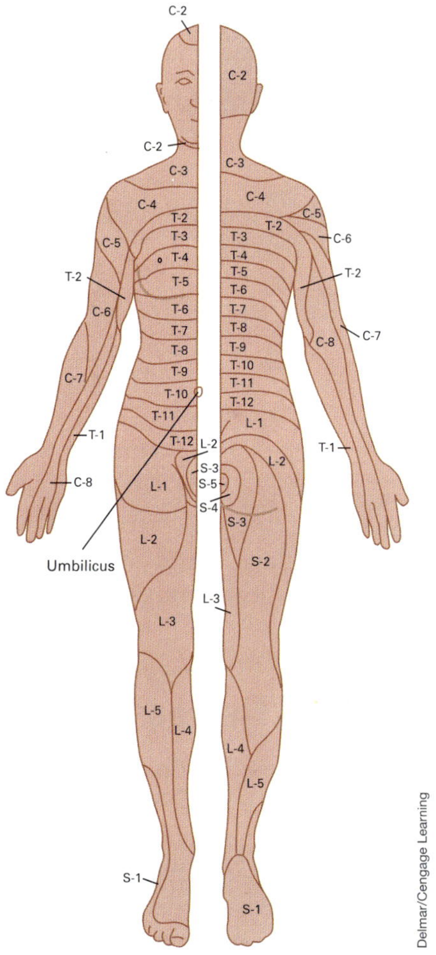

FIGURE 15–3 Spinal nerves and dermatomes.

body needed to respond to stressors such as increasing the heart rate or blood pressure—the fight-or-flight response.

Twelve pairs of cranial nerves control sensation and movement in the area of the head and neck (Table 15–1). Thirty-one pairs of spinal nerves are divided into 8 cervical, 12 thoracic, 5 lumbar, 5 sacral, and 1 coccygeal. Each spinal nerve innervates designated areas, called dermatomes, of the skin (Figure 15–3). Each of the spinal nerves sends sensory impulses from the body organs and surfaces to the spinal cord for transmission to the brain and returns motor impulses from the brain to the spinal cord and then to the muscles.

COMMON SIGNS AND SYMPTOMS

Common signs and symptoms of nervous system disorders include headache, nausea, vomiting, weakness, mood swings, and fever. Symptoms specific to the nervous system include the following:

- Disturbance in motor function (or ability to move), including:
  1. Stiffness in the neck, back, or extremities
  2. Inability to move any part of the body
  3. Seizures or convulsions
  4. Paralysis

- Disturbance in sensory function (or ability to sense or feel), including:
  1. Visual difficulties
  2. Inability to speak
  3. Paralysis
- Alteration in mental alertness or cognitive function, including:
  1. Extreme or prolonged drowsiness
  2. Stupor, unconsciousness, or coma
  3. Amnesia or extreme forgetfulness

DIAGNOSTIC TESTS

A neurologic examination includes testing motor, sensory, and mental function. This examination is often performed on any individual presenting with an injury to the head, neck, or spinal column or exhibiting neurologic symptoms. Motor testing includes checking reflexes, gait, and posture. Sensory testing includes checking the ability to feel, using pinprick or application of heat, cold, or vibration. Ability to see and smell also can be part of sensory testing. Testing of mental or cognitive function includes asking simple questions related to name, occupation, and location. Further testing might include simple math problems or questions about current events.

The most important laboratory test in a neurologic examination is the analysis of cerebrospinal fluid (CSF). The fluid is examined under a microscope to determine the presence of bacteria, leukocytes, red blood cells, neoplastic cells, and other microorganisms.

To obtain this fluid, a lumbar puncture must be performed, a procedure that consists of positioning the affected individual on his or her side in a knee–chest position to widen the vertebral disk space, inserting a spinal needle into the meningeal space around the spinal cord, and withdrawing CSF. During the procedure, a special manometer might be connected to the spinal needle so intracranial pressure (ICP) can be measured.

Because the skull is a rigid structure, any increase in the size of the brain tissue by swelling, tumor, infection, or hematoma will cause an increase in ICP. If pressure becomes too high, the brain will herniate or move downward through the foramen magnum, the only opening available. When this occurs, coma and rapid death can occur because this places pressure on vital centers in the brain stem.

Radiologic examinations include X-rays of the skull and vertebral column for fractures and other abnormalities. A myelogram, or picture of the spinal cord, might be used for diagnosis of a tumor, nerve root compression, herniated nucleus pulposus (HNP), or herniated disk. Angiograms can help determine vessel occlusion and hematomas in individuals exhibiting symptoms of cerebrovascular accident or stroke.

Electroencephalography (EEG) measures electrical brain activity. A damaged area of the brain might exhibit abnormal electrical activity as might occur with cerebrovascular accident and epilepsy. EEG is also used to determine brain death.

Computerized tomography (CT) and magnetic resonance imaging (MRI) scanning are both valuable tools to assess the anatomy of the brain and spinal cord.

COMMON DISEASES OF THE NERVOUS SYSTEM

The diseases of the nervous system can range from mild to severe, depending on the particular condition. Age-related factors can influence the severity of the disease, but many nervous system disorders can affect the individual at any age.

Infectious Diseases

Infections of the nervous system are more common in the young but can be found in older adults as well. Early diagnosis and treatment is essential to reduce the permanent neurologic deficits that can result from the infection.

ENCEPHALITIS

- ***DESCRIPTION.*** Encephalitis is an inflammation of the brain tissue.
- ***ETIOLOGY.*** Encephalitis is caused by a variety of microorganisms, including bacteria and viruses, or as a complication of measles, chicken pox, or mumps. Such viruses can be spread also by mosquitoes and carried from animal to human or from human to human.
- ***SYMPTOMS.*** Symptoms include headache, elevated temperature, and a stiff neck and back but can progress to lethargy, mental confusion, and even coma.

■ ***DIAGNOSIS.*** Encephalitis is usually diagnosed by finding the causative agent in spinal fluid obtained by lumbar puncture.

■ ***TREATMENT.*** Treatment is supportive. Antiviral medication might be effective in some types of encephalitis, but prognosis is guarded because some forms of encephalitis have a high mortality rate. Severe encephalitis can leave the individual with permanent neurologic impairment.

■ ***PREVENTION.*** Prevention is related to avoiding transmission of the disease by mosquitoes. Activities include avoiding outdoor activity when mosquitoes are active—usually near or after dark—wearing protective clothing with long sleeves and long pants, and using repellents that contain DEET.

MENINGITIS

■ ***DESCRIPTION.*** Meningitis is inflammation of the meninges, the covering of the brain and spinal cord.

■ ***ETIOLOGY.*** Meningitis can be caused by anything that causes an inflammatory response, including bacteria, viruses, fungi, and toxins such as lead and arsenic. Some forms of meningitis are more contagious and more lethal than other forms of the disease. The most common cause of meningitis is bacterial invasion by *Neisseria meningitides*. Bacteria and viruses usually reach the meninges after invading and infecting other parts of the body such as the middle ear, sinuses, and upper respiratory tract; or they can be carried to the meninges in the blood, as in septicemia.

■ ***SYMPTOMS.*** Symptoms of meningitis often include a sudden onset of high fever, severe headache, photophobia (fear of light), and a stiffness in the neck that resists bending the neck forward or sideways (**nuchal rigidity**). As the disease progresses, drowsiness, stupor, seizures, and coma might occur.

■ ***DIAGNOSIS.*** Diagnosis is usually confirmed by finding the causative agent in the spinal fluid obtained by lumbar puncture.

■ ***TREATMENT.*** Antibiotic treatment of bacterial meningitis is usually quite effective. Other treatments include antipyretics; anticonvulsive medications; and a quiet, dark environment. If untreated, meningitis can be fatal, especially in infants, children, and older individuals. It can cause permanent neurologic damage in children, leading to hearing loss, learning and developmental challenges, and epilepsy. Good hand washing practices can help prevent the spread of the disease.

■ ***PREVENTION.*** Good hand washing helps reduce exposure to infectious organisms. Avoiding those who are infected is also a preventive activity.

POLIOMYELITIS

■ ***DESCRIPTION.*** Poliomyelitis, or polio, is a viral infection affecting the brain and spinal cord. Polio was a major crippling and life-threatening disease affecting children prior to the development of a vaccine in the 1960s. Immunization programs since that time have virtually eliminated the disease in the United States.

■ ***ETIOLOGY.*** The poliomyelitis virus enters the body through the mouth and nose. It crosses the gastrointestinal tract into the blood and then travels to the brain and spinal cord. The virus is spread by oropharyngeal secretions and by infected feces.

■ ***SYMPTOMS.*** Symptoms of polio include muscle weakness, neck stiffness, and nausea and vomiting. As the disease progresses, muscles atrophy and deteriorate. Muscles of the arms, legs, and respiratory system can become paralyzed.

■ ***DIAGNOSIS.*** Diagnosis is made by clinical examination and confirmed by culturing the virus from the throat, feces, or spinal fluid.

■ ***TREATMENT.*** Treatment is supportive and includes analgesics and bed rest during the acute phase. Long-term physical therapy and limb braces might be needed. If the respiratory system is involved, mechanical ventilation might be necessary.

Ten to 40 years after the initial polio attack, many survivors experience postpolio syndrome (PPS), characterized by further weakening of muscles that were previously affected by the polio infection. Symptoms can include joint pain, fatigue, and increasing skeletal deformities such as scoliosis. The problems caused by PPS usually mirror the severity of the original polio attack. If the original attack was not severe, the PPS condition is usually not bad. PPS tends to affect females more often than it does males. This is not an infectious condition and it is rarely life-threatening.

■ ***PREVENTION.*** The most effective prevention is with polio vaccine.

HEALTHY HIGHLIGHT

Polio Vaccine Precautions

There are three distinct polioviruses, designated as types 1, 2, and 3. Dr. Jonas Salk developed an injectable vaccine against only one form of polio, so that vaccine is called a monovalent vaccine. It used dead virus to stimulate the production of antibodies against polio. Dr. Albert Sabin later developed an oral vaccine (trivalent oral polio Vaccine [TOPV]) against all three forms of the virus; that vaccine is, therefore, called a trivalent vaccine and is a live vaccine using weakened virus to stimulate antibody production.

Immunosuppressed individuals must follow precautions with polio vaccines. Immunosuppressed individuals include those who are:

- Affected with chronic disease.
- Taking chemotherapy.
- Receiving radiation treatments.
- Taking immunosuppressive medications for organ transplants.
- On long-term steroid treatment.

Precautions for immunosuppressed individuals include the following:

- Do not take the live trivalent vaccine because this can lead to contracting polio.
- Do not change diapers or come in contact with feces of children recently treated with TOPV.
- Do not come in contact with nasal secretions or vomitus of children recently treated with TOPV.

TETANUS

DESCRIPTION. Tetanus is a highly fatal infection of nerve tissue.

ETIOLOGY. Tetanus disease is caused by the *Clostridium tetani* bacterium. The effect of the toxin produced by this bacterium on the CNS leads to voluntary, or skeletal muscle, contraction.

SYMPTOMS. The first symptom is typically a stiffness of the jaw, commonly called lockjaw, and is due to strong jaw muscle contractions. This disease affects both the musculoskeletal system and the nervous system.

More detailed information about tetanus is found in Chapter 6, "Musculoskeletal System Diseases and Disorders."

RABIES

DESCRIPTION. Rabies is an often fatal encephalomyelitis.

ETIOLOGY. Rabies is caused by a virus and primarily affects animals such as dogs, cats, foxes, raccoons, squirrels, and skunks but can be transmitted to humans through a bite by an infected animal. Like tetanus, this virus travels slowly to the spinal cord and brain, so the location of the bite is significant. Incubation time is from 1 to 3 months. Shorter incubation times are related to the position of the bite, making bites to the face and neck more serious than those to the extremities.

SYMPTOMS. Symptoms of rabies include fever, pain, paralysis, convulsions, and rage. In animals, a change in temperament is often noticed. Wild animals can become friendly, and family pets can become aggressive. Another classic symptom is spasm and paralysis of the muscles of swallowing. The sight of water or attempting to drink water causes throat spasms, leading to **hydrophobia** (hydro = water, phobia = fear). Inability to swallow also causes a drooling of frothy saliva, an identifying symptom in animals.

■ ***DIAGNOSIS.*** Diagnosis is based on a history and physical exam, observing for symptoms of muscle spasms, stiffness, and pain. Laboratory tests are not helpful with diagnosis.

■ ***TREATMENT.*** Treatment of rabies includes immediate washing of the area with soap and water, followed by medical attention. A series of antirabies injections must be given before the virus has had time to reach the brain. Any animal bite needs to be investigated immediately. The biting animal should be confined and placed under observation for symptoms of rabies, and viral cultures should be obtained. If the animal cannot be captured and must be killed, care should be taken not to destroy the head because the brain must be examined for presence of disease. If the animal cannot be found, the injured individual will need to take the series of injections immediately.

There is no cure for rabies. Treatment is palliative and includes strong muscle relaxants to reduce convulsions. Untreated cases end with severe convulsions and respiratory arrest. Death usually occurs within 2 to 5 days after onset of symptoms.

■ ***PREVENTION.*** Prevention of rabies begins with vaccination of family pets and education of children in recognizing and avoiding animals with rabid symptoms.

SHINGLES

■ ***DESCRIPTION.*** Shingles is an acute viral disease, fairly common in the elderly, with approximately 50% of people over age 80 having an episode of shingles.

■ ***ETIOLOGY.*** Shingles is caused by herpes zoster, the same virus that causes chicken pox. The only difference between chicken pox and shingles is the level of the affected individual's immunity. Chickenpox usually appears in children with little or no immunity, and shingles occurs in adults with limited immunity. It is thought that herpes zoster virus is a chicken pox virus that has been dormant, usually for years, after recovery from chicken pox. This virus tends to flare up or become active during periods of stress or immunosuppression caused by other disease processes, trauma, and aging.

■ ***SYMPTOMS.*** Shingles is characterized by an itching, painful, red rash, and small vesicles or blisters that

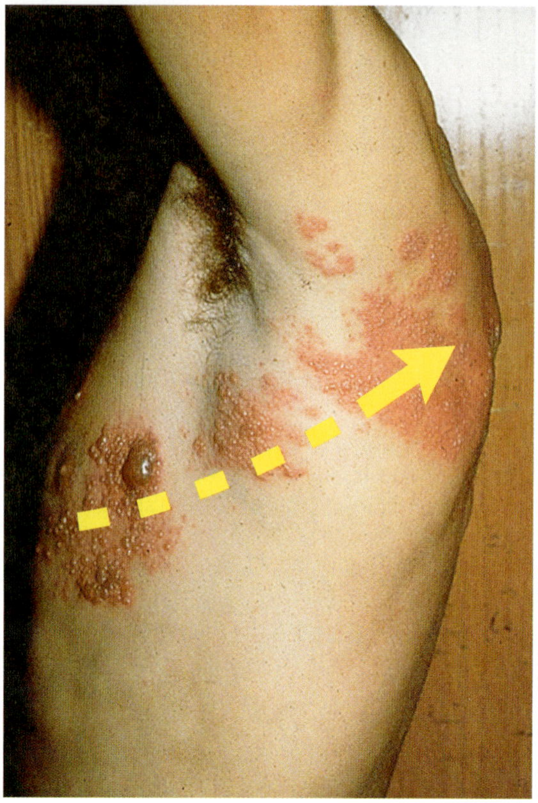

FIGURE 15–4 Shingles: vesicles follow a nerve pathway.

follow the course of a sensory nerve (Figure 15–4). The resulting neuritis or inflammation of the nerve results in a stabbing, sharp pain that usually is more severe at night. Symptoms can last from 10 days to several weeks. The pattern of rash and blisters usually appears on the body trunk and runs toward the midline but also can appear on the face, causing severe conjunctivitis.

■ ***DIAGNOSIS.*** Diagnosis is made on the basis of the appearance of lesions. A viral culture or blood test for the herpes virus can be performed to confirm the diagnosis.

■ ***TREATMENT.*** Treatment is symptomatic and involves administration of antiviral medication, analgesics, and antipruritics (medications to reduce itching).

■ ***PREVENTION.*** Zostavax®, a vaccine to prevent shingles, has been available for individuals over age 60 since it was licensed by the Food and Drug Administration (FDA) in 2006. The vaccine is not a treatment for shingles.

Vascular Disorders

Vascular disorders of the nervous system can be quite severe, causing long-term debility. Some vascular disorders can be prevented or reduced in severity by lifestyle changes.

CEREBROVASCULAR ACCIDENT (CVA)

■ ***DESCRIPTION.*** CVA commonly called a stroke, usually occurs in people over 50 years of age and is a major cause of death in this age group.

■ ***ETIOLOGY.*** CVA is due to poor blood supply to the brain. A common causative factor is arteriosclerosis. A CVA is to the brain what a heart attack is to the heart—lack of blood flow to the brain causes brain tissue death. The three common causes of poor blood supply or lack of blood flow are:

Cerebral thrombus a clot in a brain artery and the most common cause of vessel occlusion. Thrombus formation usually occurs in an area where the vessel is narrowed by arteriosclerosis. Symptoms usually appear gradually until blood flow is inadequate.

Cerebral embolism usually due to a small piece of a thrombus or arterial plaque breaking loose and traveling in the artery until it wedges and occludes the vessel. Symptoms usually appear quite suddenly.

Cerebral hemorrhage the rupture of an artery, filling the surrounding brain tissue with blood. Cerebral hemorrhage is usually due to hypertension and arteriosclerosis (See "Arteriosclerosis and Atherosclerosis" in Chapter 8, "Cardiovascular System Diseases and Disorders."), which cause the vessel to tear and hemorrhage. Another cause of cerebral hemorrhage is a weakened artery due to an aneurysm. Symptoms are very sudden with hemorrhage.

■ ***SYMPTOMS.*** When an area of the brain loses blood supply, the individual suddenly loses consciousness and can die or have permanent neurologic disability. About one third of individuals with a CVA die. Some survive without functional disability, and others might have mild, moderate, or severe disability (Figure 15–5). The symptoms of CVA are numerous, depending on the area of the brain affected and the severity of the occlusion or hemorrhage. Common symptoms include **dysphasia** (dis-FAY-zee-ah; dys = difficulty, phasia = speaking), **dysphagia** (dis-FAY-jee-ah; dys = difficulty, phagia = swallowing), **hemiparesis** (HEM-ee-par-EE-sis; hemi = one half, paresis = paralysis), confusion, and poor coordination.

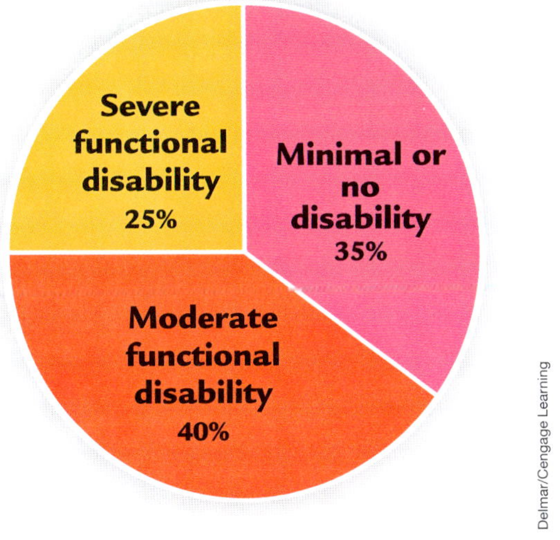

FIGURE 15–5 CVA: prognosis for individuals surviving CVA/stroke.

■ ***DIAGNOSIS.*** Diagnosis of CVA is made and confirmed by physical examination, EEG, and CT or MRI scan. One indicator of the location of brain damage is shown by the pattern of hemiparesis, if present. Hemiparesis affecting the left side is indicative of right-sided brain injury, whereas hemiparesis affecting the right side is indicative of left-sided brain injury. Symptoms of right- and left-sided brain damage vary to some degree (Figure 15–6).

■ ***TREATMENT.*** Treatment of CVA depends on the severity of the stroke and the symptoms. Anticoagulant and hypertensive medications can be given to control the formation of clots and to lower blood pressure. For those individuals with physical disability, a rehabilitation program, including the needed services of physical therapy and speech therapy, must be set up early and continued until the individual has gained maximum potential.

■ ***PREVENTION.*** Prevention of stroke is directed toward avoiding risk factors that include:

1. Smoking
2. High-fat diet
3. Obesity
4. Lack of exercise

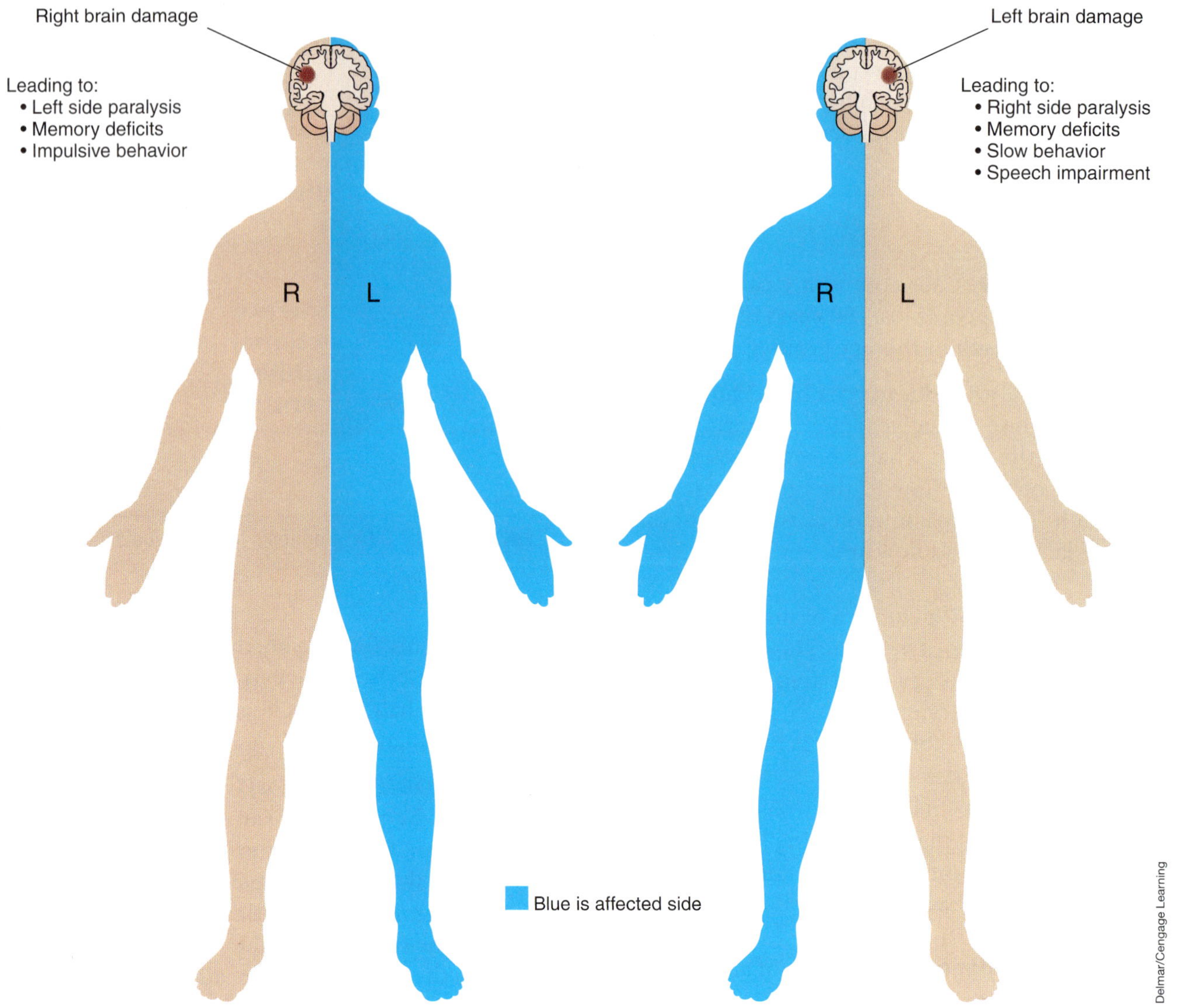

FIGURE 15–6 Symptoms of right and left CVA vary to some degree.

These factors also play a role in arteriosclerosis, a main cause of CVA.

Early detection and treatment of occluded arteries can aid in prevention of some types of CVA. Carotid artery screening involves a physician auscultating the carotid arteries and listening for vessel narrowing. As blood rushes through a narrowed vessel, a rushing sound called a bruit (BREW-ee) can be heard. Ultrasound imaging can also be performed to determine the condition of the vessel. Surgical intervention to open the vessel might prevent CVA and includes removal of plaque in the carotid arteries to improve blood flow and reduce the risk of a thrombus. This surgical procedure is called a **carotid endarterectomy**.

TRANSIENT ISCHEMIC ATTACK (TIA)

■ ***DESCRIPTION.*** TIAs are sudden, mild mini-strokes.

■ ***ETIOLOGY.*** TIAs are due to insufficient blood supply to the brain. They can serve as a warning of an impending stroke and are often due to artery narrowing by arteriosclerotic plaque.

■ ***SYMPTOMS.*** Symptoms, like those of CVA, depend on the area of the brain that is affected. Some common symptoms are weakness of an arm, leg, or both; dizziness; slurred speech; and a mild loss of consciousness. Total loss of consciousness usually does not occur. Symptoms usually subside within a few minutes to an hour.

■ ***DIAGNOSIS.*** Symptoms can be completely resolved by the time medical advice is sought. The diagnosis is made on the medical history and physical examination including a neurological exam. Blood pressure is also checked for hypertension. A stethoscope may be placed over neck veins (auscultation) to determine blood flow irregularities. Arteriograms can locate suspected vessel blockage or occlusion. A CT scan of the head might also be part of the diagnostic testing.

■ ***TREATMENT.*** Arteriograms showing blocked blood flow can be followed up with surgery to open vessels or bypass blockage. Carotid endarterectomy is one of the more common surgeries to correct blood flow for TIA.

■ ***PREVENTION.*** To stop smoking is the best preventive measure. Knowing risk factors and living a healthy lifestyle are also helpful preventive measures.

Functional Disorders

Functional disorders of the nervous system include degenerative disk disease, headache, epilepsy, and Bell's palsy. These conditions, although varying in severity, are some of the most common problems of the system. The cause of the disorder might be found, but in many cases, it is unknown. Treatment of structural disorders is directed toward the relief of symptoms and assisting the individual in maintaining maximum function in activities of daily living.

DEGENERATIVE DISK DISEASE

■ ***DESCRIPTION.*** Degenerative disk disease is actually a degeneration, or wearing away, of the intervertebral disk of the musculoskeletal system, but the results so severely affect the neurologic system that it will be considered in this chapter.

■ ***ETIOLOGY.*** The wearing away of the disk between the vertebrae of the back allows the vertebrae to bump or rub against each other. As these vertebrae move closer together, the opening for the spine and nerve roots becomes smaller, causing pressure on the nerves. The condition of narrowing of nerve root openings in the spinal column is called **spinal stenosis** (stenosis = narrowing).

■ ***SYMPTOMS.*** Common symptoms include difficulty walking, radiating pain in the back and in one or both legs. This pain often follows the nerve path and can be **intractable** (difficult to stop or control). Degenerative disk disease usually affects older individuals but can be related to trauma or congenital defects in younger individuals.

■ ***DIAGNOSIS.*** Diagnosis is made on the basis of clinical history, X-ray, myelography, CT, or MRI.

■ ***TREATMENT.*** Treatment initially involves resting the back and legs. A back brace might be beneficial. Long-term treatment involves analgesics, anti-inflammatory medications, and exercise to ease the pain. A laminectomy, surgery to remove part of the vertebrae and widen the nerve root opening, can be the treatment of choice. In severe cases, surgery to fuse the vertebrae and free the nerve root can be performed. Often, older individuals affected with degenerative disk disease and spinal stenosis are not medically stable enough to endure surgery.

■ ***PREVENTION.*** Since degenerative disc disease primarily affects the elderly due to the aging process, many cases cannot be prevented. Moderate exercise, especially daily walking programs, and good nutrition can help slow or stop painful symptoms.

HEADACHE

■ ***DESCRIPTION.*** Headache, or **cephalalgia** (SEF-ah-LAL-jee-ah; cephal = head, algia = pain), is one of the most common disorders of humans. It is usually a symptom of another disease rather than a disorder in and of itself. Disorders that typically have headaches as a symptom can include sinusitis, meningitis, encephalitis, hypertension, anemia, constipation, premenstrual tension, and tumors, to name only a few. Most headaches are not related to disease but are basically caused by two mechanisms:

- Tension on the facial, neck, and scalp muscles
- Vascular changes in arterial size (dilation or constriction) of the vessels inside the head

■ ***ETIOLOGY.*** Many factors produce headaches, including allergies, stress, noise, toxic fumes, lack of sleep, and alcohol consumption.

■ ***SYMPTOMS.*** Headaches can be acute or chronic and can affect different areas of the head. The pain can range from mild to unbearable and incapacitating; it can be constant or intermittent and might be described as pressure, throbbing, or stabbing. Interestingly, brain tissue does not contain sensory nerves, so the sense of pain must come from the pain receptors in the meninges, facial tissue, or scalp. Some of the more common types of headaches include:

Tension headache caused by stress, strain, and tension on the facial, neck, and scalp muscles. Pain is typically in the occipital area.

Cluster headache can be caused by stress, emotional trauma, or unknown reasons. These headaches occur at night after falling asleep. The pain is generally a severe, throbbing pain behind the nose and one eye. The skin in this area becomes reddened, and the nose and eye water. The pain generally subsides after 1 or 2 hours but might recur several times during the night.

Postlumbar puncture headache a severe headache affecting up to 40% of individuals, following a lumbar puncture. It is thought to be due to leakage of spinal fluid through the needle puncture site. This type of headache is often prevented by positioning the individual flat in bed without a pillow for 2 or 3 hours following this procedure.

Migraine headache a severe, incapacitating headache commonly accompanied by nausea, vomiting, and visual disturbances. Individuals affected by migraines can experience a visual **aura**, a sensation that precedes the event, including flashing light, dim vision, or photophobia. This type of headache can begin in adolescence and diminish in intensity and frequency with age. Migraine headaches occur twice as often in women than in men. The cause is still unknown, although they tend to run in families, suggesting some type of inheritance pattern. Some foods that trigger migraines are chocolate, wine, and cheese. It is also thought that these are vascular headaches caused by altered arterial blood flow.

■ ***DIAGNOSIS.*** Diagnosis of the cause of headache depends on individual history and physical examination. Testing can include X-ray, EEG, and MRI and CT scans.

■ ***TREATMENT.*** Headache treatment depends on the cause, severity, and frequency of occurrence. Often, lifestyle changes such as improvements in diet, sleep, and exercise, help. Pain medications may be over the counter, such as acetaminophen (Tylenol) or ibuprofen. Prescription pain medication and anti-nausea medications might also be needed.

■ ***PREVENTION.*** Diet and lifestyle changes along with stress reduction are measures that can help prevent headaches. Severe headaches might require prescription medication.

EPILEPSY

■ ***DESCRIPTION.*** Epilepsy is a chronic disease of the brain, characterized by intermittent episodes of abnormal electrical activity in the brain, activity that might be compared to an arrhythmia of the heart.

■ ***ETIOLOGY.*** The cause of epilepsy can be due to brain tumors, neurologic disease, or scar tissue in the brain due to trauma or stroke. More commonly, the cause cannot be determined during the individual's life or even on autopsy.

COMPLEMENTARY AND ALTERNATIVE THERAPY

Acupuncture for Migraine Headaches

This study assessed the effectiveness of using traditional Chinese medicine (TCM) acupuncture therapy for the treatment of migraines in patients who do not have an aura with the headache. Acupuncture has been used in Chinese medicine for centuries but is recently becoming more common in Western medical therapies for pain relief. The research compared the TCM method to other types of acupuncture and mock acupuncture treatments. TCM acupuncture was found to be effective in relieving the pain and nausea associated with migraine headaches.

Source: Facco, et al. (2008).

GLIMPSE OF THE FUTURE

Cost-Saving Acupuncture for Headaches

The cost-saving benefits of acupuncture treatment for headaches may put this therapy ahead of other treatment modalities currently being used. This research study compared the costs of treating primary headaches in patients with the costs associated with treating the headaches with acupuncture. The patients were adults who suffered from headaches at least two times per month. Initially, the costs were higher for the group receiving acupuncture. However, after factoring in all direct and indirect costs over time, it was concluded that acupuncture therapy was a cost-effective treatment in patients with primary headaches. This alternative treatment might be more commonly recommended to patients in the future since it has been shown to be cost-effective.

Source: Witt, et al. (2008).

SYMPTOMS. The most noted symptom of epilepsy is a convulsive seizure. A **convulsion** is an abnormal muscle contraction. A **seizure** is actually a sudden attack, but it is commonly used to indicate a convulsive seizure. Not all seizures are characterized by convulsions, and not all convulsions are due to epilepsy. Convulsions can occur in a nonepileptic individual due to conditions such as excessive temperature (hyperpyrexia), hypoglycemia, hypocalcemia, and drug or alcohol toxicity.

The most common types of seizures are:

- **Petit Mal** These seizures are also called absence seizures and commonly occur in children; they are often outgrown during puberty, but they can last a lifetime. These seizures consist of a brief change in the level of consciousness without convulsions. The involved individual might show symptoms of blank staring, blinking, twitching of the eyes or mouth, or all these. The individual might remain seated or standing with loss of awareness of surroundings. Often, the seated individual appears to have only a loss of attention or absentmindedness. Episodes often last only a few seconds but can occur multiple times during the day.
- **Grand Mal** These seizures are the type most often thought of as epilepsy. They are characterized by convulsions, loss of consciousness, urinary and fecal incontinence, and tongue biting. Epileptic individuals often perceive an aura with grand mal seizures, allowing time to lie down or call for support. Auras can include tingling of the fingers, ringing in the ears, and visual disturbances. Grand mal seizures often begin with a crying out as the contraction of the respiratory muscles forces exhalation, followed by generalized rhythmic contractions of the skeletal muscles of the body, arms, and legs. Contractions can last 1 to 2 minutes, but consciousness will return more slowly. The involved individual is often weak, drowsy, and confused and has no memory of the seizure event.
- **Status epilepticus** is a life-threatening event, a state of continued convulsive seizure with no recovery of consciousness. This is a medical emergency because treatment is needed to prevent cerebral anoxia and possible death.

DIAGNOSIS. Diagnosis of epilepsy is made on the basis of EEG, CT, and cerebral angiograms. EEG can reveal altered brain activity; CT can indicate alteration in brain structure, including tumors; and cerebral angiograms can reveal alteration in blood flow. Blood tests can be performed to indicate disorders of hypoglycemia and drug or alcohol toxicity.

TREATMENT. Anticonvulsive medications are the treatment of choice for epilepsy. Close monitoring and adjustment of medications are needed to get the best effect. Medications are effective in preventing or reducing seizures 80% of the time. Education and emotional support of the affected individual and family members are necessary because this disease is often feared due to lack of education. The goal for epileptic individuals should be maintenance of a normal lifestyle.

PREVENTION. Because the cause of epilepsy in many cases is not clear, it is not possible to prevent it. In the case of epilepsy brought on by head injury,

HEALTHY HIGHLIGHT

First Aid for Seizures

A seizure is a sign of a malfunction of some part of the brain's electrical system. Most seizures in individuals diagnosed with epilepsy are not emergencies, but they could be in others. It is always wise to call for assistance (medical personnel) when unsure.

In the event of a seizure, complete the following steps:

- Look for a medical ID.
- Loosen tight clothing.
- Protect the individual from harm or nearby hazards.
- Protect the head by placing a cushion or padding under it.
- Do not attempt to place a tongue blade, any hard object, or your fingers in the individual's mouth.
- Turn the individual to a side-lying position.
- Avoid tightly restraining the individual.
- Stay with the individual until other assistive personnel arrive.
- Reassure the individual and offer assistance as consciousness returns.

prevention measures include wearing a seat belt in the car and a helmet when riding a motorcycle, ATV, bike, or horse or while skating or skiing.

BELL'S PALSY

■ ***DESCRIPTION.*** Bell's palsy is a disease affecting the facial nerve (seventh cranial nerve), causing unilateral (one-sided) paralysis of the face. It commonly occurs in individuals 20 to 60 years of age. Bell's palsy can affect either side of the face, and both genders are affected equally. There appears to be an increased risk for pregnant women, and those with an upper-respiratory infection, influenza, and diabetes.

■ ***ETIOLOGY.*** This disease is idiopathic, but possible causes include autoimmune problems and viral disease.

■ ***SYMPTOMS.*** Symptoms include a drooping weakness of the eye and mouth, with inability to close the affected eye and drooling of saliva. The affected individual is unable to whistle or smile and has a distorted facial appearance (Figure 15–7).

■ ***DIAGNOSIS.*** Diagnosis is made on the basis of clinical history and symptoms. An electromyography can be completed to measure voluntary muscle movement and determine the extent of nerve weakness. An MRI scan is helpful also.

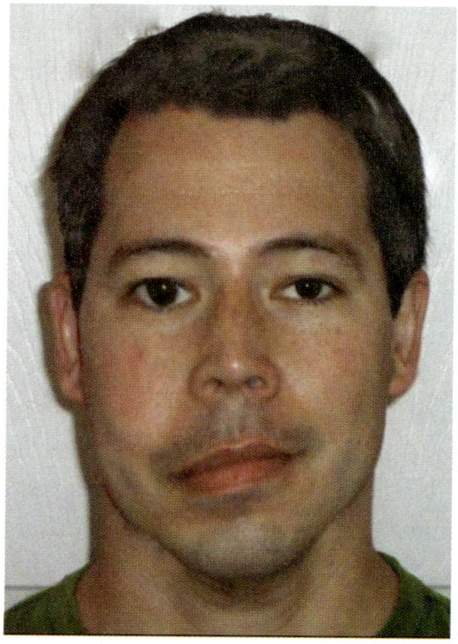

Courtesy of Mark L. Kuss

FIGURE 15–7 Facial appearance of Bell's palsy.

■ ***TREATMENT.*** Treatment includes analgesics and anti-inflammatory medications. If the individual is unable to close the affected eye, protection of the eye with a patch and artificial tear medication might be needed. Warm, moist heat, electrical nerve stimulation, and massage can be prescribed to prevent facial muscle atrophy. Prognosis for Bell's palsy is good, with most cases resolving spontaneously in 2 to 8 weeks.

Plastic surgery might be prescribed to correct the facial deformities caused by chronic disease.

PREVENTION. There are no known preventive measures.

PARKINSON'S DISEASE

Parkinson's disease is a slow, progressive brain degeneration, usually developing in individuals in their late 50s and 60s. Parkinson's affects men more often than it does women.

The cause is unknown, but individuals with Parkinson's have been found to have a deficiency of the neurotransmitter dopamine in the brain.

Classic symptoms include the following:

- Rigidity and immobility of the hands and a very slow speech pattern
- A fine tremor in the hands described as a pill rolling motion of the fingers
- An expressionless facial appearance with a fixed stare and infrequent blinking called Parkinson's facies (fay-SHEEZ)
- An abnormal bent-forward posture that includes a bowed head and flexed arms (Figure 15–8)

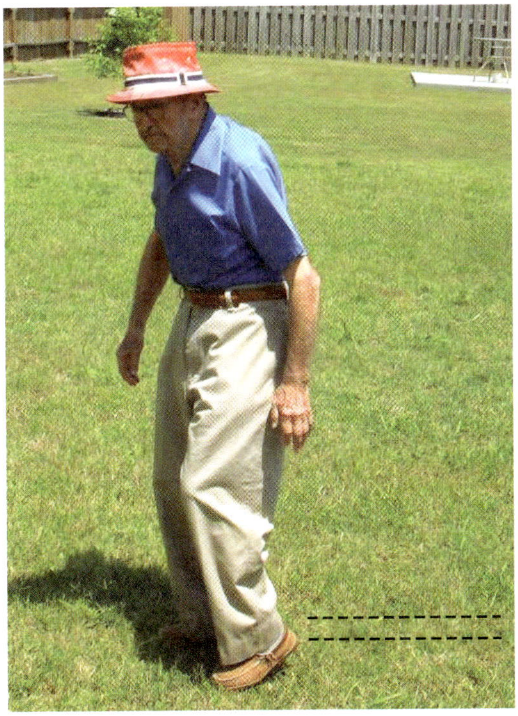

Courtesy of Larry J. Butler.

FIGURE 15–8 Classic posture in Parkinson's disease.

- A peculiar gait of short, fast-running steps due to the abnormal posture that makes the individual tend to stumble forward, leading to frequent falls

Treatment of Parkinson's is symptomatic. Dopamine replacement medications can be used; they do not stop the progression of the disease, but they might help with symptoms. Psychological support and physical therapy for muscle soreness are also helpful.

Dementias

Dementia (dee-MEN-she-ah) is a loss of mental ability due to the loss of neurons or brain cells caused in several ways. One of the most common dementias is senile (old) dementia and is related to degeneration of cells with aging. The most common cause of senile dementia is Alzheimer's disease. Therefore, Alzheimer's and senile dementia are often used synonymously, but in reality, an individual can have senile dementia without Alzheimer's. Vascular dementia also can be considered a form of senile dementia because it tends to occur in older individuals.

ALZHEIMER'S DISEASE

DESCRIPTION. Alzheimer's (ALTZ-high-merz) disease is a form of dementia characterized by the death of neurons and replacement of these neurons by microscopic plaques. It is the most common cause of dementia among older people. The disease usually affects individuals 70 years of age and older. The number of cases increases with age, with an estimated 50% of individuals over age 85 affected.

ETIOLOGY. The cause of Alzheimer's disease is unknown, but factors being considered are heredity, viral infection, autoimmunity, and aluminum toxicity. Research also shows a higher rate of Alzheimer's in individuals with a history of head trauma.

SYMPTOMS. Symptoms of the disease begin with mild mental impairment characterized by loss of short-term memory, inability to concentrate, and slight changes in personality. As the disease progresses, the affected individual struggles with communication skills, uses meaningless words, and cannot form sentences. Increased forgetfulness, along with the difficulties in communication, lead to irritability and agitation. In the final stages, which can take 5 to 10 years to develop, the affected individual's mental and physical capabilities are severely affected. The affected individual becomes restless, disoriented, incontinent, hostile, and combative and is totally dependent on a caregiver. Death is usually due to a secondary cause such as infection.

■ ***DIAGNOSIS.*** Diagnosis cannot be positively made except from autopsy. Initially, a diagnosis can be made on the basis of symptoms after ruling out other brain diseases. In the final stage of the disease, CT or MRI scans might reveal the characteristic brain atrophy and microscopic plaques.

■ ***TREATMENT.*** Treatment is supportive because there is no known cure for Alzheimer's disease. As the individual's capabilities decline, care is focused on safety and maintaining adequate nutrition, hydration, and personal hygiene. Mobility and mental capabilities are supported for as long as possible. Emotional support of family members and caregivers is of primary concern.

■ ***PREVENTION.*** According to the Alzheimer's Research and Prevention Foundation, there is some proof that preventive measures should include avoiding a diet high in trans-fat and saturated fat, especially red meats. Other prevention activities include taking high-potency multiple vitamins and minerals that include folic acid, vitamin E, and at least 2,000 mg of vitamin C.

VASCULAR DEMENTIA

■ ***DESCRIPTION.*** Vascular dementia is caused by atrophy and death of brain cells due to decreased blood flow.

■ ***ETIOLOGY.*** Atherosclerotic plaque is the common cause of decreased blood flow and is common with aging.

■ ***SYMPTOMS.*** Because the atherosclerotic plaques develop slowly, so do symptoms, which progress so slowly that they often go unnoticed by family members until they become quite severe. Symptoms include changes in memory, personality, and judgment. Irritability, depression, and sleeplessness also can occur. Personal hygiene is lacking and is often the sign that alerts family members to the condition. The affected individual can become disoriented and lost in familiar surroundings.

■ ***DIAGNOSIS.*** Diagnosis is made on the basis of a history and physical and blood flow testing. Arteriograms of the carotid and cerebral arteries will reveal narrowing of vessels, stenosis, and arteriosclerotic plaques.

■ ***TREATMENT.*** Treatment is aimed at increasing blood flow to the brain. If the cerebral arteries are involved or narrowed, medications may help improve blood flow. Carotid artery plaques can be surgically cleaned by a carotid endarterectomy (END-ar-ter-ECK-toh-me; endo = inside, arter = artery, ectomy = excision of). Prognosis depends on the effectiveness of treatment and the amount of brain cell death. If treatment is not possible or effective, or if a large amount of brain tissue has been lost, the affected individual will become progressively more demented and might need institutionalization for care.

■ ***PREVENTION.*** The best preventive measure is to quit smoking, lead a healthy lifestyle, and control hypertension.

HEAD TRAUMA DEMENTIA

■ ***DESCRIPTION.*** Head trauma can damage any part of the brain. This term fails to capture all the symptoms and long-term disabilities that can be related to such trauma. Males experience head injuries more often than females, with the most injuries occurring in the ages of 14 to 24 years. Very young children commonly have the worst outcomes.

■ ***ETIOLOGY.*** Head trauma dementia is due to death of brain cells related to head trauma. One type is Boxer's dementia, caused by repeated blows to the head as in the sport of boxing. Other types of trauma can be those sustained in accidents, especially motor vehicle accidents, and sports-related activities. The death of brain cells can be caused by the injury itself or by edema and increased ICP, which decreases or halts blood flow to brain cells, leading to cell death.

■ ***SYMPTOMS.*** Symptoms of head trauma dementia include a prolonged or permanent decrease in mental intellect, cognitive function, or both. The affected individual might be unable to perform activities that were easily completed prior to the injury. There are often symptoms of loss of the ability to reason, remember, and show appropriate emotions and behaviors following such injury. Changes in personality are not uncommon. Chronic psychological trauma can bring about major life changes, mania, major depression, post-traumatic stress and anxiety disorders.

■ ***DIAGNOSIS.*** Diagnosis is made on the basis of history, cranial X-rays, and MRI and CT scans.

■ ***TREATMENT.*** Treatment is aimed at correcting the damage if possible, preventing further damage and maintaining the existing healthy tissue. Dead brain cells cannot be replaced, so damage is permanent. Therapy and rehabilitation are needed to regain as much function as possible. Individuals suffering severe head trauma might need institutionalization for long-term care.

■ ***PREVENTION.*** Head injury is often easy to prevent with proper use of protective equipment. Preventive activities include:

- Wearing seat belts in automobiles.
- Wearing a helmet when riding bikes, ATVs, and skateboards.
- Wearing work-related safety equipment along with hard hats when needed.
- For elderly individuals, altering the surroundings by removing rugs or furniture that might slide easily and cause falls.

SUBSTANCE-INDUCED DEMENTIA

■ ***DESCRIPTION.*** This type of dementia is often cured because the cause of the dementia is curable. In some cases of substance abuse dementia, the individual might not have dementia at all but, rather, suffer from severe depression.

■ ***ETIOLOGY.*** Substance-induced dementia is due to brain cell death caused by toxicity from drugs and toxins. This type of dementia can be caused by repeated exposure to, or use or abuse of, certain substances. Commonly, those substances include alcohol, cocaine, heroine, lead, mercury, and fumes of paints, paint thinners, and insecticides, to name only a few. Brain cell death often persists long after the exposure to the substance ends.

■ ***SYMPTOMS.*** Symptoms of mental impairment and decreased cognitive ability can be permanent and often worsen over a period of time.

■ ***DIAGNOSIS.*** Substance abuse dementia is usually difficult to diagnose. A history and physical exam along with family and caregiver history of the individual's symptoms and history are helpful. A mental health exam is often needed.

■ ***TREATMENT.*** Once properly diagnosed, treating the dementia is usually a matter of removing the toxin (drugs, alcohol, fumes, or insecticides). Depending on the degree of dementia, removing the toxin might not restore normal function.

■ ***PREVENTION.*** Avoiding the toxin prevents this type of dementia.

Sleep Disorders

Sleep may be described as a necessary state of unconsciousness. It is thought that sleep is a period of time during which the body is actively restoring and repairing itself because an increased amount of growth hormone is released during sleep. Sleep also provides a time of recuperation of mental activities. It is believed that there is an increase in metabolic rate in the brain during sleep that allows it to be more alert and efficient during waking hours.

Sleep deprivation of just one night can lead to changes in personality, lack of muscle coordination, and decreased coping ability. There is a great variability in sleep requirements among individuals and different ages: infants need 16 to 20 hours of sleep every 24 hours. This need for sleep decreases into adulthood, with adults generally requiring between 6 and 9 hours of sleep and older adults requiring even less sleep. Sleep disorders can be due to a variety of causes and can be tested by polysomnography, a procedure measuring a variety of physical variables related to sleep.

INSOMNIA

■ ***DESCRIPTION.*** According to WebMD (2007), insomnia is the most common sleep disorder in the United States, with about one third of the adult population experiencing it at some time. Insomnia is the perception or feeling of inadequate or poor sleep, the inability to fall or stay asleep, or of waking up too early in the morning. The affected individual arises physically and mentally tired, irritable, and anxious. Insomnia is more common in females and occurs increasingly with age.

■ ***ETIOLOGY.*** The cause of insomnia can be related to stress, pain, fear, depression, and cardiovascular or thyroid disorders. Drugs such as caffeine, alcohol, nicotine, and bronchodilators also can cause insomnia. Eventually, the fear of being unable to fall asleep can become a cause.

■ ***SYMPTOMS.*** The symptom is sleeplessness, often leading to fatigue and irritability. The diagnostic definition of insomnia is sleeplessness for more than one month that is interfering with the individual's social or work habits.

■ ***DIAGNOSIS.*** Diagnosis is determined by taking a careful account of an individual's sleep history. Referral to a sleep lab might help if a breathing disorder is suspected.

■ ***TREATMENT.*** Treatment consists of identifying and removing the cause(s). One can develop a sleep routine with a scheduled bedtime and awakening time, and counseling might be needed to assist the individual in managing or reducing stress and anxiety. The affected individual is encouraged not to worry about when and how much he or she sleeps and to take naps and sleep as they can rather than build up anxiety about sleeping at night. The total amount of sleep in 24 hours is more important than the sleeping schedule.

■ ***PREVENTION.*** Prevention centers on living a healthy lifestyle, balancing rest, exercise, and recreation with stress management and healthy diet.

SLEEP APNEA

■ ***DESCRIPTION.*** Sleep apnea (AP-nee-ah; a = without, pnea = breathing) is a sleep disorder characterized by periods of apnea or breathlessness.

■ ***ETIOLOGY.*** This condition occurs more frequently in men and might be related to obesity, hypertension, and airway obstruction. Alcohol ingestion and smoking also can be causative factors.

■ ***SYMPTOMS.*** The diagnostic definition of sleep apnea is more than five periods of apnea lasting for at least 10 seconds each per hour of sleep. These breathless periods are followed by sudden gasps or snorts for air. Other symptoms can include (1) excessive daytime sleepiness to the point of falling asleep during driving, work, or in the middle of a conversation; (2) extreme snoring that might not awaken the affected individual but easily awakens family members; and (3) personality changes, depression, and impotence. Sleep apnea can be divided into three categories:

- Obstructive apnea, caused by nasal obstruction
- Central apnea, caused by a disorder in the brain's respiratory control center
- Mixed apnea, a combination of both obstructive and central apnea

■ ***DIAGNOSIS.*** Diagnosis is confirmed by monitoring the affected individual during sleep for apnea and low blood oxygen levels.

■ ***TREATMENT.*** Treatment is based on cause. Obstructive types and mixed types are treated with weight-loss therapy and, if needed, surgery to correct nasal obstruction. Individuals affected by obstructive apnea also might benefit from oxygen administration, oral appliances, adjustable airway pressure devices, and continuous positive airway pressure (CPAP) devices during sleep. Central apnea is more difficult to control and might be treated with medications to stimulate breathing.

■ ***PREVENTION.*** Most cases of sleep apnea can be prevented by maintaining a healthy weight, avoiding alcohol, not smoking, and avoiding environmental smoke.

Tumors

Tumors may be classified as benign and malignant. (See Chapter 3, "Neoplasms.") Benign tumors of the brain often become malignant if surgical removal is not possible. The growth of benign tumors in the confined space of the skull places pressure on the brain tissue and blood vessels, leading to loss of function and death of normal tissue. Tumors can occur in any area of the brain and at any age, although many are fairly age-specific or commonly occur in a particular age group. Gliomas and meningiomas are most common in adults.

BRAIN TUMOR

■ ***DESCRIPTION.*** Brain tumors may be classified as primary or secondary. Primary tumors start in the brain tissue, whereas secondary tumors occur in other areas and metastasize to the brain. Brain tumors in children are commonly primary tumors. Secondary tumors are not called brain tumors; they are named after the organ of origin. In other words, breast tumor that metastasizes to the brain is still called breast cancer with metastasis to the brain. Common sites of secondary tumor that metastasize to the brain include breast and lung.

■ ***ETIOLOGY.*** The cause of primary tumors is unknown.

■ ***SYMPTOMS.*** Symptoms are varied, depending on the area involved, and include headache, vomiting, seizures, mood and personality changes, visual disturbances, and loss of memory.

■ ***DIAGNOSIS.*** Diagnosis is made on the basis of clinical history, symptoms, X-ray examinations, CT and MRI scans, and biopsy. A biopsy is the most definitive study to determine the type of tumor and the best to assist with treatment and prognosis. Further studies might be needed to determine the primary location of metastatic brain tumors.

■ ***TREATMENT.*** Treatment can include surgery, radiation, and chemotherapy. Treatment and prognosis depend on the type and location of the tumor.

■ ***PREVENTION.*** Reducing or avoiding exposure to radiation, certain medications, and head trauma can benefit prevention.

TRAUMA

Injuries to the brain, neck, and spinal cord are a main cause of disability and death. Trauma to the head can cause edema, increased ICP, hemorrhage, and infection, resulting in brain damage. Injury to the neck and spinal cord can lead to temporary or permanent paralysis.

Concussions and Contusions

■ ***DESCRIPTION.*** A concussion is the less serious of the two conditions and does not involve injury to the brain. A contusion, however, is a physical bruising of the brain tissue. Brain contusions are often accompanied by skull fractures.

■ ***ETIOLOGY.*** A blow to the head by an object, fall, or other trauma such as an automobile accident can cause a concussion or contusion.

■ ***SYMPTOMS.*** Both conditions cause a disruption of normal electrical activity in the brain, which, in turn, causes immediate unconsciousness, often described as being knocked out. This state of unconsciousness can last from a few seconds to several hours, and the affected individual often awakens with **amnesia** or loss of memory. Other symptoms are headache, blurred vision, and irritability. The individual might suddenly draw up the knees and begin vomiting.

The physical bruising of a contusion can lead to the development of a hematoma, increased ICP, and permanent brain damage. If the bruised tissue is in the area of the impact, it is referred to as a coup (COO) lesion. Coup lesions often occur with direct injury such as is incurred from a direct blow to the head. If the injury occurs on the opposite side of the brain, it is called a contracoup (CON-tra-coo) lesion, which often occurs when the head is in motion and is stopped suddenly, causing a rebound effect to the opposite side (Figure 15–9), as is often found in automobile accidents. Contracoup injuries are commonly accompanied by a coup injury at the point of impact.

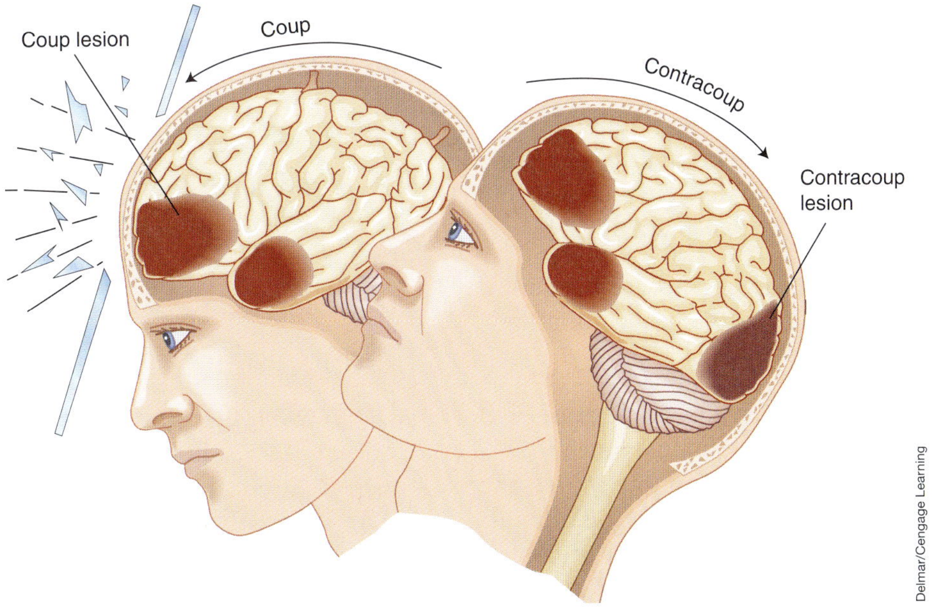

FIGURE 15–9 Coup and contracoup lesions.

■ ***DIAGNOSIS.*** Diagnosis of both conditions is made on the basis of a history of the injury, neurologic examination, cranial X-ray, and CT or MRI scans.

■ ***TREATMENT.*** Treatment of a concussion consists of bed rest in a quiet area under direct observation. The individual should be awakened every 2 to 4 hours and observed for changes in consciousness, eye pupil size, mood, and behavior. An individual suffering with a contusion should be hospitalized for continuous monitoring. Analgesic, sedative, and stimulant medications should not be given to individuals with head injuries because these medications can mask symptoms and make assessment difficult.

■ ***PREVENTION.*** Preventive actions include activities to prevent head injury such as wearing a seat belt in an automobile, wearing helmets with recreational activity, and preventing falls by removing clutter and slippery rugs.

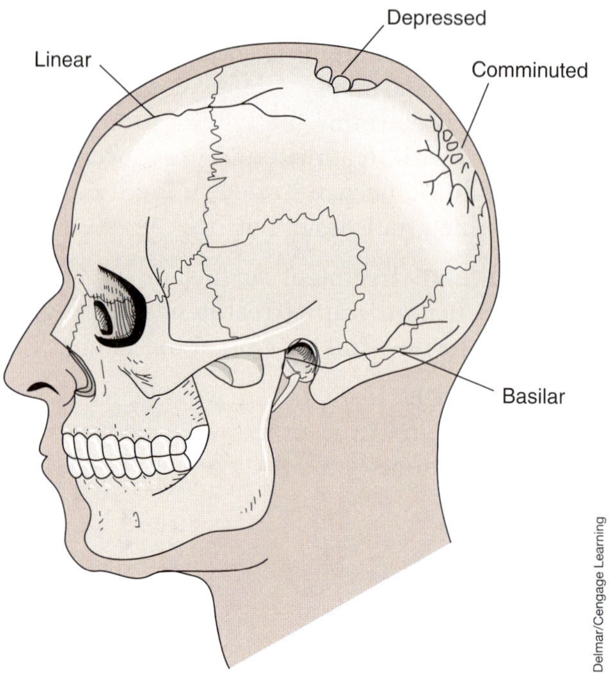

FIGURE 15–10 Common sites and types of skull fractures.

StudyWARE™ Connection

View an animation on contracoup injuries on your StudyWARE™ CD-ROM.

Skull Fractures

■ ***DESCRIPTION.*** A skull fracture is a break in a cranial (skull) bone. The greatest danger of a skull fracture is the resulting brain tissue damage (Figure 15–10). Bony fragments can cut into the brain tissue, severing a vessel and causing a hematoma. Brain damage from a fracture can be temporary or permanent.

■ ***ETIOLOGY.*** A fracture can occur with head injuries from falls, a severe blow to the head, automobile accidents, or sports injuries.

■ ***SYMPTOMS.*** The position of the fracture will cause a variety of symptoms. For instance, a fracture near the base of the skull might injure the respiratory center of the brain, causing the individual to stop breathing. Fractures in other areas can lead to hemiparesis and seizures. Another potential problem is infection of the brain tissue through the fracture site.

■ ***DIAGNOSIS.*** Diagnosis is made on the basis of clinical history, physical examination, cranial X-rays, and CT scan.

■ ***TREATMENT.*** Treatment depends on the type and position of the fracture. A craniotomy (cranio = skull, otomy = incision) might be performed to relieve ICP due to swelling. Surgical repair of the fracture might be performed if the fractured bone is pressing on the brain tissue. Protective headgear might be needed until the fracture site is healed.

■ ***PREVENTION.*** Preventive actions include practicing safety measures and avoiding risky activities to prevent head injury.

Epidural and Subdural Hematomas

■ ***DESCRIPTION.*** An epidural hematoma is a collection of blood between the skull and dura mater, the thin membrane that covers the brain. They occur more often in young adult males. A subdural hematoma is a collection of blood between the outer (dura mater) layer and the middle (arachnoid) layer. They occur twice as often as epidural hematomas.

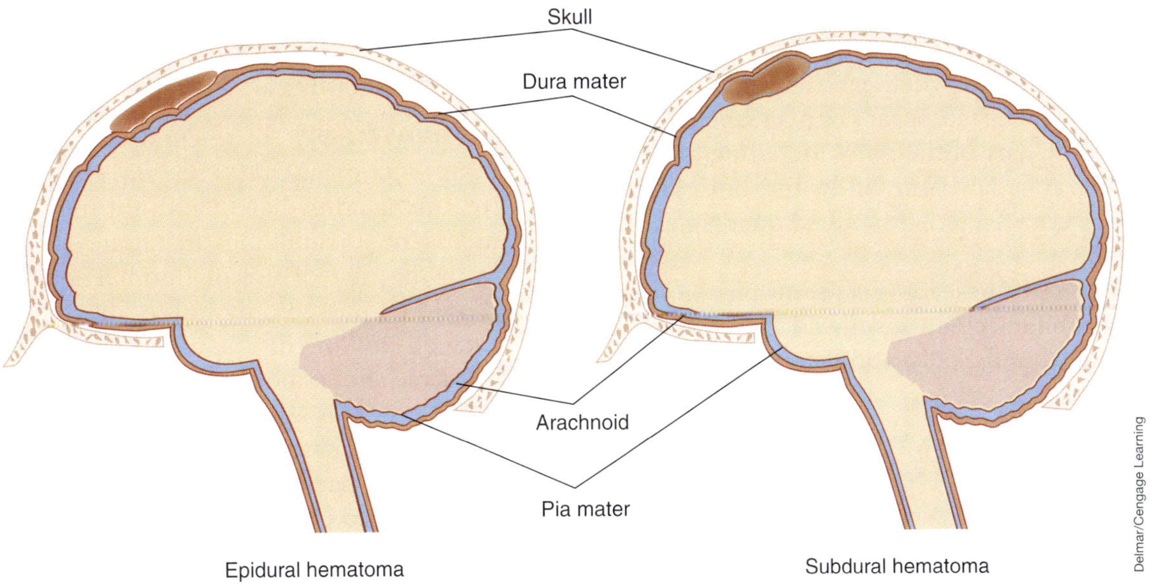

FIGURE 15–11 (A) Epidural and (B) subdural hematomas.

ETIOLOGY. A blow to the head, such as might be obtained in a fight or accident, is the common cause of an **epidural** (EP-ih-DER-al); epi = above, dural = dura, outer meninges) hematoma. Blood vessels are ruptured and hemorrhage or seep blood between the bony skull and the first, or outer, meninges, the dura mater (Figure 15–11). Blood usually collects rapidly over a period of hours, pushing the dura away from the inner bony skull.

A **subdural** (SUB-DOO-ral) hematoma is usually the result of the head hitting a stationary object, as is often seen with falls, characterized by striking the head on the floor or a solid object. Subdural hematomas are characterized by blood collecting between the outer (dura mater) layer and the middle (arachnoid) layer. Subdural hematomas generally develop more slowly over a period of days.

SYMPTOMS. Symptoms of an epidural hematoma occur within a few hours after injury and can include headache, dilated pupils, nausea, vomiting, and dizziness. As the hematoma grows, the individual might lose consciousness and develop an increase in ICP

Symptoms of a subdural hematoma are due to increased ICP. Symptoms might include hemiparesis, nausea, vomiting, dizziness, convulsions, and loss of consciousness.

DIAGNOSIS. Diagnosis of a cerebral hematoma is made on the basis of clinical history, cranial X-ray, or CT or MRI scan. Hematomas, generally, are accompanied by a skull fracture.

TREATMENT. Treatment of epidural and subdural hematomas is aimed at decreasing ICP. Pressure can be relieved by a special craniotomy called burr holes to drain the blood and **cauterization** (KAW-ter-eye-ZAY-shun; electrical burning of tissue) to stop the bleeding. If ICP is treated promptly, prognosis is good. Untreated, increased ICP can be fatal.

PREVENTION. Preventive actions include activities to prevent head injury.

Spinal Cord Injury: Quadriplegia and Paraplegia

In 1995, actor Christopher Reeve fell off a horse and severely damaged his spinal cord, leaving him paralyzed from the neck down. From then until his death in 2004, the silver screen Superman became the most famous face of spinal cord injury. (Mayo Clinic, 2007)

DESCRIPTION. The spinal cord is protected by the bony vertebral column. When this column is fractured or injured, the spinal cord also can suffer injury. The spinal cord can be injured at any level, but the mobility of the neck causes this area to be the most vulnerable. The site of the injury, the type of trauma, and the degree of injury will all play a role in determining whether paralysis will occur and whether it will be temporary or permanent. Paralysis of the lower part of the body including both legs is called paraplegia. If the body and both arms and both legs are affected, it is called quadriplegia.

■ ***ETIOLOGY.*** The leading cause of spinal cord injury is automobile accidents. Other causes are gunshot and knife wounds, falls, and recreational and sports injuries.

■ ***SYMPTOMS.*** Injury to the spinal cord can result in varying degrees of loss of movement and feeling below the area of injury. If the damage to the spinal cord is severe, there is little or no hope of regaining movement and feeling. Paralysis, initially, results in the inability to move the extremities; but with time, reflex functions might return, leading to spastic movements. Refer to Figure 15–12 while reading the following material for a better understanding of spinal cord injuries and preventive measures.

Injury to the neck is common in automobile accidents and sports accidents. Automobile accidents commonly lead to injury in the form of whiplash.

Injury to the highest level of the cervical spine (C1–C3) is usually fatal. Injuries to the cervical spine or neck area (C1–C4) can lead to **quadriplegia** (KWAD-rih-PLEE-jee-ah; quadri = four, plegia = paralysis). Quadriplegia is the loss of movement and feeling in the trunk and all four extremities with the accompanying loss of bowel, bladder, and sexual function. Other life-threatening symptoms include hypotension, **hypothermia** (hypo = low, thermia = heat or temperature), bradycardia, and respiratory problems. In some cases, respirations must be permanently assisted with mechanical ventilation. Injury to the lower cervical spine (C5–C7) can lead to varying degrees of paralysis of the arms and shoulders.

Injury to the thoracic or lumbar section of the spinal cord can lead to **paraplegia** (PARA-ah-PLEE-jee-ah; para = beyond or two like parts, plegia = paralysis), a loss of movement and feeling in the trunk and both legs. Loss of bladder, bowel, and sexual function are common. Paraplegia is often the result of a fall or an injury resulting in compression to the lower spine.

■ ***DIAGNOSIS.*** Diagnosis is made on the basis of history of the injury and physical examination along with X-rays, CT scan, MRI, and myelography.

■ ***TREATMENT.*** Treatment of suspected spinal cord injury victims includes seeking emergency medical treatment immediately and not moving the victim unless the surroundings are unsafe or life-threatening as in the case of fire or flood. The head and neck should be moved only in life threatening situations such as choking or respiratory arrest. Movement at this time should be very cautious. Emergency medical treatment is aimed at maintaining the position of the spine by limiting movement with use of special collars and backboards. The head, neck, and spine are stabilized prior to transporting in an emergency vehicle.

Hospitalization includes diagnosis and treatment of the injury, including medications, emergency surgery, and, often, immobilization with traction or traction-like devices. Much of the early treatment is aimed at preventing further spinal cord injury.

Further treatment can include surgery to realign and stabilize the bony spinal column and **decompress**, or release, pressure on the spinal cord. Early and intensive rehabilitation is necessary for the best prognosis. Generally, the earlier the treatment is begun, the better the prognosis.

During treatment, medical attention must also focus on preventing problems that arise from immobilization, including muscle wasting, contractures, decubitus (commonly called bed sores), blood clots, and urinary tract infections.

Long-term care includes rehabilitation and supportive treatment, which might include medications, electric wheelchair, computer devices, and ventilator support.

■ ***PREVENTION.*** Preventive actions include activities to prevent spinal cord injury as shown in Figure 15–12.

*Study***WARE**™ Connection

View an animation on spinal cord injuries on your StudyWARE™ CD-ROM.

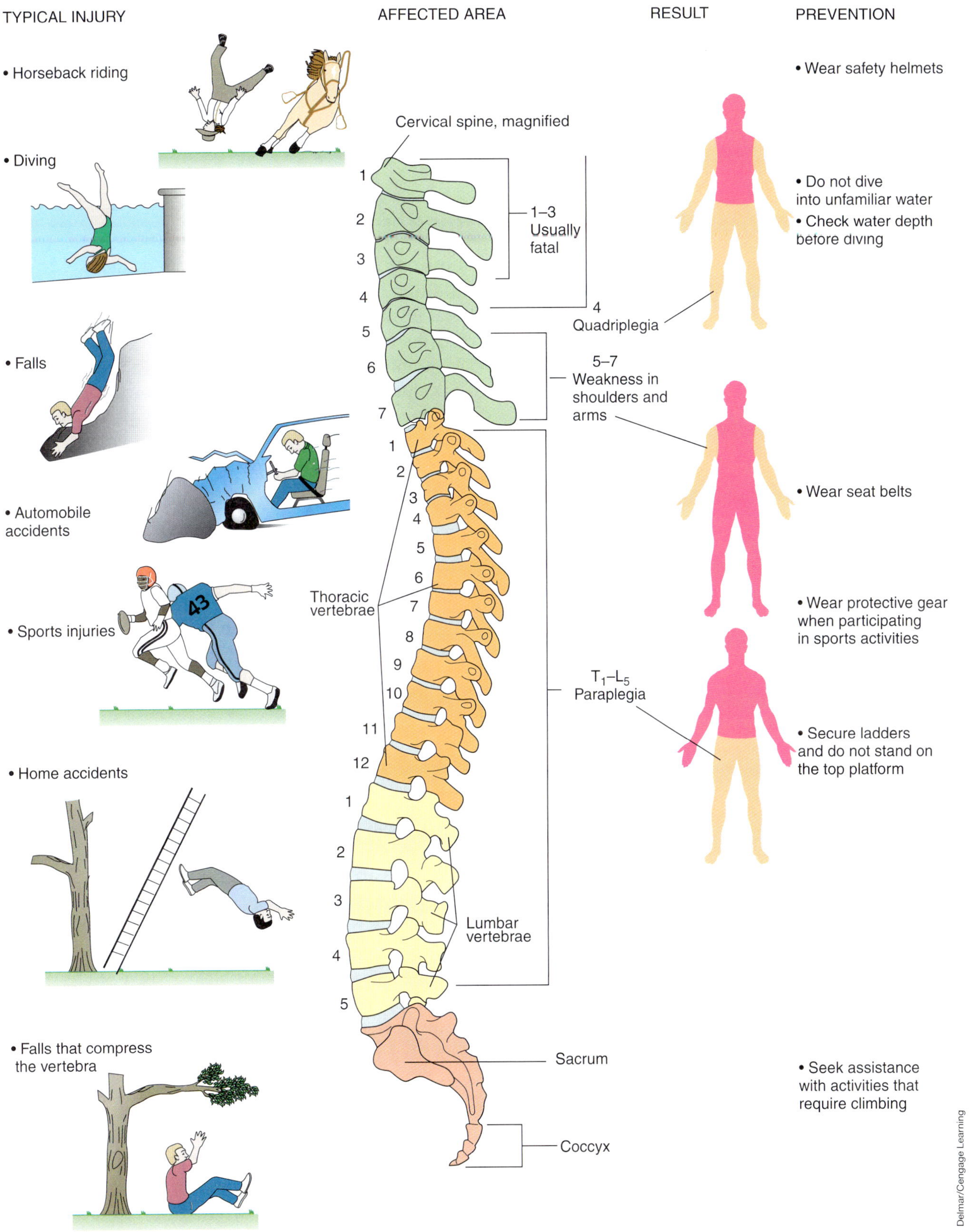

FIGURE 15–12 Spinal cord injuries.

RARE DISEASES

Although some of the disorders discussed in this section are familiar to the public due to their exposure in the media and to intensive solicitations for research, they are actually rare diseases of the nervous system, considering all the various disorders that affect this system.

Amyotrophic Lateral Sclerosis

Amyotrophic lateral sclerosis (ALS), also known as Lou Gehrig's disease, is a destructive disease of the motor, or movement, neurons. The cause of ALS is unknown, although genetic and viral-immune factors have been suggested.

ALS is characterized by atrophy of the muscles, leading to a progressive loss of movement of the hands, arms, and legs. As the disease progresses, loss of muscle function in the face and chest area leads to difficulty talking, chewing, swallowing, and breathing. Eventually, the loss of motor function causes quadriplegia.

One distinguishing factor of ALS is that there is not a loss of sensory neurons. The individual can feel the extremities, but movement is impaired. Mental function is unaffected, so the affected individual is aware of the condition and can take an active role in planning care. ALS usually affects men twice as often as it affects women, with onset of the disease after age 50.

Treatment is supportive because there is no cure for ALS. Management of respiratory complications is vital because most individuals affected with ALS die of respiratory failure. ALS is eventually fatal, with death usually occurring 4 to 6 years after onset. In some cases, affected individuals have remained active for 10 to 20 years after onset.

Guillain–Barré Syndrome

Guillain–Barré syndrome is an acute, progressive disease affecting the spinal nerves. The cause of this disease is unknown, but it is suggested to be an autoimmune disorder because the symptoms usually begin 10 to 21 days after a febrile illness such as a respiratory infection or gastroenteritis.

Early symptoms include nausea, fever, and malaise. Within 24 to 72 hours, **paresthesia** (PAR-es-THEE-see-ah; abnormal sensation, burning, tingling, or numbness), muscle weakness, and paralysis usually begin. These symptoms generally begin in the legs and move upward but can also start in the face and arms and move downward.

Guillain–Barré syndrome becomes life-threatening if respiratory muscles are involved. Symptoms can progress for several days to some weeks. When progression ceases, recovery begins and can require 3 to 12 months. Treatment is supportive. Recovery is usually complete.

Huntington's Chorea

Huntington's chorea is an inherited disease. It is a dominant gene disorder affecting 50% of all children in families in which one parent has Huntington's. This disorder does not appear until middle age, so children are often grown before the parent shows symptoms.

Symptoms of Huntington's consist of a progressive degeneration of the brain, characterized by loss of muscle control and **chorea**, a constant, jerky, uncontrollable movement. The disease also leads to mental deterioration with symptoms of personality change, moody behavior, and loss of memory. Over a period of years, dementia (total mental incapacitation) occurs.

There is no cure for Huntington's chorea. Treatment is supportive and protective with institutionalization often necessary to provide the needed care. Genetic counseling is needed in families with this inheritance pattern.

Multiple Sclerosis

Multiple sclerosis (MS) is a disease that causes demyelination of the nerves of the CNS. Myelin, remember, acts as an insulator around nerves, much like the insulation around an electric cord. Demyelination allows information to leak from the nerve pathway, leading to poor or absent nerve transmission.

The cause of MS is not clear. It is thought that a genetic predisposition plays some part because it is 15 times more likely to occur in first-degree relatives of affected persons. It is also believed that the immune system and viral infection play a part.

Symptoms caused by demyelinating lesions are muscle weakness, lack of coordination, paresthesia, speech difficulty, loss of bladder function, and visual disturbance, especially diplopia (double vision). Symptoms are varied, depending on the location of the lesions, making diagnosis difficult.

MS usually affects young adults between the ages of 20 and 40 years. It is characterized by periods of remission and exacerbation, usually over a period of several years.

Physical therapy and muscle relaxants can be helpful to maintain muscle tone and reduce spastic movement. The severity of the disease varies from individual to individual, but generally speaking, most affected individuals live a normal life span.

EFFECTS OF AGING ON THE SYSTEM

The effects of aging on the nervous system are some of the most noticeable to the older adult. With aging, there is a decrease in nervous system activity in the brain and spinal cord due to a loss of neurons and shrinkage of the hypothalamus. Research has shown that continued active use of the brain decreases this process to some extent, but some changes still occur. With these changes in the brain and spinal cord come many changes in the individual's functioning, for instance, a loss in short-term memory but not in long-term memory. There is also a slower general reaction time. The older person also might have difficulty completing fine motor skills. General touch perception is somewhat diminished, too, so the individual might have difficulty distinguishing temperature changes and pain stimuli.

Vision ability is one of the first changes the individual often notices. There is a loss of visual acuity and a decrease in peripheral vision. Some individuals also become intolerant of very bright light and have difficulty adapting to changes in light from dark to bright. Some hearing loss is a subtle process that occurs at different levels in individuals. Taste sensation also can diminish over time.

Sleep patterns are usually affected in the aging process. Generally, the older adult does not sleep as well at night but makes up for this deficit by taking short naps throughout the day or in the early evening.

SUMMARY

The nervous system is a highly complex system responsible for the individual's ability to reason, interact with other individuals, understand complex ideas, and respond both intellectually and physically. Disorders of the system usually result in symptoms involving many other systems.

Injuries to the brain, neck, and spinal cord are a main cause of disability and death nationwide. Permanent neurologic deficits are common in brain and spinal cord injuries.

Changes in the nervous system with aging result in some of the most commonly seen symptoms; losses in the senses are the most noticeable problems. Changes in vision and hearing are some of the earliest symptoms realized by the middle-aged individual. Alzheimer's disease is one of the most common disorders of the nervous system diagnosed today.

REVIEW QUESTIONS

Short Answer

1. What are the functions of the nervous system?

2. Which signs and symptoms are associated with common nervous system disorders?

3. Which diagnostic tests are most commonly used to determine the type and cause of nervous system disorders?

Matching

4. Match the disorders listed in the left column with the correct description in the right column:

_____ Encephalitis	a. inflammation of the covering of the brain and spinal cord
_____ Tetanus	b. a disorder affecting the seventh cranial nerve
_____ Meningitis	c. disruption in the electrical activity of the brain, causing unconsciousness
_____ TIA	d. blood collection between the dura mater and arachnoid layer of the brain
_____ Cephalalgia	e. physical bruising of the brain
_____ Concussion	f. infection of nerve tissue
_____ Contusion	g. disease characterized by the demyelination of nerves of the CNS
_____ Subdural hematoma	h. inflammation of brain tissue
_____ Alzheimer's disease	i. headache
_____ ALS	j. a neurodegenerative disease characterized by cognitive dysfunction
_____ MS	k. destructive disease of the motor neurons
_____ Bell's palsy	l. mild stroke

CASE STUDIES

■ Mr. Speed is a 57-year-old gentleman who has been recently diagnosed with Alzheimer's disease. He is in the early stage of the disease at this point. Mrs. Speed is quite concerned about the progression of the disease, whether Mr. Speed can still be employed, if he can be left alone for several hours at a time, and what medications he will be required to take. How would you respond to her concerns? Is there other information that would be helpful to the Speeds? Where can they find more information about Alzheimer's disease?

■ Mrs. Simpson, age 56, comes to the clinic for her yearly routine physical examination. She asks you about receiving the vaccine for shingles that she heard about on television. She thought she should get it because her sister had shingles a year ago. Mrs. Simpson stated that her sister really suffered with the disease, and she does not want to have that same experience. What can you tell her about the vaccine? Is she a candidate for Zostava®? Who should receive the vaccine? Where can she find more information about this vaccine?

*Study*WARE™ Connection

To help you learn the content in this chapter, take a practice quiz or play an interactive game on your StudyWARE™ CD-ROM.

Workbook Practice

Go to your Workbook and complete the practice questions.

BIBLIOGRAPHY

Act fast to treat ministrokes (2007). *Nursing 37*(12), 33.

Arai, N., Takahashi, T., Komori, T., Yagishita, A., & Shimizu, H. (2007). Diagnostic surgical neuropathology of intractable epilepsy. *Neuropathology 27*(6), 594–600.

Are alternative headache therapies right for you? (2006). *Nutrition Health Review: The Consumer's Medical Journal* (95), 3–8.

Aschenbrenner, D. (2008). New indication for raloxifene. *American Journal of Nursing 108*(1), 38.

Birmingham, K. (2006). Sound bite. *Nursing Older People 18*(8), 4.

Facco, E., Liguori, A., Petti, F., Zanette, G., Coluzzi, F., DeNardin, M., & Mattia C. (2008). Traditional acupuncture in migraine: A controlled randomized study. *Headache: The Journal of Head & Face Pain 48*(3), 398–407.

Fox, S., Mitchell, S., & Booth-Jones, M. (2006). Cognitive impairment in patients with brain tumors: Assessment and intervention in the clinic setting. *Clinical Journal of Oncology Nursing 10*(2), 169–176.

Hardy, J. (2008). Multiple system atrophy: Pathophysiology, treatment and nursing care. *Nursing Standard 22*(22), 50–56.

Herpes Zoster Vaccine Q & A. (2008). Centers for Disease Control and Prevention (CDC). *www.cdc.gov* (accessed March 9, 2008).

Hussar, D. (2007). New drugs 07. *Nursing 37*(8), 46–55.

Mathew, N., Kaliasam, J., & Meadors, L. (2008). Botulinum toxin type A for the treatment of nummular headache: Four case studies. *Headache: The Journal of Head & Face Pain 48*(3), 442–447.

Mathews, C., Miller, L., & Mott, M. (2007). Getting ahead of acute meningitis & encephalitis. *Nursing 37*(11), 37–41.

May is National Stroke Awareness Month. (2007). *Journal of Cardiovascular Nursing 22*(3), 156.

Mayo Clinic. (2007). Spinal cord injury. Mayo Clinic. *www.mayoclinic.com* (accessed June 2008).

McCluskey, L. (2007). Amyotrophic lateral sclerosis: Ethical issues from diagnosis to end of life. *NeuroRehabilitation 22*(6), 563–472.

New skin patch for dementia. (2007). *Nursing 37*(10), 30.

Palmieri, R. (2007). Responding to primary brain tumor. *Nursing 37*(1), 36–42.

Parkinson's care at risk from job cuts. (2006). *Nursing Standard 20*(43), 11.

Parkinson's disease. (2007). *Nursing Standard 22*(7), 51.

Parkinson's disease: New drug treats dementia. (2006). *Nursing 36*(9), 32.

Pillar 1: Diet and vitamins. (2008). Alzheimer's Research and Prevention Foundation. *www.alzheimersprevention.org* (accessed June 2008).

Poliomyelitis. Centers for Disease Control. National Center for Health Marketing. *cdcinfo@cdc.gov.* (accessed June 2008).

Ricon, F., & Sacco, R. (2008). Secondary stroke prevention. *Journal of Cardiovascular Nursing 23*(1), 34–41.

Rowe, B., Colman, I., Edmonds, M., Blitz, S., Walker, A., & Sheldon, H. (2008). Randomized controlled trial of intravenous dexamethosone to prevent relapse in acute migraine headaches. *Headache: The Journal of Head & Face Pain 48*(3), 333–340.

Sandman L., Bolmsjo, I., & Westergren, A. (2008). Ethical considerations of refusing nutrition after stroke. *Nursing Ethics 15*(2), 147–159.

Stroke detection training to help nurses save lives. (2007). *Nursing Standard 22*(14–16), 10.

Thomure, A. (2006). Helping your patient manage Parkinson's disease. *Nursing 36*(8), 20–21.

Trojan, D., & Cashman, N. (2005). Post-poliomyelitis syndrome. *Muscle Nerve 31*(1), 6–19.

Vacca Jr., V. (2007). Autonomic dysreflexia. *Nursing 37*(9), 72.

Vitiello, M. (2007). Growing old should not mean sleeping poorly: Recognizing and properly treating sleep disorders in older adults. *Journal of the American Geriatrics Society 55*(11), 1882–1883.

WebMD (2007). Understanding insomnia. *www.Webmd.com/sleepdisorders* (accessed June 2008).

Witt, C., Reinhold, T., Jena, S., Brinkhaus, B., & Willich, S. (2008). Cost-effectiveness of acupuncture treatment in patients with headache. *Cephalalgia 28*(4), 334–345.

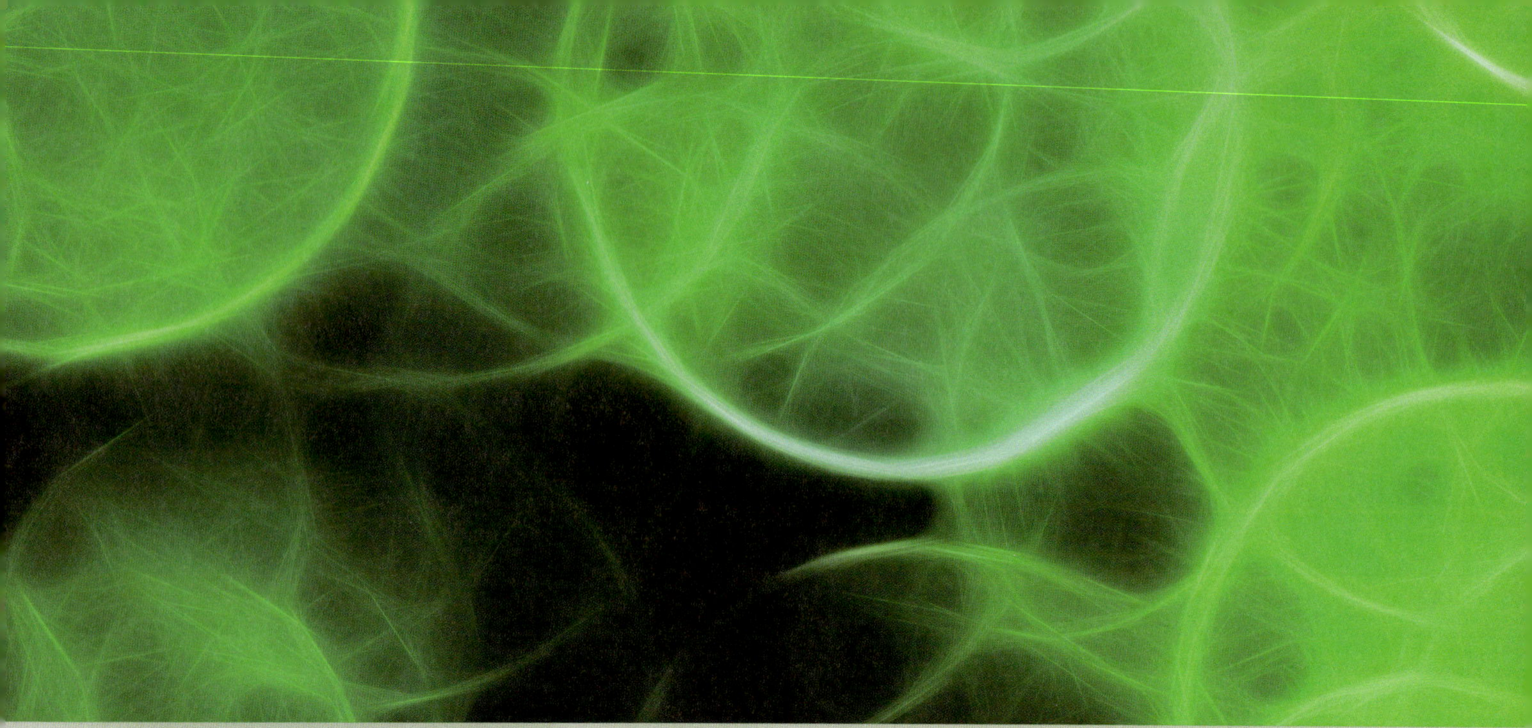

OUTLINE

- Anatomy and Physiology
  - *Eye*
  - *Ear*
- Common Signs and Symptoms
- Diagnostic Tests
  - *Diagnostic Tests of the Eye*
  - *Diagnostic Tests of the Ear*
- Common Diseases of the Eye
  - *Refractive Errors*
  - *Inflammation and Infection*
  - *Cataract*
  - *Glaucoma*
  - *Nystagmus*
  - *Strabismus*
  - *Macular Degeneration*
  - *Diabetic Retinopathy*
  - *Color Blindness or Color Deficiency*
- Common Diseases of the Ear
  - *Infection*
  - *Deafness*
  - *Motion Sickness*
- Trauma
  - *Corneal Abrasion*
  - *Retinal Detachment*
  - *Ruptured Tympanic Membrane*
- Rare Diseases
  - *Retinoblastoma*
  - *Ménière's Disease*
- Effects of Aging on the System
- Summary
- Review Questions
- Case Studies
- Bibliography

KEY TERMS

Amblyopia (p. 341)
Angiography (p. 335)
Audiometry (p. 335)
Cerumen (p. 333)
Diplopia (p. 341)
Enucleation (p. 351)
Mastoidectomy (p. 346)
Myringotomy (p. 344)
Ophthalmoscope (p. 334)
Otalgia (p. 344)
Otoscope (p. 335)
Photophobia (p. 339)
Prosthesis (p. 347)
Pruritus (p. 345)
Purulent (p. 345)
Radial keratotomy (p. 337)
Stapedectomy (p. 347)
Suppurative (p. 344)
Tinnitus (p. 346)
Tonometry (p. 335)
Topical (p. 339)
Tympanoplasty (p. 344)
Tympanostomy (p. 344)
Vertigo (p. 344)

16

Eye and Ear Diseases and Disorders

LEARNING OBJECTIVES

Upon completion of the chapter, the learner should be able to:

1. Define the terminology common to the eye and ear.
2. Discuss the basic anatomy and physiology of the eye and ear.
3. Identify the important signs and symptoms associated with common eye and ear disorders.
4. Describe the common diagnostics used to determine the type and cause of eye and ear disorders.
5. Identify common disorders of the eye and ear.
6. Describe the typical course and management of the common eye and ear disorders.
7. Describe the effects of aging on the eye and ear and the common disorders associated with aging of these organs.

OVERVIEW

The eyes and ears are the major sensory organs of the body. They are extremely important to most individuals to maintain quality of life and ease of functioning. However, although sensory deficits affect many people adversely, a high-quality lifestyle is still possible after sensory losses. Individuals with visual and hearing impairment learn to function extremely well in activities of daily living. Disorders of the sensory organs are frequently the result of other system problems. Early detection of vision or hearing impairment can prevent permanent loss of these senses. ■

ANATOMY AND PHYSIOLOGY

The eye and ear are sensory organs that perform highly complex functions in the individual. They each are unique in their structure and function.

Eye

The eyeball is the sensory organ of sight located in the bony orbit of the skull. It is about 1 inch in diameter and consists of extraocular and intraocular structures (Figure 16–1). The extraocular structures include the following:

- Muscles that hold the eyeball in place and facilitate movement of the eyeball
  - Superior and inferior rectus—move eye up and down
  - Medial and lateral rectus—move eye toward the nose and toward the temple
  - Superior and inferior oblique—move the eye to the right and left vertically
- Cranial nerves that innervate the eye and its structures
  - Optic (II)
  - Oculomotor (III)
  - Trochlear (IV)
  - Trigeminal (V)
  - Abducens (VI)
  - Facial (VII)
- Eyelids that cover the anterior portion of the eyeball, regulate light entering the eye, protect the eye, and lubricate the eye
- Conjunctivae (clear transparent membranes) to protect the eye from foreign objects
- Lacrimal glands (tear glands) to clean and moisten the eye

The intraocular structures consist of some parts of the eye that are visible externally and some parts visible only through an ophthalmoscope. The intraocular structures include the following:

- Sclera—white area covering the outside of the eye except over the pupil and iris
- Cornea—clear tissue covering the pupil and iris
- Iris—round disk of smooth and radial muscles giving the eye its color
- Pupil—round opening in the iris that changes size as the iris reacts to light and dark
- Anterior chamber—space between the cornea and iris/pupil that is filled with clear fluid called aqueous humor
- Posterior chamber—space between the iris and lens that is filled with aqueous humor
- Lens—clear fibers enclosed in a membrane that refract and focus light to the retina

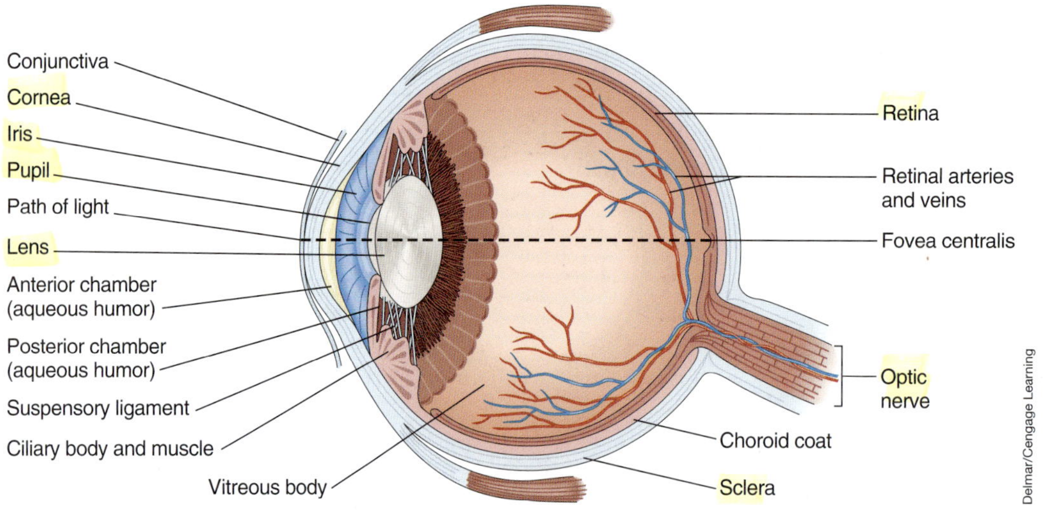

FIGURE 16–1 The eyeball: cross-sectional view.

- Posterior cavity—the space in the posterior two thirds of the eyeball, filled with a thick, gelatinous material called vitreous humor
- Posterior sclera—white opaque layer covering the posterior part of the eyeball
- Choroid layer—the layer containing blood vessels between the sclera and retina
- Retina—the inner layer of the posterior part of the eye that receives the light rays (visual stimuli)

The mechanism of vision occurs after impulses leave the retinae and travel through the optic nerves to the brain. At the optic chiasm, the nerve fibers cross and continue to the thalamus. These fibers synapse with other neurons that send the impulses to the right and left visual area of the occipital lobe of the brain. Because the tracts cross at the optic chiasm, the stimuli coming from the right visual fields are translated in the visual area of the left occipital area, and the stimuli coming from the left visual fields are translated in the visual area of the right occipital lobe (Figure 16–2).

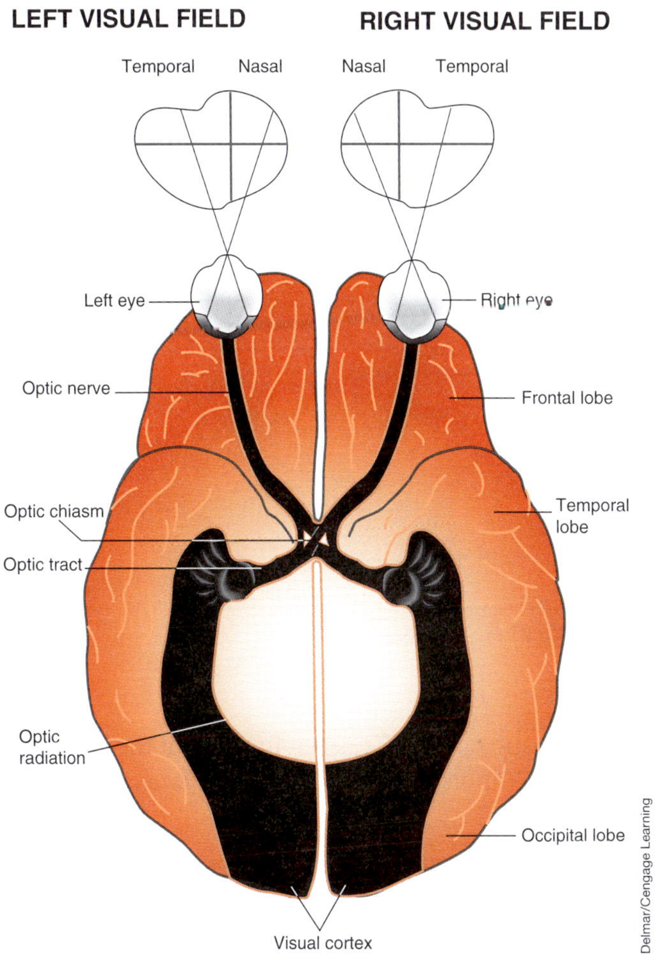

FIGURE 16–2 The visual pathways of the eye.

StudyWARE™ Connection

View an animation about the structures of the eye on your StudyWARE™ CD-ROM.

Ear

The structures of hearing and equilibrium are divided into the external ear, the middle ear, and the inner ear (Figure 16–3). The external ear includes the pinna (auricle) and the external auditory canal. The pinna is mostly cartilaginous tissue with a small amount of adipose tissue in the earlobe. The external auditory canal is about 1 inch long and contains hair and wax (**cerumen**, se-ROO-men) producing glands. The external ear and middle ear are separated by the tympanic membrane (eardrum).

The middle ear, also called the tympanic cavity, is a small space containing three bones: the malleus (hammer), incus (anvil), and stapes (stirrup). Next to the stapes is the oval window that leads to the inner ear.

The inner ear is the most sophisticated part of the ear and is responsible for both hearing and equilibrium (balance). It consists of a fluid-filled space housing the vestibule, the semicircular canals, the round window, and the cochlea. The structures in the vestibule maintain equilibrium during movement of the head. The semicircular canals assist the body in adjusting to changes in direction, and the movement of fluid in this area can cause symptoms of dizziness. The cochlea is the organ of hearing.

The outer ear (pinna) picks up sound waves sent through the external auditory canal to the tympanic membrane. The membrane vibrates in reaction to the sound waves striking it. These vibrations pass through the three tiny middle ear bones, through the oval window, and into the fluid in the cochlea. Receptor cells respond and transfer the sounds into electrical impulses that travel to the brain through

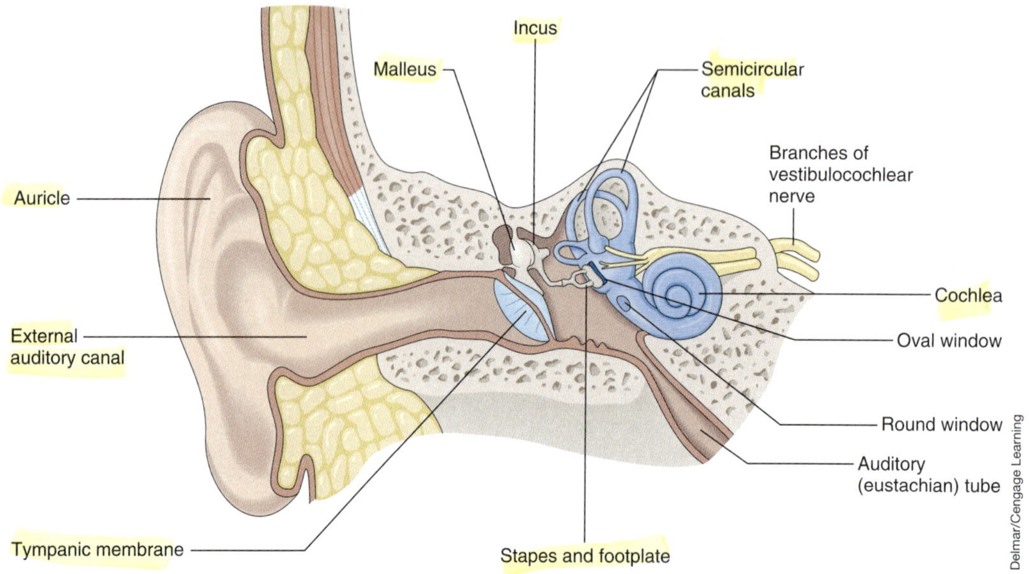

FIGURE 16–3 The ear.

the acoustic nerve. The receiving area of the brain for auditory impulses is in the temporal lobe.

> **StudyWARE™ Connection**
>
> View an animation about the structures of the ear on your StudyWARE™ CD-ROM.

COMMON SIGNS AND SYMPTOMS

Common signs and symptoms of eye disease that need medical attention include:

- Pain or burning in or around the eye
- Decreased visual acuity or ability to see
- Any visual disorder such as seeing flashes of light
- Eye redness

Common signs and symptoms of ear disease that need medical attention include:

- Otalgia (oh-TAL-gee-ah; oto = ear, algia = pain; ear pain)
- Deafness
- Vertigo (VER-tih-go; dizziness)
- Tinnitus (tin-EYE-tus; ringing in the ears)

DIAGNOSTIC TESTS

Diagnostic Tests of the Eye

An **ophthalmoscope** (aft-THAL-moh-skope; ophthalm = eye, scope = instrument used to look) is the instrument used for a basic examination of the eye. During an ophthalmoscopy (ophthalm = eye, oscopy = procedure to look), the fundus, or interior aspect of the eye, is examined. The retina, vessels, and optic disk of the eye can be visualized easily.

Visual acuity is measured by the use of a Snellen chart (Figure 16–4). The chart contains lines of letters in varying sizes with predetermined numbers at the end of each line. The predetermined numbers indicate the distance from which an individual with normal vision can see that particular line of letters. Normal vision is expressed as 20/20 and is considered normal vision for an individual viewing a particular line of the chart from 20 feet away.

For testing, the individual is positioned 20 feet from the chart, or this distance can be simulated with reflective mirrors. During the testing, one eye is covered, allowing measurement of each eye separately. The smallest line of letters the individual can read is noted, and the predetermined numbers at

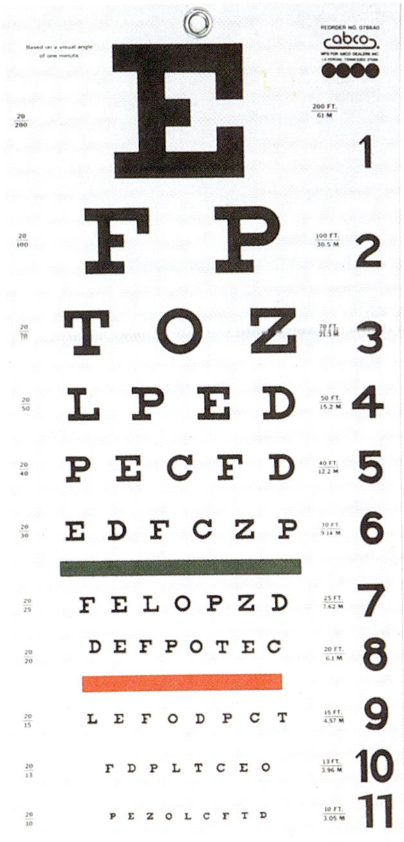

Delmar/Cengage Learning

FIGURE 16–4 The Snellen chart.

the end of that line are recorded in a fraction. The first number, 20, expresses the fact that the individual is tested from 20 feet, and the second number expresses the distance an individual with normal vision could view those same images. For example, 20/220 means that the tested individual can see at 20 feet what most people can see at 220 feet.

Diagnostic testing includes tonometry, slit-lamp examination, and retinal angiography. **Tonometry** (toh-NOM-eh-tree; tono = tone or pressure, metry = measurement) measures the pressure inside the eye and is therefore useful in determining the presence of glaucoma. A slit-lamp examination uses a microscope to magnify the surface of the eye by directing a beam of light, narrowed to a slit, at the cornea. Instilling fluorescein dye in the eye prior to the examination can improve visualization of eye disorders. A slit-lamp examination is helpful in determining corneal abrasions, keratitis, and cataracts. **Angiography** (AN-jee-OG-rah-fee; angio = vessel, graphy = procedure to record) is used to discover vessel disease and problems with blood flow to the eye. For this test, fluorescein dye is injected into a vein, usually in the arm, and after the dye fills the vessels of the eye, X-rays show the vessels. Vascular disorders such as those caused by diabetic retinopathy can be visualized.

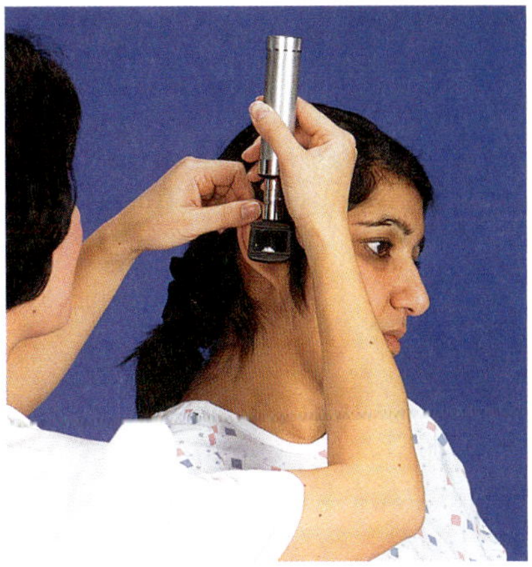
Delmar/Cengage Learning

FIGURE 16–5 Otoscopy.

Diagnostic Tests of the Ear

An **otoscope** (OH-toh-skope; oto = ear, scope = instrument to look) is the instrument used to examine the ear. During an otoscopy (oto = ear, scopy = procedure to look), or otoscopic examination (Figure 16–5), the external canal and tympanic membrane can be visualized easily. Otitis externa and a ruptured tympanic membrane can be diagnosed using the otoscope.

The basic test for hearing is called **audiometry** (AW-dee-OM-eh-tree; audio = sound, metry = measure). During the test, sound is delivered in varying levels, or decibels, through a headset to each ear separately. The greater the amount of sound needed for the individual to hear or recognize it, the greater the amount of deafness or hearing loss.

COMMON DISEASES OF THE EYE

The most common problem of the eyes is a decrease in visual acuity, the ability to see clearly. The most common cause of poor visual acuity is refractive errors. Other common problems include those related to inflammation or infection, which usually affects the outer eye because of its contact with the environment. Other eye disorders are clouding of the lens (cataract), increased inner eye pressure (glaucoma), altered eye movement (nystagmus, strabismus), degenerative disorders (such as macular degeneration), secondary disease (diabetic retinopathy), and hereditary disorders (color blindness).

Refractive Errors

■ ***DESCRIPTION.*** Refractive errors are those caused by the eye's inability to focus images correctly on the retina. Approximately one third of the population is affected by refractive errors.

■ ***ETIOLOGY.*** The cause of refractive errors is unknown, although some run in families, suggesting an inheritance pattern. Although these disorders affect individuals of all ages, incidence increases with age. There are four common types of refractive errors:

- Myopia (my-OH-pee-ah) is commonly called nearsightedness or shortsightedness. Individuals with myopia can see nearby objects but have difficulty seeing distant objects. Light entering the eye of a myopic individual falls short of the retina due to the eyeball being abnormally long from front to back (Figure 16–6). Myopia can be treated with prescriptive lenses, radial keratotomy (RK), automated lamellar keratoplasty (ALK), laser-assisted in-situ keratomileusis (LASIK), and implantable contact lenses (ICL) surgery (as described in the section titled, "Treatments").
- Hyperopia (HIGH-per-OH-pee-ah) is commonly called farsightedness. Individuals with hyperopia can see objects that are far away but have difficulty seeing close objects. Light entering the eye of a hyperoptic individual falls too far past the retina due to the eyeball being abnormally short from front to back (see Figure 16–6). Hyperopia can be treated with prescriptive lenses, CK, ALK, laser epithelial keratomileusis (H-LASEK), and thermal keratoplasty.
- Presbyopia (PRES-bee-OH-pee-ah; presby = old age) is hyperopia that is age-related. It is not due to the shape of the eyeball but, rather, is related to the inability of the aging lens to focus light rays properly. When the eye focuses on a distant object, the muscles of the eye pull the lens into a flatter shape. As the eye focuses on nearby objects, the muscles relax, allowing the lens to return to a more spherical shape. In presbyopia, the lens does not return to the normal shape, causing light rays to

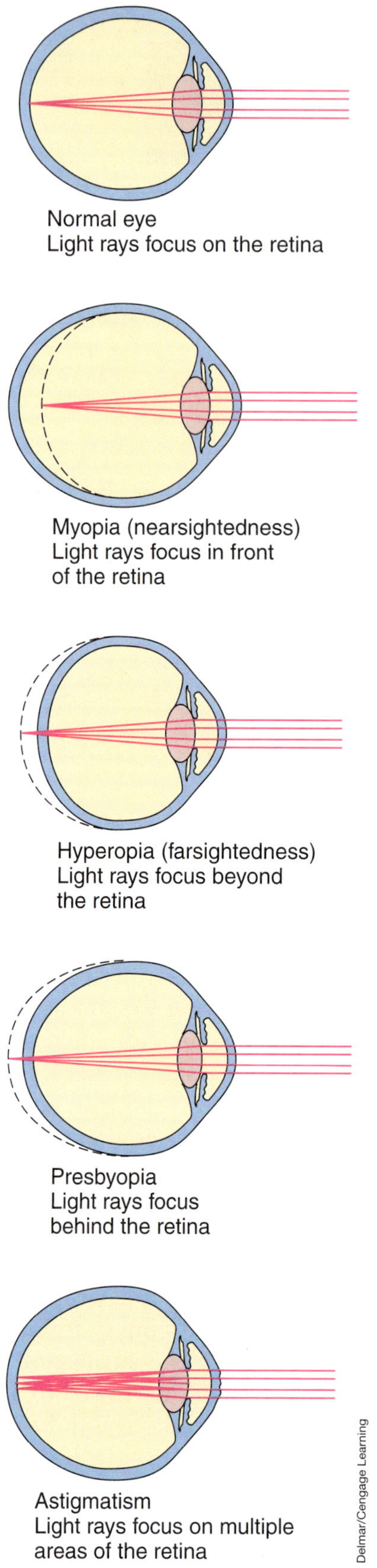

FIGURE 16–6 Normal eye vision, myopia, hyperopia, presbyopia, and astigmatism.

fall beyond the retina (see Figure 16–6). Presbyopia usually affects individuals aged 40 or older and can be corrected with reading glasses, bifocals, CK, and monovision LASIK.

- Astigmatism (ah-STIG-mah-tizm) is an irregularity in the surface of the cornea, causing light rays to spread over the retina rather than focus properly on part of the retina (see Figure 16–6). This refractive error can lead to blurred or fuzzy vision, often described as seeing halos around objects. Astigmatism can be treated with prescriptive lenses or LASIK.

SYMPTOMS. Common symptoms of refractive errors include squinting, blurred vision, headaches, and rubbing of eyes.

DIAGNOSIS. Tests for visual acuity include an ophthalmoscopic examination to look inside the eye and the individual reading a Snellen chart.

TREATMENT. Refractive errors are commonly corrected with prescriptive eyeglasses or contact lenses. Surgical treatments include:

- **Radial keratotomy** (**RK**) (KER-ah-TOT-oh-me; kerato = cornea, otomy = incision) is a procedure to correct myopia. Incisions are made in a radial fashion in the cornea to flatten the cornea, shortening the length of the eyeball and correcting the refractive error (Figure 16–7). Approximately 66% of the individuals undergoing this procedure are able to see clearly without corrective lenses.
- **Automated lamellar keratoplasty (ALK)** is a surgery using a device called a microkeratome to separate and remove a thin disc of cornea. The thickness of the disc removed determines the change in the refractive error.
- **Laser-assisted in-situ keratomileusis (LASIK)** uses an excimer laser to change the shape of the cornea permanently. After cutting and lifting an outer portion of the cornea, pulses from a computer-controlled laser vaporize a midsection of the cornea to flatten the curvature.
- **Implantable contact lenses (ICL)** permanently implant contact lenses into the eye. An advantage of ICL over surgeries that flatten the cornea is that overcorrection or undercorrection can be remedied by replacing the contact lens with the correct prescription.
- **Conductive keratoplasty (CK)** surgery uses mild heat from radio waves to shrink connective tissue

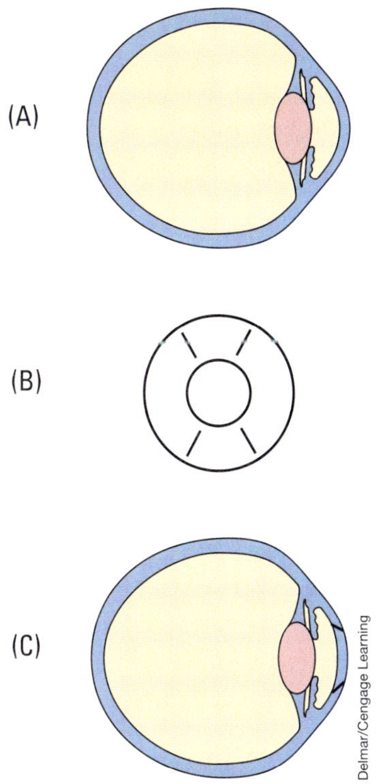

FIGURE 16–7 Radial keratotomy. (A) Cross-section of the eye prior to surgery. (B) Small incisions are made in the cornea from the middle outward. (C) This causes the cornea to become flatter, thereby improving vision.

(collagen) around the edge of the cornea. This circular pattern acts like a belt that tightens around the cornea, causing it to bulge or steepen the center of the cornea, thus lengthening the too-short eyeball.

- **Laser epithelial keratomileusis (H-Lasek)** surgery loosens the surface area of the cornea and pushes it to the side; a laser reshapes the inner layer of the cornea, and then the outer surface is replaced.
- **Thermal keratoplasty (TK)** uses heat to change the shape of the cornea by shrinking collagen fibers.
- **Monovision** surgery adjusts or fits one eye to see at a distance, leaving the other eye unadjusted for seeing close up, such as is needed for reading. (Normally, the eyes work equally to look at an object, a process called binocular vision.) The monovision idea is easy to achieve also with contact lenses in that one lens can be left out, allowing one eye to be corrected while the other is not.

LASIK surgeons are capable of producing monovision in presbyopic patients by purposefully adjusting one eye to see nearsighted. This technique does not work in all cases because some individuals cannot become accustomed to monovision. Monovision can affect depth perception and should be avoided by individuals such as airplane pilots, professional drivers, and some athletes.

■ ***PREVENTION.*** There are no preventive measures for refractive errors.

Inflammation and Infection

Inflammation of the eye and related structures is commonly caused by infectious microorganisms. Internal infections, or infection affecting the inside of the eye, are rare and are usually related to trauma; more common are inflammations or infections of the surface of the eye and its related structures. Eye infections are commonly caused by viruses and bacteria and can be secondary to allergies, trauma, and upper respiratory infections. Microorganisms can reach the eye from the individual's hands and contaminated washcloths and towels. Good hand washing and cleanliness are preventive measures.

CONJUNCTIVITIS

■ ***DESCRIPTION.*** Conjunctivitis is an inflammation of the conjunctiva, the pink membrane lining the inner eyelids (Figure 16–8).

■ ***ETIOLOGY.*** Conjunctivitis can be caused by excessive exposure to wind, sun, heat, and cold. The eyelids become red and swollen.

■ ***SYMPTOMS.*** Affected individuals might complain of excessive tearing, itching, burning, and pain. An acute, contagious bacterial infection of the conjunctiva is called pinkeye, which can become epidemic among school-aged children.

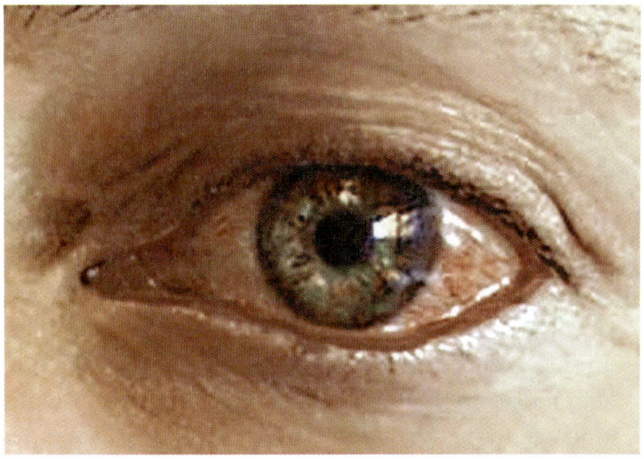

Courtesy of Mark L. Kuss

FIGURE 16–8 Conjunctivitis.

■ ***DIAGNOSIS.*** Diagnosis is usually simple because of obvious symptoms and is confirmed by a medical history and physical examination of the eye. If infection is a consideration, a swab of eye drainage can be obtained for a bacterial culture and sensitivity test.

■ ***TREATMENT.*** Treatment includes warm compresses, anti-inflammatory medications, and analgesics to relieve pain. If a culture identifies a microorganisms, antibiotic ointment or drops might be needed.

■ ***PREVENTION.*** Good hygiene measures, including frequent hand washing, use of protective eye wear, avoiding allergens such as dust and pollen, and using a clean tissue to remove drainage in the eye can prevent most cases.

BLEPHARITIS

■ ***DESCRIPTION.*** Blepharitis is inflammation of the edge of the eyelid, including the eyelash follicles and glands.

■ ***ETIOLOGY.*** Blepharitis can be caused by bacterial infection and allergic reaction to smoke, dust, or chemicals. Seborrhea, a disorder of the sebaceous gland, or oil-secreting gland, also can cause blepharitis.

■ ***SYMPTOMS.*** Affected individuals might complain of itching and burning and a feeling of something in the eye. The eyelids appear red, swollen, and crusted.

■ ***DIAGNOSIS.*** A routine examination of the eye with a slit-lamp microscope is usually all that is needed for diagnosis.

■ ***TREATMENT.*** Treatment is directed toward removal of the cause and can include antibiotics, allergy medication, or treatment for seborrhea.

■ ***PREVENTION.*** Good eyelid hygiene and a regular cleaning routine usually controls blepharitis. Eyelid hygiene includes frequent hand and face washing, warm water soaks on the eyelids, and eyelid and eyelash cleansing with warm water and baby shampoo. Good eyelid hygiene is very important upon awakening due to the secretions that accumulate on the eyelids during sleep.

KERATITIS

DESCRIPTION. Keratitis is inflammation of the cornea, usually unilateral, affecting only one eye.

ETIOLOGY. A frequent cause of keratitis is infection by herpes simplex virus secondary to an upper respiratory infection involving cold sores (herpes simplex). Allergies and contact lens can also lead to this condition.

SYMPTOMS. Symptoms include pain, **photophobia** (photo = light, phobia = fear), and excessive tearing.

DIAGNOSIS. A slit-lamp examination of the surface of the cornea will confirm the diagnosis.

TREATMENT. Treatment can include antibiotic ointment or drops to treat or prevent infection, analgesics for pain, and an eye patch to treat photophobia.

PREVENTION. Preventing trauma and avoiding unnecessary touching and rubbing of the eye help prevent keratitis.

STYE (HORDEOLUM)

DESCRIPTION. A stye, or hordeolum (hor-DEE-oh-lum), is an inflammatory infection of a sebaceous (oil-secreting) gland of the eyelid (Figure 16–9) at the base of a hair follicle or eyelash.

ETIOLOGY. Most styes are caused by staphylococcus bacteria and are often seen in blepharitis. They are also found more frequently in individuals who have diabetes and seborrhea.

SYMPTOMS. A tender, painful, red bump, often resembling a pimple, is located at the base of an eyelash or inside the eyelid. Often there is swelling or edema along the entire lid. Purulent drainage can come from the eyelash line or on the conjunctival surface of the eye.

DIAGNOSIS. Diagnosis is made on the basis of examination of the eye and presence of symptoms.

TREATMENT. Warm compresses may relieve pain, help localize the infection, and promote drainage. Styes usually form a soft spot, open, and drain and heal without further treatment. In some cases, styes may need to be incised to promote drainage and healing. In chronic conditions, **topical** (placed on the skin) antibiotic or systemic (taken by mouth or injection) antibiotic may be needed.

PREVENTION. Good eyelid and eye hygiene are preventive measures.

Cataract

DESCRIPTION. A cataract is a clouding of the lens of the eye (Figure 16–10).

ETIOLOGY. Cataracts develop from a change in metabolism and nutrition within the lens, most commonly from aging. Approximately 60% of all individuals 70 years of age or older will have clouding of a lens. Cataracts also can be caused by trauma, birth defects, and other diseases such as diabetes mellitus. Cataracts usually develop very slowly in one or both eyes.

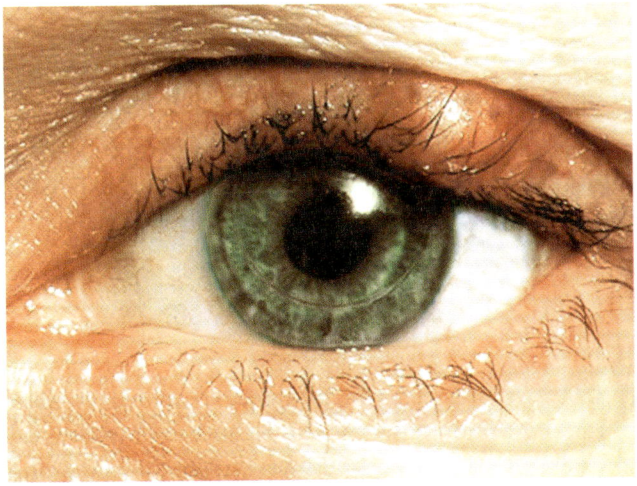

Courtesy of Mark L. Kuss

FIGURE 16–9 Stye (hordeolum).

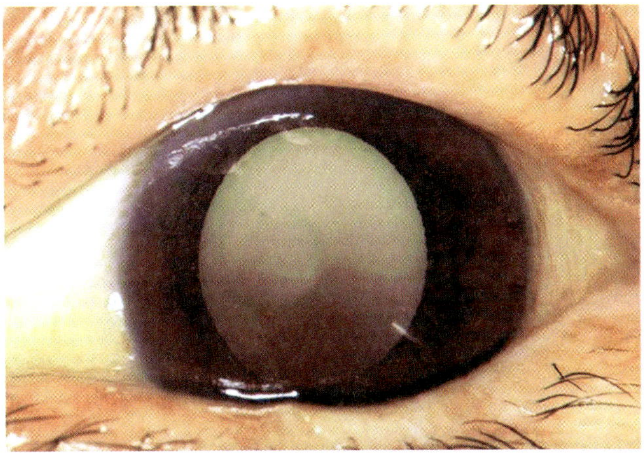

Courtesy of Mark L. Kuss

FIGURE 16–10 Cataract.

■ ***SYMPTOMS.*** The main symptom is a decrease in visual acuity or a complaint about not being able to see clearly. Other symptoms include blurred vision, glare, and a decrease in color perception. In advanced cases, the cataract can be seen through the pupil, giving the pupil a white, cloudy appearance.

■ ***DIAGNOSIS.*** Diagnosis is confirmed by slit-lamp examination.

■ ***TREATMENT.*** Cataracts are commonly treated with surgery, which involves removing the cloudy lens and replacing it with a clear artificial lens (Figure 16–11). This surgery, commonly called cataract extraction with placement of intraocular lens, is routinely performed as outpatient surgery. Postoperative prognosis is usually good.

■ ***PREVENTION.*** There are no known preventive measures.

Glaucoma

■ ***DESCRIPTION.*** Glaucoma is a common condition characterized by excessive pressure inside the eye from the fluid inside the eye, known as aqueous humor, which is produced constantly by blood. It circulates through the eye and is reabsorbed into the bloodstream.

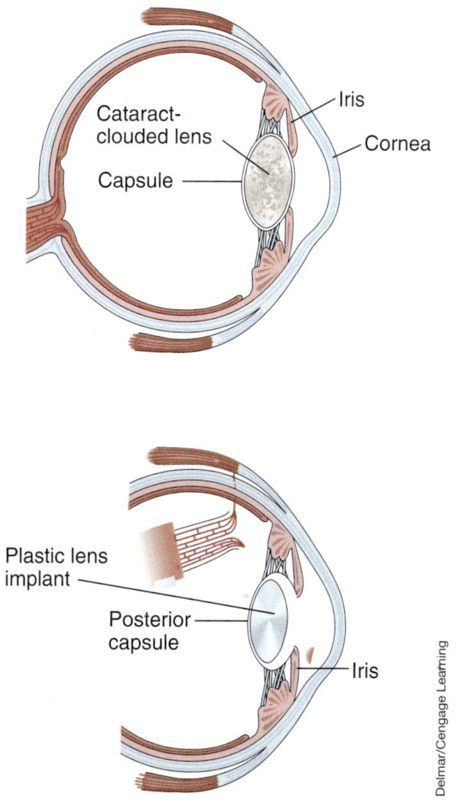

FIGURE 16–11 Cataract extraction with placement of intraocular lens.

■ ***ETIOLOGY.*** Excessive pressure inside the eye occurs if too much fluid is produced or does not drain properly. There are several forms of glaucoma, including open angle and closed angle glaucoma.

■ ***SYMPTOMS.*** Generally speaking, glaucoma progresses slowly, might or might not be symptomatic and rarely affects individuals under age 40. Increased pressure inside the eye for a continued period of time can lead to damage of the optic nerve and blindness, and permanent damage is often done before symptoms occur. For this reason, intraocular pressure should be checked on an annual basis.

■ ***DIAGNOSIS.*** Diagnosis is made on the basis of an ophthalmic examination and tonometry revealing an increase in intraocular pressure.

■ ***TREATMENT.*** Early treatment is essential to prevent permanent blindness. Depending on the form of glaucoma, treatment can include use of eye drops or surgery. Both are directed toward either reducing the amount of aqueous humor produced or improving the drainage.

■ ***PREVENTION.*** Regular eye examination with monitoring of eye pressure to discover glaucoma before any damage is done is the best preventive measure.

Nystagmus

■ ***DESCRIPTION.*** Nystagmus (nis-TAG-mus) is a constant, involuntary movement of the eyes that might be unnoticed by the affected individual. Movement can be vertical, horizontal, circular, or a combination of these. One or both eyes might be affected.

■ ***ETIOLOGY.*** Nystagmus might be the result of brain tumors, disease, alcohol abuse, or congenital defects. Diseases that cause nystagmus include Ménière's disease and multiple sclerosis.

■ ***SYMPTOMS.*** Abnormal eye movement as described.

■ ***DIAGNOSIS.*** It is usually easy to diagnosis nystagmus but difficult to diagnose the cause. Computerized tomography (CT) scan, magnetic resonance imaging (MRI), myelogram, angiography, and spinal tap might be needed to confirm the cause of the condition.

COMPLEMENTARY AND ALTERNATIVE THERAPY

Herbals for Eyes

Nutritional supplements and herbal products have shown some evidence that they can be beneficial for the eyes. In addition to proper rest, leafy greens and even herbal teas may be of some benefit. Kale and spinach contain lutein, which may reduce the individual's risk for developing cataracts or macular degeneration. The goji berry is often used to reduce blurriness. Patients should always report to their ophthalmologist if they are taking any herbal or nutritional supplements to boost their eye health.

Source: How do I boost my eye health (2008).

■ ***TREATMENT.*** Treatment is directed toward correction of the underlying cause. Congenital nystagmus is often untreatable and permanent.

■ ***PREVENTION.*** Prevention is aimed at curing or preventing the cause.

Strabismus

■ ***DESCRIPTION.*** Strabismus (strah-BIZ-mus) is a disorder in which the eyes fail to look in the same direction at the same time (Figure 16–12). Strabismus is often incorrectly referred to as lazy eye and as crossed eye or cockeye.

■ ***ETIOLOGY.*** Strabismus is the result of muscle weakness in one or both eyes. The affected eye can deviate upward or downward, but more commonly, it looks inward (convergent strabismus) or outward (divergent strabismus). Strabismus commonly occurs in children and requires early intervention to prevent **amblyopia** (AM-blee-OH-pee-ah), a decrease in the vision of the affected eye due to a lack of visual stimuli.

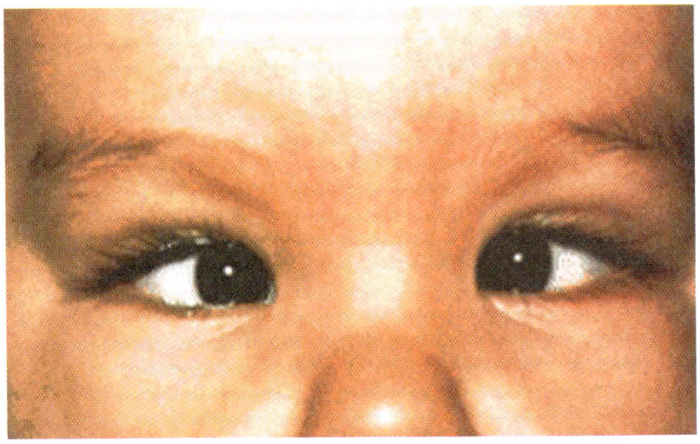

FIGURE 16–12 Strabismus.

■ ***SYMPTOMS.*** The primary symptom of strabismus is **diplopia** (dih-PLOH-pee-ah), or double vision, and altered eye movement.

■ ***DIAGNOSIS.*** A cover test is helpful in diagnosis. This involves covering each of the eyes while the individual is looking at an object. The straight eye will continue to look at the object when the opposite eye is covered. When the straight eye is covered, the strabismic eye will shift or straighten to fixate on the object.

■ ***TREATMENT.*** Treatment often consists of covering the normal eye in an effort to force the affected eye to function. Eye exercises and corrective lenses also can be ordered. The earlier the treatment is begun, the better. If correction is not made by the age of 6 or 7, the visual impairment can be permanent. Surgical intervention might be needed to correct strabismus.

■ ***PREVENTION.*** Strabismus cannot be prevented, but complications can be prevented with early detection and proper treatment.

Macular Degeneration

■ ***DESCRIPTION.*** Macular degeneration is a degeneration of the macular area of the retina, which is important in seeing fine detail.

■ ***ETIOLOGY.*** The cause of this degeneration can be due to the effects of drugs, but the most common cause is age. Risk factors include farsightedness, light

GLIMPSE OF THE FUTURE

The Food and Drug Administration approved research trials for vascular endothelial growth factor (VEGF) treatment of age-related macular degeneration (AMD). There have been some promising results thus far from the use of the anti-VEGF agents in treating AMD. The Phase III trial is using VEGF Trap, which prevents the growth of new blood vessels into a tumor. It belongs to the family of drugs called angiogenesis inhibitors (agents that stop blood vessel growth). Researchers are looking forward to evaluating the results of the trials, hoping that VEGF Trap may simplify the current treatment for AMD.

Source: Ciulla (2007).

eye color, and cigarette smoking. This disease is the leading cause of visual impairment in individuals 50 years of age and older.

■ ***SYMPTOMS.*** The primary symptom is a loss of central vision. Peripheral vision and color perception are unaffected. The disease generally develops slowly and painlessly, and both eyes are usually affected. As the disease progresses, reading and activities that require fine, detailed vision become impossible. There can be a complete loss of central vision, but generally, blindness does not occur.

■ ***DIAGNOSIS.*** Diagnosis is made on the basis of fluorescein angiography and routine examination.

■ ***TREATMENT.*** Vision might be improved in some cases by laser surgery.

■ ***PREVENTION.*** Since the most common cause is due to aging, this condition cannot always be prevented. Some activities aid prevention and include smoking cessation, eating foods high in antioxidants, eating fish regularly, wearing sunglasses that block ultraviolet light, managing other diseases such as cardiovascular disease and hypertension, and getting regular eye exams.

Diabetic Retinopathy

■ ***DESCRIPTION.*** Diabetic retinopathy (RET-ih-NOP-ah-thee; retino = retina, opathy = disease) is a complication of diabetes and the leading cause of blindness in the United States (National Eye Institute, 2008). This condition can happen to any individual with Type 1 or Type 2 diabetes. The longer the individual has diabetes, the more likely the development of diabetic retinopathy.

■ ***ETIOLOGY.*** Diabetes mellitus causes vascular changes in the retina that lead to a decrease in visual acuity. These changes include capillary aneurysms (also called microaneurysms), microhemorrhages, venous dilation, and new vessel growth (Figure 16–13). The affected vessels tend to bleed easily into the retina and produce scarring.

■ ***SYMPTOMS.*** Retinal scarring decreases visual acuity and can ultimately cause permanent blindness.

HEALTHY HIGHLIGHT

Foods to Help Dry Eyes

Dry eye syndrome (DES) can be helped by using artificial tears but also by eating a healthy diet. Studies have shown that people with DES often have low levels of omega-3 fatty acids in their food choices. Some of the foods that contain these include walnuts, flaxseeds, beans, fish, olive oil, and winter squash. Other supplements that help DES are the antioxidant vitamins C and E, agents that can be naturally found in vegetables, fruits, and plants. Antioxidants are also synthesized in the body and are essential to the immune system. They can be found in vegetables, fruits, legumes, and whole-grain foods.

Source: Eperjesi & Bartlett (2006).

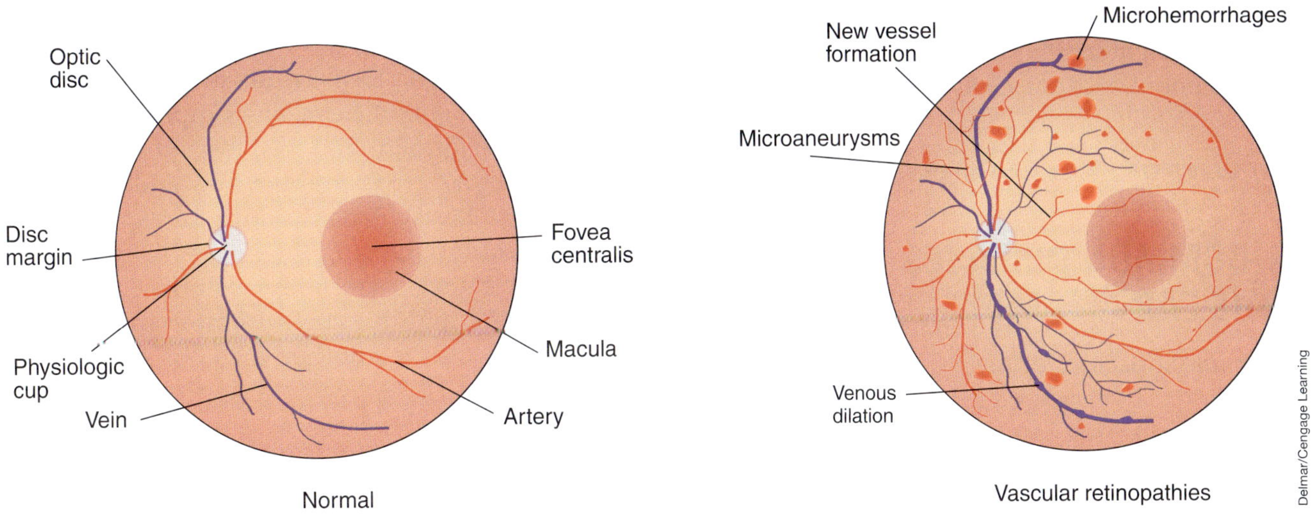

FIGURE 16–13 Vascular changes caused by diabetic retinopathy.

These vascular changes tend to occur in both eyes and are more extensive in uncontrolled diabetes or in individuals whose blood sugar is not controlled. Diabetic retinopathy can be asymptomatic in the early stages, but as the disease progresses, symptoms include blurred vision, poor night vision, floating spots in the visual field, and vision loss.

■ ***DIAGNOSIS.*** This condition is best diagnosed with a dilated-eye exam to allow the physician to see abnormal blood vessels, blood or fatty deposits in the retina, retinal detachment, and damage to the nerve tissue, all symptoms of diabetic retinopathy.

■ ***TREATMENT.*** Laser photocoagulation treatment is usually effective, but the condition tends to recur and might need repeated treatment.

■ ***PREVENTION.*** Prevention is directed toward controlling blood sugar levels to reduce the retinopathy. Other preventive methods include monitoring and controlling blood pressure and cholesterol levels, not smoking, reducing stress, and getting regular eye examinations.

Color Blindness or Color Vision Deficiency

■ ***DESCRIPTION.*** Normal ability to see colors diminishes with age due to the progressive yellowing of the lens. Colors become less intense, and the colors of green and blue often become more difficult to distinguish. Difficulty in distinguishing colors also can occur in young individuals affected with color vision deficiency (CVD).

■ ***ETIOLOGY.*** Color blindness also commonly occurs as an inherited, X-linked disorder that affects approximately 1 in 10 males. It is rarely seen in females.

■ ***SYMPTOMS.*** There are three main kinds of color vision defects. Red–green color vision defects are the most common, occur more often in men, and affect the ability to distinguish between red and green. The other major types are blue–yellow defects and complete absence of color vision.

■ ***DIAGNOSIS.*** CVD can be diagnosed using color plates or charts. A common plate is the Ishihara color plate shown in Figure 16–14.

■ ***TREATMENT.*** There is no known treatment or cure for color blindness. Interestingly, affected individuals might be sought to perform military duties that

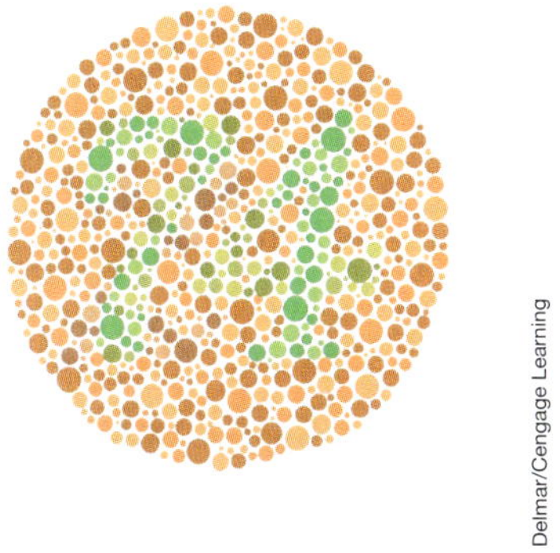

FIGURE 16–14 Ishirara Color Test Plate. The numeral "74" should be clearly visible to viewers with normal color vision.

include the discovery of camouflage. Color-blind individuals might exhibit an uncanny ability to see through camouflage, especially that using shades of green.

■ ***PREVENTION.*** There are no preventive measures.

COMMON DISEASES OF THE EAR

The common diseases of the ear include infections and conditions of decreased hearing or total hearing loss. Gradual hearing loss can be due to a primary ear disorder, such as an infection, or secondary to a disease or injury.

Infection

The ear and related bony structures are commonly subject to infection. The middle ear is connected to the nasopharynx by way of the Eustachian tube, making it easily accessible to bacteria that cause throat and respiratory infections. The external ear is open to the external environment, allowing infection from air and water. The bony mastoid process connects with the middle ear and is subject to infections affecting the middle ear. Ear infections are more common in infants and children.

OTITIS MEDIA

■ ***DESCRIPTION.*** Otitis media is inflammation in the middle ear. It usually affects infants and young children and is commonly called middle-ear infection, but it might not necessarily be an infection. The middle ear is normally filled with air, but when this area fills with fluid, inflammation occurs. For this reason, otitis media is classified by the type of fluid that fills the ear. Fluid types are:

Serous

■ ***ETIOLOGY.*** The fluid is clear and can be due to a Eustachian tube obstruction, allergy, or change in middle-ear pressure, as occurs with air flight, that allows clear serous fluid to accumulate in the middle ear. This fluid accumulation causes inflammation of the middle ear but without infection.

■ ***SYMPTOMS.*** Symptoms are usually mild and include a feeling of fullness in the ear and conductive hearing loss.

Suppurative

■ ***ETIOLOGY.*** The fluid is pus due to a bacterial infection in the middle ear. The **suppurative** (SUP-you-RAY-tiv; formation of pus) form of otitis media is often due to bacteria entering the middle ear, usually from the Eustachian tube during an upper respiratory infection. Blowing the nose forcefully often drives respiratory bacteria through the Eustachian tube into the middle ear. Swimming in contaminated water can be another cause of suppurative infection.

■ ***SYMPTOMS.*** Symptoms include varying degrees of **otalgia** (oh-TAL-gee-ah; ot = ear, algia = pain), nausea, vomiting, fever, chills, **vertigo** (VER-tih-go; dizziness), and conductive hearing loss.

The structure and position of the Eustachian tube is an important factor with either type of otitis media. If the Eustachian tube is narrower, shorter, more horizontally placed than normal, or all three of these conditions, the individual is more prone to otitis media. Infants and young children normally have narrower and more horizontally placed Eustachian tubes, thus predisposing them to otitis media. As the child grows, the tube becomes more vertical, which explains why children often outgrow ear infections.

■ ***DIAGNOSIS.*** Diagnosis is made on the basis of otoscopy revealing a bulging tympanic membrane or eardrum (Figure 16–15). The normally pearly colored tympanic membrane is red and swollen. If the tympanic membrane is ruptured, a culture of the fluid can be performed; otherwise, cultures are not obtainable. An elevated white blood cell count is also indicative of infection.

■ ***TREATMENT.*** Treatment for both types of otitis media includes analgesics for pain and decongestants to promote drainage. Suppurative otitis media requires antibiotic therapy.

Chronic otitis media, both forms, might need surgical removal of fluid by **myringotomy** (MIR-in-GOT-oh-me; myringo = eardrum, tomy = incision into) to prevent rupture of the tympanic membrane, permanent hearing loss, and possible mastoiditis. To prevent further accumulation of fluid and to relieve pressure, **tympanostomy** (TIM-pan-OSS-toh-me; tympano = eardrum, ostomy = new opeing) tubes, commonly called pediatric ear (PE) tubes, can be placed through the tympanic mebrane during a procedure called a **tympanoplasty**

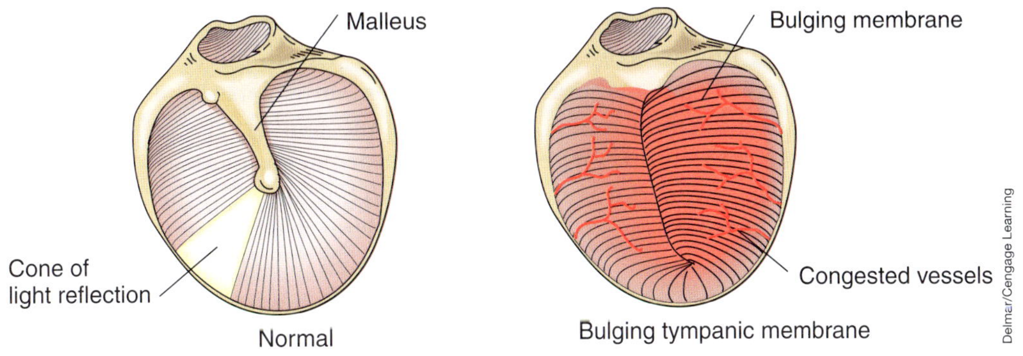

FIGURE 16–15 Bulging tympanic membrane indicative of otitis media.

(TIM-pah-no-PLASTY; tympano = eardrum, plasty = surgical repair) (Figure 16–16). Tubes commonly fall out after several months but can be removed after 6 months to a year. Prognosis for both types of otitis media is good if given prompt treatment. Chronic untreated otitis media, however, can lead to severe ear damage and permanent hearing loss. Prevention of complications is directed toward prevention and prompt treatment of upper respiratory infections and otitis media.

■ ***PREVENTION.*** Avoiding bottle feeding, smoking environments, and group child care are all preventive measures. Babies who are breast-fed, cared for in their homes, and kept in nonsmoking environments have fewer bouts of otitis media.

OTITIS EXTERNA

■ ***DESCRIPTION.*** Otitis externa, also called swimmer's ear or external otitis, is an inflammation of the external ear canal.

■ ***ETIOLOGY.*** This disease commonly affects swimmers who spend many hours in the water. Other causes include trauma to the ear canal, such as can occur when attempting to scratch or clean the ear canal, and when swimming in contaminated water. The condition often is due to bacterial or fungal infection. Wearing headphones also creates a favorable environment for the growth of microorganisms.

■ ***SYMPTOMS.*** Symptoms of otitis externa include an inflamed ear canal with extreme pain, fever, **pruritus** (proo-RYE-tus; itching), and hearing loss. The ear also might drain clear or **purulent** (PYOU-roo-lent; containing pus) fluid.

■ ***DIAGNOSIS.*** Diagnosis is made on the basis of an otologic examination. If an infection is suspected, a culture and sensitivity test might be needed.

■ ***TREATMENT.*** Treatment includes keeping the ear canal clean and dry and giving analgesics for pain and antibiotics if an infection is detected.

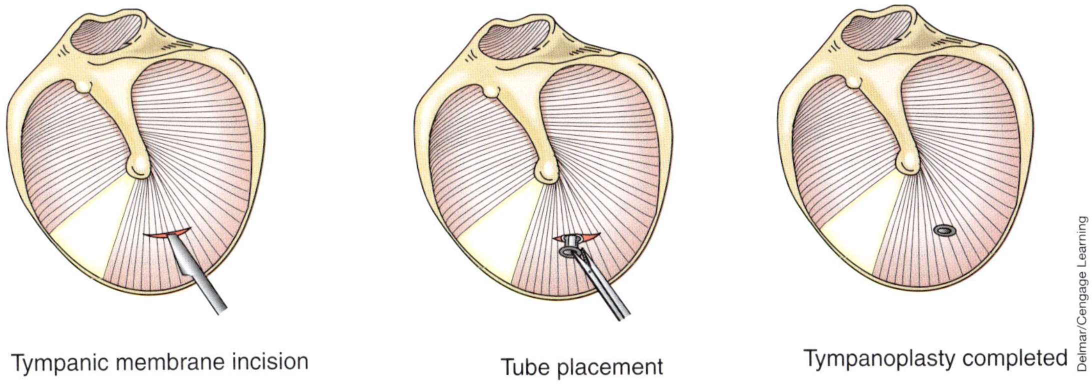

FIGURE 16–16 Tympanoplasty.

■ ***PREVENTION.*** Prevention includes wearing earplugs while showering or swimming to keep the external canal clean and dry. Decreasing the amount of time headphones are worn and keeping foreign objects out of the ears also can be helpful. Otitis externa tends to be a recurring disease that can eventually become chronic and cause hearing loss.

MASTOIDITIS

■ ***DESCRIPTION.*** Mastoiditis (MAS-toy-DYE-tis) is inflammation of the mastoid bone or process. This bone is porous or honeycombed in appearance and located behind the ear. This condition commonly affects children and is usually the result of a middle-ear infection. Prior to antibiotics, this was a leading cause of death in children. With current diagnosis and treatment regimens, it is less common and rarely dangerous.

■ ***ETIOLOGY.*** Acute mastoiditis is usually the result of a middle-ear infection commonly caused by streptococcus.

■ ***SYMPTOMS.*** Symptoms include **tinnitus** (tin-EYE-tus; ringing in the ears), otalgia (oh-TAL-gee-ah; ot = ear, algia = pain), fever, and headache. The mastoid also can become swollen and painful, and ear drainage can be present.

■ ***DIAGNOSIS.*** Diagnosis is made on the basis of examination and otoscopy, (OH-TOS-koh-pee; oto = ear, scopy = procedure to look into), X-ray of the mastoid bone, CT scan, and bacterial cultures.

■ ***TREATMENT.*** Mastoiditis generally responds to antibiotic therapy. Severe or chronic mastoiditis might need surgical treatment with a **mastoidectomy** (MAS-toy-DECK-toh-me; ectomy = removal or excision) to prevent complications and preserve hearing.

■ ***PREVENTION.*** Prompt and thorough treatment of ear infections reduces the risk of developing mastoiditis.

Deafness

Deafness, or loss of hearing, is a common disease affecting millions of Americans. There are multiple reasons for deafness, but most causes fall into two basic categories: conductive and sensory. Conductive deafness is caused by external or middle-ear disorders that decrease or stop conduction of sound to the inner ear. Conductive disorders include impacted cerumen, otosclerosis, and a ruptured tympanic membrane. Sensory deafness is the result of cochlear or auditory nerve damage that impairs the ability of sound to be carried to the brain. Sensory deafness is often related to damaging noise levels and ototoxic medications.

IMPACTED CERUMEN

■ ***DEFINITION.*** Cerumen is the soft, yellow-brown secretion produced by the external ear, commonly called ear wax.

■ ***ETIOLOGY.*** Impacted cerumen is a common cause of conductive hearing loss. If cerumen accumulates and becomes impacted (pressed firmly) in the ear canal, it can cause tinnitus and temporary deafness. An abnormal amount of cerumen can build up in the ear due to skin dryness, excessive hair in the ear, or a narrow ear canal. Another cause of buildup is due to excessive dust in the ear, which occurs among construction workers, farmers, and cabinetmakers, to name a few.

■ ***SYMPTOMS.*** The common symptom is a partial loss of hearing. Itching, tinnitus and pain can also be symptoms.

■ ***DIAGNOSIS.*** An otologic examination will confirm the diagnosis.

■ ***TREATMENT.*** Cerumen is normally washed out of the ear during routine showering and shampooing. Impacted cerumen is often removed with ear irrigations. This condition tends to recur, so routine examination should be performed.

■ ***PREVENTION.*** Placing two to three drops of mineral oil into the ear once a week, allowing it to remain for three to four minutes, and then rinsing it out with warm water is a preventive method.

OTOSCLEROSIS

■ ***DESCRIPTION.*** Otosclerosis (OH-toh-skleh-ROH-sis; oto = ear, scler = hardening, osis = condition) is a condition characterized by bony fixation of the small bones of the middle ear. This fixation prevents the bones from conducting vibrations from the eardrum to the inner ear, causing a conductive hearing loss. Otosclerosis occurs more commonly in females than

HEALTHY HIGHLIGHT

Removing Impacted Cerumen

Impacted cerumen should be softened and removed gently in the following manner.

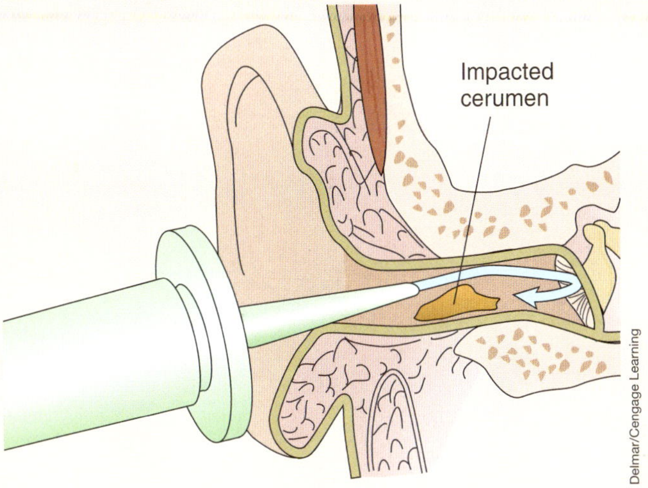

1. Warm mineral oil or glycerin by holding it between the hands or placing the bottle in a cup of warm water.
2. Check the temperature to ensure that it is not too hot. It should be lukewarm.
3. Drop two or three drops of oil in the ear canal.
4. Gently irrigate the ear canal by using a bulb syringe filled with lukewarm water.
5. Aim the water flow toward the top of the ear canal, not toward the eardrum.
6. Continue to irrigate until the impacted cerumen is removed. This can take 10 to 15 minutes.
7. Repeat steps 1–6 until the impacted cerumen is removed.

in males; it usually affects females under the age of 35 and can be aggravated by pregnancy.

■ ***ETIOLOGY.*** The cause of otosclerosis is unknown, but there is evidence of familial tendency, suggesting a hereditary cause.

■ ***SYMPTOMS.*** The primary symptom is slow hearing loss that continues to worsen.

■ ***DIAGNOSIS.*** Diagnosis is made on the basis of physical examination, audiogram, and otoscopy.

■ ***TREATMENT.*** A common treatment for otosclerosis is a **stapedectomy** (STAY-peh-DECK-toh-me; stape = stapes, ectomy = removal or excision of). A stapedectomy involves removal of the stapes bone in the middle ear and replacement with a **prosthesis** (pros-THEE-sis; an artificial part) (Figure 16–17). Hearing is generally improved soon after surgery. If a stapedectomy is not an option for the affected individual, a hearing aid might improve hearing.

■ ***PREVENTION.*** Otosclerosis cannot be prevented.

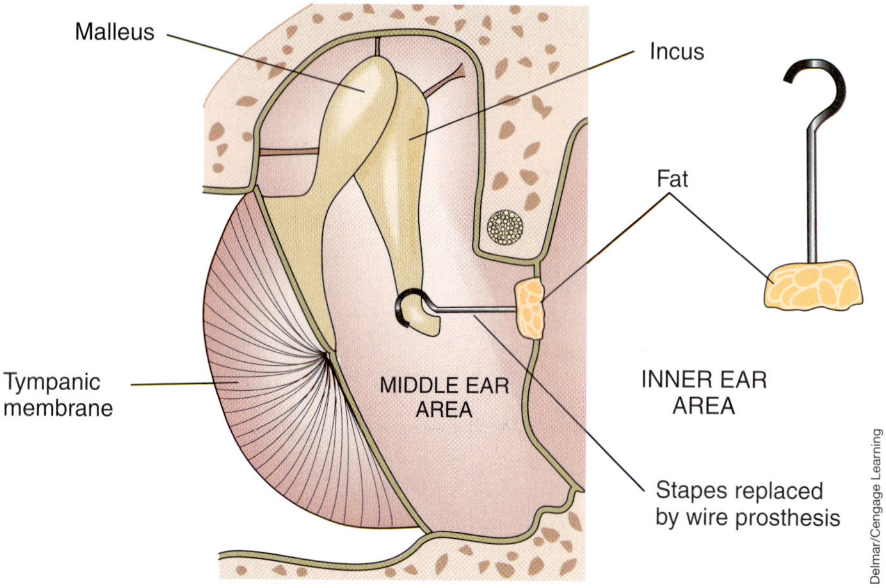

FIGURE 16–17 Stapedectomy with wire prosthesis.

SENSORINEURAL DEAFNESS

■ ***DESCRIPTION.*** Sensorineural deafness is a type of sensory deafness due to damage to the cochlea or the auditory nerve.

■ ***ETIOLOGY.*** There are many causes of this condition; some are congenital, or inherited, whereas others are acquired. Acquired causes are more common and include stroke, tumors, certain medications, infections, diseases, and trauma. The most common trauma is due to exposure to loud noise. Occupational noise, including that from heavy machinery, jackhammers, and airplane engines, can lead to deafness. Teenagers and young adults are at high risk due to the popularity of playing loud music, especially while using personal ear buds, and attending music concerts that use large amplifiers.

■ ***SYMPTOMS.*** The primary symptom is a gradual loss of hearing.

■ ***DIAGNOSIS.*** Diagnosis is made on the basis of audiometry.

■ ***TREATMENT.*** Sensorineural deafness caused by cochlear or auditory nerve damage is often permanent. Treatment is limited to use of hearing aids or cochlear implants.

A hearing aid is a tiny microphone, amplifier, and speaker in one device. It fits in the external ear and increases volume to the internal ear.

A cochlear implant is an electronic device that is implanted behind the ear. It directly stimulates the auditory nerve fibers to increase hearing.

■ ***PREVENTION.*** Prevention is aimed at avoiding the cause if possible. Reducing the amount of noise and protecting the ears by using protective earphones and earplugs is beneficial.

PRESBYCUSIS

■ ***DESCRIPTION.*** Presbycusis (PRES-beh-KOO-sis; presby = old age, cusis = hearing) is a progressive sensory hearing loss related to aging.

■ ***ETIOLOGY.*** The cause of presbycusis is from degenerative changes in the organs of hearing.

■ ***SYMPTOMS.*** Onset of symptoms is gradual and usually begins after age 50. Initially, there is a loss of hearing of high tones, but as hearing loss progresses, lower tones become difficult to hear as well. In affected individuals, the speech of others might seem mumbled or slurred, and conversations might be difficult to hear, especially against background noise.

■ ***DIAGNOSIS.*** Diagnosis is made after physical examination and medical history to rule out other causes of hearing loss. An audiogram confirms the diagnosis.

■ ***TREATMENT.*** Use of a hearing aid can be helpful initially, but as the hearing declines, aids might become less useful.

■ ***PREVENTION.*** Much of the hearing loss caused by trauma and noise can be prevented. Avoiding activities with damaging noise levels and wearing ear muffs or ear plugs to protect the ears are helpful preventive measures.

Motion Sickness

■ ***DESCRIPTION.*** Motion sickness is the nauseated feeling some individuals experience when traveling by automobile, boat, or airplane.

■ ***ETIOLOGY.*** The cause of motion sickness is abnormal movement of the organs of balance—the semicircular canals—that are located in the inner ear. These semicircular canals are accustomed to traveling in a horizontal plane, but movement in a vertical plane, as in a boat or bumpy airplane ride, produces an abnormal sensation in these organs, leading to motion sickness. Watching motion on a widescreen picture also can cause motion sickness, even though the individual is not actually moving.

■ ***SYMPTOMS.*** Symptoms of motion sickness include varying degrees of nausea, vomiting, diaphoresis, and vertigo. Fortunately, motion sickness usually subsides when movement stops.

■ ***DIAGNOSIS.*** A history and description of symptoms is usually adequate to diagnose this condition. Laboratory testing is usually not needed.

■ ***TREATMENT.*** Antihistamine medications are generally used to treat and prevent this condition. These medications appear to work by calming the stimulation of the inner ear. Meclizine (Antivert, Dramamine) can treat symptoms. Motion sickness can also be relieved or reduced by lying down and closing the eyes.

■ ***PREVENTION.*** Meclizine is also helpful in prevention of motion sickness if taken at least one hour prior to travel.

Scopolamine is the most commonly prescribed preventive medication. It is available in a skin patch (Transderm Scop) that is applied behind the ear; the medication is then slowly absorbed into the skin. To be most effective, this patch should be placed at least 4 hours in advance of the motion activity. Effects of the patch last up to 3 days.

Promethazine, Dimenhydrimate, and Cyclizime are all preventive medications when take prior to the motion activity.

Other considerations that might decrease the effect or prevent the occurrence of motion sickness include:

- Avoiding heavy meals prior to a trip.
- Finding a seat in the most stable area of the boat or plane.
- During automobile rides, making frequent stops for short walks in the fresh air.
- Not reading while traveling.
- Avoiding stuffy areas, especially those with odors such as cigarette smoke.
- Trying to stay cool with plenty of fresh air when possible.
- Avoiding too much heat.

TRAUMA

Corneal Abrasion

■ ***DESCRIPTION.*** The cornea, the transparent outer layer of the eye, is subject to trauma because of its position.

■ ***ETIOLOGY.*** Corneal abrasions can be caused by:

- Trapping a foreign object such as sand or sawdust between the eyelid and the cornea.
- Contact lenses that do not fit properly, are dirty or scratched, or are worn for too long a time period.
- Accidentally poking a finger in the eye.
- Extreme light, as with welding.

■ ***SYMPTOMS.*** Symptoms are often delayed, occurring 12 to 18 hours after the trauma, and include severe pain, tearing, and photophobia.

■ ***DIAGNOSIS.*** Diagnosis is made on the basis of history and visual examination. Abrasions can be stained easily with fluorescein and viewed with a slit lamp.

■ ***TREATMENT.*** Treatment includes removal of the foreign body and administration of antibiotic ointment or drops to prevent infection. Analgesic medications for pain might be prescribed. A pressure dressing can be applied to the eye to keep the eyelid from moving against the cornea and to reduce the pain of photophobia. Interestingly, the pain caused by corneal abrasion comes from the inside of the eyelid rubbing over the abrasion on the cornea. The cornea does not have sensory nerves.

■ ***PREVENTION.*** Abrasions can often be avoided by use of protective eyewear.

Retinal Detachment

■ ***DESCRIPTION.*** This is a disorder of the eye in which the retina peels away from the underlying tissue. Detachment usually starts in a small area but can quickly lead to detachment of the entire retina. If this occurs, blindness can occur. Retinal detachment is a medical emergency.

■ ***ETIOLOGY.*** Retinal detachment often occurs with trauma, diabetes, and other retinopathies that cause an opening or hole in the retinal layer. This opening allows fluid from the vitreous humor to leak between the retina and choroid layer. The fluid lifts or floats the retina away from the choroid (Figure 16–18).

■ ***SYMPTOMS.*** Because the retina has no sensory nerves, this condition is painless. The individual experiences loss of vision in the affected area with symptoms of blurred vision, flashes of light, and floating spots. As more of the retina detaches, the symptoms become more pronounced.

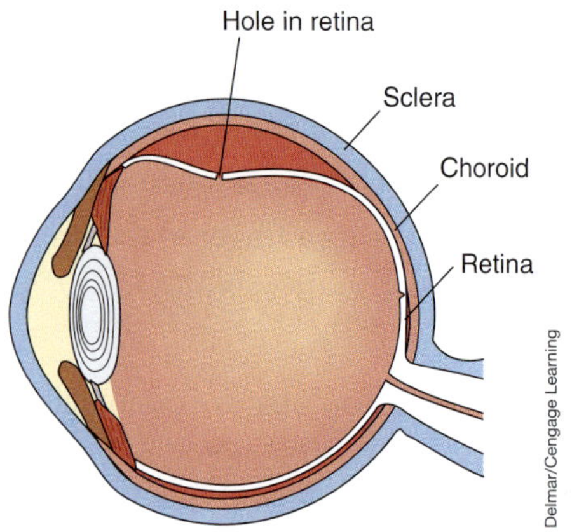

FIGURE 16–18 Retinal detachment.

■ ***DIAGNOSIS.*** Ophthalmoscopic examination will readily show the detachment.

■ ***TREATMENT.*** Surgery is the usual treatment to seal the opening and reattach the retina to the choroid layer. This can be done using laser technology. The retina usually regains function unless extreme detachment has occurred.

■ ***PREVENTION.*** Most cases cannot be prevented, although prompt treatment of the cause, when known, does reduce risk. Some eye injuries cause damage to the retina that lead to detachment. Prevention of these injuries by wearing safety glasses, sports glasses, or goggles also reduces risk.

Ruptured Tympanic Membrane

■ ***DESCRIPTION.*** A ruptured tympanic membrane, also called perforated eardrum, is a tear or hole in the tympanic membrane. This thin membrane separates the ear canal from the middle ear and vibrates when sound waves strike it, starting the process of hearing.

■ ***ETIOLOGY.*** The most common causes include severe middle-ear infection or trauma from inserting something, such as a pencil, into the ear canal.

■ ***SYMPTOMS.*** Symptoms include pain, partial loss of hearing, and usually bloody or purulent drainage. The main risk of a ruptured membrane is from infection.

■ ***DIAGNOSIS.*** Diagnosis can be confirmed by otoscopy.

■ ***TREATMENT.*** Treatment can include antibiotics to prevent infection and surgical patching of the membrane with a tissue graft. Minimal hearing loss is associated with a ruptured tympanic membrane.

■ ***PREVENTION.*** Getting prompt and thorough treatment for middle-ear infection and keeping the ears free of foreign objects are preventive measures.

RARE DISEASES

Retinoblastoma

Retinoblastoma is a malignant tumor of the eye. It occurs during infancy and childhood and tends to be hereditary. Often, both eyes are affected. Retinoblastomas grow as intraocular masses that fill the eye and can extend into the optic nerve. The mass is usually recognized by a white light reflex seen at the pupil (cat's eye). Untreated retinoblastoma is fatal. With treatment, 90% of affected children survive. Treatment includes **enucleation** (removal of the eyeball), radiation, and chemotherapy.

Ménière's Disease

Ménière's disease usually affects individuals between the ages of 40 and 60. The cause is unknown, although predisposing factors appear to include middle-ear infections and head trauma. Ménière's disease is a chronic disease of the inner ear characterized by tinnitus, vertigo, progressive hearing loss, and a feeling of fullness in the ear.

Acute attacks can last from a few hours to several days with symptoms of nausea, vomiting, diaphoresis, and vertigo. Treatment for acute attacks includes medications to control nausea and vomiting. A low-salt diet, diuretics, antihistamines, and cessation of smoking are usually effective for long-term treatment. Surgery can be performed if the disease does not respond to treatment, but a major complication of surgery is permanent deafness.

EFFECTS OF AGING ON THE SYSTEM

The effects of aging on the sensory organs are significant. Changes in vision begin in middle age and progress through the older adult years. The change is obvious in most people, beginning with the inability to read small print or to see well in low light. These changes affect the older adult's ability to function well in society and often cause social isolation and dependence on others.

Vision changes begin around age 40 and continue through the life span. Inability to focus on near objects, diminishing color perception, some sensitivity to light, and decreased visual acuity are all normal physiologic changes that occur during the aging process. Although the changes vary among individuals, most persons have about a 20/70 visual acuity by age 65. Glaucoma and cataracts are common problems of older adults, reducing even further their ability to see. In the diabetic older person, retinopathy is a very common problem that often eventually leads to blindness. Arcus senilis is an opaque, grayish ring at the periphery of the cornea that frequently occurs in an older person. It results from fatty granule deposits in, or hyaline degeneration of, the lamellae and cells of the cornea (Figure 16–19).

Hearing changes in the older adult affect the ability to perceive what is heard and might affect behavior, personality, and attitudes. Many hearing problems can be corrected but, because of financial constraints or social concerns, are not attended to. The inability to hear often affects the individual's ability to communicate and interferes with one's social life and independence. In some instances, speaking in a clear, concise manner to someone with such hearing loss is more beneficial than raising one's voice.

As the individual ages, the tympanic membrane becomes thinner and less flexible, reducing the conduction of sound. This is a conductive hearing loss associated with aging. If there has been damage to the eighth cranial nerve, the individual has a sensorineural loss. If both types of hearing loss are present, it is called a mixed hearing loss.

The slow but gradual loss of hearing called presbycusis affects more men than women and is

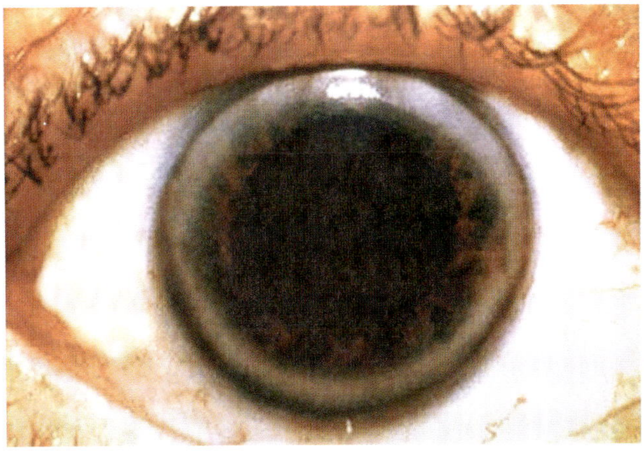

Courtesy of Mark L. Kuss

FIGURE 16–19 Arcus senilis.

due to degenerative changes in neurons, the bones of the middle ear, and the cochlea. High-pitched sounds become the most difficult to hear at first, but gradual loss of low-pitched sounds also occurs eventually.

Other hearing conditions apparent in the older adult include otosclerosis, tinnitus, and Ménière's disease. Although some of these can begin in younger life, they are most commonly detected in later years.

SUMMARY

The sensory organs of the body are often regarded as the most important to the individual to maintain quality of life. Visual and hearing impairments are often correctable, especially if diagnosed early in the degenerative period. Other system diseases such as diabetes often affect the sensory organs and can destroy their ability to function. Some of the most common disorders of the eyes include myopia, presbyopia, hyperopia, diabetic retinopathy, cataracts, and glaucoma. The most common diseases of the ear include tinnitus, otitis media, conduction loss, otosclerosis, and Ménière's disease. In the older adult, sensory organ disorders are common. Some losses of vision and hearing occur naturally through the aging process, whereas others are a result of other system diseases. Diagnosis and treatment of vision and hearing losses should be implemented early to prevent some of the complications of sensory dysfunction.

REVIEW QUESTIONS

Short Answer

1. What are some of the most common problems affecting the eyes?

2. What are some of the most common problems affecting the ears?

3. What diagnostic tests are used to diagnose or evaluate eye disorders?

4. What diagnostic tests are used to diagnose or evaluate ear disorders?

Fill in the Blanks

5. ____________ is the chronic inflammation of the eyelid.
6. The lay term for ____________ is pinkeye.
7. Extreme sensitivity to light is called ____________.
8. Another term for nearsightedness is ____________.
9. Farsightedness is also called ____________.
10. A common eye disorder that occurs with aging is called ____________.

11. The main symptom of a cataract is the gradual ___________ of vision.

12. In ___________, aqueous humor is produced faster than it can be drained.

13. Sudden flashes or spots before the eyes can be a sign of ___________.

14. Flushing the eye with large amounts of water is the best immediate treatment for a ___________ of the eye.

15. The cranial nerves that control the muscles of eye movement include ___________, ___________, and ___________.

16. Within the ear, the organ of hearing is the ___________.

17. The major symptom of ear disorders is ___________.

18. Buzzing or ringing in the ear(s) is called ___________.

19. Pediatric ear tubes can be placed through the tympanic membrane during a procedure called ___________.

20. ___________ is also commonly called swimmer's ear.

21. The most common cause of a progressive hearing loss is ___________.

22. The surgical treatment for progressive otosclerosis is a ___________.

23. Vertigo is the common complaint of an individual with ___________.

24. The slow but gradual loss of hearing common in the older adult is called ___________.

25. Chronic otitis media can result in perforation of the ___________.

CASE STUDIES

- Ms. Tesar is a 52-year-old woman who has been doing intricate needlework for years. She has exhibited her work in many fairs and received awards for her unique original patterns. While having lunch with her one day, she confides that she is having difficulty seeing the eye of the needle while trying to thread it. She is also having some difficulty drawing the minute details of the patterns. She has noticed, however, that she can see a little better if she holds the needle out away from her while threading it rather than holding it close, as she was used to doing. Having just completed a unit on vision and hearing disorders in your Human Disease course, you think you can explain what is probably occurring with Ms. Tesar's eyesight. What would you tell her about this problem? How would you explain the natural changes that occur with aging? Would you recommend she make an appointment to have her eyes checked?

- Suzie Lindquist is a friend who has suffered from motion sickness for several years. What medications might help her? What other suggestions could you could give her to decrease the frequency of her motion sickness problems?

StudyWARE™ Connection

To help you learn the content in this chapter, take a practice quiz or play an interactive game on your StudyWARE™ CD-ROM.

Workbook Practice

Go to your Workbook and complete the practice questions.

BIBLIOGRAPHY

Aslam, S., Shethm H., & Vaughan, A. (2007). Emergency management of corneal injuries. *Injury 38*(5), 594–597.

Blepharitis. (2008) University of Michigan, Kellogg Eye Center. *www.kellogg.umich.edu* (accessed June 2008).

Bruce, A., O'Day, J., McKay, D., & Swan, P. (2007). Normal tension glaucoma. *Optician 234*(6124), 59.

Ciulla, T. (2007). Targeting VEGF: The VEGF trap clinical trials. *Review of Ophthalmology 14*(12), 50–54.

Color Blindness. (2008). University of Maryland Medical Center. *www.umm.edu* (accessed June 2008).

Eperjesi, F., & Bartlett, H. (2006). New perspectives on the investigation and treatment of dry eye syndrome, Part 2. *Optician 231*(6051), 30–33.

Faag, C., Bergenuis, J., & Forsberg, C. (2007). Symptoms experienced by patients with peripheral vestibular disorders: Evaluation of the Vertigo Symptom Scale for clinical application. *Clinical Otolaryngology 32*(6), 440–446.

Gurney, M. (2007). A poke in the eye. *Nursing Older People 19*(10), 3.

Harvey, E., Dobson, V., Miller, J., & Clifford-Donaldson, C. (2008). Changes in visual function following treatment of astigmatism-related amblyopia. *Vision Research 48*(6). 773–787.

Hayden, E. (2008). Battle over eye medicine gives drug maker a dose of reality. *Nature Medicine 14*(2), 108.

Holland, G. (2008). AIDS and ophthalmology: The first quarter century. *American Journal of Ophthalmology 145*(3), 497–508.

How do I boost my eye health? (2008). *Natural Health 38*(6), 28.

Laser Eye Surgery. (2008). Mayo Clinic. *www.mayoclinic .org* (accessed June 2008).

Lazaridis, E., & Saunders, J. (2008). Can you hear me now? A genetic model of otitis media with effusion. *Journal of Clinical Investigation 118*(2), 471–474.

Lelong, A., Fairley, J., & Padgham, N. (2007). Sudden hearing loss. *Clinical Otolarygology 32*(5), 391–394.

Mastoiditis. (2008). University of Maryland Medical Center. *www.umm.edu* (accessed June 2008).

McCabe, B. (2007). Autoimmune sensorineural hearing loss. *Annals of Otology, Rhinology & Laryngology 116*(12), 585–589.

Middleton, E., Sinason, M., & Davids, Z. (2008). Blurred vision due to psychological difficulties: A case study. *Eye 22*(2), 316–317.

Mills, L. (2007). Irrigating ears safely. *Practical Nurse 33*(4), 42–47.

Motion Sickness. (2007). MedicineNet,Inc. *www.medicinenet .com* (accessed June 2008).

National Eye Institute. (2006). Diabetic retinopathy. National Eye Institute. www.nei.nih.gov (accessed June 2008). Then move between Motion and Otitis.

Otitis Media. (2008). National Institute on Deafness and Other Communication Disorders. *www.nidcd.nih.gov* (accessed June 2008).

Refractive Eye Surgery. (2004). Penn State Milton S. Hershey Medical Center. *www.hmc.psu.edu/healthinfo.htm* (accessed June 2008).

Retinal Detachment. (2007). WebMD. *www.webmed.com* (accessed June 2008).

Snow, M. (2007). Keeping an eye on infectious keratitis. *Nursing 37*(11), 60–61.

Travelers' Health: Yellow Book. (2007). Centers for Disease Control and Prevention (CDC). *www.cdc.gov* (accessed March 12, 2008).

Villasenor, I. (2007). Bioactivities of iridoids. *Anti-inflammatory & Anti-allergy Agents in Medicinal Chemistry 6*(4), 307–314.

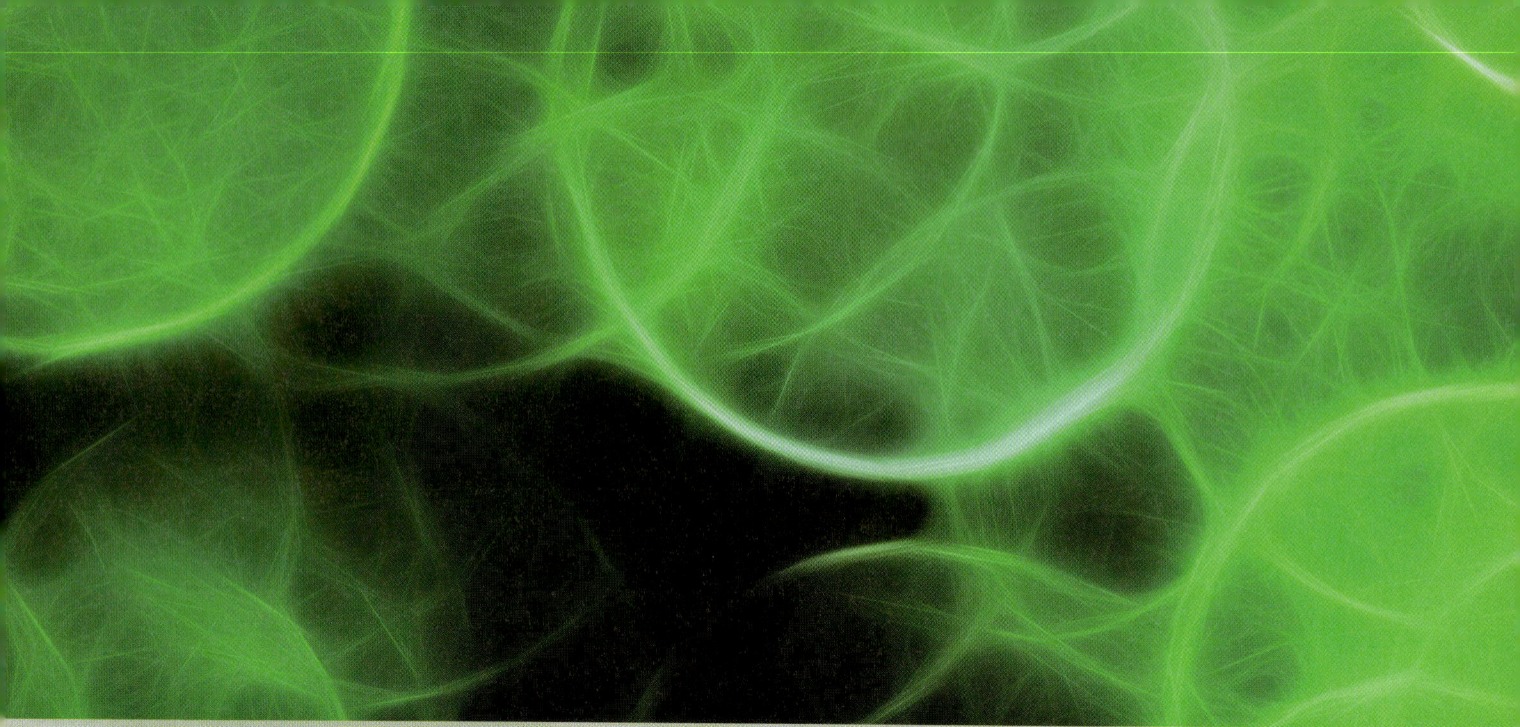

OUTLINE

- Anatomy and Physiology
  - *Female Anatomy and Physiology*
  - *Male Anatomy and Physiology*
- Common Signs and Symptoms
- Diagnostic Tests
- Common Diseases of the Reproductive System
  - *Female Reproductive System Diseases*
  - *Diseases of the Breast*
  - *Disorders of Pregnancy*
  - *Male Reproductive System Diseases*
  - *Sexually Transmitted Diseases (STDs)*
  - *Sexual Dysfunction*
- Trauma
  - *Rape*
- Rare Diseases
  - *Vaginal Cancer*
  - *Puerperal Sepsis*
  - *Hydatidiform Mole*
- Effects Of Aging on the System
- Summary
- Review Questions
- Case Studies
- Bibliography

KEY TERMS

Bimanual examination (p. 360)
Carcinoma in situ (p. 370)
Cervicitis (p. 367)
Chancre (p. 383)
Cryptorchidism (p. 381)
Cystoscopy (p. 362)
Cytologic (p. 360)
Digital rectal examination (p. 362)
Dilatation and curettage (D&C) (p. 360)
Dysmenorrhea (p. 367)
Dyspareunia (p. 367)
Dysuria (p. 377)
Eclampsia (p. 376)
Ectopic (p. 367)
Endometritis (p. 367)
Gumma (p. 384)
Hysterosalpingogram (p. 361)
Impotent (p. 381)
Laparoscopy (p. 360)
Leukorrhea (p. 367)
Mammography (p. 361)
Mammoplasty (p. 373)
Mastectomy (p. 373)
Multiparity (p. 376)
Nocturia (p. 378)
Oophoritis (p. 367)
Orchiectomy (p. 379)
Panhysterectomy (p. 367)
Phimosis (p. 386)
Preeclampsia (p. 376)
Primigravid (p. 376)
Prophylactic (p. 372)
Puerperal (p. 372)
Pyuria (p. 377)
Rapid Plasma Reagin (RPR) (p. 361)
Salpingitis (p. 367)
Septicemia (p. 367)
Sterility (p. 380)
Trichomonas (p. 366)
Venereal Disease Research Laboratory (VDRL) (p. 361)

17

Reproductive System Diseases and Disorders

LEARNING OBJECTIVES

Upon completion of the chapter, the learner should be able to:

1. Define the terminology common to the reproductive system and the disorders of the system.
2. Discuss the basic anatomy and physiology of the reproductive system.
3. Identify the important signs and symptoms associated with common reproductive system disorders.
4. Describe the common diagnostics used to determine the type and cause of reproductive system disorders.
5. Identify common disorders of the reproductive system.
6. Describe the typical course and management of the common reproductive system disorders.
7. Describe the effects of aging on the reproductive system and the common disorders associated with aging of the system.

OVERVIEW

The reproductive system is a complex system of structures with a variety of physiological functions. Some parts of the reproductive system are endocrine glands (ovaries and testes) with purpose throughout a person's lifetime, whereas other parts are strictly involved in procreation for a specific time during the individual's life span. Disorders of the system are common at all ages and can range from mild to severe, especially if not diagnosed early in the development of the disorder. Changes in the system during the aging process have both physiological and psychosocial implications. ■

ANATOMY AND PHYSIOLOGY

The reproductive system is quite different between the male and female. Although the anatomy and physiological features have a few commonalities, there are enough differences to discuss them separately.

Female Anatomy and Physiology

The female reproductive system consists of external structures that include the vulva, labia majora, labia minora, clitoris, vestibule, hymen, vaginal orifice, and vestibular glands. Internal structures include the ovaries, fallopian tubes, uterus, cervix, and vagina (Figure 17–1). The ovaries secrete the female sex hormones, estrogen and progesterone, and produce ova, the reproductive cells, within the graafian follicles (microscopic sacs). After a follicle releases an ovum, it develops into a corpus luteum, created by the luteinizing hormone from the pituitary gland. The corpus luteum secretes estrogen and progesterone. The fallopian tubes are ducts that carry the ova (eggs) from the ovaries to the uterus.

The uterus is a pear-shaped muscular structure lying above the bladder in the pelvis. It measures only about 2 inches by 3 inches in the nonpregnant state. The lower part of the uterus is called the cervix (neck); the inner layer of the uterus is the endometrium. During menstruation, part of this layer is sloughed off and passed through the vagina and vaginal orifice. The vagina is the structure that receives the penis during intercourse and becomes the birth canal during delivery of the fetus.

The hormones secreted by the ovaries are estrogens and progesterone. Secretion occurs in response to the effects of the follicle-stimulating hormone (FSH) and the LH produced by the anterior pituitary gland. Estrogen affects the development of secondary sex characteristics (characteristics occurring at puberty), changes in the endometrium, and growth of the uterus and vagina. Progesterone affects the development of the endometrium, assists in the development of the placenta, causes enlargement of the breasts during pregnancy, prevents ova from being produced during pregnancy, and assists in the development of cells in the mammary glands.

The menstrual cycle is the process of secretion of hormones, the preparation of the endometrium for the implantation of the fertilized egg, and, if the egg is not implanted, the sloughing of the layer with bleeding from torn capillaries. The cycle runs for about 28 days but varies among individuals. The start of the menstrual flow is the first day of the cycle and usually lasts about 4 to 5 days. After that, estrogen is secreted

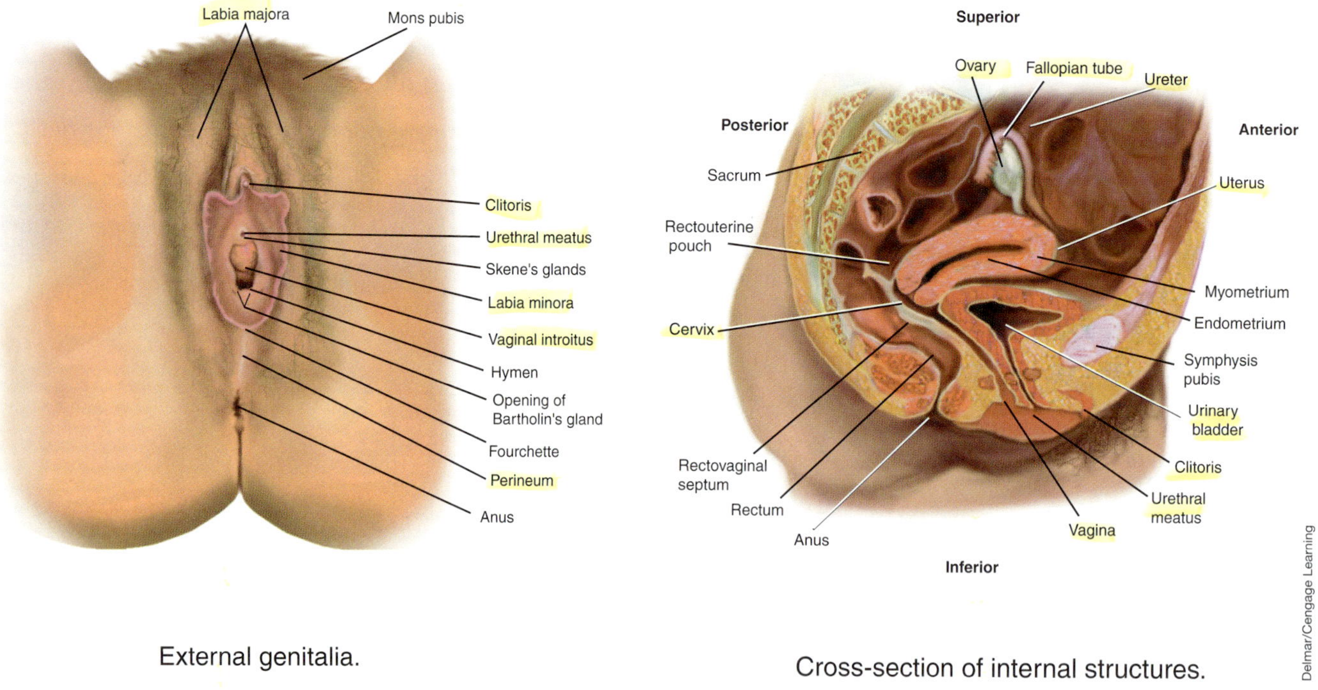

FIGURE 17–1 The female reproductive system.

until the Graafian follicle matures and ruptures, about halfway through the cycle. Progesterone is then secreted by the corpus luteum. As the corpus luteum ages, progesterone levels decline, causing menses and the beginning of the next cycle. Pregnancy will sustain progesterone levels, maintaining the endometrium. The menstrual cycle can begin (menarche) in females as young as 10 years of age but typically begins at age 11 or 12. The cessation of the cycle is called menopause, which usually occurs between ages 40 and 50 but also varies with the individual.

The female breasts are located between the second and seventh ribs over the pectoralis major muscle of the chest. They are usually almost symmetrical and might be small or very large, depending on the individual's structure, body weight, and other factors. Endocrine secretions during menstruation and pregnancy affect the breast size and composition. The breasts show little sign of development until puberty, when, over a 2- to 3-year period, the breasts change from the flattened preadolescent stage to full breast maturity. As the female enters menopause, the breasts begin to atrophy and become more relaxed with a reduction in size.

The female breasts consist of three types of tissue: glandular, fibrous, and adipose (fat). The structure of the breast includes the nipple, areola, lactiferous ducts, lobules lined with milk-producing glands called acini, and fibrous dividers (septa). The breast also contains a network of lymph glands that drains the lymph and returns it to the circulatory system.

StudyWARE™ Connection

View an animation on the female reproductive system on your StudyWARE™ CD-ROM.

Male Anatomy and Physiology

The male reproductive system includes the external organs, scrotum and penis, and the internal organs, testes, epididymis, vas deferens, urethra, seminal vesicles, bulbourethral glands, and the prostate (Figure 17–2). The penis houses the urethra, a tube

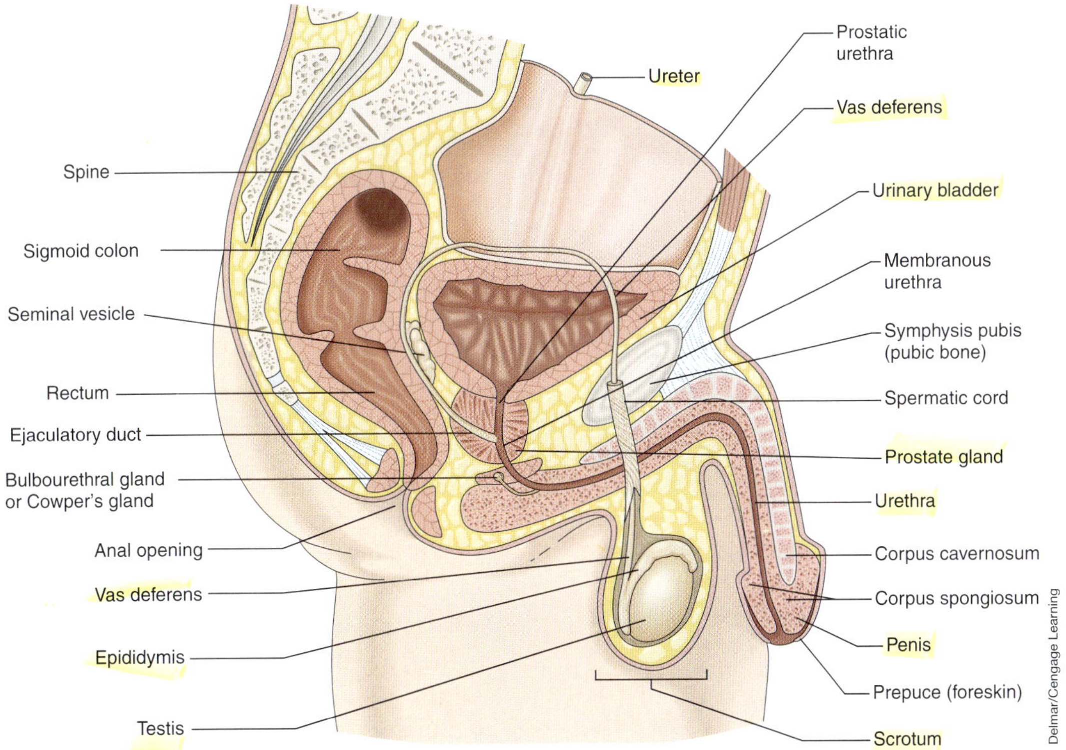

FIGURE 17–2 The male reproductive system.

that carries urine from the bladder and semen from the ejaculatory duct. At the tip of the penis is the prepuce (foreskin). The penis is composed of erectile tissue and arteries that dilate during sexual arousal, causing the penis to become erect for the purpose of intercourse. The scrotum is a sac that hangs below the penis and holds the testes. The testes secrete testosterone (the male sex hormone) and produce sperm (the reproductive cells). Testosterone is responsible for the changes occurring during puberty and secondary sex characteristics in the male.

The epididymis is the duct leading from each testis to the vas deferens, the excretory duct. The vas deferens from each testis extends up into the abdomen, where it connects to create the ejaculatory duct that opens into the urethra. The seminal vesicles sit behind the bladder near the neck. They secrete fluid that is part of the thick, white secretion called semen. The prostate gland and bulbourethral glands also secrete fluid that becomes part of the semen.

StudyWARE™ Connection

View an animation on the male reproductive system on your StudyWARE™ CD-ROM.

COMMON SIGNS AND SYMPTOMS

Common signs and symptoms of female reproductive system diseases and disorders include:

- Abdominal and pelvic pain.
- Fever and malaise.
- Abnormal vaginal drainage.
- Burning, itching, or both of the genitals.
- Pain during sexual intercourse.
- Any change in breast tissue.
- Abnormal discharge from the nipple.

Common signs and symptoms of male reproductive system diseases and disorders include:

- Urinary disorders, including frequency, dysuria, nocturia, and incontinence.
- Pain in the pelvis, groin, or reproductive organs.
- Lesions on the external genitalia.
- Swelling or abnormal enlargement of the reproductive organs.
- Abnormal penile drainage.
- Burning, itching, or both of the genitals.

DIAGNOSTIC TESTS

Physical examination of the female reproductive system to aid in diagnosis of diseases begins with a pelvic examination that includes inspection of the external genitalia, visual examination of the vagina and cervix through a speculum or instrument used to spread and hold the vaginal wall in an open position (Figure 17–3), and palpation of female internal organs by **bimanual examination**. A bimanual (two-handed) examination is so named because the physician places one hand on the abdomen and inserts fingers of the other hand into the vagina to feel the female organs between the two hands. A bimanual rectal examination allows palpation of the posterior aspect of the uterus and the rectum.

The most common test of the female reproductive system is the Papanicolaou (Pap smear) of the cervix (see Figure 17–3). Pap smears are **cytologic** (sigh-toe-LAWG-ic; cyto = cell, logic = study) examinations to discover cervical cancer. If an abnormal Pap smear is obtained, follow-up can involve a cervical biopsy that entails taking a small piece of tissue from the cervix for microscopic examination. A special type of biopsy, called a cone biopsy, refers to taking a cone-shaped piece of cervical tissue including the cervical os and endocervical lining. The diagnosis of endometrial cancer is best discovered by obtaining tissue for biopsy during a **dilatation and curettage** (KYOU-reh-TAHZH) (D&C). This procedure involves a light surgical sedative, dilation of the cervix (dilatation), and scraping (curettage) of the uterine endometrial tissue. D&C is also commonly performed for abnormal uterine bleeding and following a spontaneous abortion.

A **laparoscopy** (LAP-ah-ROS-ko-pee; laparo = abdomen, scopy = scope procedure), or looking inside the abdominal cavity with a lighted scope (Figure 17–4), is commonly used to view the female organs for abnormalities, to diagnose endometriosis, and perform a tubal ligation. To determine the size, position, and patency of the uterus and fallopian

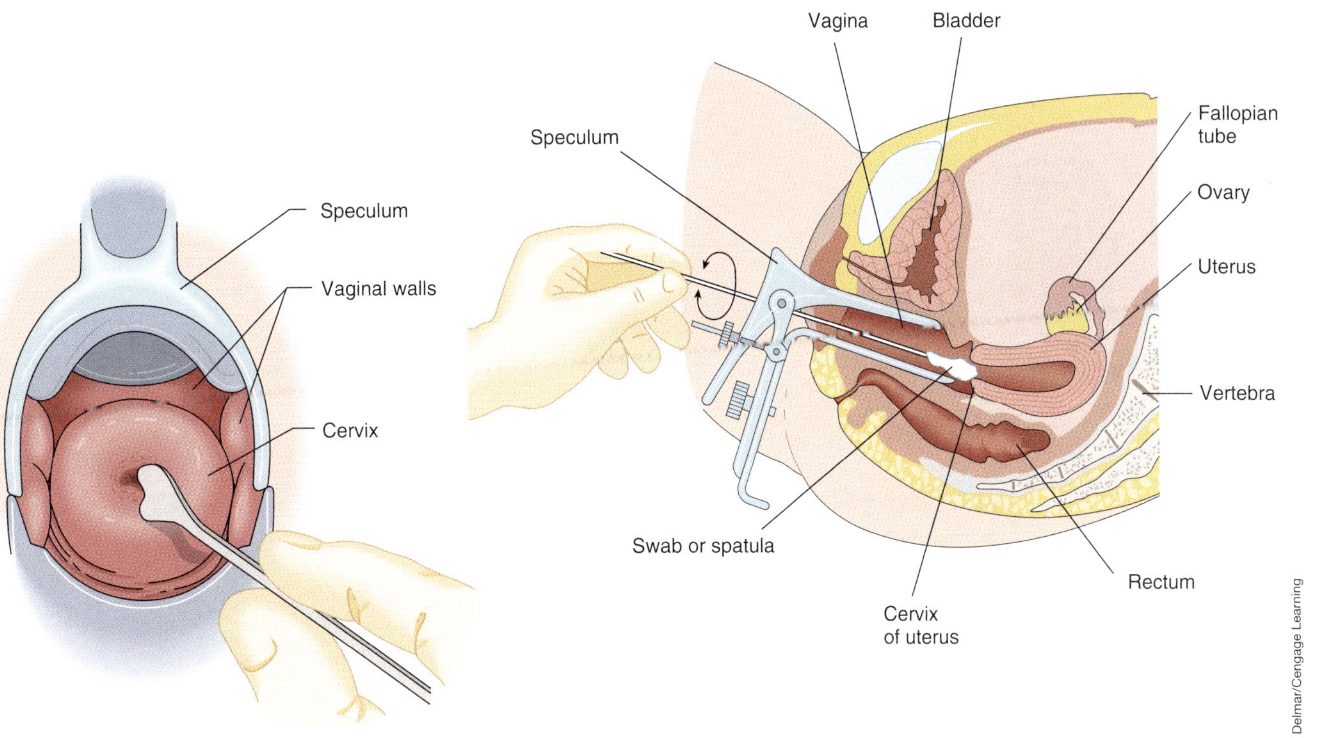

FIGURE 17–3 Use of a speculum and obtaining a Pap smear.

tubes, a **hysterosalpingogram** (hystero = uterus, salpingo = fallopian tubes, gram = picture), or X-ray, of these organs can be obtained. During a hysterosalpingogram, a small tube is passed through the cervix and a radiopaque dye is injected. As the dye fills the uterus and fallopian tubes and spills into the abdominal cavity, X-rays are taken to show patency, or openness, of the tubes. This procedure is commonly done as part of infertility testing.

Laboratory tests to determine reproductive diseases include microscopic examination and culture and sensitivity of secretions or drainage from the vagina and genital lesions to determine the presence of infection. Blood tests to measure hormone levels, including estrogen and progesterone, are also common. Other blood testing includes **venereal disease research laboratory (VDRL)** and **rapid plasma reagin (RPR)** test for syphilis.

Mammography (mam-OG-rah-fee; mammo = breast, ography = procedure to take a picture) is an X-ray or radiologic examination of breast tissue (Figure 17–5) to determine the presence of cysts or tumors. Digital mammography is a newer technique that takes an electronic image of the breast and stores it in a computer for the radiologist to view. If an abnormal mass is discovered during mammography, further diagnostic techniques include fine-needle aspiration and incisional biopsy.

Ultrasound can be performed on the pelvis to determine the presence of tumors and pregnancy

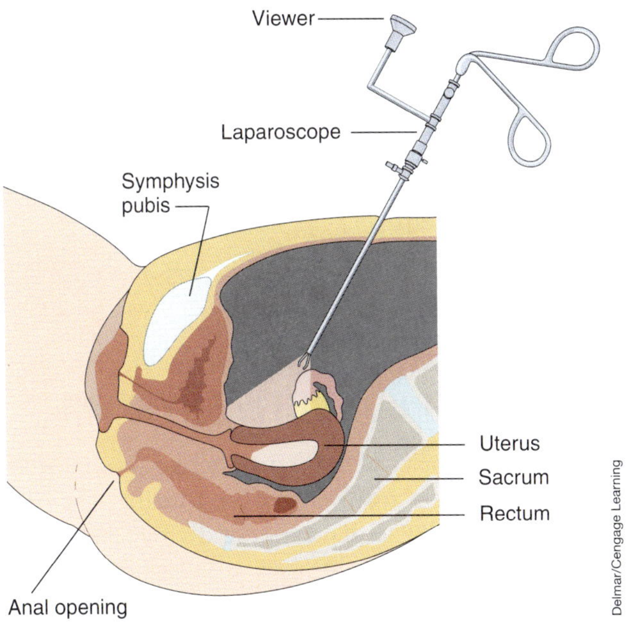

FIGURE 17–4 Laparoscopy.

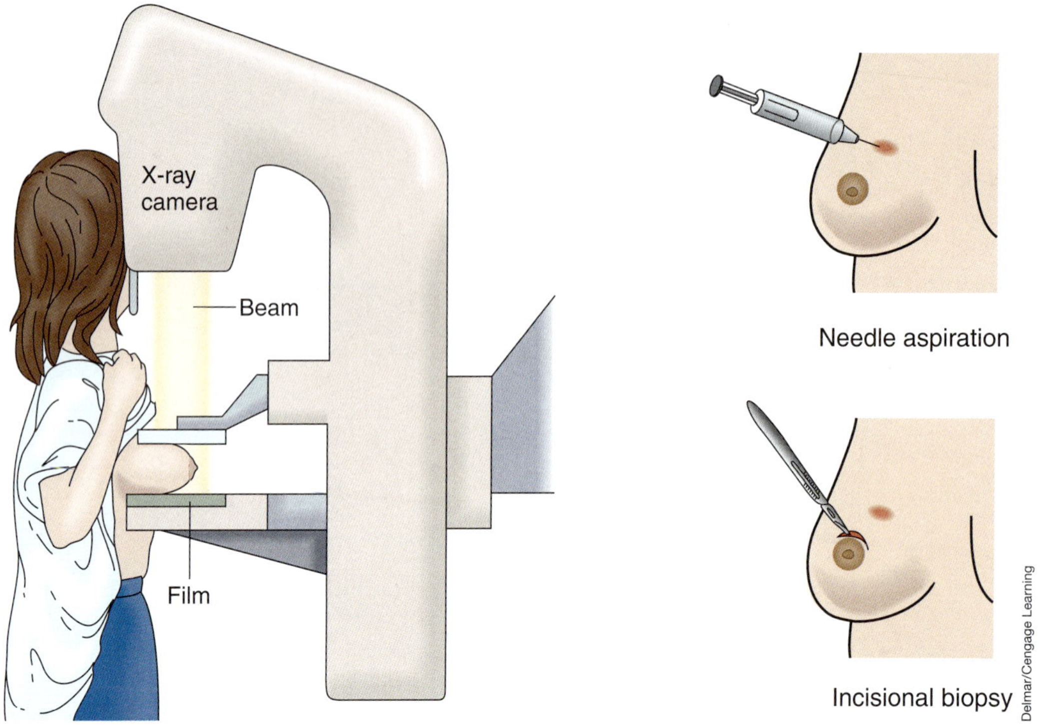

FIGURE 17–5 Mammography, needle aspiration, and incisional biopsy.

and to visualize pelvic organ position and size. Benign breast cysts can be differentiated from solid tumors by ultrasonography.

Physical examination of the male reproductive system includes visual examination of the external genitalia for tumors, lesions, or penile drainage. The testes are palpated to determine presence of tumors. A **digital rectal examination** allows the physician to feel the prostate (Figure 17–6) for abnormal enlargement (hypertrophy or hyperplasia) and tumors.

A **cystoscopy** (sis-TOS-koh-pee; cysto = bladder, oscopy = scope procedure) is performed to view the urethra and bladder with a lighted scope to evaluate the size of the prostate and the degree of obstruction the gland is placing on the urethra.

Biopsy of the male reproductive organs commonly involves the prostate and the testicle. Both procedures are performed to determine malignancy. To obtain a prostatic biopsy, a fine needle is guided through the rectum and into the prostate. A testicular biopsy involves the use of local anesthetic and a fine needle to withdraw a small piece of tissue. Testicular biopsy also can be used to evaluate sperm production.

Laboratory tests used in the determination of diseases of the male reproductive system include cultures and sensitivities of penile drainage, lesions, and urine to determine the presence of infection. A blood test called a prostate-specific antigen (PSA) is helpful in the detection of prostate cancer. PSA levels also assist in determining effectiveness of prostate cancer treatment. Urine estrogen levels can assist in the diagnosis of testicular cancers.

Specific laboratory tests used for infertility testing include microscopic examination of semen to perform a sperm count, to check sperm viability or ability to survive, and to look for abnormally shaped sperm. Blood tests for the hormones testosterone and LH are also used.

COMMON DISEASES OF THE REPRODUCTIVE SYSTEM

Common diseases of the reproductive system involve those affecting both sexes, including the pregnant female. These diseases are divided into female reproductive system diseases, diseases of the breast, disorders of pregnancy, male reproductive system diseases, sexually transmitted diseases (STDs), and sexual dysfunction.

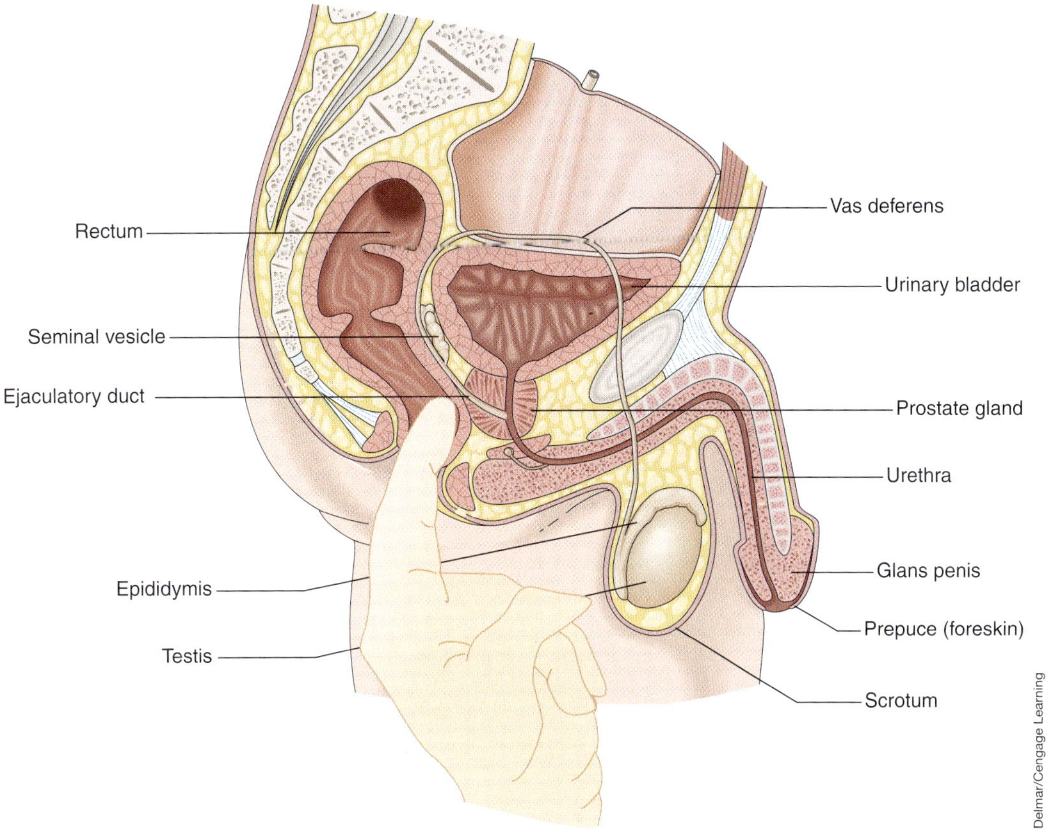

FIGURE 17–6 Digital rectal examination.

Female Reproductive System Diseases

The female reproductive system is affected by numerous diseases and disorders caused by inflammation, infection, tumors, cysts, and hormonal imbalances. Diseases can range from mild to life-threatening. Common symptoms include pain and abnormalities in the menstrual cycle.

MENSTRUAL ABNORMALITIES

DESCRIPTION. Menstrual abnormalities are a common problem in the ovulating female.

ETIOLOGY. Causes of menstrual abnormalities vary, as does treatment. Common abnormalities include premenstrual syndrome, amenorrhea, dysmenorrhea, menorrhagia, and metrorrhagia. A short description of these disorders follows.

PREMENSTRUAL SYNDROME

DESCRIPTION. Premenstrual syndrome, commonly called PMS, is a group of symptoms occurring prior to the onset of menses.

ETIOLOGY. The cause of PMS is uncertain, but research has shown an increase in PMS with rapid hormonal changes in estrogen levels that occur during the menstrual cycle. Other causes might be related to vitamin deficiencies and psychological disturbances. In the past, PMS was thought to be entirely due to emotional factors and stress, but it is now known to have a true physical cause.

SYMPTOMS. Symptoms of PMS usually begin mid-cycle with ovulation and increase in severity until a few hours after the onset of menses. PMS symptoms can affect virtually every system of the body and include headache, nausea, and back and joint pain. An increase in water retention can cause edema, bloating, weight gain, and breast tenderness and engorgement. Psychological symptoms can include irritability, mood swings, depression, and sleep disturbances. Symptoms of PMS vary significantly from one individual to another. It is unknown why some females have severe, disabling PMS, whereas others are virtually unaffected.

■ ***DIAGNOSIS.*** Diagnosis is difficult because the cause of this disorder is not clearly understood. A thorough history and physical examination might help determine the correlation of the onset of symptoms in relation to the menstrual cycle. Thyroid testing along with tests for dysmenorrhea and endometriosis aid in ruling out other causes. Because depression is common, some women might undergo psychological testing to rule out psychiatric disorders and confirm that the depression is related to PMS.

■ ***TREATMENT.*** Due to the variation in symptoms, treatment must be individualized because affected individuals have differing symptoms and respond differently to treatment. Dietary changes might be helpful and include avoidance of caffeine, chocolate, nicotine, sugar, salt, and alcohol. Developing a regular exercise program of brisk walking or swimming can be beneficial. Medications might be helpful and include diuretics, analgesics, and progesterone.

■ ***PREVENTION.*** PMS cannot be prevented, but certain activities can reduce the symptoms. These activities include quitting smoking, limiting caffeine, taking daily calcium (1,200 mg) and vitamin B_6 (50 mg), exercising, eating a balanced diet, and reducing stress.

AMENORRHEA

■ ***DESCRIPTION.*** Amenorrhea (ah-MEN-oh-REE-ah; a = without, menorrhea = menstruation) is the absence of menstrual periods. Primary amenorrhea is defined as not having menses by age 18. This can be caused by hormonal disorders, malformation or absence of female organs, pregnancy, or anorexia. Secondary amenorrhea is the absence of menses for 6 months or more in a female who has had regular cycles.

■ ***ETIOLOGY.*** Causes include hormonal imbalance, emotional upset, depression, malnutrition, excessive fitness training, ovarian tumor, and pregnancy.

■ ***DIAGNOSIS.*** Diagnosis is made on the basis of a physical examination and hormonal blood and urine studies.

■ ***TREATMENT.*** Treatment depends on cause. If no abnormalities are present, hormone administration will usually begin the menstrual cycle in primary amenorrhea.

■ ***PREVENTION.*** Preventive measures include adequate nutrition, exercise, and stress reduction.

DYSMENORRHEA

■ ***DESCRIPTION.*** Dysmenorrhea (DIS-men-oh-REE-ah; dys = difficult, menorrhea = menses) is painful or difficult menses, one of the most common gynecological disorders.

■ ***ETIOLOGY.*** Causes of dysmenorrhea include pelvic infections, cervical stenosis, endometriosis, and unknown causes.

■ ***SYMPTOMS.*** Symptoms include dull to severe cramping pain in the pelvic area and low-back pain. Pain also might radiate into the upper back, thighs, and genitalia. Pain associated with cervical stenosis and endometriosis often occurs in females prior to childbearing and is often relieved after the birth of a child. Prognosis is good if the cause can be found and treated.

■ ***TREATMENT.*** Oral contraceptives can be effective in reducing dysmenorrhea because they regulate and decrease menstrual flow. Nonsteroidal anti-inflammatory medications are helpful in reducing inflammation and pain. Application of a heating pad to the pelvic area also might be helpful.

MENORRHAGIA

■ ***DESCRIPTION.*** Menorrhagia (MEN-oh-RAY-jee-ah; meno = menses, orrhagia = bursting forth, abnormal, excessive) is excessive or prolonged menstrual flow.

■ ***ETIOLOGY.*** Cause can be due to uterine tumors, pelvic inflammatory disease (PID), and hormone imbalances.

■ ***TREATMENT.*** Treatment is related to cause and can include surgery to remove tumors, antibiotics to treat PID, and hormone therapy for hormone imbalances.

METRORRHAGIA

■ ***DESCRIPTION.*** Metrorrhagia (MET-roh-RAY-jee-ah; metro = uterus, orrhagia = bursting forth, abnormal, excessive) is abnormal bleeding between menstrual periods.

■ ***ETIOLOGY.*** The cause is commonly due to hormonal imbalance, leading to an abnormal thickening and shedding of the endometrial tissue.

■ ***TREATMENT.*** Treatment can be a D&C, returning the endometrium to normal and ending metrorrhagia.

MENOPAUSE

■ ***DESCRIPTION.*** Menopause is the natural halting of menstruation.

■ ***ETIOLOGY.*** Menopause is not a disease but rather a normal physical change related to aging, but many women consider menopause a disorder because they commonly have physical and psychological symptoms. Menopause usually takes place between the ages of 40 and 50 years. As a female ages, the ovaries produce less estrogen, causing cessation of ovulation and menstruation. This process can be surgically induced by removal of both ovaries (bilateral oophorectomy).

■ ***SYMPTOMS.*** Common physical symptoms of menopause include hot flashes, night sweats, and vaginal dryness. Some women also experience psychological symptoms of depression, sleep disorders, and decreased libido (sex drive). Hormonal changes brought about by menopause increase a woman's risk of cardiac disease and osteoporosis.

■ ***DIAGNOSIS.*** The blood testing for presence of FSH aids in diagnosis of menopause.

■ ***TREATMENT.*** Hormone replacement therapy has been the treatment of choice for more than 60 years for prevention of hot flashes and vaginal dryness in menopausal women. In the mid-1980s, estrogen also was approved as preventive treatment of heart disease and osteoporosis.

More recently, in 2002, a federally funded Women's Health Initiative (WHI) prematurely halted a hormone study, finding that hormone therapy did not protect against heart disease and actually led to a slight increase in risk of heart attacks, breast cancer, strokes, and blood clots. This same study reported benefits of reduced risk of bone fractures and colon cancer in women using hormone replacement.

Since the release of this study, many unanswered questions and much confusion about hormone therapy remain. Benefits of hormone replacement include relief or prevention of hot flashes and vaginal dryness and decreased risk of bone fractures and colon cancer. The question is whether these benefits outweigh the risk of heart attack, breast cancer, stroke, and blood clots. Each individual has different risk levels depending on a variety of factors, including family history, individual health history, the amount of hormone medication prescribed, and the length of time this medication is taken.

As with all medications, the decision to use hormone therapy is an individual one based on review of the individual woman's health needs. The decision should be made only after detailed discussion with the physician, regarding the risks and benefits of therapy. For more information, search *www.hormone.org*.

■ ***PREVENTION.*** There are no preventive measures.

VAGINITIS

■ ***DESCRIPTION.*** Vaginitis (VAJ-ih-NIGH-tis) is inflammation of the vagina.

■ ***ETIOLOGY.*** Vaginitis is a very common disease caused by a variety of microorganisms. It is not dangerous but is irritating and uncomfortable and often leads to a bladder infection.

■ ***SYMPTOMS.*** Symptoms of vaginitis are burning, itching, and swelling of the vagina and external genitalia. A white cottage cheese–appearing discharge is common with Candida vaginitis.

■ ***TREATMENT.*** The key to proper treatment of vaginitis is to determine the correct cause of the infection. Yeast infections that occur more often than four times a year need physician treatment. Abstaining from sexual intercourse until the condition has healed is recommended primarily to decrease the risk of reinfection.

■ ***PREVENTION.*** Preventive activities include keeping the vaginal area clean and dry; wearing cotton underwear to help absorb moisture; always wiping genital area front to back; avoiding excessive douching; avoiding deodorized tampons; eating yogurt especially, if taking antibiotics; removing and replacing tampons as directed; and decreasing intake of sweets and alcohol. The most common types of vaginitis include the following.

CANDIDA VAGINITIS

■ ***DESCRIPTION.*** Candida vaginitis is a type of fungus or yeast vaginitis that normally cohabits with lactobacillus bacteria in the vagina, maintaining vaginal normal flora. (See Chapter 4, "Inflammation and Infection," for more details on normal flora.)

■ ***ETIOLOGY.*** If the balance between the candida and the lactobacillus is disturbed, the affected individual develops a candida vaginitis, the most common type of vaginitis, commonly called a yeast infection. To maintain normal healthy vaginal flora, sufficient estrogen must be produced to enhance the growth of lactobacilli, a beneficial, normal flora bacterium. Lactobacilli aids in the production of lactic acid, causing a lower vaginal pH of 4 or 4.5. This acid environment is also a deterrent to the growth of harmful microorganisms.

Use of tampons, diaphragms, condoms, spermiacides, vaginal douche, and deodorant sprays can easily upset the normal flora of the vagina and lead to vaginitis. Antibiotic use commonly kills lactobacilli and can lead to severe vaginitis. Candida infection is usually not spread by sexual transmission except in severe cases.

■ ***TREATMENT.*** Home remedies include douching with 1 teaspoon of vinegar in one gallon of water and eating yogurt or adding the yogurt in the douche to restore the normal flora. Over the counter, vaginal antifungal ointments and tablets such as clotrimazole (Gyne-Lotrimin, Femcare) and miconazole are beneficial in most cases. Oral antifungal medications such as fluconazole (Diflucan) might be needed for more severe cases.

TRICHOMONAS VAGINITIS

■ ***ETIOLOGY.*** Trichomonas (TRICK-oh-MOH-nas) vaginitis is a parasitic vaginitis that is commonly transmitted during sexual intercourse.

■ ***TREATMENT.*** Both sexual partners must be treated with an oral antiparasitic medication to eradicate the infection.

ATROPHIC VAGINITIS

■ ***ETIOLOGY.*** Atrophic vaginitis commonly occurs postmenopausal and is caused by a decrease in secretion of estrogen, which is needed to maintain the vaginal lining. Without an adequate supply, the lining becomes more susceptible to infection.

■ ***TREATMENT.*** Treatment often includes estrogen therapy and the use of adequate lubrication during sexual intercourse to prevent injury to the vaginal lining.

■ ***DIAGNOSIS.*** Diagnosis is usually confirmed by microscopic examination of vaginal secretions, revealing the presence of the infecting organism.

OTHER FEMALE REPRODUCTIVE SYSTEM DISEASES AND DISORDERS

ENDOMETRIOSIS

■ ***DESCRIPTION.*** Endometriosis (EN-doh-ME-tree-OH-sis; endo = inside, metri = uterus, osis = condition of) is the abnormal growth of endometrial tissue outside the uterus. Endometrial tissue might flow retrograde during menses and escape into the abdominopelvic cavity through the fallopian tubes or, even worse, escape into the blood supply and be carried to sites all over the body.

■ ***ETIOLOGY.*** The cause of retrograde flow is unknown, but use of tampons might be a causative factor. For this reason, the use of tampons is discouraged. Common sites of endometrial implantation include the ovaries, fallopian tubes, abdominal wall, and intestine. Other sites of implantation include the urinary bladder, the diaphragm, nerves and ligaments of the back, and the vulva, to name only a few (Figure 17–7).

This endometrial tissue continues to act under the influence of hormones, thickening and bleeding with menstrual cycles, causing irritation and inflammation of normal tissue surrounding the implanted endometrial tissue, thus causing the development of

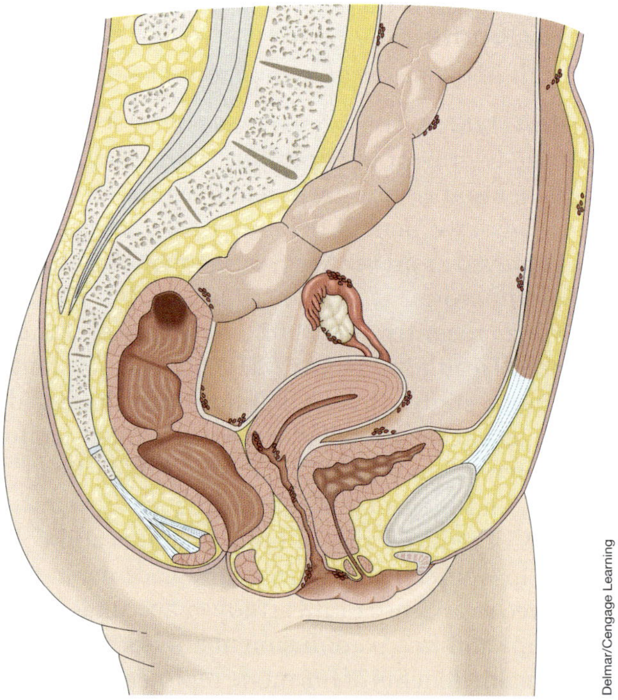

FIGURE 17–7 Endometriosis—common sites of endometrial implants.

a special blood-filled cyst (chocolate cyst), scar tissue, and adhesions.

SYMPTOMS. This bleeding of endometrial tissue in the abdominopelvic cavity and other **ectopic** (eck-TOP-ick, out of normal place) areas causes **dysmenorrhea** (DIS-men-oh-REE-ah; dys = painful, menorrhea = menses), beginning a few days before menses and extending several days into the menstrual cycle. There might be a constant cramping pain in the low back, pelvis, and vagina. Affected individuals, usually females of childbearing age, also might experience heavy menses and **dyspareunia** (DIS-pah-ROO-knee-ah; painful sexual intercourse).

The primary complication of endometriosis is infertility. Other complications include ectopic pregnancy and spontaneous abortion.

DIAGNOSIS. Diagnosis is made on the basis of history and pelvic examination. A laparoscopy will confirm the diagnosis and allow visualization of the extent of the condition.

TREATMENT. Treatment depends on the affected individual's age and desire to have children. Young females wishing to have children should not delay childbearing. Treatment with various hormonal medications might be helpful in younger individuals. Pregnancy, nursing, and menopause will not cure the condition but do cause a remission in symptoms because the abnormal tissue shrinks when menstrual hormones are halted. In severe cases, a total, or **panhysterectomy** (removal of ovaries, fallopian tubes, and uterus), might be indicated.

PREVENTION. Endometriosis cannot be prevented, primarily because the etiology is not well understood. Long-term birth control hormones might prevent the condition from worsening.

PELVIC INFLAMMATORY DISEASE

DESCRIPTION. PID is an inflammation of some or all of the pelvic reproductive organs. It can be mild to severe and might involve the cervix (**cervicitis**), the inner lining of the uterus (**endometritis**), fallopian tubes (**salpingitis**), and ovaries (**oophoritis**).

ETIOLOGY. This inflammation is commonly due to infection by bacteria that ascend from the vagina and travel upward to the pelvic cavity. Bacteria can be introduced into the female reproductive system during childbirth, miscarriage, abortion, or other gynecologic procedures. The most common cause of PID is sexually transmitted disease, including gonorrheal and chlamydial infection. Young, sexually active females, and those who use intrauterine devices (IUDs), are most at risk of developing PID.

SYMPTOMS. Symptoms are typical of an infection and include fever, chills, pain in the pelvic area, and **leukorrhea** (LOO-koh-REE-ah; leuk = white, orrhea = flow or discharge), a white, usually foul-smelling vaginal discharge.

DIAGNOSIS. Diagnosis is made on the basis of a pelvic examination including a positive culture of vaginal discharge.

TREATMENT. Treatment includes antibiotic therapy, analgesics, and bed rest. Without proper treatment, the infection can become **septicemic** (SEP-tih-SEE-mic; septic = dirty or contaminated, emia = blood), or blood-borne, and life-threatening. Inflammation of the reproductive organs can lead to the development of scar tissue and adhesions that can cause the complications of infertility and ectopic pregnancy.

PREVENTION. PID can usually be prevented by practicing safe sex with proper use of condoms. This will reduce but not eliminate risk of contracting STDs, the primary cause of the disease. Monogamous sexual relationships and abstinence also help prevent STDs.

OVARIAN CYST

DESCRIPTION. Ovarian cysts are commonly benign, fluid-filled sacs on or near the ovary (Figure 17–8).

ETIOLOGY. There are two types of cysts: physiologic—those caused by a normally functioning

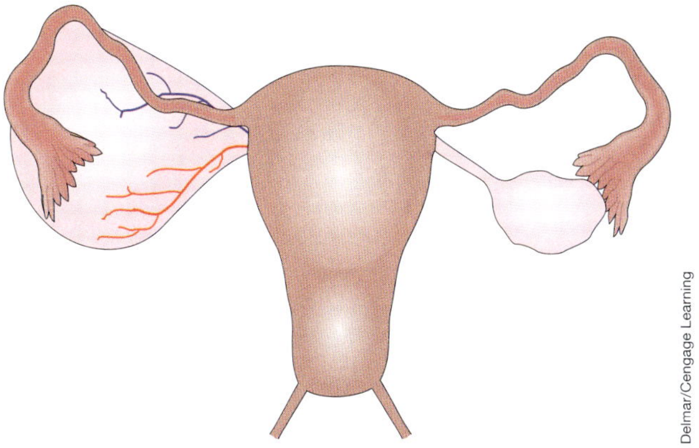

FIGURE 17–8 Ovarian cyst.

ovary—and neoplastic, an abnormal type not related to the function of the ovary. Physiologic cysts are the most common and can become very large (grapefruit size) before producing symptoms.

■ ***SYMPTOMS.*** Symptoms include low back pain, pelvic pain, and dyspareunia. Acute, extreme pain, nausea, and vomiting can occur if the ovary becomes twisted from the weight of the cyst.

■ ***DIAGNOSIS.*** Diagnosis is made on the basis of history, pelvic examination, and ultrasound.

■ ***TREATMENT.*** Treatment depends on the type and size of the cyst. Small physiologic cysts usually do not need treatment and often resolve spontaneously. Oral contraceptive medication can be given for several months to help resolve physiologic tumors of various sizes. Large cysts or those of questionable type are often viewed by laparoscopy, during which the cyst can be removed or drained. Determination should be made of the type of cyst because cancerous cysts need immediate treatment.

■ ***PREVENTION.*** Anything that prevents ovulation, such as birth control hormones, breast feeding, pregnancy, and menopause, reduce the risk of ovarian cysts.

FIBROID TUMOR

■ ***DESCRIPTION.*** Leiomyomas, commonly called fibroid tumors, are benign tumors of the smooth muscle of the uterus (Figure 17–9). They are the most common tumor of the female reproductive system, occurring in one out of five women over age 35.

■ ***ETIOLOGY.*** The cause of fibroid tumors is unknown, but it is known that these tumors are stimulated by estrogen and, thus, tend to occur during reproductive years and regress or calcify after menopause. They often appear in multiples and vary in size from small to quite large. Small fibroids are often asymptomatic.

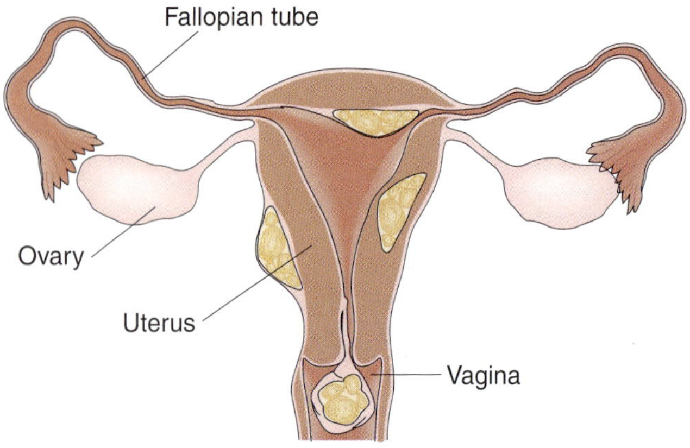

FIGURE 17–9 Fibroid tumors.

■ ***SYMPTOMS.*** Symptoms include abnormal uterine bleeding, excessive menstrual bleeding, and pain.

■ ***DIAGNOSIS.*** Diagnosis is made on the basis of pelvic examination and ultrasound.

■ ***TREATMENT.*** Treatment depends on the individual's age and desire for childbearing. Fibroids can be removed surgically, but in older individuals, a hysterectomy is often the treatment of choice. A new technology called high-intensity focused ultrasound (HIFU) that uses sound waves to destroy tumors can be used to treat the uterine fibroids (see the Complementary and Alternative Therapy box on p. 380).

■ ***PREVENTION.*** Fibroid tumors cannot be prevented. Estrogen therapy and oral contraceptives do increase risk of developing these tumors.

TOXIC SHOCK SYNDROME

■ ***DESCRIPTION.*** Toxic shock syndrome (TSS) is a severe, life-threatening illness found almost exclusively in menstruating females using tampons.

■ ***ETIOLOGY.*** TSS is thought to be caused by *Staphylococcus aureus*, a normal flora bacterium of the skin that produces an increased amount of toxin when in contact with the synthetic fibers found in tampons.

■ ***SYMPTOMS.*** Symptoms include the sudden onset of high fever, vomiting, diarrhea, and a dropping blood pressure.

■ ***DIAGNOSIS.*** Diagnosis is made on the basis of history of tampon use and symptoms. Complete blood count (CBC), chest X-ray, and electrocardiogram (EKG) may be completed to rule out other serious conditions.

■ ***TREATMENT.*** Treatment includes intravenous fluids to counteract shock and antibiotics to treat the infection. Untreated or delayed treatment may be fatal.

■ ***PREVENTION*** The best preventive measure is to avoid use of tampons. If this is not a good option, proper tampon usage helps reduce risk. Proper usage includes:

- Good hand washing to decrease the number of bacteria on the individual's hands prior to tampon insertion
- Avoiding super absorbent tampons
- Changing the tampon every 2 to 3 hours.

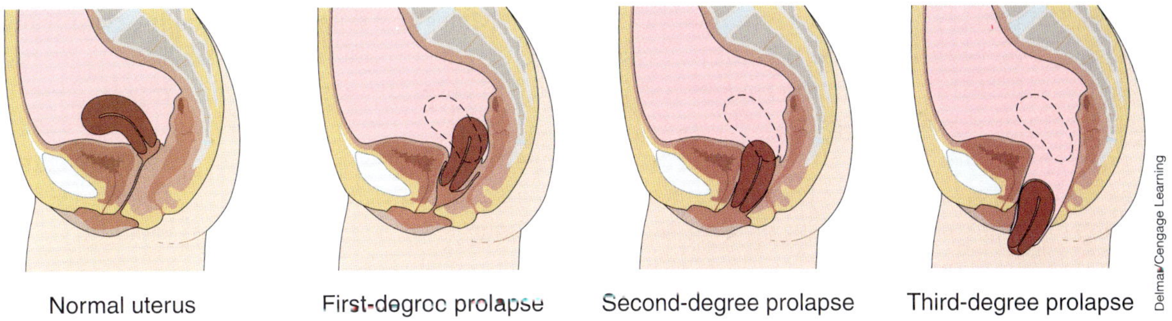

FIGURE 17–10 Uterine prolapse—varying degrees.

UTERINE PROLAPSE

■ ***DESCRIPTION.*** Uterine prolapse occurs when the uterus drops or protrudes downward into the vagina. There are varying degrees of prolapse (Figure 17–10).

■ ***ETIOLOGY.*** Prolapse is commonly due to aging and childbirth because these weaken the pelvic floor muscles.

■ ***SYMPTOMS.*** Symptoms include heaviness in the pelvic area; urinary stress, incontinence, or dysuria; and low back pain. With a complete prolapse, one can easily see the uterus bulging out of the vaginal opening. Although quite uncomfortable, this condition is not an emergency or even a health risk unless there is bleeding or an inability to urinate.

■ ***DIAGNOSIS.*** Diagnosis is made on the basis of a pelvic examination.

■ ***TREATMENT.*** A hysterectomy is often the surgical treatment of choice, depending on the woman's age and desire to bear children.

■ ***PREVENTION.*** This condition might not be preventable. Preventive behavior includes not smoking, maintaining a healthy weight, exercising daily, performing Kegel exercises to strengthen pelvic floor muscles, and controlling coughing.

CYSTOCELE

■ ***DESCRIPTION.*** Cystocele (SIS-toh-seel; cysto = urinary bladder, cele = hernia) is the herniation, or protrusion, of the urinary bladder through the anterior vaginal wall (Figure 17–11).

■ ***ETIOLOGY.*** Cystocele is often due to weakening of or trauma to the pelvic muscles related to aging and childbirth.

■ ***SYMPTOMS.*** Symptoms include pelvic pressure, urinary urgency, frequency, and incontinence.

■ ***DIAGNOSIS.*** Diagnosis is made on the basis of a pelvic examination.

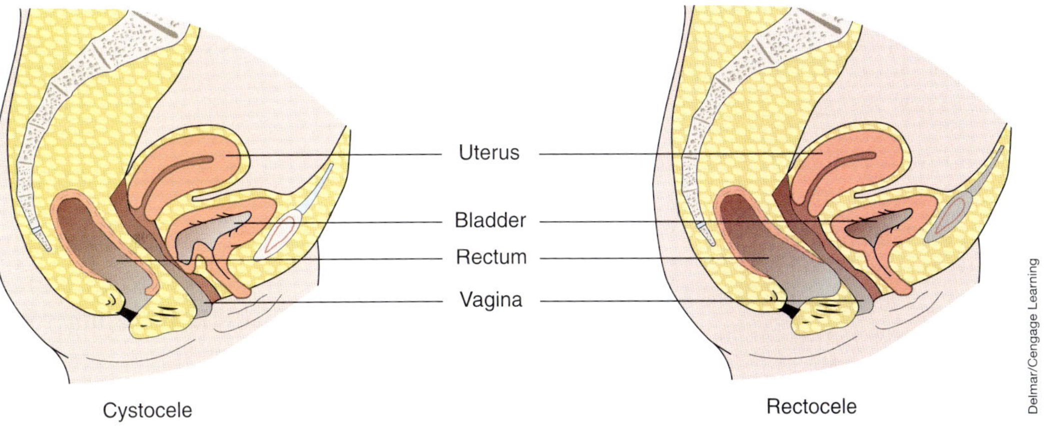

FIGURE 17–11 Cystocele and rectocele.

■ ***TREATMENT.*** Treatment depends on the degree of herniation. Strengthening the pelvic floor muscles with exercise can be beneficial. The specific exercise (Kegel exercise) is performed by contracting the pelvic floor muscles (this group of muscles is tightened to cut off urine flow) and releasing the muscles several times a day. If the cystocele is large or exercise is ineffective, surgery (anterior colporrhaphy) might be necessary.

■ ***PREVENTION.*** Preventive activities include not smoking, controlling coughing, avoiding heavy lifting, maintaining a healthy weight, controlling constipation, and performing Kegel exercises.

RECTOCELE

■ ***DESCRIPTION.*** Rectocele is the herniation or protrusion of the rectum through the posterior vaginal wall (see Figure 17–11).

■ ***ETIOLOGY.*** Rectocele, like a cystocele, is due to trauma to this area during childbirth.

■ ***SYMPTOMS.*** Symptoms include discomfort, constipation, and fecal incontinence.

■ ***DIAGNOSIS.*** Diagnosis is made on the basis of a physical examination.

■ ***TREATMENT.*** Treatment commonly is surgical repair (posterior colpoplasty). Often, the affected individual needs both a cystocele repair and a rectocele repair, called an anterior–posterior, or A&P, repair.

■ ***PREVENTION.*** Preventive activities include not smoking, avoiding coughing, maintaining a healthy body weight, and performing Kegel exercises.

CERVICAL CANCER

■ ***DESCRIPTION.*** Cervical cancer is the fifth-leading cause of cancer-related death in females. This cancer usually begins with **carcinoma in situ**—neoplastic cells that sit on the basement membrane and have not invaded into deeper tissue. As the cancer progresses, ulceration and cervical bleeding occur.

■ ***ETIOLOGY.*** Human papillomavirus (HPV) has been determined to be the cause of essentially all cervical cancer. There are over 60 types of HPV. Some types cause warts on the hands and feet of children, whereas other types cause genital warts. Several types of HPV do not cause warts but cause changes to the cells in the cervix, leading to cervical cancer.

HPV is generally acquired through sexual contact. Condoms cannot prevent the spread of HPV because it is found on all genital tissues of the infected individual. Males and females are usually asymptomatic with HPV infection. Discovery of HPV is usually made when cervical changes are found with a Pap smear. It is very difficult to trace exposure to the virus because it can lie dormant on the cervix for 20 years before it causes changes to the cells of the cervix. Activities that increase risk of HPV infection include:

- Beginning sexual intercourse at an early age. This activity generally results in an increase in the number of sex partners over the individual's lifetime.
- Having multiple sexual partners. Studies show that approximately 40% of young, sexually active females carry HPV in their vaginas. Presumably, a similar percentage of males are infected.

One fact in support of these identified risk factors is that females who abstain from sexual intercourse throughout life do not get cervical cancer.

HPV infection does not cause cervical cancer in all females. Most women who have evidence of HPV on their cervix never get cervical cancer. Studies suggest that whether a female will develop cervical cancer depends on a variety of factors acting together with HPV infection. These factors include:

- **Decreased resistance to infection.**
- **Smoking** Women who smoke concentrate nicotine in their cervix, which harms the cells.
- **Sexual intercourse with males who smoke** Men also concentrate nicotine in their genital secretions and can bathe the cervix with these chemicals during intercourse.
- **Marriage to a male whose previous spouse was diagnosed with cervical cancer** Females married to men whose former spouse was diagnosed with cervical cancer are at greater risk of also developing cervical cancer.
- **Obesity.**
- **Excessive alcohol consumption.**

■ ***SYMPTOMS.*** Development of cervical cancer is usually slow, and symptoms of abnormal cervical bleeding are easily noticed, leading to early detection of this form of cancer.

■ ***DIAGNOSIS.*** Diagnosis of cervical cancer is made on the basis of a Pap smear.

■ ***TREATMENT.*** Treatment is usually surgical removal of the tumor. If metastasis has occurred, surgery is often followed by radiation therapy. If the tumor has spread into adjacent tissues, a complete hysterectomy might be performed. Untreated, the tumor becomes inoperable and fatal.

■ ***PREVENTION.*** Cervical cancer is one of the few preventable cancers. Regular Pap smear testing aids in identifying precancerous cells, allowing treatment prior to cancer development. Other activities to reduce risk include not smoking, limiting the number of sexual partners, using condoms, following up on abnormal Pap tests, and, if under 27 years old, getting the HPV vaccine.

The HPV vaccine is recommended for 11- to 12-year-old girls and can be given to girls as young as 9. The vaccine is also recommended for 13- to 26-year-old girls and women who have not yet received or completed the vaccine series. The vaccine helps protect against four types of HPV: two types that cause 70% of cervical cancer cases, and two more types that cause 90% of genital warts cases.

UTERINE CANCER

■ ***DESCRIPTION.*** Uterine cancer develops in the inner lining of the uterus, the endometrium, and spreads into the uterine wall. Uterine cancer also may be called endometrial cancer.

■ ***ETIOLOGY.*** This type of cancer usually occurs in postmenopausal females who have never had children. Increased risk factors include infertility, obesity, and prolonged estrogen stimulation as occurs with hormone replacement therapy.

■ ***SYMPTOMS.*** The symptoms of uterine cancer include abnormal bleeding, which is quite noticeable in postmenopausal females and usually leads to early detection of this form of cancer.

■ ***DIAGNOSIS.*** Diagnosis is made on the basis of visual examination and endometrial biopsy.

■ ***TREATMENT.*** Treatment is very successful, if the cancer is discovered in its early stages, and includes surgical removal of the ovaries and uterus, combined with radiation therapy.

■ ***PREVENTION.*** Most cases are not preventable, but reducing risk factors is helpful. Risk reduction includes a history of taking oral contraceptives or birth control pills and taking hormone therapy with progestin after menopause. Other activities to reduce risk include not smoking and maintaining a healthy weight.

OVARIAN CANCER

■ ***DESCRIPTION.*** Ovarian cancer is quite common and often fatal.

■ ***ETIOLOGY.*** The cause of ovarian cancer is unknown, and the ovaries' position deep in the pelvis make discovery of this tumor difficult. Often, extensive metastasis will occur before noticeable symptoms present.

■ ***SYMPTOMS.*** Symptoms include a feeling of pressure on the bladder, low abdominal or pelvic pain, and a general feeling of ill health.

■ ***DIAGNOSIS.*** Diagnosis is made on the basis of physical examination and visualization of the mass during an exploratory laparoscopy.

■ ***TREATMENT.*** Treatment depends on the stage of the cancer and often includes a complete hysterectomy, radiation, and chemotherapy. Prognosis is good with early detection, but as stated previously, this is not the usual case. If metastasis has occurred, this cancer can be fatal in 1 to 2 years. The only preventive measure is early detection through annual gynecologic exams.

■ ***PREVENTION.*** Activities that lower risk include a history of taking oral contraceptive (birth control pills), bearing at least one child, and breast feeding for at least 1 year. An interesting fact about preventive activities is that having a tubal ligation reduces risk more than having a hysterectomy. The reason for this is unknown.

Diseases of the Breast

Diseases of the breast are quite common, affecting one in eight women in the United States and ranging from mild to life-threatening. Breast self-examination and mammography are important methods of screening for cancer. Although women are most often affected with breast diseases, men also can be affected. Any change from normal in tissue shape or appearance in males or females should be called to the attention of a physician.

FIBROCYSTIC DISEASE

■ ***DESCRIPTION.*** Fibrocystic disease of the breast is the most common breast disorder of premenopausal females between the ages of 30 and 55.

■ ***ETIOLOGY.*** It is thought the development of cysts is linked to estrogen levels.

■ ***SYMPTOMS.*** This disorder is characterized by:

- An irregular, lumpy feeling in the breast, usually in the upper outer quadrant area of the breast.
- Breast discomfort that is persistent or occurs on and off, typically peaking around the menstrual period and receding afterward.
- Breast often feeling heavy, full, and tender.
- A tendency to run in families.

Fibrocystic disease causes an increased risk of cancer approximately one-and-a-half times that of the normal population. Multiple cysts also make detection of neoplasm more difficult. For these reasons, affected females need to perform monthly breast self-examinations routinely and have yearly mammograms. Females with severe fibrocystic disease and at high risk of breast cancer might decide to have a **prophylactic** (preventive) mastectomy.

■ ***DIAGNOSIS.*** Diagnosis is made primarily by feeling, or palpation, of lumpy areas in the breast. Breasts that have many areas of fibrocystic disease can be difficult to palpate and to mammogram properly. In this case, breast ultrasound can be helpful. If there is a suspicious area, a needle or surgical biopsy can be performed to confirm diagnosis.

■ ***TREATMENT.*** Measures to decrease breast pain due to fibrocystic disease include elimination of caffeine in the diet, reduction of salt intake, the use of a mild diuretic the week prior to menstruation, and the use of mild analgesics. For severe cases, hormonal therapy with synthetic androgen might be helpful.

■ ***PREVENTION.*** This condition is often not preventable, but decreasing dietary fat and caffeine can be helpful. A recent researcher has shown a strong correlation between wearing brassieres and fibrocystic lumps, with 90% of the women in the study finding improvement in symptoms when they stopped wearing their brassieres (Reed, 2008).

MASTITIS

■ ***DESCRIPTION.*** Mastitis (mas-TYE-tis; mast = breast, itis = inflammation) is inflammation of the breast tissue and is a broad term covering a variety of diseases and disorders. The type of mastitis commonly thought of is **puerperal** (pyou-ER-pier-al; childbirth) mastitis.

■ ***ETIOLOGY.*** Puerperal mastitis occurs when bacteria from the nursing baby's mouth or mother's hands enter the breast tissue through the nipple and cause infection.

■ ***SYMPTOMS.*** Symptoms include redness, heat, swelling, pain, and, often, bloody discharges from the nipple.

■ ***DIAGNOSIS.*** Diagnosis is made on the basis of symptoms.

■ ***TREATMENT.*** Treatment includes antibiotics, application of heat, analgesics, and a firm support brassiere to decrease discomfort.

■ ***PREVENTION.*** Preventive measures include complete emptying of the breast when breast feeding. The baby should completely empty one breast before the other is offered.

BREAST CANCER

■ ***DESCRIPTION.*** Breast cancer is an adenocarcinoma (adeno = gland, carcinoma = cancer) of the breast ducts. It is the most common neoplasm affecting breast tissue and occurs in one out of eight females. It is second only to lung cancer as the leading cause of cancer-related deaths in females in the United States (Imaginis, 2008). Monthly breast self-examinations and routine mammograms are a must for early detection of breast cancer.

■ ***ETIOLOGY.*** The cause of breast cancer is unknown, but possible identified risk factors include:

- Age 40 and over.
- Family member affected with breast cancer.
- Onset of menses before age 13.
- Menses continuing after age 50.
- Nullipara (nuh-LIP-ah-rah; nulli = none or no, para = births).
- First child after age 30.
- Obesity.
- Chronic breast disease.
- Brassiere wear time.

■ ***SYMPTOMS.*** Symptoms of breast cancer include a nontender lump of varying size. These occur most often in the upper outer quadrant of the breast, near the axillary area. The lump might cause a dimpling of the skin, or the nipple might be retracted. Often, there are no visual symptoms.

■ ***DIAGNOSIS.*** Diagnosis is made on the basis of the presence of the lump, mammogram, and biopsy. A biopsy is the definitive test and can be performed by aspiration or surgery. Prognosis is good if the lump is found early. However, metastasis is common and usually affects the lungs, liver, brain, and bone. If metastasis has occurred, the prognosis can be poor.

■ ***TREATMENT.*** Treatment is usually surgical removal of the mass or the breast (**mastectomy**: mas-TECK-toh-me; mast = breast, ectomy = excision), followed by chemotherapy, radiation therapy, or both. Carcinoma spreads through the lymphatic system, so removal of the lymph nodes and lymph vessels is a common procedure. Several types of surgical procedures are performed for breast cancer, depending on the location, size, and metastasis of the tumor. Commonly, these types of surgery include:

- Lumpectomy, involving removal of the lump only.
- Simple or total mastectomy, involving removal of the breast and nipple.
- Modified radical mastectomy, involving removal of the breast, nipple, and lymph nodes.
- Radical mastectomy, involving removal of the breast, nipple, lymph nodes, and underlying chest (pectoral) muscles (Figure 17–12).

Mastectomy surgery not only causes an alteration in the physical image but also can lead to a variety of psychological disorders for a female. For this reason, many women decide to have reconstructive surgery (mammoplasty) performed along with the mastectomy in an effort to reduce the physical and psychological trauma. **Mammoplasty** (MAM-oh-PLAS-tee; mammo = breast, plasty = surgical repair or restructuring) involves reconstruction of the breast with plastic surgery and prosthetic breast implants or skin flaps.

Many new postmastectomy or postlumpectomy treatments are reducing the rate of recurrence of the disease. Depending on the type of breast cancer, medications that target the specific problem (such as hormones, protein receptors, or blood vessel problems) are having a positive impact on the disease.

■ ***PREVENTION.*** Preventive measures include reducing identified risk factors. Several researchers have supported the theory of a relationship between brassiere wear time and breast cancer.

Researchers at Harvard School of Public Health published a medical journal article on breast cancer risk. Their research supported the fact that women who did not wear brassieres had a 60% lower rate of breast cancer than women who did wear brassieres. Explanations included that the tightness of the brassiere slows lymphatic flow. Lymph fluid helps dilute and wash away cellular toxins. A second explanation is that brassieres hold heat, thus increasing the temperature of breast tissues, a possible cause of increased cancer (Reed, 2008).

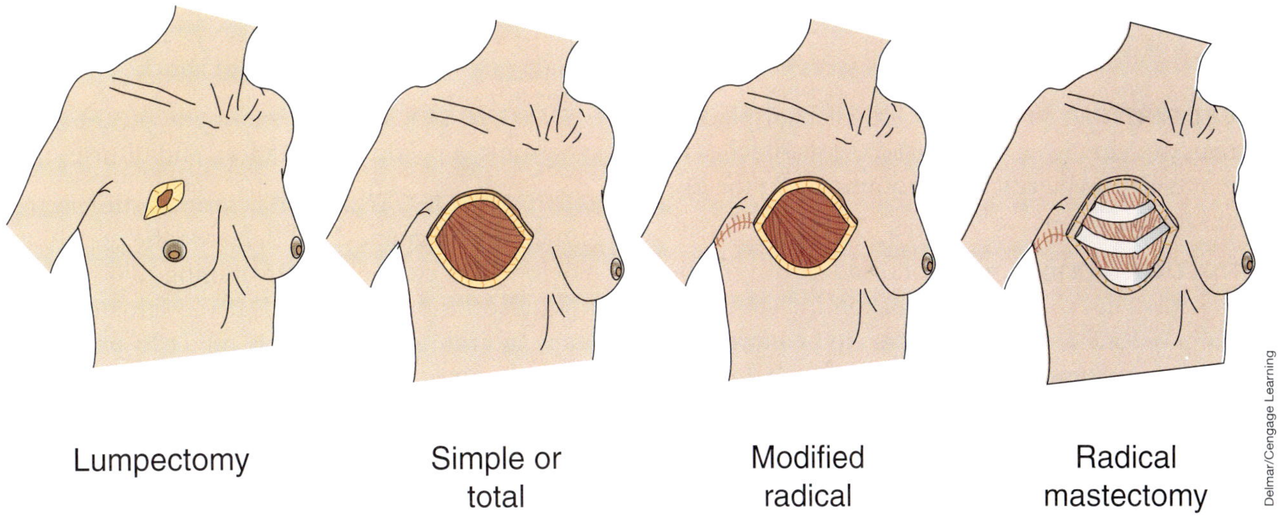

FIGURE 17–12 Types of mastectomy.

GLIMPSE OF THE FUTURE

Improving Treatments for Breast Cancer

Tamoxifen is a drug that is frequently used for treatment of breast cancer and for breast cancer prevention in women at increased risk. It interferes with the activity of the female hormone estrogen. Although it is effective for some types of breast cancer, tamoxifen has several significant side effects. Recent research is looking at the use of taurine (an organic acid found mostly in bile but also in other tissues in the body) to overcome some of the serious side effects of tamoxifen. Although the laboratory research is being conducted on mice, some studies have shown taurine can be beneficial in protecting the individual from the adverse effects of tamoxifen. Since the benefits of tamoxifen treatment have been shown to outweigh the risks, it will continue to be used. However, in the future, other adjunct therapies such as taurine may be added to the treatment plans for individuals taking tamoxifen.

Source: Parvez, et al. (2008).

The book, *Dressed to Kill: The Link Between Breast Cancer and Bras*, reports results of a study of 4,600 women, half of whom had breast cancer and half who did not. Authors found that the more hours per day that a bra is worn, the higher the rate of breast cancer, and women who did not wear a bra have a dramatically reduced rate of breast cancer.

Disorders of Pregnancy

Pregnancy is a normal condition of developing a fetus in the female body. However, disorders of pregnancy range from mild to life-threatening, sometimes risking the lives of the mother and the fetus. For this reason, the importance of prenatal care cannot be stressed enough.

ECTOPIC PREGNANCY

■ ***DESCRIPTION.*** Ectopic (eck-TOP-ick; displaced) pregnancy occurs when a fertilized ovum attaches to tissue outside the uterus, most commonly in the fallopian tubes.

■ ***ETIOLOGY.*** Strictures, adhesions, and scarring of the fallopian tubes due to PID, inflammation, infection, and structural defects can cause the tube to be narrowed, allowing microscopic-sized sperm to travel up the tube and fertilize the ovum, whereas the larger ovum is unable to travel down the tube and implant normally in the uterus. Other ectopic sites include the ovary, intestine, and outside wall of the uterus (Figure 17–13).

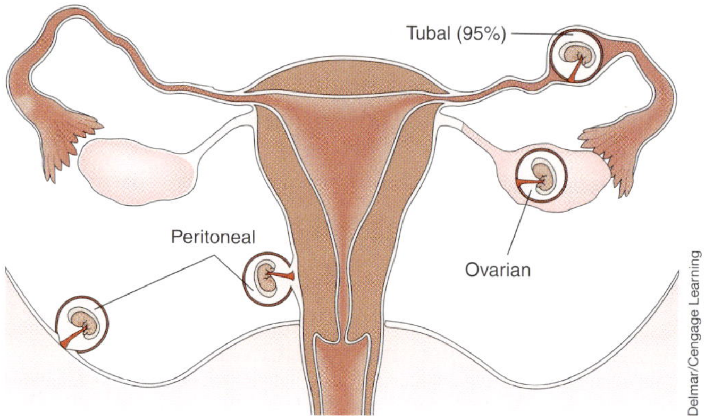

FIGURE 17–13 Sites of ectopic pregnancy

■ ***SYMPTOMS.*** Symptoms of ectopic pregnancy include acute pelvic pain, vaginal bleeding, and a positive pregnancy test. If large blood vessels are ruptured, bleeding can be heavy, and the affected female might show symptoms of shock.

■ ***DIAGNOSIS.*** Diagnosis is made on the basis of symptoms, a pelvic examination, and ultrasound.

■ ***TREATMENT.*** Treatment is prompt surgery to terminate the pregnancy and decrease the possibility of shock, which can be life-threatening. Blood replacement also might be needed. If the female wants to bear children, every effort is made to preserve the affected ovary and tube.

■ ***PREVENTION.*** Two preventive measures are to not smoke and to practice safe sex. Those who smoke, or who have smoked in the past, are at higher risk of ectopic pregnancy. Practicing safe sex lowers the risk of STD, the most common cause of this condition.

SPONTANEOUS ABORTION (MISCARRIAGE)

DESCRIPTION. Spontaneous abortion is the natural termination of pregnancy before the fetus is able to live on its own. This type of abortion is commonly called miscarriage.

ETIOLOGY. The cause of spontaneous abortion is unknown. It is believed that it might be due to infection, drug use by the pregnant mother, abnormal fetal development, or an incompetent cervix (one that dilates prematurely). Approximately one in every six pregnancies ends with spontaneous abortion, and 75% of these occur in the first 12 weeks. The risk is higher during a woman's first pregnancy.

SYMPTOMS. Symptoms of miscarriage include vaginal bleeding, cramping, and pelvic pain, usually in the first trimester of pregnancy. If bleeding is severe, shock is of major concern.

DIAGNOSIS. Diagnosis is made on the basis of symptoms and pelvic ultrasound.

TREATMENT. Bed rest is the treatment of choice if bleeding is not severe. Bed rest is continued until spotting stops. If the individual is hemorrhaging and showing signs of shock, hospitalization might be needed to control hemorrhage and give blood replacement. After spontaneous abortion begins, its progression is difficult to stop. A surgical D&C can be performed to remove any tissue remaining in the uterus after the abortion.

PREVENTION. There is no way to prevent spontaneous abortion, but activities to reduce risk include not smoking, eating healthy foods, monitoring and controlling chronic diseases, and taking folic acid prior to becoming pregnant.

MORNING SICKNESS

DESCRIPTION. Morning sickness is the nausea and vomiting associated with pregnancy, usually occurring in the first trimester of pregnancy.

ETIOLOGY. The cause of morning sickness is unknown, but it is thought to be due to hormonal changes related to pregnancy. It is also believed that hunger might play some part in the cause.

SYMPTOMS. Morning sickness, as its name implies, usually occurs in the morning, but it also can occur later in the day. Approximately 50% of pregnant females experience varying degrees of morning sickness.

DIAGNOSIS. Morning sickness is diagnosed by symptoms in a pregnant female.

TREATMENT. Treatment is not necessary unless there is excessive vomiting, which can lead to dehydration and weight loss. This condition is then termed *hyperemesis gravidarum*. No antiemetic (anti = against, emetic = vomiting) medication has been approved by the Food and Drug Administration (FDA) for morning sickness, and taking medications at this time in pregnancy can lead to fetal abnormalities.

PREVENTION. Morning sickness might not be preventable, but activities that might help reduce morning sickness include:

- Eating something light such as soda crackers before getting out of bed in the morning.
- Eating dry foods before drinking liquids.
- Eating several small meals during the day instead of three large ones.
- Avoiding fatty foods such as fried foods, butter, and margarine.
- Resting after meals.

HYPEREMESIS GRAVIDARUM

DESCRIPTION. Hyperemesis (hyper = excessive, emesis = vomiting) gravidarum is excessive vomiting during pregnancy.

ETIOLOGY. The cause is unknown but is thought to be due to an increased production of chorionic gonadotropin by the fetus. This thought is supported by the fact that hyperemesis gravidarum occurs more often in pregnancies with multiple fetuses.

SYMPTOMS. This condition can lead to dehydration, weight loss, and possible electrolyte imbalances in the mother and baby. The condition is not usually life threatening, but prompt medical attention is needed to preserve the health of the mother and baby.

DIAGNOSIS. Diagnosis is made on the basis of symptoms.

TREATMENT. Severe cases can be treated with intravenous fluids and by withholding all foods and oral fluids. Most cases subside by the second trimester of pregnancy.

PREVENTION. This condition cannot be prevented. Vomiting might be lessened by maintaining a healthy diet, eating dry foods, taking several small meals throughout the day, getting adequate sleep, reducing stress, and eating soda crackers before rising from bed in the morning.

TOXEMIA

DESCRIPTION. Toxemia is a condition usually appearing in the third trimester of pregnancy. The name of this condition is misleading because there is no toxin in the blood, but it was once thought that the fetus produced a toxin that led to toxemia.

ETIOLOGY. The cause of toxemia is unknown, but it does tend to occur more frequently in:

- Individuals with poor prenatal care.
- **Primigravid** (PRE-mih-GRAV-id; primi = first, gravid = pregnancy) females younger than 20 years of age and older than 30.
- Individuals with poor nutritional intake.
- Those who are hypertensive prior to becoming pregnant.
- **Multiparity** (mul-TIP-ah-rah-tee; multiple births), especially in individuals who have had five or more pregnancies.

SYMPTOMS. Toxemia is characterized by hypertension, sudden weight gain, proteinuria (protein = blood protein, urina = urine), and edema in the face, hands, and feet. It is also called **preeclampsia** (PREE-ee-KLAMP-see-ah). The individual with toxemia is preeclamptic before convulsions occur. Toxemia or preeclampsia, if untreated or unresolved, can progress into **eclampsia** (eh-KLAMP-see-ah), a condition characterized by all the symptoms of toxemia or preeclampsia plus convulsions. Eclampsia can lead to abruptio placentae and become life-threatening to the mother and baby.

DIAGNOSIS. Diagnosis is made on the basis of symptoms.

TREATMENT. Treatment includes frequent monitoring of blood pressure, weight, and urine protein as part of prenatal care. If symptoms of toxemia occur, a low-salt diet and antihypertensive medications might be recommended. If toxemia becomes severe, hospitalization in a quiet environment with frequent monitoring and administration of antihypertensive medications is the usual therapy to prevent convulsions. Prognosis is good because delivery of the baby or termination of the pregnancy resolves the problem.

PREVENTION. This condition is not preventable, but good prenatal care and good nutrition greatly reduce the risk of toxemia.

ABRUPTIO PLACENTAE

DESCRIPTION. Abruptio placentae is the sudden separation of the placenta from the uterus prior to or during labor (Figure 17–14).

ETIOLOGY. Often, the cause is unknown, but convulsions, trauma, multiple births, and chronic hypertension are known causes.

SYMPTOMS. The degree of separation determines the symptoms. A partial separation during labor might be asymptomatic, whereas a complete separation prior to labor can be life-threatening to the mother and baby. Symptoms of a complete separation can include severe abdominal pain with large amounts of vaginal bleeding (hemorrhage), shock, a decrease in fetal heart tones, and a decrease in fetal activity. Complete separations are a medical emergency because these can lead to maternal death from hemorrhage and death of the baby from a lack of oxygen and nutrition.

DIAGNOSIS. Diagnosis is usually made on the basis of clinical history because there is not time for other testing.

TREATMENT. Treatment is prompt delivery, either vaginally or by surgical cesarean section (C-section). Blood replacement also might be needed.

PREVENTION. Abruptio placentae is often not preventable. Controlling risk factors such not smoking, preventing maternal trauma such as that caused by domestic violence, and avoiding substance abuse are all helpful in reducing risks.

PLACENTA PREVIA

DESCRIPTION. Placenta previa is the abnormal positioning of the placenta in the lower uterus, often near or over the cervical os or opening (see Figure 17–14). If the placenta is totally over the os, it is a complete placenta previa; partial covering is a partial placenta previa.

ETIOLOGY. The cause of this condition is unknown. Some risk factors include multiparity, maternal age over 35, and previous uterine surgery.

SYMPTOMS. The affected individual has symptoms of painless, bright red vaginal bleeding during the third trimester of pregnancy. Vital signs can

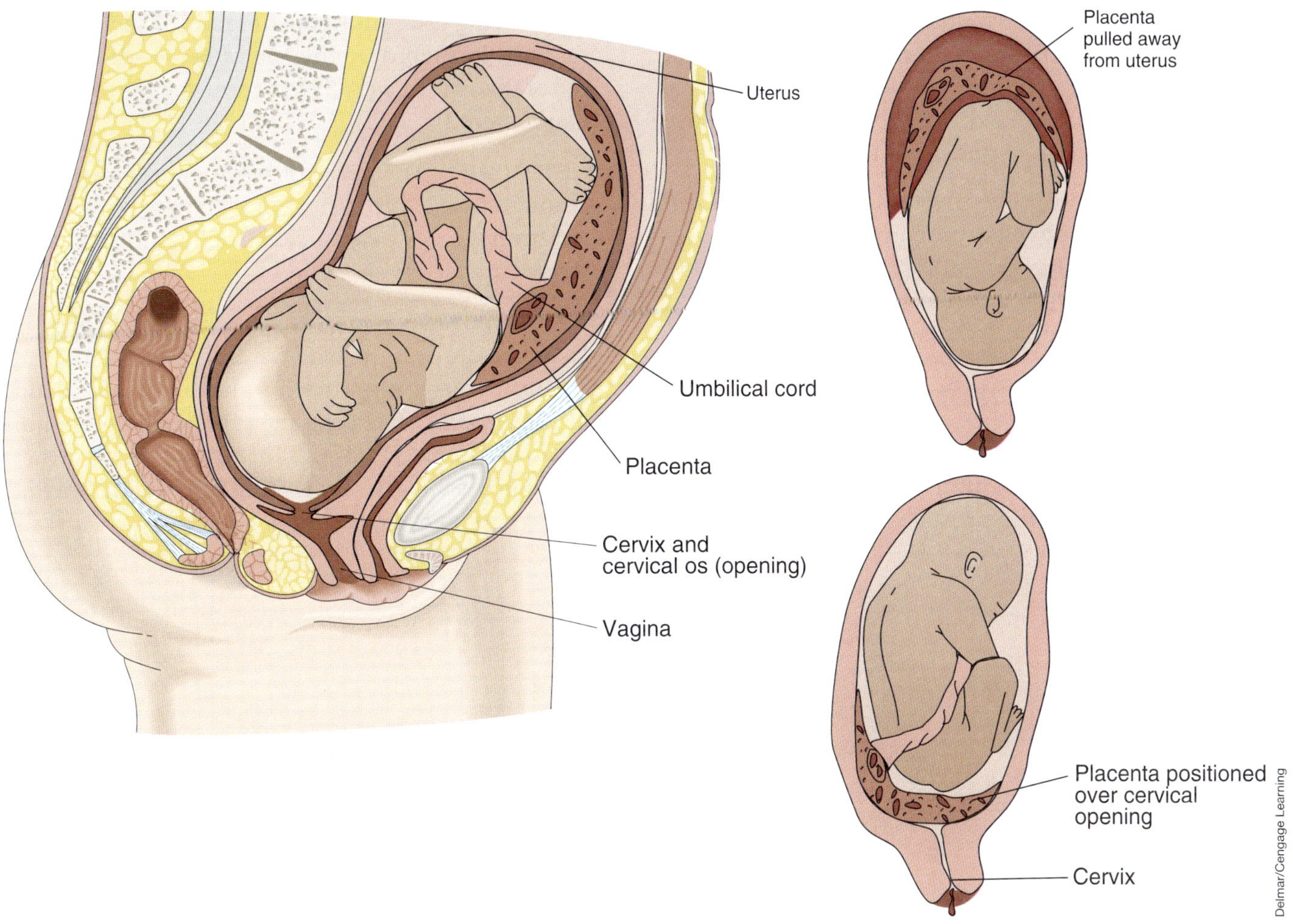

FIGURE 17–14 (A) Normal uterine pregnancy, (B) abruptio placentae, and (C) placenta previa.

indicate shock if the bleeding is severe. Placenta previa can be life-threatening to the mother due to hemorrhaging and to the baby due to anoxia.

■ ***DIAGNOSIS.*** Diagnosis is made by pelvic ultrasound.

■ ***TREATMENT.*** Vaginal delivery might be possible if the mother is asymptomatic or if bleeding is not severe. Severe maternal bleeding or fetal anoxia is reason to perform an emergency C-section.

■ ***PREVENTION.*** Because the cause is unknown, prevention is not possible.

Male Reproductive System Diseases

The most common diseases affecting the male reproductive system include infection and diseases affecting the prostate. The positional relationship of the male urinary bladder and the prostate cause the male to experience urinary symptoms when the prostate is affected with disease.

PROSTATITIS

■ ***DESCRIPTION.*** Prostatitis (PROS-tah-TYE-tis; prost = prostate, itis = inflammation) is inflammation of the prostate gland. This condition is more common in men over 50 years of age.

■ ***ETIOLOGY.*** Cause can be unknown or the result of a urinary tract infection or infection by STDs.

■ ***SYMPTOMS.*** Symptoms include **dysuria** (dis-YOU-ree-ah; dys-painful, uria = urination), **pyuria** (pye-YOU-ree-ah; py = pus, uria = urine), fever, and low back pain.

■ ***DIAGNOSIS.*** Diagnosis is made on the basis of a urinalysis, urine culture, and digital rectal examination.

■ ***TREATMENT.*** Treatment depends on cause but often includes antibiotic therapy with penicillin. Warm sitz baths, increased fluid intake, and analgesics also can be prescribed. Prognosis is good because prostatitis usually responds well to treatment.

■ ***PREVENTION.*** Preventive activities include not smoking, drinking plenty of fluids, seeking early treatment for urinary symptoms, and practicing good hygiene by keeping the penis clean. This takes extra effort in an uncircumcised male.

BENIGN PROSTATIC HYPERPLASIA

■ ***DESCRIPTION.*** Benign prostatic hyperplasia (BPH) is also called benign prostatic hypertrophy, the enlargement of the prostate due to normal cells overgrowing and enlarging (Figure 17–15). BPH is common in men over the age of 60. Approximately 50% of males over age 65 have some degree of prostate enlargement.

■ ***ETIOLOGY.*** The cause of BPH is unknown, but it is thought to be due to hormonal changes, including alterations in testosterone, estrogen, and androgen levels associated with aging.

■ ***SYMPTOMS.*** The enlargement of the prostate places pressure on the bladder and prostatic urethra, causing urinary obstruction and a variety of urinary symptoms. The primary symptoms of BPH are **nocturia** (nock-TOO-ree-ah; noc = night, uria = urination), or frequently getting up at night to void, inability to start urination, a weak urinary stream,

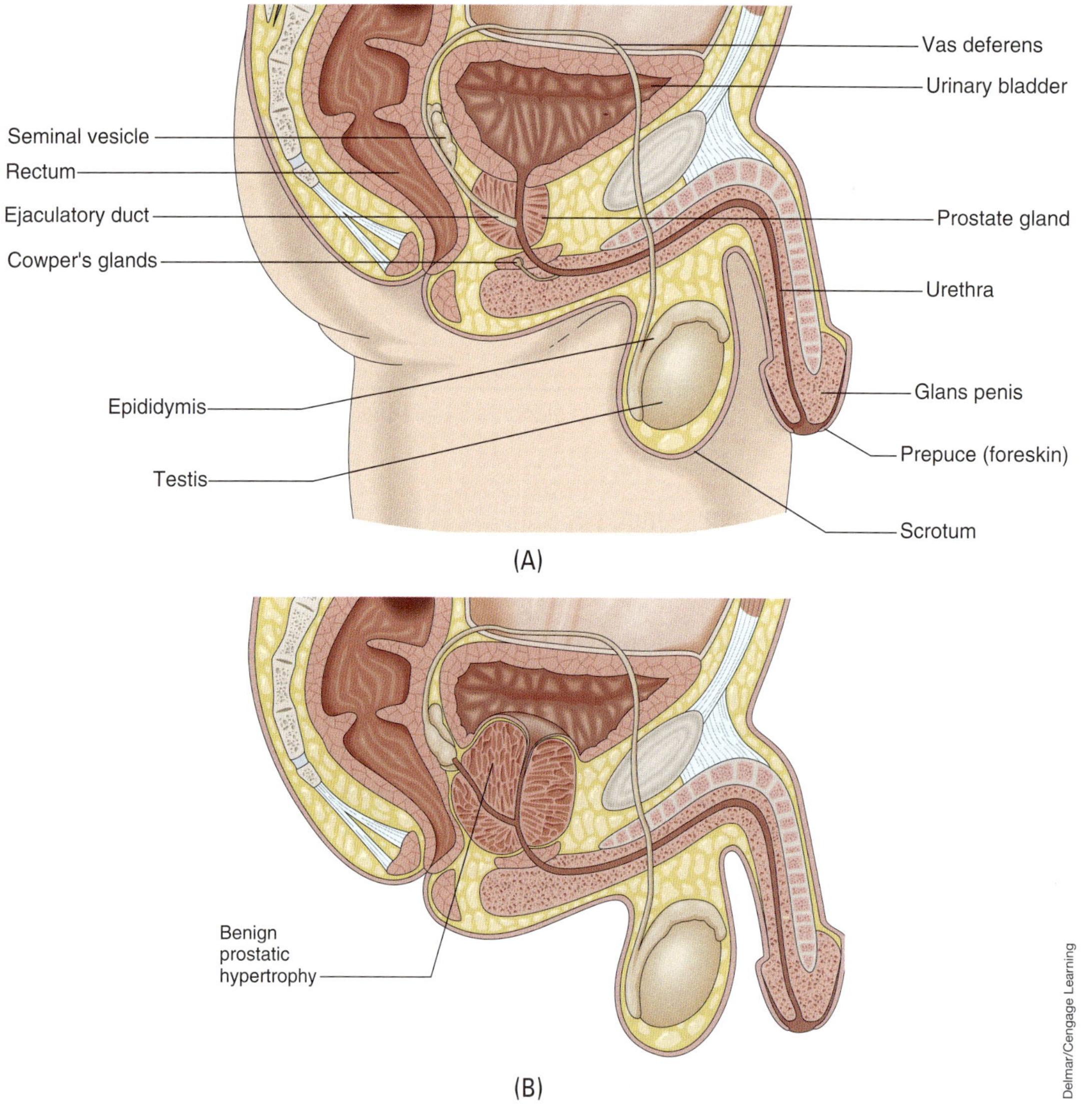

FIGURE 17–15 Normal and enlarged prostate. (A) normal. (B) benign prostatic hypertrophy or hyperplasia (enlarged).

and inability to empty the bladder. The inability to empty the bladder often causes the excess urine to fill the ureters, leading to hydroureter, hydronephrosis, and frequent urinary tract infections.

■ ***DIAGNOSIS.*** Diagnosis is made on the basis of symptoms and digital rectal examination revealing an enlarged prostate.

■ ***TREATMENT.*** Treatment is symptomatic and might include prostatic massage, sitz baths, and catheterizations. Regular sexual intercourse can be helpful in reducing prostatic congestion. Surgery to resect or decrease the size of the prostate is one common treatment. This procedure is called a transurethral (trans = through, urethral = urethra) resection of the prostate (TURP). This procedure is performed, as the name indicates, through the urethra. No surgical incision is needed. During a TURP, the surgeon uses a cystoscope to chisel away the excess prostate tissue causing the urinary obstruction (Figure 17–16).

■ ***PREVENTION.*** There are no known preventive measures for BPH. An annual prostate exam is recommended for males after age 40. Some people believe that regular ejaculation will help prevent prostate enlargement, but there is no scientific proof of this belief.

PROSTATIC CARCINOMA

■ ***DESCRIPTION.*** Prostatic carcinoma is a neoplasm of the prostate gland that commonly affects men after age 50. It is the second most common cause of cancer-related death in men; lung cancer is first.

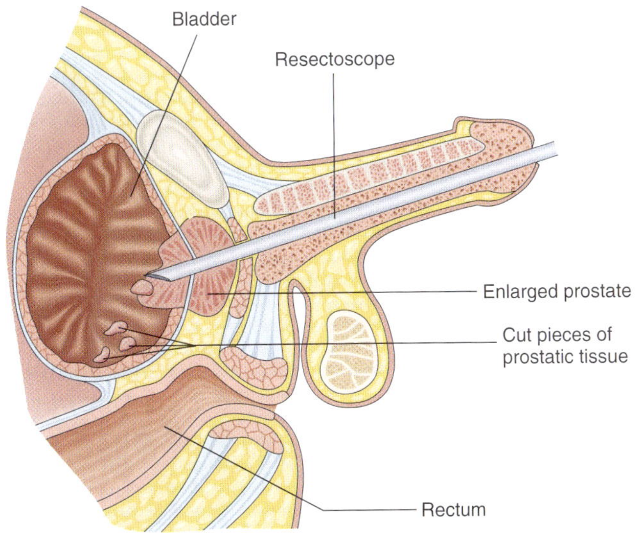

FIGURE 17–16 Transurethral resection of prostate (TURP).

■ ***ETIOLOGY.*** The cause of this cancer is unknown, although some believe that testosterone levels are involved. A puzzling fact with this theory is the great racial inequity in incidence of prostatic cancer. Caucasian men are affected with prostatic cancer 10 times more often than Oriental men. This fact leads to the belief that environmental and lifestyle factors are involved. Diets high in fat are also believed to be associated with an increase in prostate cancer. It is known that incidence does increase with age.

This adenocarcinoma grows in the outer layer of the prostate and often does not cause symptoms until it has metastasized. Common sites of metastasis include the bones of the spine and pelvis.

■ ***SYMPTOMS.*** Symptoms, when present, are similar to BPH as the urethra becomes obstructed.

■ ***DIAGNOSIS.*** Digital rectal examination will reveal a hard, abnormal mass. A blood test measuring PSA will be elevated with prostatic cancer. A serum PSA test result of 2.0 to 5.5 might be within the normal range, depending on the patient's age. Biopsy is the definitive test.

■ ***TREATMENT.*** Treatment depends on the age and physical condition of the affected individual and the degree of metastasis. If the tumor has not metastasized, complete removal and cure can be accomplished with a prostatectomy. If metastasis has occurred, treatment might involve hormone therapy to slow the growth of the neoplasm. Hormone therapy might include:

- Administration of estrogen to counteract testosterone.
- Surgical **orchiectomy** (OR-kee-ECK-toh-me; orchi = testicle, ectomy = removal), removal of the testicles to halt testosterone production.
- A combination of both treatments.

Much controversy exists over the benefits of hormone therapy. Many urologists do not believe an orchiectomy improves the survival rate of the affected individual. Chemotherapy and radiation treatments also might be beneficial treatments. The prognosis of prostatic carcinoma varies, depending on the age of the affected individual and the degree of spread. If the individual is older than 60 years of age, he will probably outlive the cancer and die of some other disease process. Younger individuals and those with extensive metastasis do not have as

COMPLEMENTARY AND ALTERNATIVE THERAPY

New Technology Treatment for Prostate Cancer

The use of alternative therapies for prostate cancer is increasing. One new technology being used is called high-intensity focused ultrasound (HIFU). This procedure uses sound waves that create intense heat to destroy solid tumors with very minor damage to the surrounding tissues. HIFU is currently being used to treat uterine fibroid tumors in the United States because it is FDA approved for that treatment. It is not approved in the United States for treatment of prostate cancer but is approved in Europe and many other countries for this treatment. HIFU is also used in other countries for tumors of the kidney and liver. It is being used in clinical trials in the United States at the present time.

Source: Saul (2008).

positive a prognosis. Overall, 50% to 75% of affected individuals live 5 years or more.

■ ***PREVENTION.*** There are no preventive measures, although getting an annual prostate examination is recommended for early detection.

EPIDIDYMITIS

■ ***DESCRIPTION.*** Epididymitis (EP-ih-did-ih-MY-tis; epididym = epididymis, itis = inflammation) is inflammation of the epididymis.

■ ***ETIOLOGY.*** Common causes include prostatitis, urinary tract infection, mumps, and STD such as chlamydia, syphilis, and gonorrhea. Epididymitis is one of the most common diseases of the male reproductive tract and usually affects only one epididymis (unilateral).

■ ***SYMPTOMS.*** Symptoms include a swollen, hard, and painful epididymis, often accompanied by severe scrotal pain and swelling. Scrotal discomfort makes walking difficult, and the affected individual might walk straddle-legged to protect the scrotum.

■ ***DIAGNOSIS.*** Diagnosis is made on the basis of symptoms, urinalysis, and urine culture.

■ ***TREATMENT.*** Prompt, appropriate antibiotic therapy is usually very effective. A delay in treatment can lead to complications of scarring and **sterility** (inability to impregnate a female, related to sperm quality or quantity). Other treatment includes bed rest, analgesics, use of a scrotal support, and avoidance of alcohol, spicy foods, and sexual stimulation.

■ ***PREVENTION.*** Prevention is aimed at cause and includes sexual abstinence, or use of condoms during sexual intercourse to decrease the risk of infection with STDs, and prompt treatment of causative infections.

ORCHITIS

■ ***DESCRIPTION.*** Orchitis (or-KYE-tis, orch = testis, itis = inflammation) is inflammation of one or both testes, usually due to bacterial or viral infection or trauma.

■ ***ETIOLOGY.*** Viral mumps is the most common cause of orchitis in the adult male. Commonly, orchitis occurs in conjunction with or as a complication of epididymitis.

■ ***SYMPTOMS.*** Symptoms include swelling, pain and tenderness of one or both testes, fever, and malaise.

■ ***DIAGNOSIS.*** Diagnosis is made on the basis of symptoms, blood testing, and urinalysis.

■ ***TREATMENT.*** Treatment depends on cause. If the cause is bacterial, antibiotic therapy is usually effective. Orchitis caused by mumps is treated symptomatically and includes bed rest and analgesic and antipyretic medications. A scrotal support might be helpful. Prognosis is good, although atrophy of the involved testicle does occur 50% of the time. If both testes are involved, sterility can occur.

■ ***PREVENTION.*** Prevention is aimed at causative factors and includes mumps vaccination and prevention of infection from STDs.

TESTICULAR TUMORS

■ ***DESCRIPTION.*** Testicular tumors commonly affect young males aged 20 to 35 and are the most common type of cancer for this age group. Testicular tumors rarely occur in males over age 40.

■ ***ETIOLOGY.*** The cause of this cancer is unknown, but predisposing factors include individuals who have been affected by **cryptorchidism** (krip-TOR kih dizm; crypt = hidden, orchid = testicle, ism = condition), or undescended testicle, and an inguinal hernia as a child. Cryptorchisdism increases the risk of developing testicular tumor by 10-fold (American Cancer Society, 2008c).

■ ***SYMPTOMS.*** The primary symptom of a testicular tumor is a painless mass felt in the testicle.

■ ***DIAGNOSIS.*** Diagnosis is made on the basis of palpation of a testicular mass and confirmation by biopsy.

■ ***TREATMENT.*** Treatment commonly includes surgery (orchiectomy), followed by chemotherapy and radiation. Because there is no direct lymphatic connection between the testes, testicular tumors do not usually spread from one testicle to the other. Surgical removal of the affected testis is often the treatment of choice. This procedure leaves the unaffected testis, and the male is not rendered sterile or **impotent** (inability to achieve or maintain a penile erection).

Metastatic testicular cancers can be treated with radical surgery involving removal of both testes and adjacent lymph nodes. This surgery might or might not affect impotency, but it will cause sterility. Males wishing to father children might elect to bank sperm prior to surgery so to father children at a later date by artificial insemination. If discovered early, prognosis of testicular tumor is good, with an approximately 90% cure rate. If metastasis has occurred, the prognosis is poor.

■ ***PREVENTION.*** There are no preventive measures for testicular cancer because most of the risk factors are unavoidable, such as age, race, and conditions occurring at birth. The best method of controlling spread of the disease is to discover the tumors prior to metastasis; the American Cancer Society (ACS) recommends a testicular exam as part of a routine annual checkup.

CRYPTORCHIDISM

■ ***DESCRIPTION.*** Cryptorchidism is a condition commonly referred to as an undescended testicle. As the unborn male fetus develops, the testes appear first

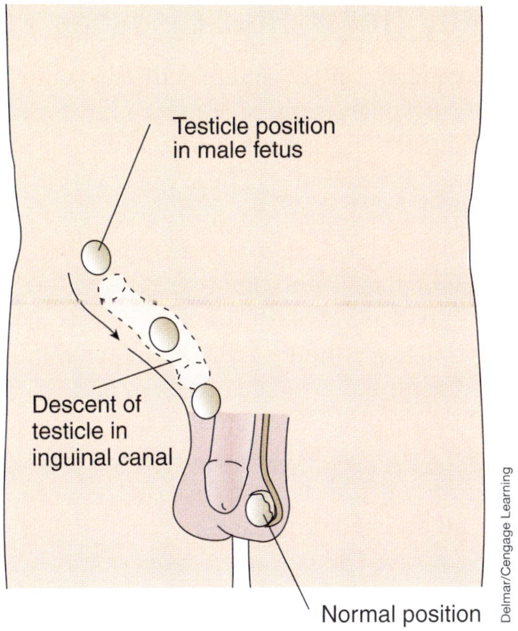

FIGURE 17–17 Cryptorchidism—pathway and common sites of hidden testis.

in the abdominal cavity. As the fetus grows and develops, the testes should move downward through the inguinal canal and into the scrotum.

■ ***ETIOLOGY.*** If this process does not occur properly, the testes might become lodged in any position in the abdominal cavity (Figure 17–17). Premature birth is a common cause of cryptorchidism and is usually time limited. The failure of both testes to descend is uncommon.

■ ***SYMPTOMS.*** Primary symptom is an undescended testis.

■ ***DIAGNOSIS.*** Diagnosis is made on the basis of physical examination noting an undescended testis.

■ ***TREATMENT.*** If a testis remains undescended into childhood, surgical intervention is necessary to move and secure the testis in the scrotum. This surgery is usually performed during infancy or prior to the age of 5. If the testis is left in the abdominal cavity, it will not function properly, but this will not affect potency or sterility because one testis can maintain adequate male hormone levels. If both testes are undescended, the male will be sterile. Men who have an undescended testicle at birth are at increased risk of developing testicular cancer in both testes (Husmann, 2003).

■ ***PREVENTION.*** There is no way to prevent this condition because the cause is still unknown.

Sexually Transmitted Diseases

STDs, formerly called venereal diseases, include a group of many diseases that are spread by intimate or sexual contact. The spread of STD is at an epidemic level in the United States. These infections are transmitted from one person to another by contact with infected skin, blood, semen, and vaginal secretions during vaginal, anal, and oral sex.

Treatment of STDs commonly consists of identifying sex partners and treating the infected individuals concurrently to avoid reinfection, or a ping-pong effect, of passing the infection back and forth between involved individuals. Follow-up testing is needed after treatment to ensure that the disease has been eradicated in all infected individuals.

Prevention of STDs is best achieved by avoiding intimate contact with infected individuals. Other precautions include use of a condom during sexual intercourse, avoiding multiple sex partners, avoiding sex with someone with an unknown sexual history, and avoiding the use of alcohol that can impair judgment concerning a sexual encounter.

ACQUIRED IMMUNODEFICIENCY SYNDROME

Acquired immunodeficiency syndrome (AIDS) is a blood-borne infection commonly transmitted sexually. AIDS is the most dreaded disease of modern society and has reached global epidemic proportion. Currently, there is no cure for this immunodeficiency disease that predisposes the affected individual to a multitude of opportunistic diseases. Prevention is imperative and must include health and AIDS education. For more details about AIDS, see Chapter 5, "Immune System Diseases and Disorders."

HEPATITIS

Hepatitis B and C can be spread by sexual intercourse and are, therefore, considered STDs. For more information, see Chapter 12, "Liver, Gallbladder, and Pancreatic Diseases and Disorders."

GENITAL HERPES

■ ***DESCRIPTION.*** Genital herpes is an extremely painful, recurring viral infection characterized by multiple, blister-like lesions (Figure 17–18). The incidence of genital herpes in the United States is increasing at a frightening rate, with one in every five individuals currently infected (CDC, 2002).

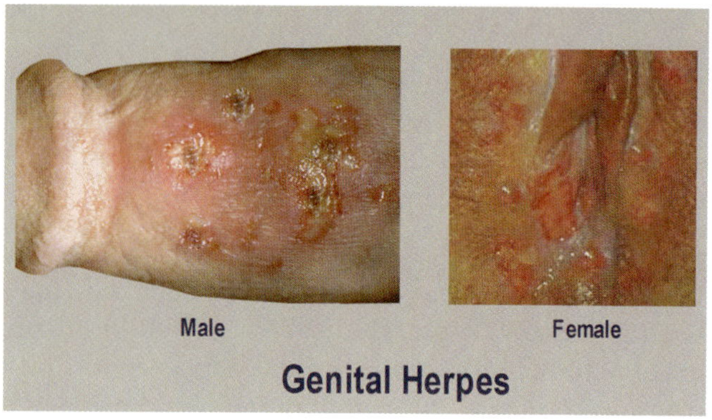

FIGURE 17–18 Genital herpes.

■ ***ETIOLOGY.*** Genital herpes is caused by herpes simplex virus (HSV) type II. (Herpes viruses are discussed in detail in Chapter 18, "Integumentary System Diseases and Disorders.") This is a highly contagious virus transmitted by intimate contact between two mucous membrane surfaces. HSV II is commonly spread by sexual intercourse but can be spread also to the lips by oral–genital exposure or by self-infection with the hands by touching an infected area and then touching the lips, genitals, or eyes. Extreme care should be taken to avoid infection of the mucous membranes of the eyes.

Herpes disease cannot be cured. The virus remains dormant in the tissues until activated by stress or lowered immunity. Sunlight, fever, emotional stress, and menses are common activators of the herpes virus.

■ ***SYMPTOMS.*** When activated, the virus produces blisters that enlarge, rupture, and ulcerate. The lesions are extremely painful, especially during sexual intercourse. Severe itching and painful urination (dysuria) are common. Genital herpes infection in the male commonly produces blisters on the glans penis, the shaft of the penis, scrotum, and inner thighs.

Lesions in the female commonly appear on the vulva, vagina, inner thighs, and rectal area. Childbirth in a female with active herpes infection is fatal to the infant 50% of the time. If the infant survives, major neurologic and ophthalmic complications usually occur. For this reason, delivery by C-section is performed in mothers with active genital herpes.

Herpes lesions generally last between one and 3 weeks but can recur weekly, monthly, or yearly.

■ ***DIAGNOSIS.*** Diagnosis is made on the basis of the presence of characteristic lesions and a positive viral culture of active lesions.

■ ***TREATMENT.*** Treatment is symptomatic and involves antiviral medications to reduce symptoms.

Sitz baths, ice therapy, analgesics, and keeping the lesions clean and dry can help with the discomfort. Females with genital herpes should have Pap smears every 6 months because they are eight times more likely to develop cervical cancer.

PREVENTION. Avoid intimate contact with infected individuals.

GONORRHEA

DESCRIPTION. Gonorrhea, also known as clap, is one of the most common STDs in the United States. It is a highly contagious, STD.

ETIOLOGY. Gonorrhea is caused by the *Neisseria gonorrhoeae* bacterium. The transmission of gonorrhea is often difficult to control because the infected individual, either male or female, might be asymptomatic. In this case, the infected individual is a carrier of the infection and might unknowingly spread the infection.

Infants born to mothers with gonorrhea run the risk of developing gonorrheal eye infection, which can lead to blindness. To prevent infant blindness, it is a common practice, and is state law in some instances, to treat all newborns' eyes with a prophylactic antibiotic or silver nitrate drops at birth.

SYMPTOMS. This bacterial infection causes inflammation of mucous membranes of the genital and urinary systems in both males and females. In males, symptoms include urethritis with purulent discharge from the penis, dysuria, and urinary frequency. Females commonly show signs of cervicitis with purulent vaginal discharge, dysuria, urinary frequency, genital itching, and a burning pain.

DIAGNOSIS. Diagnosis of gonorrhea is made on the basis of a culture of secretions.

TREATMENT. Treatment with antibiotics, including penicillin, tetracycline, and ceftriaxone, is usually effective. Untreated gonorrhea can lead to life-threatening, systemic infections such as meningitis and endocarditis. Arthritis and sterility are also common in both the untreated male and female.

PREVENTION. Avoid intimate contact with infected individuals.

SYPHILIS

DESCRIPTION. Syphilis is a serious STD. If untreated, it has a much worse outcome than gonorrhea because it can become a chronic, life-threatening disease.

ETIOLOGY. Syphilis is caused by the *Treponema pallidum* bacterium. It is spread by sexual or intimate contact with contagious lesions. As soon as exposure occurs, these bacteria rapidly penetrate the skin or mucous membrane and gain access to the vascular system, producing a systemic infection.

SYMPTOMS. Syphilis progresses through three distinct stages with characteristic signs and symptoms. The stages are primary, secondary, and tertiary.

PRIMARY

SYMPTOMS. This stage is marked by the appearance of a painless, highly contagious lesion called a **chancre** (SHANG-ker) (Figure 17–19) that occurs at the site of bacterial entry and usually appears several weeks after contact. It can vary in appearance from pimple-like to an ulcerated sore. In the male, the chancre usually appears on the head of the penis. In the female, the chancre commonly appears on the vulva, although it can be hidden inside the vaginal cavity and, thus, go unnoticed. The chancre can appear also at other sites in both sexes, including on the lips, fingers, anus, and tongue. Even without treatment, the chancre commonly disappears in 10 to 30 days, often leading to the false conclusion that the disease is cured. Lymphadenopathy, or sore swollen lymph nodes, is common.

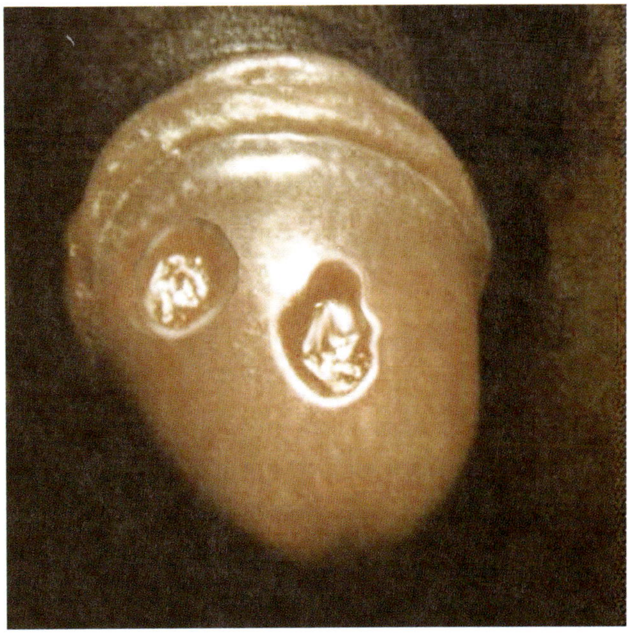

Courtesy of Mark L. Kuss

FIGURE 17–19 Syphilis chancre.

■ ***TREATMENT.*** The disease is highly contagious during this stage but is easily cured with antibiotic therapy.

SECONDARY

■ ***DESCRIPTION.*** After the chancre heals, a period of rest occurs that can last from 6 weeks to 1 year.

■ ***SYMPTOMS.*** During this time, the bacteria rests and then rapidly grows and multiplies, causing the characteristic rash of secondary syphilis. This rash can appear in any area of the body such as on the palms, the soles of the feet, and in the mouth, or it can spread over the entire body. The rash does not itch and might be erroneously diagnosed as mumps, chicken pox, or ringworm. The individual is highly contagious during this stage. If mouth sores are present, kissing can spread the disease.

■ ***TREATMENT.*** During this stage, it can be easily diagnosed based on a blood test and easily treated with antibiotics.

The primary and secondary stages are often combined and called early syphilis.

TERTIARY (LATE OR LATENT)

■ ***DESCRIPTION.*** If secondary syphilis is untreated, the bacterial organisms withdraw into single or multiple sites in the body and become dormant. The length of this dormant time ranges from 1 to 20 years. During this time, the infected individual can be unaware of the infection. Blood testing even might show negative results. The disease at this time is less contagious to others but is dangerous for the infected individual.

■ ***SYMPTOMS.*** Bacteria invade organs throughout the body, producing a characteristic soft gummy lesion called **gumma** (GUM-mah). Symptoms vary, depending on the organs attacked. Common problems include aortic aneurysm, heart failure, mental disorders, insanity, deafness, blindness, paralysis, and death.

■ ***TREATMENT.*** Tertiary syphilis can be cured with antibiotic treatment, but the effects of the lesions are irreversible.

Syphilis in pregnant females can cause spontaneous abortion or death of the infant. Infants that survive commonly have numerous defects, including physical and mental deformities, blindness, and deafness. Pregnant females should be tested for syphilis early because syphilis can be cured with antibiotic treatment during the first five months of pregnancy, thus preventing infection in the unborn child.

■ ***DIAGNOSIS.*** Diagnosis is made on the basis of blood tests, VDRL, and RPR.

■ ***PREVENTION.*** Avoid intimate contact with infected individuals.

CHLAMYDIAL INFECTION

■ ***DESCRIPTION.*** Chlamydial infection is very common in the United States and is one of the most damaging of the STDs. It is often called the silent STD because infected individuals can be asymptomatic until dangerous complications occur. Chlamydial infection is the leading cause of PID and is a major cause of female infertility.

■ ***ETIOLOGY.*** Chlamydial infection is due to the *Chlamydia trachomatis* bacterium.

■ ***SYMPTOMS.*** Males with chlamydial infection are usually symptomatic with drainage from the penis, burning and itching with urination due to urethritis, and epididymitis. Symptomatic females experience vaginal drainage with burning and itching of the genital area. Abdominal pain and dyspareunia can be indicative of PID.

■ ***DIAGNOSIS.*** Diagnosis is made on the basis of cytologic (microscopic examination of cells) examination for the bacteria.

■ ***TREATMENT.*** Treatment with antibiotic therapy is effective. Prognosis is good if treatment occurs prior to the onset of complications. Untreated males can suffer with severe epididymitis, causing sterility.

■ ***PREVENTION.*** Avoid intimate contact with infected individuals.

TRICHOMONIASIS

■ ***DESCRIPTION.*** Trichomoniasis is a fairly common STD, affecting approximately 10% of all sexually active individuals.

■ ***ETIOLOGY.*** Trichomoniasis is caused by a protozoan, *Trichomonas vaginalis.*

■ ***SYMPTOMS.*** Most infected individuals are asymptomatic, resulting in extensive spread of the infection. If symptoms occur in the male, they commonly include urethritis, epididymitis, and prostatitis. Infected females, when symptomatic, have itching and burning of the genital area and a green, frothy vaginal drainage.

■ ***DIAGNOSIS.*** Diagnosis is made on the basis of microscopic examination of vaginal or penile secretions revealing the presence of the causative organism.

■ ***TREATMENT.*** Treatment with an antiparasitic medication is usually very effective.

■ ***PREVENTION.*** Avoid intimate contact with infected individuals.

GENITAL WARTS

■ ***DESCRIPTION.*** Genital warts, or venereal warts, are one of the most common types of STDs. As the names suggests, these warts affect the warm, moist tissues of the genital area.

■ ***ETIOLOGY.*** Genital warts are due to infection with the HPV (Figure 17–20). Mode of transmission is usually through sexual contact, but autoinoculation, or self-inoculation, is also possible. These viral lesions commonly appear 1 to 6 months after exposure to an infected individual.

■ ***SYMPTOMS.*** Warts can be asymptomatic or cause tenderness in the affected area. The amount of discomfort is related to the size, location, and number of warts present. Size of genital warts might be very small, about the size of a ballpoint pen tip, or they might multiply into large clusters as wide as 3 or 4 inches in diameter. They can appear as small, flesh-colored bumps or have a stacked-up, cauliflower-like appearance.

In the male, warts are usually located on the head of the penis but also can be found along the penile shaft and around the anus. In the female, these lesions commonly appear around the vaginal opening and can spread to the perianal area.

Pregnancy tends to cause the warts to grow more rapidly and even reach a point of occluding the vaginal canal, thus making a C-section necessary. Cervical cancer is also more common in females with genital warts.

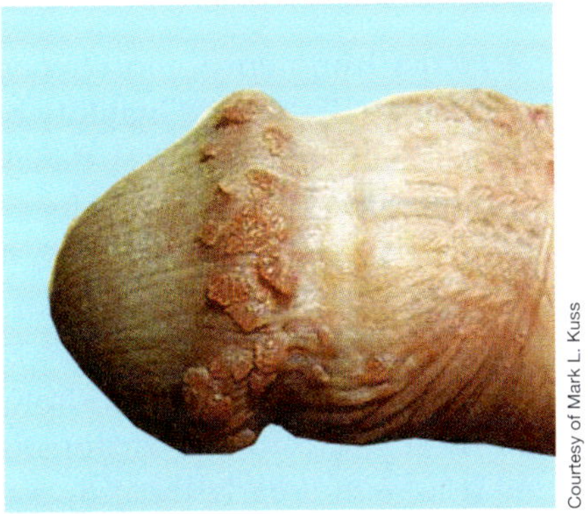

FIGURE 17–20 Genital warts.

■ ***DIAGNOSIS.*** Diagnosis is made on the basis of visualization of the warts and biopsy to rule out carcinoma.

■ ***TREATMENT.*** Treatment is commonly surgical or chemical removal of the infected tissue. Surgical removal does not mean cure because recurrence of genital warts is common.

■ ***PREVENTION.*** Avoid intimate contact with infected individuals.

Sexual Dysfunction

A brief description of the most common sexual dysfunctions is provided in this section. Sexual dysfunction, whether due to physical or psychological conditions, can limit the ability of the individual to reproduce and to develop a close, nurturing sexual relationship with a significant other.

The human sexual cycle progresses through stages of arousal, sexual intercourse, and climax and ends with feelings of pleasure and relaxation. Any disorder that interrupts this cycle can be considered a sexual dysfunction.

Diagnosis of sexual dysfunction depends on general examination including a complete medical history, a sexual history including details of the dysfunction, a physical examination, and laboratory testing as indicated.

Psychological disorders leading to sexual dysfunction might need treatment by psychological counselors. Success in counseling often depends on both partners participating and maintaining a patient and sensitive attitude toward each other.

DYSPAREUNIA

■ ***DESCRIPTION.*** Dyspareunia is a condition of experiencing pain or discomfort with sexual intercourse. It can affect both males and females, although it is more common in women. Dyspareunia is not considered a disease but, rather, a symptom of a psychological or physical disorder.

■ ***ETIOLOGY.*** Dyspareunia for both sexes can be related to physical or psychological conditions. In females, common physical conditions causing dyspareunia include an intact hymen, vaginal deformity, insufficient lubrication, sensitivity to spermicide, presence of an STD, bladder infection, pelvic inflammatory disease, and endometriosis.

In the male, common physical conditions causing dyspareunia include penile deformity, presence of an STD, **phimosis** (figh-MOH-sis), or an abnormally tight foreskin (Figure 17–21), prostatitis, and epididymitis.

Psychological conditions in both sexes that might lead to dyspareunia include a history of past sexual abuse, anxiety, guilt, and fear of pregnancy.

■ ***SYMPTOMS.*** The pain can be mild or severe and appear in the pelvis, genitals, or low back. Females might feel pain specifically in the clitoris, labia, or vagina.

■ ***DIAGNOSIS.*** Diagnosis is made on the basis of general examination including a description of the type of pain and the time of occurrence.

■ ***TREATMENT.*** Treatment depends on cause and can include instructions on extended foreplay, use of lubricating jelly, and manual stretching of the vaginal opening prior to intercourse. Infections need to be treated appropriately. Surgery might be needed to correct deformities, remove tumors, and treat endometriosis. Psychological conditions might need to be addressed with counseling.

■ ***PREVENTION.*** Some dyspareunia, like that caused by sexual trauma or abuse, is not preventable. Activities that reduce risk for the female include avoiding vaginal yeast infections, STDs, bladder infections, and sex on days near menstruation due to increased tenderness.

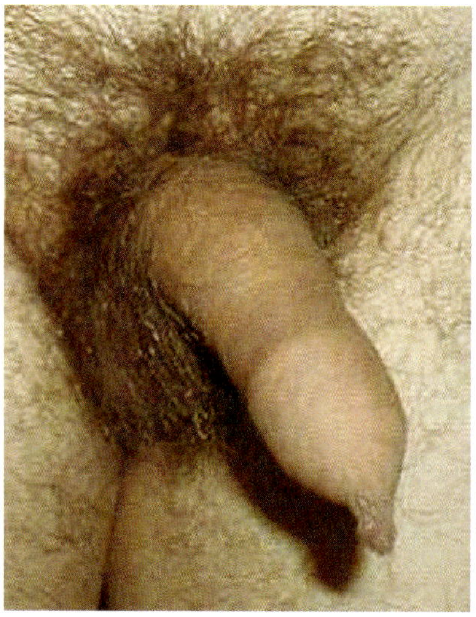
Courtesy of Mark L. Kuss

FIGURE 17–21 Phimosis.

FEMALE AROUSAL–ORGASMIC DYSFUNCTION

■ ***DESCRIPTION.*** Female arousal–orgasmic dysfunction, also called *frigidity*, is the lack of sexual desire or responsiveness in a female.

■ ***ETIOLOGY.*** Frigidity is seldom caused by physical conditions, but neurological disturbances such as those experienced with diabetes mellitus and multiple sclerosis can produce this condition. More commonly, frigidity is due to psychological conditions, including stress, depression, fatigue, past sexual abuse, guilt, and anxiety.

■ ***SYMPTOMS.*** Common signs include the inability to produce and maintain adequate vaginal lubrication and vasocongestive response, indicative of sexual arousal. The primary symptom is an inability to reach orgasm.

■ ***DIAGNOSIS.*** Diagnosis is based on the history or complaint of an inability to reach orgasm.

■ ***TREATMENT.*** A physical examination to rule out physical disorders or disease is the first step in treatment. Psychological disorders might require the couple to visit a qualified specialist in sex therapy to identify and treat the cause.

■ ***PREVENTION.*** Education on healthy sex attitudes and sexual stimulation techniques will minimize problems. Couples who are able to communicate feelings and sexual needs effectively to one another are most likely to prevent this disorder.

IMPOTENCE

■ ***DESCRIPTION.*** Impotence, more recently called erectile dysfunction (ED), is the inability of the male to achieve or maintain an erection sufficient to complete sexual intercourse. Impotence does not affect fertility or the ability to produce offspring. It is a common disorder, affecting approximately half of all men over 40 years of age.

Interestingly, recent research has shown that ED might be the first indicator of cardiovascular disease, making it a helpful early warning for impending heart attacks, stroke, and death. There is a strong relationship between ED and high cholesterol, high blood pressure, and angina. One author suggests that the increase in sales of ED medications is an indicator of the growth of cardiovascular disease in men (Fuhrman, 2008).

■ ***ETIOLOGY.*** ED is primarily caused by vascular insufficiency in the penis. Common causes are physical problems caused by endocrine disorders affecting testosterone levels; drug and alcohol abuse; neurologic disorders; spinal cord injury; urologic disorders; extensive pelvic surgery such as radical prostatectomy; diabetes mellitus; arteriosclerosis, which reduces blood flow; and certain medications such as diuretics, antihypertensives, and vasodilators.

Impotence is also caused by psychological factors, but these are not as common as physical problems. Psychological factors include depression, stress, guilt, sexual anxiety, sexual trauma, and disagreeable relationships.

■ ***SYMPTOMS.*** The only symptom is the inability of the male to achieve or maintain an erection sufficient to complete sexual intercourse.

■ ***DIAGNOSIS.*** Diagnosis is made on the basis of a medical history, sexual history, and physical examination including review of medications and laboratory testing.

■ ***TREATMENT.*** Treatment is based on diagnosis and might be as simple as a change in medications or involved and include psychological counseling and behavior modification. Systemically untreatable physical disorders can be treated with implantation of an inflatable penile implant. Erections also can be achieved artificially by use of external vacuum devices and injections into the penis with vasodilator medications.

■ ***PREVENTION.*** In some cases, ED is not preventable. However, preventive activities are those that control cardiovascular disease and diabetes, including not smoking, eating a healthy diet, maintaining a healthy body weight, and exercising.

PREMATURE EJACULATION

■ ***DESCRIPTION.*** Premature ejaculation, also known as rapid ejaculation or rapid climax, is expulsion of seminal fluid during foreplay, prior to complete erection or immediately after the beginning of sexual intercourse. Some researchers define premature ejaculation with time limits such as within 2 minutes of penetration, whereas others do not use time and simply state that premature ejaculation occurs any time a lack of control interferes with emotional and sexual well-being of both partners. This disorder is the most common sexual problem in males, especially in young males.

■ ***ETIOLOGY.*** The cause of this disorder is usually psychological rather than physical in nature. Common psychological causes include, but are not limited to, guilt, anxiety, and negative feelings or dislike for the sexual partner. Physical causes are rare but can include neurologic disorders, prostatitis, and urethritis.

■ ***SYMPTOMS.*** The only symptom is premature ejaculation.

■ ***DIAGNOSIS.*** Diagnosis is made on the basis of a medical history, sexual history, and a physical examination. Clinicians will consider factors that might lead to premature ejaculation such as duration of excitement, age of client, and frequency of sexual activity. Although the client's complaint of premature ejaculation might not meet all definitions, many clinicians diagnose premature ejaculation based on the client's feeling that the lack of control interfered with emotional and sexual well-being.

■ ***TREATMENT.*** Treatment is based on the diagnosis and can include sex therapy and instruction for both partners in techniques that help delay ejaculation. Control of male stimulation is important during lovemaking to allow the female time to reach orgasm and allow penetration into the vagina before ejaculation occurs. It is important for both partners to understand that this condition is reversible with treatment. In some cases, various medications might help slow arousal and thus delay ejaculation.

■ ***PREVENTION.*** Premature ejaculation can be prevented by masturbating and achieving orgasm several hours prior to intercourse.

INFERTILITY

■ ***DESCRIPTION.*** Infertility is the inability of a couple to achieve pregnancy after 1 year of unprotected sexual intercourse.

■ ***ETIOLOGY.*** Infertility can be due to male or female disorders or a combination of both. It was once thought that female disorders were the primary cause of infertility, but currently, male, female, and combination disorders are fairly equal in occurrence. Approximately 1 in 10 couples experiences difficulty with infertility. Of that group, it is estimated that half will eventually be able to have a child. Common causes of infertility in the female include:

- Presence of STD.
- Hormonal disorders.
- Abnormality of reproductive organs.
- Endometriosis.
- Scarring from PID or blockage of fallopian tubes.
- Development of vaginal antibodies that kill sperm.

Common causes of infertility in the male include:

- Presence of STD.
- Chronic genitourinary infection or blockage of the tract.
- Structural abnormalities.
- Hormone imbalances.

DIAGNOSIS. Diagnostic testing for the female can include a complete medical and gynecologic history and examination. Hormone levels are determined by blood testing. Ovary function and ovulation can be evaluated by recording daily basal body temperatures. The structure of the uterus and patency (openness) of the fallopian tubes can be determined by a hysterosalpingogram. Endometriosis and other pelvic conditions can be assessed by visualization during a laparoscopy.

Diagnostic testing for the male can include a complete medical history and physical examination with semen analysis. Blood testing for endocrine or hormone imbalances can be beneficial. A urinalysis might assist in determination of the presence of infection.

TREATMENT. Treatment is based on cause with the common goal of achieving pregnancy. Treatment can include surgery to correct anatomical abnormalities or remove blockages or medication therapy to correct endocrine or hormone imbalances and treat infection. Fertility drugs, artificial insemination with husband sperm (AIH), artificial insemination with donor semen (AID), and in vitro fertilization (IVF) can be beneficial in complicated cases.

PREVENTION. Many cases of infertility cannot be prevented. The following activities, however, might improve the chance of pregnancy:

- Do not smoke. Smoking reduces sperm count and increases miscarriage.
- Do not drink. Alcohol is toxic to sperm, disrupts hormone balances, and increases risk of miscarriage.
- Eat a healthy diet. Females should increase folic acid intake through dietary selection or supplements.
- Avoid excessive exercise. Excessive exercise can cause low sperm counts in men due to increased heat around the testicles and can lead to menstrual disorders in the female.
- Check with your physician to ensure that any medications, including herbal remedies, are not affecting fertility.
- Avoid STDs. These diseases can damage the reproductive system and cause infertility.
- Maintain proper body weight to reduce the possibility of hormone imbalance

TRAUMA

Rape

Rape is sexual intercourse (vaginal or anal) without consent or against the will of the involved individual. Victims of rape can be any age and of either sex, but

COMPLEMENTARY AND ALTERNATIVE THERAPY

Potential Dangers of Herbal Treatment for Infertility

Although it is probably very rare, cases of lead poisoning have been found in persons who have taken herbal preparations for infertility. In this particular case, the individual reported symptoms of severe abdominal pain, which was eventually diagnosed as lead poisoning. The individual had been taking herbal medicines for treatment of infertility. The herbal products were analyzed and found to contain high levels of lead. The public should be aware that unbranded herbal products should be avoided or taken with extreme caution.

Source: Menezes, et al. (2007).

it is primarily an act violating females. The crime of rape occurs at an alarming rate, but many cases are unreported because the victim often feels embarrassed, ashamed, and guilty. Rape is a crime of violence more than of sexual passion. An acquaintance, date, spouse, or an unknown individual can carry out rape. Recent publicity has been devoted to date-rape drugs or medication that is placed in a drink and renders the individual unconscious to the point of becoming an easy victim.

Signs and symptoms of rape can include, but are not limited to, torn clothing, disheveled appearance, bruises, and lacerations around the mouth, breasts, genitals, and rectum. Semen might be found on the inner thighs, in the vaginal cavity, and around the genital and rectal area if the victim has not bathed, showered, or douched after the act.

Diagnosis is made on the basis of history and physical examination. Special attention should be given to the emotional condition of the victim. Emergency guidelines are aimed at protecting the victim against disease and pregnancy and collecting legal evidence if the victim decides to press charges against the perpetrator. Gathering of criminal evidence is best if the individual has not bathed, showered, or douched, although, often, because the victim feels dirty and violated, these cleansing activities are performed immediately and prior to reporting the crime.

Sex crime evidence gathering can involve collecting samples of clothing, hair, scrapings from under fingernails, pubic hair, semen samples, and taking pictures of areas of trauma. Sexual assault nurse examiners (SANEs) are often called in to collect the evidence and counsel the victim. These nurses have been educated and certified in the forensic specialty of sexual assault.

Recovery from rape is difficult. Crisis intervention counselors are needed, and follow-up is very important. Individuals involved with the victim need to be nonjudgmental, affirm that the individual is a victim, and assure the individual that this act of violence was not deserved.

RARE DISEASES

Vaginal Cancer

Vaginal cancer is a rare form of cancer that occurs in the daughters of mothers who used the synthetic hormone diethylstilbestrol (DES) to prevent spontaneous abortion. Symptoms include leukorrhea and bloody vaginal drainage. Diagnosis is made on the basis of a Pap smear and biopsy. Treatment usually consists of surgery, chemotherapy, and radiation.

Puerperal Sepsis

Puerperal (pyou-ER-pier-al; after childbirth) sepsis is an infection of the endometrium, usually with streptococcus bacteria, following childbirth. Other names for puerperal sepsis include puerperal fever and childbed fever. In the 1800s, the cause and spread of this infection was unknown, and it was common for puerperal sepsis to sweep through maternity wards and kill most of the new mothers.

Symptoms of puerperal sepsis include chills, fever, and abdominal and pelvic pain. The modern use of aseptic technique has made this infection uncommon in most of the world except for special instances when asepsis is not properly carried out. Without prompt and effective antibiotic treatment, this condition is often fatal.

Hydatidiform Mole

Hydatidiform mole is the formation of grape-like cysts in the uterus that fill the uterus and give indications of pregnancy. There is no fetus, although HCG levels get abnormally high. The cause of hydatidiform mole may be a genetic abnormality.

Toward the end of the third month, the affected individual might have symptoms of bright red vaginal bleeding, nausea, and vomiting. Diagnosis is made on the basis of symptoms and no fetal heart tones. Treatment is a surgical D&C to remove the abnormal tissue. Because individuals affected with hydatidiform mole are at higher risk for a certain type of carcinoma (choriocarcinoma), the individual should have frequent follow-up examinations.

EFFECTS OF AGING ON THE SYSTEM

As the female ages, changes in the reproductive system might seem more distinct than in the male. The pubic hair becomes thin and gray, and the external structures become less elastic and appear more wrinkled and sagging. The internal organs shrink in size, vaginal secretions diminish, and there is less elasticity of the vagina. Although sexual stimulation is still important, as in the male, it can take increased stimulation and the aid of a vaginal lubricant to enhance sexual intercourse. Using vaginal hormone cream might be recommended to reduce the dryness and improve the mucosal tone of the vagina. Some cancers of the female reproductive system such as cancer of the uterus and ovaries are more common in the older adult. Women over age 65 should be screened regularly for these disorders.

As the female enters menopause, the breasts also begin to atrophy and become more relaxed with a reduction in size. Women over age 50 are at increased risk for breast cancer. They should have yearly clinical exams as well as a mammogram.

As the male ages, production of testosterone and the formation of sperm decreases. The size of the testes also can diminish, but the functional ability of the male for sexual intercourse and reproduction continues. There is some loss of elasticity of the penis and scrotum, causing them to appear more wrinkled and sagging, and some thinning and graying of the pubic hair. Although the male is still able to have an erection, sometimes it takes greater stimulation to achieve this. The ejaculation amount also might be diminished. The prostate slowly enlarges in most men, beginning around age 50. This prostatic hypertrophy can cause problems with urination. The prostate is also a common site for cancer development in the older male. Routine rectal examination of the prostate and laboratory levels of PSA should be completed by all adult males over age 50.

SUMMARY

The reproductive system is a highly complex, multifunction system. It has important physiologic functions but is also very important in social relationships between individuals. Both procreation and the relationship and intercourse aspects of the system can be altered when disorders develop in the system. Common disorders of the system in the female include infections, inflammation, infertility, fibrocystic disease, pregnancy abnormalities, STDs, and cancer. In the male, common disorders include infections, STDs, impotence, and cancer. Signs and symptoms of reproductive disorders in both sexes can include pain, discharge, lesions, and abnormal enlargement of tissue. Changes occurring in the system in the older adult often affect the individual's ability to perform sexual intercourse satisfactorily. Other changes include decrease in hormone secretion, loss of elasticity of tissues, diminished lubricating secretions, and increased risk for cancer development.

REVIEW QUESTIONS

Short Answer

1. What are some of the common reproductive system disorders in the:

a. Female?

b. Male?

2. What are the common signs and symptoms of reproductive system disorders in the:

a. Female?

b. Male?

True or False

3. T F Endometriosis is an ectopic occurrence of endometrial tissue.

4. T F A hernia of the bladder into the vagina is called a urethrocele.

5. T F Vaginal infections are very uncommon.

6. T F TSS is characterized by high fever.
7. T F Intermittent painless bleeding is the most common symptom of cervical cancer.
8. T F Leiomyoma is a metastatic tumor of the uterus.
9. T F A Pap smear should be performed every 2 years on a female who is not high risk.
10. T F PMS is probably caused by a hormone imbalance.
11. T F Phimosis is a narrowed opening of the prepuce.
12. T F Epididymitis is usually caused by an infection from the bladder.
13. T F STDs are not common in the male reproductive system.
14. T F The best preventive measure for testicular cancer is the monthly self-examination.
15. T F One of the symptoms of BPH is urinary retention.
16. T F An orchiectomy is the removal of the prostate gland.
17. T F Cancer of the prostate can be detected early by the PSA test.
18. T F The testosterone hormone is secreted by the prostate gland.
19. T F There is some loss of elasticity of the penis and scrotum during the aging process.
20. T F It might take increased stimulation and the aid of a vaginal lubricant to enhance sexual intercourse between the older adult male and female.

CASE STUDIES

■ Charles Roberts is a 63-year-old man who has been having difficulty urinating. He states he tends to get up at least twice a night to void and has some difficulty getting the stream started. Is this a problem? He is basically quite healthy and does not have a family physician. He asks for your advice about this. What should you tell Mr. Roberts? Are there other questions you should ask him before giving him any information? How could you explain the effects of aging to him? Should he make an appointment with a physician?

■ Janice Simmonds is a 53-year-old first-grade school teacher. At the present time, she is single but dates on a fairly regular basis. She has been an active person all of her life. Janice has played on a tennis team for 20 years and works out at the local athletic club. She considers herself to be in great shape for her age and has never been concerned about any possible health problems. Her past laboratory history includes an average routine cholesterol level, normal blood sugar, and normal blood pressure. Her mother is still living and well, but her aunt died at age 69 of breast cancer. Her father is also living and well. Janice does not consider herself at risk for any major health problems. Do you agree with her? Would you consider her at risk for breast cancer? If so, what risk factors can you identify? Is she also at risk for cervical cancer? What routine clinical examinations should she have based on her age and gender?

StudyWARE™ Connection

To help you learn the content in this chapter, take a practice quiz or play an interactive game on your StudyWARE™ CD-ROM.

Workbook Practice

Go to your Workbook and complete the practice questions.

BIBLIOGRAPHY

American Cancer Society. (2008a). Cancer statistics 2006. *www.cancer.org* (accessed March 2008).

American Cancer Society. (2008b). Detailed guide: Breast cancer. *www.cancer.org* (accessed March 2008).

American Cancer Society. (2008c). Detailed guide: Testicular cancer. *www.cancer.org* (accessed March 2008).

Anderson, M., McKee, D., Yukes, J., Alvarez, A., & Karasz, A. (2008). An investigation of douching practices in the botanicas of the Bronx. *Culture, Health & Sexuality 10*(1), 1–11.

Aschenbrenner, S. (2008). A new indication for raloxifene. *American Journal of Nursing 108i*(1), 38.

Billups, K. L., Edina, M. N., Kaiser. D., et al. (2003). Erectile dysfunction as an early indicator of systemic oxidative stress and endothelial dysfunction. *Journal of Urology 169*:323.

Bohnenkamp, S., LeBaron, V., & Yoder, L. (2007a). The medical-surgical nurse's guide to ovarian cancer: Part I. *MEDSURG Nursing 16*(4), 259–266.

Bohnenkamp, S., LeBaron, V., & Yoder, L. (2007b). The medical-surgical nurse's guide to ovarian cancer: Part II. *MEDSURG Nursing 16*(5), 323–331.

Bukovsky, A., & Caudle, M. (2008). Immune physiology of the mammalian ovary: A review. *American Journal of Reproductive Immunology 59*(1), 12–26.

Canderelli, R., Leccesse, L., Miller, N., & Unruh-Davidson, J. (2007). Benefits of hormone replacement therapy in postmenopausal women. *Journal of the American Academy of Nurse Practitioners 19*(12), 635–641

Centers for Disease Control and Prevention. (2002). *Tracking the hidden epidemics.* Atlanta, GA: Centers for Disease Control and Prevention.

Centers for Disease Control and Prevention. (2007). United States cancer statistics. *www.cdc.gov/uscs/* (accessed June 2008).

Chemotherapy in epithelial ovarian cancer. *Clinical Journal of Oncology Nursing 11*(2), 211–216.

Dirksen, S., & Epstein, D. (2008). Efficacy of an insomnia intervention on fatigue, mood and quality of life in breast cancer. *Journal of Advanced Nursing 61*(6), 664–675.

Dobie, M. (2007). Cancer drugs right on target. *Nursing Standard 21*(18), 29.

Elghblawi, E. (2007). Polycystic ovary syndrome and female reproduction. *British Journal of Nursing 16*(18), 1118–1121.

Erectile dysfunction and inflammation linked to diabetes. (2006). *Nursing Standard 20*(50), 16–17.

Esteva, F., & Hortobagyi, G. (2008). Gaining ground on breast cancer. *Scientific American 298*(6), 58–65.

Feldman, D., Bosl, G., Sheinfels, J., & Motzer, R. (2008). Medical treatment of advanced testicular cancer. *JAMA 299*(6), 672–684.

Fleming, R. M. (2000). The effect of high-protein diets on coronary blood flow. *Angiology 51*(10), 817–826.

Fuhrman, J. (2008). Health disease and impotence. Spotlight on men's health. *www.drfuhrman.com* (accessed June 2008.)

Hsieh, C. C., & Trichopoulos, D. (1991). Breast size, handedness and breast cancer risk. *European Journal of Cancer 27*:131–135.

Husmann, D. (2003). Cryptorchidism and its relationship to testicular neoplasm and nicrolithiasis. *Urology 66*(2), 424.

Hydzik, C. (2007). Implementation of intraperitoneal chemotherapy for the treatment of ovarian cancer. *Clinical Journal of Oncology Nursing 11*(2), 221–225.

Imaginis. Breast cancer statistics on incidence, survival, and screening. (2008). Imaginis. *www.imaginis.com* (accessed June 2008).

Lajiness, M. (2007). Megestrol acetate for the treatment of hot flashes in men undergoing hormone ablation therapy or orchiectomy. *Urologic Nursing 27*(6), 556–557.

Locklear, T., Doyle, B., Perez Sanchez, A., Laurito-Gomez, J., Brenes, J., Yue, H., & Mahady, G. (2007). Alternative therapies from Costa Rica for the management of PMS and dysmenorrheal: Justica pectoralis Jacq.: Mechanisms of action. *FASEB Journal 21*(5), A436.

Marin, K., Oleszewski, K., & Muehlbauer, P. (2007). Intraperitoneal chemotherapy: Implications beyond ovarian cancer. *Clinical Journal of Oncology Nursing 11*(6), 881–889.

Martin, V. (2007). Ovarian cancer: An overview of treatment options. *Clinical Journal of Oncology Nursing 11*(2), 201–207.

Menezes, G., D'Souza, H., & Venkatesh, T. (2007). Lead poisoning as a result of infertility treatment using herbal remedies. *Archives of Gynecology & Obstetrics 275*(4), 279–281.

National Cancer Institute Fact Sheet. (2008). Digital vs. film mammography in the digital mammographic imaging screening trial (DMIST): Questions and answers. *www.nci.nih.gov* (accessed March 2008).

Newton, K., Reed, S., LaCroix, A., Grothaus, L., Ehrlich, K., & Guiltinan, J. (2006). Treatment of vasomotor symptoms of menopause with black cohosh, multibotanicals, soy, hormone therapy or placebo. *Annals of Internal Medicine 145*(12), 869–W244.

Orgasmic dysfunction. (2008). National Institutues of Health. *www.nim.nih.gov* (accessed June 2008).

Parvez, S., Tabassum, H., Banerjee, B., & Raisuddin, S. (2008). Taurine prevents tamoxifen-induced mitochondrial oxidative damage in mice. *Basic & Clinical Pharmacology & Toxicology. 102*(4), 382–387.

Perez-Lopez, F. (2007). Vitamin D: The secosteroid hormone and human reproduction. *Gynecological Endocrinology 23*(1), 13–24.

Reb, A. (2007). Transforming the death sentence: Elements of hope in women with advanced ovarian cancer. *Oncology Nursing Forum 34*(6), E70–E81.

Reed, R. L. (2008). Prevention and treatment of fibrocystic breast disease. Natural Health and Longevity Resource Center. *www.all-natural.com* (accessed June 2008).

Ridner, S., & Dietrich, M. (2008). Self-reported comorbid conditions and medication usage in breast cancer survivors with and without lymphedema. *Oncology Nursing Forum 35*(1), 57–63.

Sadeghinejad, H., & Watson, R. (2008) Premature ejaculation: Current medical treatment and new directions. *Journal of Sexual Medicine 5*:1037–1050.

Safarinejad, M. R., & Hosseine, S. Y. (2006) Pharmacotherapy for premature ejaculation. *Current Drug Therapy 1*:37–46.

Saul, S. (January 18, 2008). Despite doubts, cancer therapy draws patients. *New York Times 157*(54193), A1–A11.

Shaw, J. (2008). Diagnosis and treatment of testicular cancer. *American Family Physician 77*(4), 469–474.

Singer, S. R., & Grismaijer, S. (1995). *Dressed to kill: The link between breast cancer and bras*. Boulder, CO: Avery Press.

Solomon, H., Han, J. W., & Jackson, G. (2003). Erectile dysfunction and the cardiovascular patient: Endothelial dysfunction is the most common denominator. *Heart 89*:251–254.

Stiffler, D., Haase, J., Hosei, B., & Barada, B. (2008). Parenting experiences with adolescent daughters when mothers have breast cancer. *Oncology Nursing Forum 35*(1), 113–120.

Tatum, T. (2007). One practitioner's experience with counseling and testing women at risk for hereditary breast and ovarian cancer syndrome. *Oncology Nursing Forum 34*(2), 496–497.

Torpy, J. (2008). Testicular cancer. *JAMA 299*(6), 718.

Ufema, J. (2008). What's left is real. *Nursing 38*(1), 23.

Wurn, B., Wurn, L., King, C., Heuer, M., Roscow, A., Hornberger, K., & Scharf, E. (2008). Treating fallopian tube occlusion with a manual pelvic physical therapy. *Alternative Therapies in Health & Medicine 14*(12), 18–23.

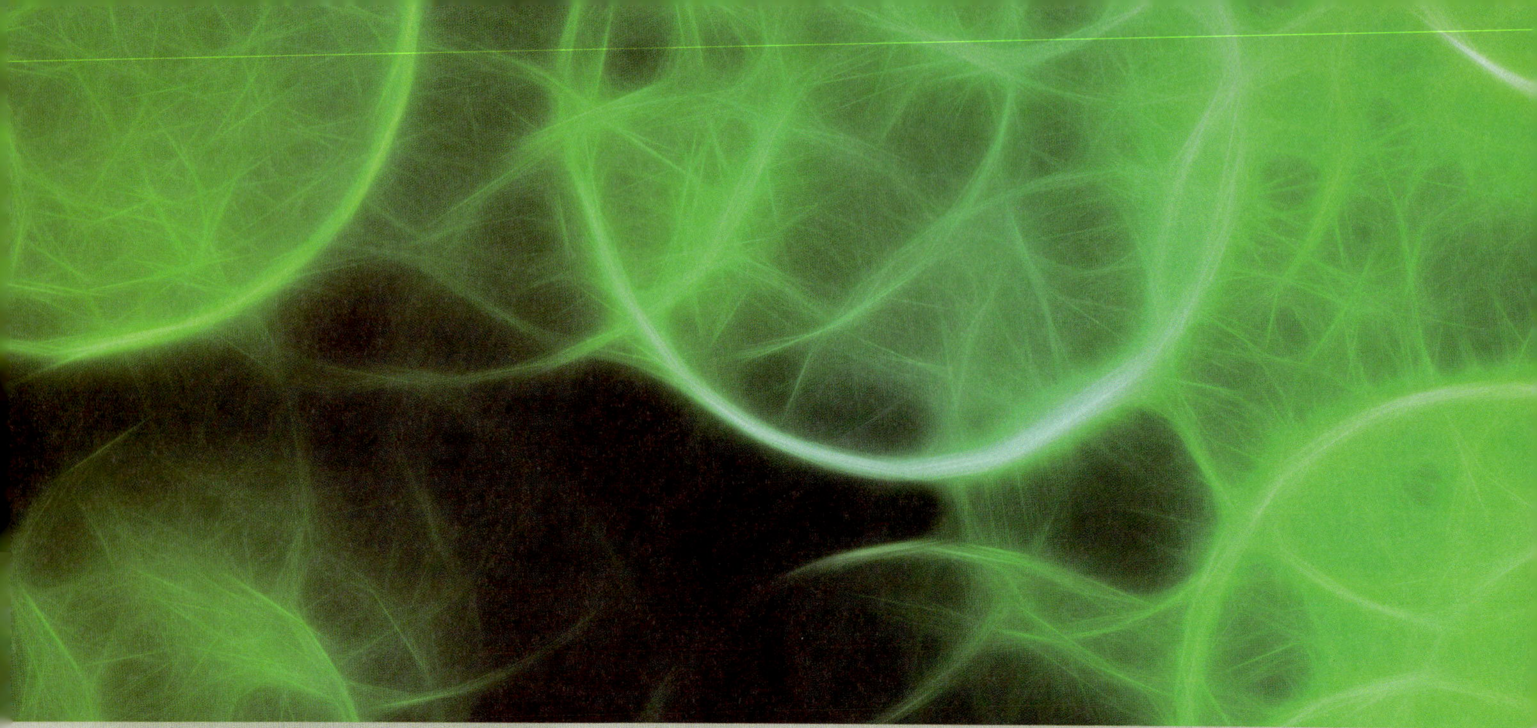

OUTLINE

- Anatomy and Physiology
- Common Signs and Symptoms
- Diagnostic Tests
- Common Diseases of the Integumentary System
  - *Infectious Diseases*
  - *Metabolic Diseases*
  - *Hypersensitivity or Immune Diseases*
  - *Idiopathic Diseases*
  - *Benign Tumors*
  - *Premalignant and Malignant Tumors*
  - *Abnormal Pigmented Lesions*
  - *Diseases of the Nails*
  - *Diseases of the Hair*
- Trauma
  - *Mechanical Skin Injury*
  - *Thermal Skin Injury*
  - *Electrical Injury*
  - *Radiation Injury*
  - *Pressure Injury*
  - *Insect and Spider Bites and Stings*
- Rare Diseases
  - *Elephantiasis*
- Effects of Aging on the System
- Summary
- Review Questions
- Case Studies
- Bibliography

KEY TERMS

Abrasion (p. 418)
Alopecia (p. 417)
Avulsion (p. 419)
Blunt trauma (p. 418)
Comedones (p. 407)
Contusion (p. 418)
Erythema (p. 397)
Exacerbation (p. 397)
Frostbite (p. 420)
Hirsutism (p. 417)
Incision (p. 419)
Keratin (p. 397)
Laceration (p. 419)
Lesion (p. 397)
Paronychia (p. 416)
Pilonidal cyst (p. 409)
Pruritus (p. 397)
Pustules (p. 401)
Sebum (p. 396)
Ulcer (p. 402)
Vesicles (p. 399)
Wheals (p. 410)
Xerosis (p. 425)

18

Integumentary System Diseases and Disorders

LEARNING OBJECTIVES

Upon completion of the chapter, the learner should be able to:

1. Define the terminology common to the integumentary system and the disorders of the system.
2. Discuss the basic anatomy and physiology of the integumentary system.
3. Identify the important signs and symptoms associated with common integumentary system disorders.
4. Describe the common diagnostics used to determine the type and cause of integumentary system disorders.
5. Identify common disorders of the integumentary system.
6. Describe the typical course and management of the common integumentary system disorders.
7. Describe the effects of aging on the integumentary system and the common disorders associated with aging of the system.

OVERVIEW

The integumentary system is composed of all the skin and its layers. The skin is also known as the largest organ of the body. It makes up about 15% of the total body weight. The skin is the first line of defense against disease. Many diseases of the integumentary system are the result of other body or system disorders. For instance, measles is a viral disease of the respiratory system, but it is characterized by the maculopapular rash seen on the skin. Skin disorders such as psoriasis are traumatic to the individual because of the obvious lesions and the effect it has on body image. Skin disorders range from mild to severe and acute to chronic. ■

ANATOMY AND PHYSIOLOGY

The skin is the largest organ of the body. It is a large, durable, and pliable organ and is the first line of protection for the body against invading organisms. The skin also provides a sense of touch, heat and cold, and pain and helps stabilize temperature and fluid and electrolyte balance. The skin is composed of two layers: the epidermis and the dermis, with a subcutaneous (hypodermis) level (Figure 18–1).

The epidermis, or outer layer, is composed of five layers: the stratum corneum, stratum lucidum, stratum granulosum, stratum spinosum, and stratum basale. The cells of the epidermis are called stratified squamous epithelial cells. Most of these are keratinocytes; the others are melanocytes that produce melanin, the pigment that darkens the skin and gives it color. The dermis is the deeper layer, consisting of connective tissue and a variety of cell types. Blood vessels traverse the dermal layer to provide nutrients and oxygen, regulate heat, and remove waste products. Nerves also form a network in the dermis to provide the sensations of heat, cold, pain, and touch.

The subcutaneous layer is composed of connective tissue containing fat cells and blood vessels and protects the body against cold. The amount of fat varies considerably with the individual.

Embedded in the dermis and extending to the epidermis are the sebaceous, apocrine, and eccrine sweat glands. The sebaceous glands produce oil called **sebum**. The apocrine sweat glands are located in the underarms (axillae), around the nipples of the breasts, and around the umbilicus, anus, and genital areas. These glands are inactive until puberty and initiate their function with hormonal changes at that time. Their secretions are odorless, but bacteria that accumulate in these areas cause the smell referred to as body odor. Both the sebaceous glands and the apocrine glands secrete through the hair follicles. The eccrine sweat glands are found throughout the body surfaces and secrete through the skin pores to help the body regulate heat. Some electrolytes are also lost through these sweat glands.

The hair follicles are found in the dermal layer and extend through the epidermis. They grow in cycles, which vary with the individual, with an average growth of about 1 cm per month. Hair loss occurs continually but is not usually obvious until a large amount is lost and not replaced. Testosterone, the male hormone, influences hair growth, especially

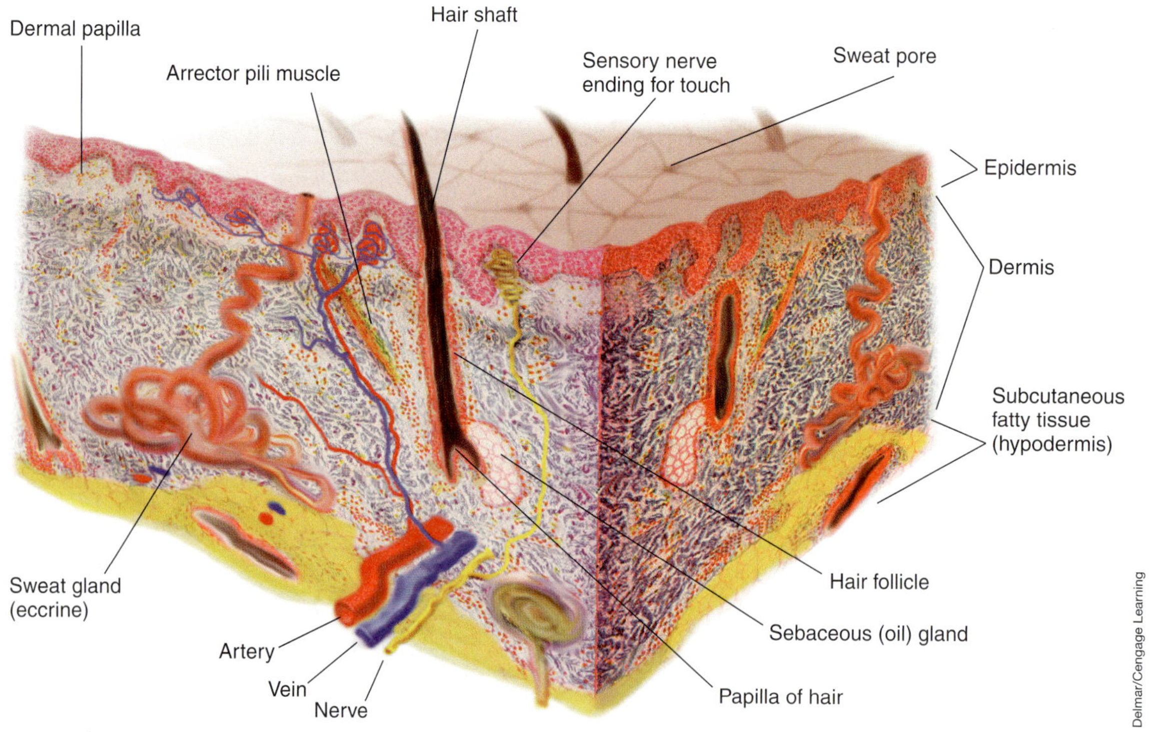

FIGURE 18–1 The structures of the skin.

at puberty when hair begins to appear in the axillae and groin. It also triggers the male's baldness later in life. Generally, soft, tiny hairs cover most of the body, and terminal hairs (stiffer, longer, and often darker) are found on the scalp, axillae, groin, eyebrows, and eyelashes of both sexes and the face and trunk of males.

The nails are composed of **keratin** (epidermal cells in a tight web). Fingernails grow more rapidly than toenails, but they are composed of the same material. The thickness and growth rate of the nail varies with the individual. Health status, nutrition, and other factors can influence nail strength and growth.

> *Study***WARE**™ Connection
>
> View an animation about skin on your StudyWARE™ CD-ROM.

COMMON SIGNS AND SYMPTOMS

Common signs and symptoms of integumentary diseases include the following:

- Skin **lesion** (LEE-zhun). A lesion is a very broad term meaning any discontinuity or abnormality of tissue. Lesions can be hard, soft, flat, raised, large, small, reddened, crusted, fluid-filled, or pus-filled, to name only a few characteristics (Figure 18–2).
- Pain.
- **Pruritus** (proo-RYE-tus) or itching.
- Edema (swelling).
- **Erythema** (ER-oh-THEE-mah) or skin redness.
- Inflammation.

DIAGNOSTIC TESTS

There are numerous skin diseases; several have very characteristic lesions, leading to an easy diagnosis. However, many exhibit the same or similar types of lesions and symptoms, making diagnosis difficult. Biopsy might be used in diagnosing nodules and chronic lesions. Culture and sensitivity are effective in determining the presence of bacterial infections. Blood tests are helpful, especially if there is concern about a systemic infection or metabolic disorder. Diagnosis and identification of fungal and parasitic infections can be determined by using cultures and microscopic smear examinations.

COMMON DISEASES OF THE INTEGUMENTARY SYSTEM

The numerous diseases and disorders of the integumentary system often make diagnosis of skin disorders quite difficult because several diseases can be characterized by the same type or similar types of lesions. Common diseases include infections; metabolic, hypersensitivity, and idiopathic disorders; and tumors and can be categorized according to cause.

Infectious Diseases

Skin infections are quite common and usually contagious, so care must be taken to prevent spread from one area of the body to another and from one person to another. Most infections are not serious unless systemic involvement occurs. Infections of the skin can be caused by viruses, bacteria, fungi, and parasites.

VIRAL DISEASES

Viral skin diseases can be acute or chronic. Acute viral diseases commonly affect children and usually resolve spontaneously, but many viral infections become lifelong with periods of remission and **exacerbation** (flaring up).

HERPES

DESCRIPTION. Herpes is a large family of viruses, including:

1. Cold sores and fever blisters (Herpes simplex 1 or HSV-1).
2. Genital herpes (Herpes simplex 2, HSV-2, or herpes genitalis).
3. Chicken pox (herpes varicella).
4. Shingles (herpes zoster).

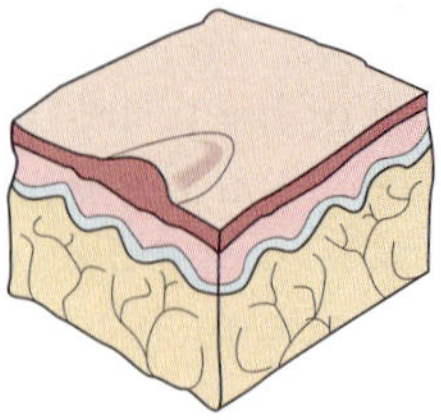

A **papule** is a small solid raised lesion that is less than 0.5 cm in diameter.

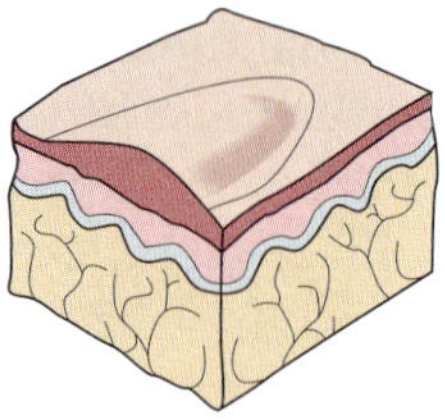

A **plaque** is a solid raised lesion that is greater than 0.5 cm in diameter.

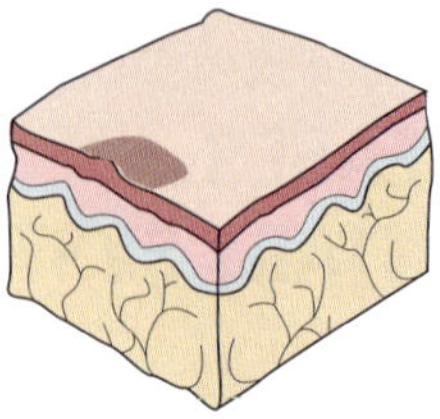

A **macule** is a flat discolored lesion that is less than 1 cm in diameter.

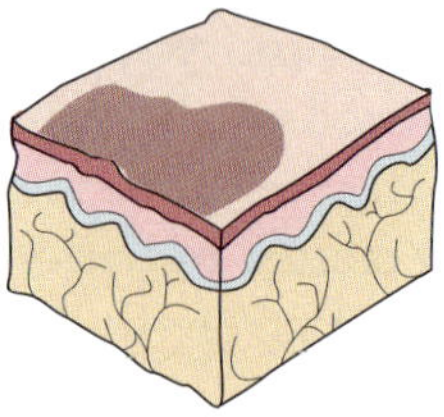

A **patch** is a flat discolored lesion that is greater than 1 cm in diameter.

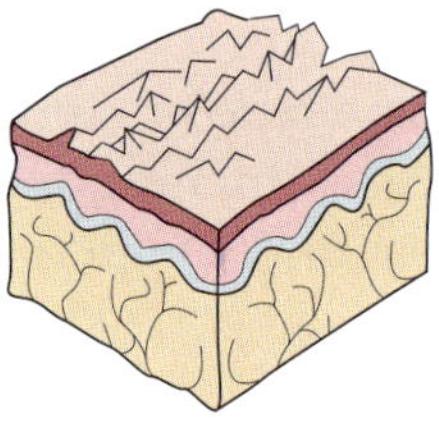

A **scale** is a flaking or dry patch made up of excess dead epidermal cells.

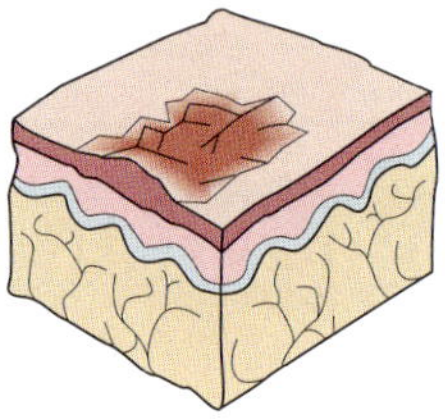

A **crust** is a collection of dried serum and cellular debris.

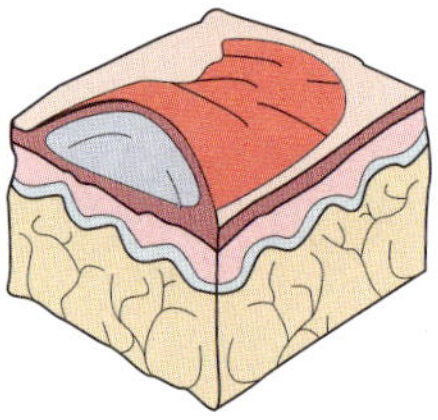

A **wheal** is a smooth, slightly elevated swollen area that is redder or paler than the surrounding skin. It is usually accompanied by itching.

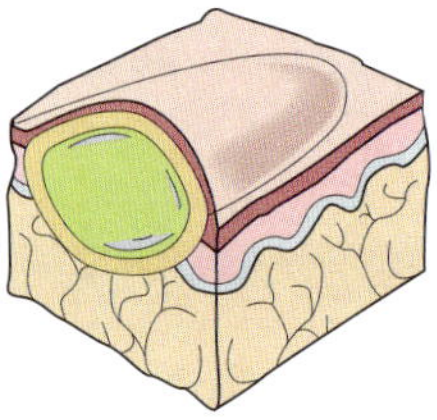

A **cyst** is a closed sack or pouch containing fluid or semisolid material.

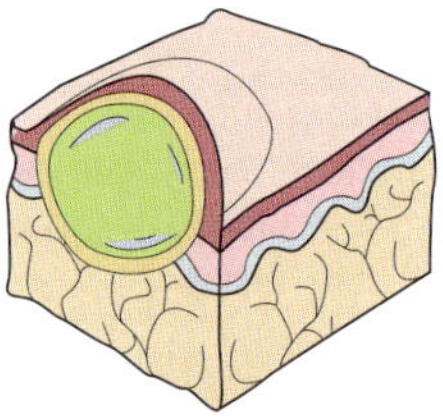

A **pustule** is a small circumscribed elevation of the skin containing pus.

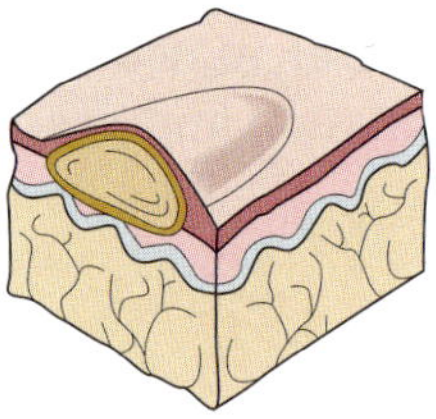

A **vesicle** is a circumscribed elevation of skin containing fluid that is less than 0.5 cm in diameter.

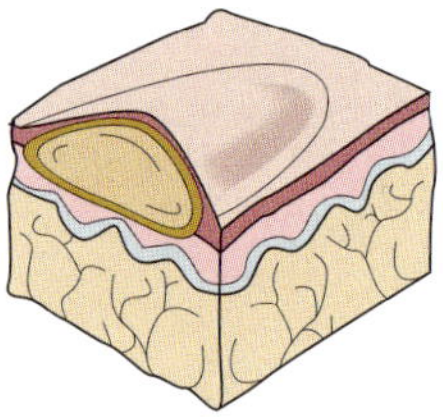

A **bulla** is a large vesicle that is more than 0.5 cm in diameter.

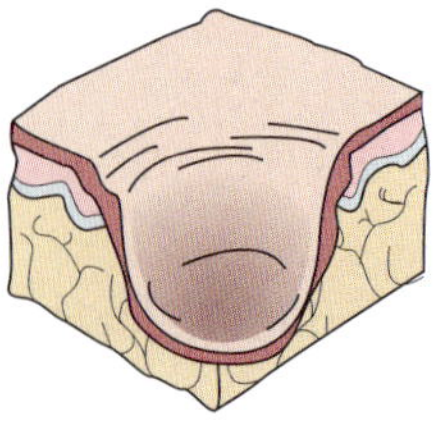

An **ulcer** is an open sore or erosion of the skin or mucous membrane resulting in tissue loss.

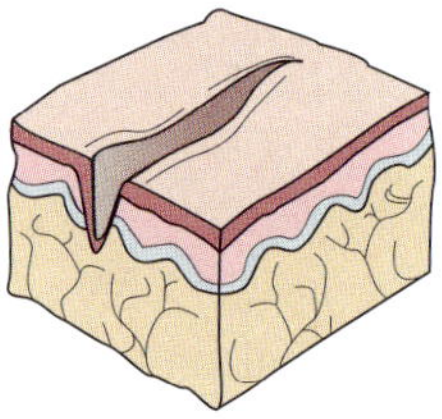

A **fissure** of the skin is a groove or crack-like sore.

FIGURE 18–2 Skin lesions.

5. Other, rarer, herpes are ocular herpes, herpes simplex encephalitis, and neonatal herpes simplex. These cases can lead to blindness and high levels of morbidity and mortality, respectively.

Herpes simplex is very common and often appears on the mouth, nose, buttocks, and genitals. The herpes simplex viruses (HSV-1 and HSV-2) appear identical under a microscope, cause the same type of lesions, and, clinically, cannot be separated. Both can infect the mouth or genitals. Usually, HSV-1 appears above the waist and HSV-2 appears below the waist.

- **Herpes simplex type 1** Commonly called fever blisters and cold sores because febrile conditions and the common cold often bring about an exacerbation. The vesicles commonly appear around the lips and nose (Figure 18–3). Lesions appearing around the lips can be further identified as herpes labialis (labia = lip), and those occurring in conjunction with a fever can be further identified as herpes febrilis.
- **Herpes genitalis (herpes simplex type 2)** Commonly called genital herpes. This is a highly contagious disease and is spread by direct contact. Genital herpes can be a sexually transmitted disease, but transmission is not limited to sexual contact. Autoinoculation with the hands is also possible by touching the lips and then the genitals and vice versa. Herpes genitalis is discussed in detail in Chapter 17, "Reproductive System Diseases and Disorders."
- **Herpes varicella** Commonly called chicken pox. This is an acute, highly contagious childhood disease. Varicella is discussed in detail in Chapter 20, "Childhood Diseases and Disorders."
- **Herpes zoster** Commonly called shingles. The virus that causes chicken pox in children causes zoster in adults. It is characterized by painful lesions that follow the course of a spinal nerve. Zostavax is the vaccine for shingles, but it is recommended for only adults over age 60. More detailed information can be found in Chapter 15, "Nervous System Diseases and Disorders."

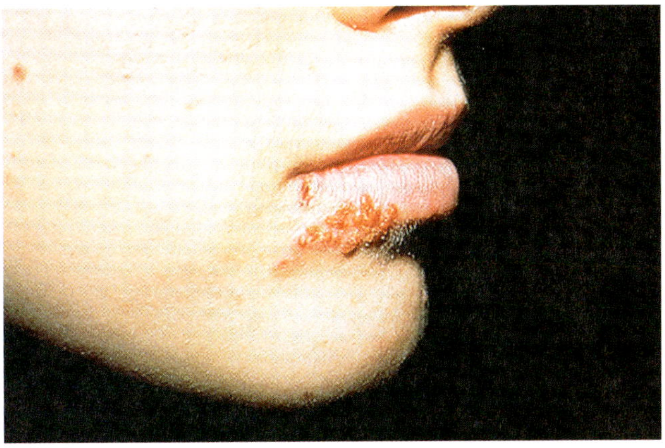

Courtesy of Robert A. Silverman, MD, Pediatric Dermatology, Georgetown University

FIGURE 18–3 Herpes simplex virus 1.

SYMPTOMS. Herpes is characterized by inflammation of the skin and clusters of fluid-filled **vesicles** (VES-ih-kul). The infection is painful, embarrassing, and often recurrent.

DIAGNOSIS. Diagnosis is made by observation of vesicles, positive viral culture, and blood testing for herpes antibodies.

TREATMENT. The virus is treatable but remains in the affected individual's body for life. Some type of balance between the host and the virus exists, with periods of viral remission and exacerbation. The virus exacerbates, or flares up, often during times of decreased immunity as occurs with stress. Valacyclovir, acyclovir, and famciclovir are approved to treat herpes genitalis but are also used for oral herpes. Penciclovir cream can also be prescribed for oral herpes.

PREVENTION. Prevention of simplex viruses includes avoiding skin-to-skin contact with anyone showing signs of infection. Use of a condom helps prevent herpes genitalis. Vaccination in children and those over 60 helps prevent varicella and zoster, respectively. In general, maintaining a healthy immune system by making healthy lifestyle choices helps reduce risk.

VERRUCAE (WARTS)

DESCRIPTION. Verrucae, or warts, a chronic skin condition, usually occur in multiples that can differ in size, shape, and appearance. They can appear at any age but more commonly affect children. The most common types are:

- **Common warts** Predominantly appear on the hands and fingers of children (Figure 18–4). These lesions are contagious and are spread by scratching and direct contact. Although unsightly, they are usually painless and harmless and often

COMPLEMENTARY AND ALTERNATIVE THERAPY

Amino Acid Treatment for Herpes

There has been some information distributed through the Internet and supplemental health literature about the benefit of taking lysine, an essential amino acid, for genital herpes. Although some reports state there is evidence that taking lysine supplements can reduce the number of outbreaks the individual suffers from, most of the research does not support this treatment as being effective. In fact, taking large doses of lysine may even cause other metabolic problems to develop in the individual. Individuals taking lysine for herpes treatment should report this to their physicians and be watching for potential adverse side effects.

Source: American Social Health Association (2008).

disappear spontaneously. Common warts occurring in adults should be called to the attention of a physician to ensure that they are not skin cancers.

- **Plantar warts** Appear on the sole of the foot. This wart usually grows inward, is smooth on the sole of the foot, and feels like a hard lump. Plantar warts contain small, clotted blood vessels that appear like dark splinters inside the wart and give it a cauliflower-like appearance (Figure 18–5). This wart commonly causes pain with walking; thus, surgical removal is often the treatment of choice.
- **Genital warts** A sexually transmitted disease. They are highly contagious and often need to be removed surgically. More detailed information can be found in Chapter 17.

■ ***ETIOLOGY.*** A verruca is caused by the papillomavirus affecting the keratin cells of the skin, causing cellular hypertrophy.

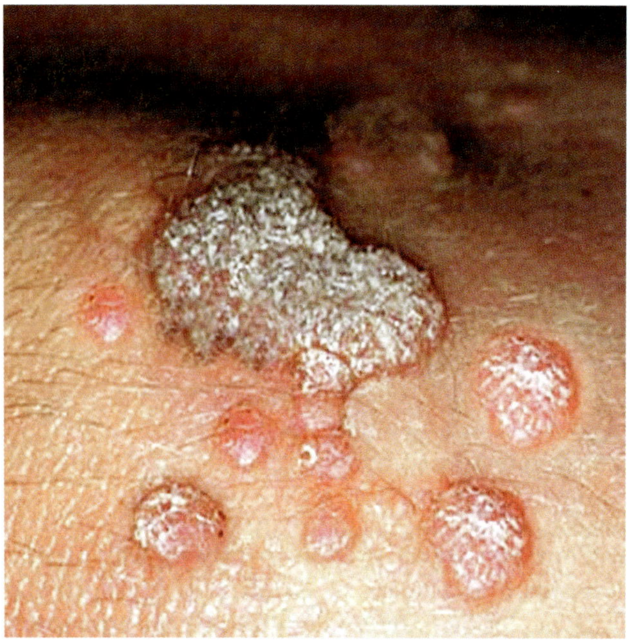

FIGURE 18–4 Verrucae (warts).

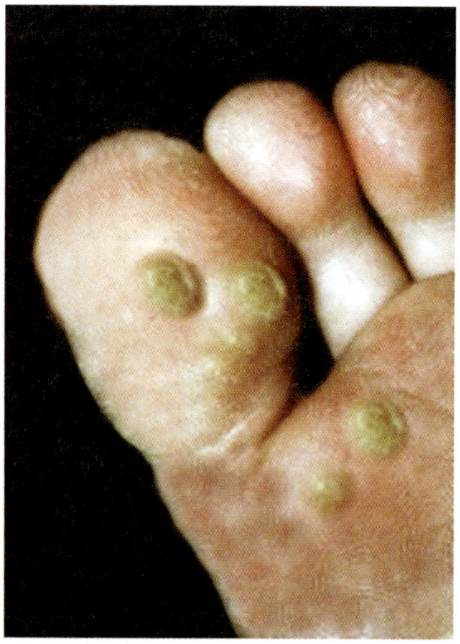

FIGURE 18–5 Plantar warts.

■ ***SYMPTOMS.*** The only symptom is a painless, often rough-surfaced skin lesion appearing on any surface of the body but primarily on the fingers and hands.

■ ***TREATMENT.*** Treatment depends on the location of the verruca. Warts on the finger and hands are commonly treated topically with over-the-counter medications. The best topical medications are those containing salicylic acid such as Trans-Ver-Sal, Sal-Acid Plaster, or Sal-Plant Gel. Genital and plantar warts are commonly removed surgically. Verrucae are often resistant to treatment, and recurrence is frequent.

■ ***PREVENTION.*** The best prevention is to avoid skin-to-skin contact with those infected with verruca.

MEASLES

Measles is a highly contagious childhood disease that causes a characteristic maculopapular skin rash. For more information on measles, see Chapter 20.

BACTERIAL DISEASES

Bacterial skin infections are often highly contagious and affect individuals who are immunosuppressed or who practice poor personal hygiene. These skin infections are generally caused by normal flora bacteria and are treated effectively with antibiotics.

IMPETIGO

■ ***DESCRIPTION.*** Impetigo is a highly contagious skin disease. It is one of the most common skin infections of children and usually affects the face and hands.

■ ***ETIOLOGY.*** Impetigo is caused by streptococcus and staphylococcus bacteria.

■ ***SYMPTOMS.*** Impetigo is characterized by the appearance of vesicles and **pustules** (PUS-tyouls; small pus-filled lesion) that rupture, producing a yellow crust over the lesions. Impetigo occurs more readily in those with poor hygiene, anemia, and malnutrition.

■ ***DIAGNOSIS.*** Diagnosis is confirmed by symptoms and a positive bacterial culture of the infected lesion.

■ ***TREATMENT.*** Treatment includes washing and drying the affected area several times a day and applying antibiotic ointment. More serious conditions might also require oral antibiotics.

■ ***PREVENTION.*** Prevention is aimed at good personal hygiene, including frequent hand washing. Those with anemia and malnutrition need treatment to cure those conditions also.

FOLLICULITIS

■ ***DESCRIPTION.*** Folliculitis is inflammation and infection of the hair follicle and can occur anywhere on the skin.

■ ***ETIOLOGY.*** Folliculitis usually starts when hair follicles are damaged by shaving or friction from clothing. The damaged hair follicle then becomes infected with staphylococcus bacteria.

■ ***SYMPTOMS.*** Common symptoms include rash, itching, and the formation of pimples or small pustules surrounding the hair (Figure 18–6) that can also open, drain, and crust over. This condition commonly occurs in young men and affects the neck, groin, thighs, buttocks, beard, and scalp.

■ ***DIAGNOSIS.*** Diagnosis is based on physical examination of pustules and condition of the skin. Cultures can reveal bacterial or fungal infection.

■ ***TREATMENT.*** Warm, moist compresses help ease the pain and promote drainage of the pustules. Daily cleansing of the area with an antiseptic cleanser and application of antibiotic or antifungal creams for several weeks usually cures the condition. Severe or chronic cases might need additional treatment with oral antibiotics.

■ ***PREVENTION.*** Preventive measures include reducing friction from clothing, keeping skin clean and dry, avoiding bathing with dirty or contaminated

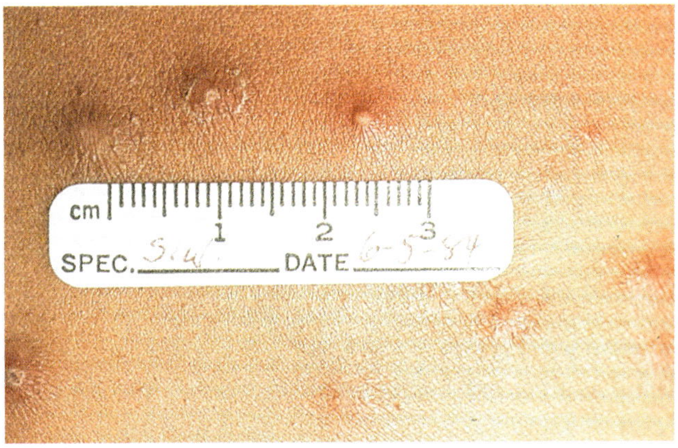

Courtesy of Robert A. Silverman, MD, Pediatric Dermatology, Georgetown University

FIGURE 18–6 Folliculitis.

washcloths, and avoiding shaving the area until the infection is healed.

ABSCESS, FURUNCLE, CARBUNCLE

■ ***DESCRIPTION.*** There are some differences in these lesions. An abscess is a localized collection of pus occurring in any tissue of the body, including the skin. Abscesses commonly occur around sites of trauma, embedded foreign material such as splinters, and hair follicles.

A small abscess occurring in the tissues of the skin is a furuncle, commonly called a boil. Furuncles generally occur around a hair follicle and can develop during an acute case of folliculitis. Boils can develop in any hairy area of the body, with common sites including the skin of the neck, back, and buttocks.

Carbuncles are larger abscesses and involve several interconnected furuncles. These lesions arise in a cluster of hair follicles and have multiple drainage sites. Needless to say, carbuncles are much larger than furuncles and are less common.

■ ***ETIOLOGY.*** These lesions are commonly caused by the pyogenic, normal flora bacteria, staphylococcus. Predisposing factors for these lesions include a lowered immunity due to the presence of other diseases and poor personal hygiene.

■ ***SYMPTOMS.*** Abscess, furuncle, and carbuncle are all characterized by inflammation, infection, and the formation of a capsule to wall off and prevent the spread of infection. All of these encapsulated lesions are extremely painful, usually develop a soft spot or come to a head, and need to be opened or surgically drained.

■ ***DIAGNOSIS.*** Diagnosis is based on history and physical examination of the lesion.

■ ***TREATMENT.*** Warm, moist compresses usually relieve pain and promote spontaneous drainage. If spontaneous opening and drainage does not occur, surgical opening and drainage might be necessary. Antibacterial or antifungal medications are usually prescribed to treat infection.

■ ***PREVENTION.*** Nothing can prevent these lesions, although using antibacterial soaps can help reduce bacterial count on the skin and thus aid in prevention.

CELLULITIS

■ ***DESCRIPTION.*** Cellulitis is a diffuse, or spreading, inflammation of the skin and subcutaneous tissue. It commonly appears on the lower legs but can affect any part of the body.

■ ***ETIOLOGY.*** Cellulitis is a bacterial infection commonly caused by streptococcus and staphylococcus. These bacteria are common bacteria of the skin (normal flora). Cellulitis often appears in open areas of the skin and can be the extension of a wound, **ulcer**, insect bite, blister, burn, or other skin infection.

■ ***SYMPTOMS.*** Cellulitis is characterized by pain, redness, swelling, warmth, and tenderness of the involved skin. Other symptoms might include headaches, fever, or chills. In advancing cases, red streaks can develop and travel from the affected area.

■ ***DIAGNOSIS.*** Medical history and physical examination of the involved area is helpful in diagnosis. If the leg is involved, an ultrasound can be performed to rule out deep vein thrombosis.

■ ***TREATMENT.*** Treatment is generally treated successfully with oral antibiotics. Analgesics for pain and resting the affected limb or affected area also can be part of the treatment plan. In extreme cases, intravenous antibiotics might be needed. Any cellulitis involving the face can be dangerous because this has the potential of spreading into the sinuses of the skull. If pain becomes severe, necrotizing fasciitis might have developed, which will require emergency surgical treatment.

■ ***PREVENTION.*** Good hand washing, proper cleansing, and care of open areas of the skin lower the risk of cellulitis. Deep, dirty, and open wounds need prompt medical treatment to prevent cellulitis.

ERYSIPELAS

■ ***DESCRIPTION.*** Erysipelas is an acute infection of the dermis that extends into underlying fat tissue. It can affect the face, especially in children and older adults, but also affects the legs.

■ ***ETIOLOGY.*** Most cases are due to streptococcus, specifically group A streptococcus. These bacteria can come from the skin or from the affected individual's throat or nasal passages and can enter the skin through any open area such as surgical incisions, ulcers, and minor trauma.

SYMPTOMS. Symptoms include fatigue, chills, fever, headaches, and vomiting. The infected skin develops a red, warm, hard, and painful rash showing a consistency similar to an orange peel. Swelling develops rapidly and exhibits sharply demarcated, raised edges.

DIAGNOSIS. A physical examination of the classic orange-peel rash and affected skin assist in diagnosis. Tests can determine that this skin condition is not herpes zoster or contact dermatitis.

TREATMENT. Antibiotics given orally or intravenously usually resolve the condition, but it often takes weeks for the skin to return to normal. In some cases, bacteria can infect the blood, leading to endocarditis and osteomyelitis.

PREVENTION. Prevention includes maintaining healthy skin, avoiding injuries to the skin, and promptly and completely treating streptococcal infections, including strep throat.

LYME DISEASE

DESCRIPTION. Lyme disease was first discovered in 1975 in the town of Lyme, Connecticut, for which it is named. It is more prevalent in the northeast and has become the most common tick-borne disease in the United States.

ETIOLOGY. Lyme disease is caused by the *Borrelia burgdorferi* bacterium and is transmitted to humans by the bite of an infected deer or black-legged tick.

SYMPTOMS. The bacteria can affect any organ, causing a variety of symptoms and possibly delaying diagnosis. Symptoms can include flu-like symptoms, arthritis, malaise, chills, and fever. A characteristic bull's eye skin rash is a common sign. The bull's eye is a reddened circle with a lighter center and can appear days to weeks after the infected bite.

DIAGNOSIS. Lyme disease is diagnosed by a history confirming possible exposure to infected ticks and a physical examination revealing positive symptoms. Positive blood testing for antibodies confirms the diagnosis.

TREATMENT. Most cases can be treated successfully with a few weeks of antibiotics. If left untreated, the disease can cause arthritis and various neurologic and cardiovascular complications.

PREVENTION. Prevention of Lyme disease is aimed at preventing tick bites by using insect repellent; wearing long-sleeved shirts, long pants, and socks; and tucking the pants into the socks and boots when hiking or camping in grassy or wooded areas. Showering and inspecting the skin immediately after outside activities can also help prevent bites.

METHICILLIN-RESISTANT STAPHYLOCOCCUS AUREUS

DESCRIPTION. Methicillin-resistant staphylococcus aureus (MRSA) is a strain of bacteria that is resistant to the antibiotics commonly used to treat staphylococcal infections. This infection usually affects the elderly and those with other disease conditions and occurs in hospitals, nursing homes, and other health care settings and is known as health care–associated MRSA. More recently, MRSA is appearing in healthy people who might share personal items, such as athletes and students. These individuals are often in a community of people. In this case, MRSA is responsible for skin, tissue, and lung infections and is called community-associated MRSA.

In 2007, the Centers for Disease Control and Prevention published alarming information that estimated the number of MRSA infections in hospitals had doubled nationwide in a period of 6 years. Another concern identified by the CDC was that, by 2005, the number of MRSA deaths had climbed higher than the deaths caused nationwide by AIDS (CDC, 2007). These reports suggest a nationwide epidemic of MRSA, a super bug.

ETIOLOGY. *S. aureus* is commonly found on the skin of individuals, is usually harmless, and does not cause illness. This presence of bacteria without illness is called being colonized. Individuals who are colonized with MRSA can easily pass these bacteria to others.

MRSA represents a group of bacteria that have developed a resistance to antibiotic, which is a natural survival method of bacteria. However, humans have helped build this resistance by excessive and unnecessary use of antibiotics. Many individuals insist on taking antibiotics for viral conditions such as flu and the common cold, even though it has been proven that these viruses are not affected by antibiotics. This overuse helps strengthen bacteria and build their resistance.

Even when antibiotics are used properly, they do not always kill every kind of bacterium. Those that survive become resistant to that antibiotic and many others. Because bacteria reproduce rapidly, they can build family resistance faster than new antibiotics can be developed. Staph is one of the families of bacteria that have built such a resistance that currently only a few drugs are effective against them.

Prescription medications are not the only sources of antibiotics that help build resistance. Antibiotics are often used in livestock. These antibiotics not only end up in meat products but eventually end up in groundwater supply from feedlot runoff.

SYMPTOMS. Symptoms of MRSA, like other staph bacteria, often start with small red bumps that resemble pimples or boils. These can quickly cause deep abscesses or become blood-borne. As a blood-borne infection, staph bacteria can invade all organs of the body, including bones, heart, and lungs. Symptoms of sepsis include a rash over most of the body along with fever, chills, headaches, joint pain, and shortness of breath. Sepsis with MRSA can be life-threatening, and infection requires immediate medical attention.

DIAGNOSIS. Diagnosis is determined by culture and drug sensitivity testing of wound and nasal secretions for MRSA.

TREATMENT. Current treatment of MRSA is with another, quite expensive antibiotic, Vancomycin, which must be given intravenously. Even though it is currently effective, it is already showing signs that some MRSA bacteria are building resistance to this medication also.

PREVENTION. Avoiding those with active infection is helpful along with maintaining a healthy lifestyle to keep natural immunity levels high. Other activities include frequent hand washing and carrying hand sanitizer for use when hand washing is not possible. Do not share personal items such as towels, clothing, combs, and eating utensils. Keep any open wounds covered and protected. Do not share or overuse antibiotics.

Prevention in health care facilities requires complete sanitation of all surface areas, fabrics, linens, and equipment in patient areas. Alcohol has been proven to be an effective sanitizer against MRSA. Therefore, many health care facilities have installed alcohol-based skin sanitizers in patient rooms, hall ways, and utility rooms. Current best practices to prevent MRSA infection in health care settings includes frequent hand washing by all staff, testing all patients upon admission for colonization with MRSA, placing all patients in isolation until culture results are reported as negative, and thorough cleansing regimes of patient rooms and common clinical areas.

FUNGAL DISEASES

Fungal infections are very common and usually affect the nails and hair. Pathogenic fungi are called dermatophytes, which often cause the skin to itch and crack, leaving it open to bacterial infections. Fungal infections are difficult to eradicate and can cause lifelong symptoms.

TINEA (RINGWORM)

DESCRIPTION. Tinea is a term used to identify any of a number of highly contagious fungal infections of the skin. They typically affect warm, moist areas of the body, feeding on perspiration and dead skin. Types of tinea include:

- **Tinea corporis** Affects the smooth skin of the arms, legs, and body. It is characterized by red, ring-shaped patches with pale centers and is commonly called ringworm, although no worm is involved. Tinea corporis is often spread from cats to humans and is common in children.
- **Tinea pedis** The most common form of tinea infection. It is typically called athlete's foot because it is a common condition in athletes. Tinea pedis is highly contagious and can be spread by direct contact with contaminated surfaces such as locker room floors, showers, and towels. Athlete's foot affects the spaces between the toes, causing intense itching and burning. The affected skin peels, leaving painful cracks or fissures (Figure 18–7). Untreated athlete's foot can spread to the entire foot. Wearing

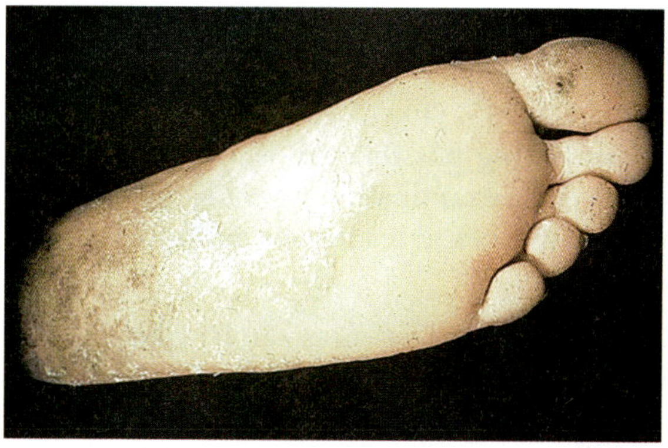

Courtesy of the Centers for Disease Control and Prevention

FIGURE 18–7 Tinea pedis.

cotton socks, alternating shoes to allow complete drying, and wearing sandals help prevent and treat the fungus.

- **Tinea cruris** Often occurs in conjunction with tinea pedis and is commonly called jock itch. It generally affects the scrotal and groin area of adult men. It tends to flare up during summer months and is aggravated by physical activity, tight-fitting jeans, and increased perspiration.
- **Tinea unguium** Involves the fingernail or toenail and is characterized by white patches in the nail. This tinea is difficult to treat because the fungus hides under the nail. Untreated, the fungus can destroy the entire nail, causing it to thicken, overgrow, turn white, and become brittle (Figure 18–8).
- **Tinea capitis** Affects the scalp, causing areas of hair loss. This tinea occurs most often in children. (See Chapter 20 for more information.)
- **Tinea barbae** Affects bearded areas of the neck and face and, thus, is commonly called barber's itch. Shaving the affected area is helpful.

■ ***ETIOLOGY.*** Tinea is caused by a variety of fungi.

■ ***SYMPTOMS.*** Symptoms include itching, cracking, and weeping of the skin.

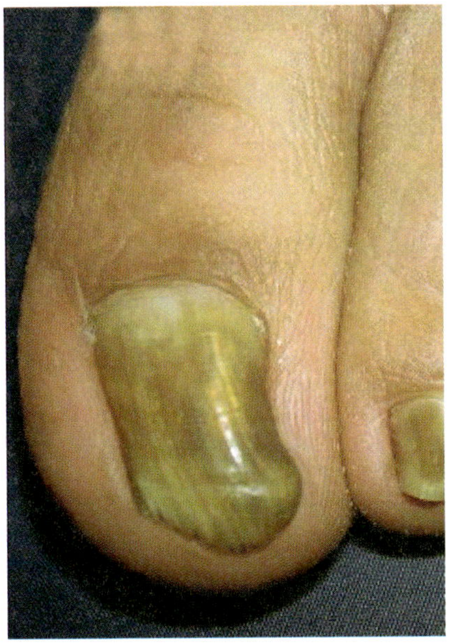

FIGURE 18–8 Tinea unguium.

■ ***DIAGNOSIS.*** Diagnosis is made on the basis of clinical appearance and microscopic examination of skin scrapings, revealing the fungi.

■ ***TREATMENT.*** Treatment includes keeping the affected area clean and dry. Antifungal agents in liquid, cream, and powder forms are effective but must be used consistently over a long period of time to eradicate the fungus. Oral prescription medications might be needed and include ketoconazole (Nizoral) and fluconazole (Diflucan). Commonly, these fungal infections recur and become a chronic problem.

■ ***PREVENTION.*** Keeping the skin healthy, clean, and dry is the most helpful preventive measure. Other measures include avoiding tight-fitting clothing and avoiding areas where fungal infection might be prevalent such as community showers and hot tubs.

CANDIDIASIS

■ ***DESCRIPTION.*** Candidiasis (KAN-dih-DYE-ah-sis) is commonly called yeast infection or thrush. This fungal infection can be superficial or systemic and potentially life threatening.

■ ***ETIOLOGY.*** Candida is a fungus that is normal flora of the skin, mouth, vagina, and intestines. It becomes an infection when some change in the body allows it to grow out of control. Taking antibiotics is a common cause of candidiasis. Antibiotic kills beneficial normal bacterial flora that help keep candidiasis under control.

Candidiasis also commonly affects individuals with chronic diseases such as diabetes mellitus, those who are on immunosuppressive medications, and those exposed to long-term water immersion such as dishwashers, bartenders, and waitresses.

■ ***SYMPTOMS.*** Symptoms of candidiasis differ, depending on the area affected. Infection in the mouth is called thrush and commonly occurs in infants. Symptoms include patches of white infection on the inner cheeks and tongue.

Candidiasis infection on an infant's bottom is commonly called diaper rash and appears as red, inflamed, and sometimes scaly rash.

Candidiasis also affects the fingernails and is called candidal onychomycosis. When it affects the area around the nail, is it paronychia. Infection between the fingers and toes often appears as itchy skin with blisters and pustules.

Candidiasis of the vagina causes vaginitis and is discussed in detail in Chapter 17.

■ ***DIAGNOSIS.*** Two primary methods for diagnosis include microscopic examination of the yeast and positive culture. A blood test and cultures might also be needed if the infection becomes blood-borne.

■ ***TREATMENT.*** Most candida infections can be treated with over-the-counter or prescription antifungal medications. Topical creams, vaginal creams, and oral medications are available. More serious infections need long-term administration of intravenous antifungal medication. Even with a variety of antifungal medication available, fungal infections are often difficult to eradicate and can become chronic in some cases.

■ ***PREVENTION.*** Keeping skin clean, dry, and free from abrasions or cuts can help prevent skin candida infections. Avoiding unnecessary antibiotics is also preventive.

PARASITIC DISEASES

Parasites are organisms that feed on a host, sometimes a human. Human parasites affecting the skin are easily spread and cause intense itching. They commonly occur in crowded living conditions with inadequate bathing facilities. The two most common skin parasites are pediculosis (lice) and scabies.

PEDICULOSIS

■ ***DESCRIPTION.*** Pediculosis is an infestation of lice. Three types of lice commonly affect humans:

1. **Head lice** Commonly spread among school-aged children and their families (Figure 18–9). See Chapter 20 for more information.
2. **Body lice** Often occur in individuals with poor hygiene practices, such as transients and the homeless. Body lice can spread disease and were responsible for the spread of typhus during war times.
3. **Pubic lice** Spread by sexual contact with an affected individual and commonly called crabs. Pubic lice infect males and females and cause intense itching in the genital area. These lice also can spread to the eyelashes and eyebrows.

■ ***ETIOLOGY.*** Lice are easily spread by direct contact with an infected individual, or they can be carried by sharing combs, brushes, towels, clothing, or bed linens. Lice are not partial to any of the socioeconomic classes and, thus, affect anyone coming in contact with them.

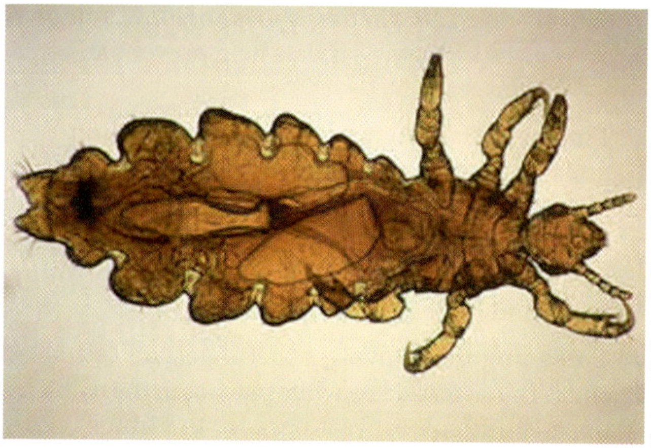

Courtesy of the Centers for Disease Control and Prevention

FIGURE 18–9 Head lice.

■ ***SYMPTOMS.*** Lice can be seen in various areas, depending on the type of insect. Head lice are located on the scalp, crab lice in the pubic area, and body lice in the folds of the skin and on the clothing. Head lice lay their eggs (nits) on the hair shaft of the head. These lice are visible, as is the nit infestation in the hair. Lice crawl on the body and feed on human blood, causing severe itching.

■ ***DIAGNOSIS.*** Diagnosis is easily made by observation of lice on the body.

■ ***TREATMENT.*** Eradicating pediculosis is difficult. Treatment includes:

- Bathing and shampooing with medicated shampoo. (Petroleum jelly can be applied to the eyelashes to kill lice.)
- Dry cleaning or washing all clothing and bed linens in hot water (140 degrees) for 20 minutes.
- Cleaning and treating furniture.

All lice on the body, clothing, bedding, and furniture must be killed to eradicate a lice infestation.

■ ***PREVENTION.*** Prevention includes avoiding contact with infested individuals and their clothing, bedding, and furniture.

SCABIES

■ ***DESCRIPTION.*** Scabies is an infestation by the itch mite.

ETIOLOGY. The mite responsible for scabies is *Sarcoptes scabiei*, a tiny (.03–.09 millimeter long), eight-legged parasite (in contrast to six-legged insects). The pregnant female mite burrows into the skin and lays her eggs in a short tunnel near the surface of the skin. The eggs hatch in 3 to 5 days; the mite matures on the surface of the skin in 2 to 3 weeks, then mates, and the cycle begins again.

Scabies mites can live off a host body for only 48 to 72 hours. Scabies is often transmitted throughout an entire household by skin-to-skin contact with an infected parent or child by hugging, holding, and sharing beds. Over a more extended period of time, relatives and close friends can also contact scabies. Sexual contact is the most common form of transmission among sexually active young people.

It is almost impossible to catch scabies by just touching or shaking hands with an infected individual. School settings, sports activities, and community shower rooms also do not provide the level of personal contact needed for transmission of the mites.

Mites cannot be picked up from animals, although cats and dogs do get mite infections. In dogs, scabies is called mange. Animal mites are different from scabies and do not infect humans but can produce a mild itch that goes away in a few days.

SYMPTOMS. The word *scabies* comes from a Latin word for scratch, the primary symptom for this condition. The action of the burrowing, along with movement of the mites within the skin, produces an intense itch that tends to be worse at night. Vesicles and pustules develop due to hypersensitivity to the bite, the mite's feces, and the presence of the ova.

Scabies are not visible with the naked eye but can be seen with a magnifying glass or microscope. The scabies burrow is visible and often appears as a slightly elevated, grayish white line. Common burrow sites are in the webs between the fingers and toes; in the folds of skin under the breast, armpits, and genital areas; on flexing surfaces of the wrist (Figure 18–10); along the belt line; and around underwear leg lines.

DIAGNOSIS. Diagnosis is made on the basis of microscopic skin examination revealing the presence of mites. Female mites can be viewed at the end of the burrowed tunnel and appear as a tiny black dot.

TREATMENT. Treatment includes application of lindane cream (Kwell) to the entire body, leaving the cream on for 8 to 14 hours before showering or bathing. All infected individuals must be treated to prevent reinfection. Itching might persist for 3 to 4 weeks after successful treatment.

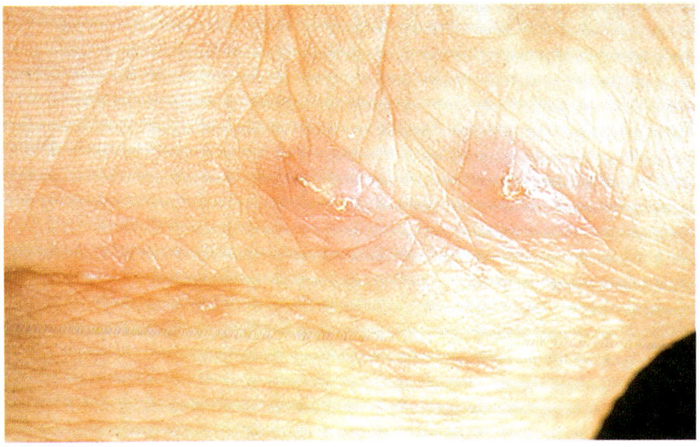

Courtesy of Robert A. Silverman, MD, Pediatric Dermatology, Georgetown University

FIGURE 18–10 Scabies.

Cleaning and treating all personal items at the same time is recommended to prevent reinfection. Wash in hot water or dry clean all clothes, bedding, and towels. Treat furniture, carpets, and rugs. Place personal items that cannot be adequately cleaned, such as stuffed animals, brushes, gloves, hats, shoes, and pillows in plastic bags and freeze overnight or starve mites by placing items in zip-locked plastic bags and storing for a couple of weeks. Mites die after a week without food.

PREVENTION. Avoiding skin-to-skin contact with an infected individual is the best preventive measure.

Metabolic Diseases

Hyperactivity of the sebaceous gland causes several skin diseases. Inflammation and infection also can play a role in these diseases, although the primary cause is metabolic.

ACNE VULGARIS

DESCRIPTION. Acne is an inflammation of the sebaceous (oil-secreting) glands and hair follicles of the skin, characterized by the formation of **comedones** (KOM-eh-dones; a plugged skin pore; the open form is a blackhead; the closed form is a whitehead). Acne vulgaris is the most common form of acne and affects a large number, or crowd (vulgus = crowd), of individuals.

■ ***ETIOLOGY.*** The cause of acne is unknown, but it can be considered a metabolic disease because it occurs at puberty during increased production of sex hormones. An increase in these hormones, especially androgen, causes an increase in the size and activity of the sebaceous glands on the face, neck, chest, and back of males and females. Other factors contributing to the development of acne are heredity, food allergies, and endocrine disorders. Many misconceptions and misinformation exist concerning acne. It is not contagious nor due to lack of cleanliness, lack of sleep, or lack or excess of sexual release or masturbation; it is not caused by venereal disease or consumption of chocolate, colas, or fried foods.

■ ***SYMPTOMS.*** Acne develops when sebaceous glands secrete excessive amounts of oil, or sebum, into a skin pore, eventually clogging the pore and causing the development of comedones. Sebaceous secretions at the opening of the pore can become oxidized and turn black, thus forming a blackhead. If bacteria enter the accumulated sebum and cause infection, the comedone becomes a whitehead or pimple. Acne can be mild to severe. Teens should be instructed to manage acne by:

- Cleansing the face and affected skin frequently with antibacterial soap to remove excess oil and bacteria.
- Avoiding the use of heavy makeup, which contributes to clogging the skin pores.
- Using over-the-counter acne creams or gels to help dry up excess oil.
- Avoiding tight-fitting clothing that traps heat.
- Showering often and especially after exercising or performing strenuous work.
- Avoiding the temptation to squeeze comedones because this can push the collected sebum farther into the skin pore, causing further inflammation and infection.

Comedones should be extracted gently, and pustules or pimples and cysts should be incised and drained.

■ ***DIAGNOSIS.*** Diagnosis is based on a history and physical examination of sebaceous lesions.

■ ***TREATMENT.*** Mild cases of acne are usually managed with proper cleansing and over-the-counter treatments. Severe cases need a treatment regimen prescribed by a dermatologist and often include cleansing with prescription medications, oral antibiotic therapy (tetracycline), steroids, and retinoic acid preparations or Retin-A. Even with proper treatment, severe cases often result in permanent skin scarring. Symptoms of acne generally subside after puberty with or without treatment.

■ ***PREVENTION.*** Following treatment activities not only treats but helps prevent acne.

SEBORRHEIC DERMATITIS

■ ***DESCRIPTION.*** Seborrheic dermatitis is a common type of dermatitis affecting the sebaceous, or oil-secreting, glands of the skin. It is not harmful or contagious but can be uncomfortable and unsightly. Seborrheic dermatitis affecting the scalp of infants is commonly called cradle cap (Figure 18–11) and usually clears by 12 months of age without treatment. Seborrheic dermatitis affecting the scalp of adults is called dandruff.

■ ***ETIOLOGY.*** The exact cause is unknown, although heredity and stress might be factors. This disease appears to run in families and appears more commonly in individuals who are obese; live with weather extremes; have other skin disorders such as acne; or have Parkinson's disease, stroke, head injury, and impaired immunity such as HIV. Individuals recovering from stressful medical conditions such as myocardial infarction or who are confined for long periods of time in nursing homes are also more prone to this

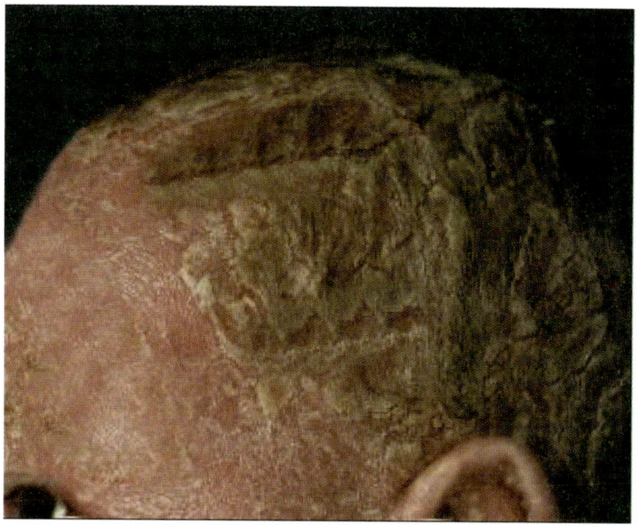

Courtesy of Mark L. Kuss

FIGURE 18–11 Seborrheic dermatitis.

condition. The disease is characterized by an increase in the production of sebum, causing inflammation in the areas of the skin with the greatest number of glands. There is no cure for this disease.

■ **SYMPTOMS.** Seborrheic dermatitis affects the scalp, eyebrows, eyelashes, skin behind the ears (postauricular area), the sides of the nose, and the middle of the chest. Affected skin is usually reddened and covered with greasy-looking, yellowish scales. The eyebrows and eyelashes of an individual with seborrheic dermatitis show dry, dirty-white scales. The affected nose area is generally reddened and itches. Mid-chest or sternal lesions are reddened and greasy-feeling. Itching might or might not be present.

■ **DIAGNOSIS.** The diagnosis is made based on physical examination of the location and appearance of the skin lesions.

■ **TREATMENT.** Treatment of the scalp involves use of over-the-counter medicated shampoo. If these are ineffective, a prescription-strength medicated shampoo might be necessary. Aggressive therapy includes the use of steroid lotion or creams.

Non-scalp areas often need to be cleaned and kept dry and treated often with antifungal or anti-itch medications. A prescription medication might be necessary if the disease is not manageable or if large areas of the body are involved.

■ **PREVENTION.** The severity of this condition can be lessened by controlling risk factors and treating appropriately.

SEBACEOUS CYST

■ **DESCRIPTION.** A sebaceous cyst is a closed sac of oily, cheese-like material located under the skin. This cyst can form anywhere on the body except in the palms of the hands and soles of the feet and commonly develop in the scalp, neck, and groin area. A special type of sebaceous cyst is a **pilonidal cyst**, which develops around a hair in the sacrococcygeal area.

■ **ETIOLOGY.** Sebaceous (seh-BAY-shus) cysts develop when a sebaceous gland becomes blocked and the sebum collects under the skin. They are often seen in individuals affected with acne, commonly result from a swollen hair follicle, and appear as slow-growing, painless lumps.

■ **SYMPTOMS.** The main symptom is the presence of the cyst. If it becomes infected, the skin will become red, warm, and tender over the area.

■ **DIAGNOSIS.** Diagnosis is made by physical examination of the cyst.

■ **TREATMENT.** No treatment is needed unless infection occurs. A warm, moist compress can be placed over the area to help relieve pain and promote drainage. Further treatment includes incising and draining the cyst, although it might tend to recur. Permanent treatment is surgical removal.

■ **PREVENTION.** There are no known measures that can prevent these cysts, but maintaining clean, healthy skin reduces in the risk of occurrence.

Hypersensitivity or Immune Diseases

Hypersensitivity diseases are those caused by an immune reaction within the body. Frequently, the cause is unknown, and treatment is symptomatic.

ECZEMA

■ **DESCRIPTION.** Eczema (ECK-zeh-mah) is an inflammation of the skin or a type of dermatitis. It is not dangerous, not contagious, and often not curable.

■ **ETIOLOGY.** Eczema is also called atopic dermatitis because it tends to occur in atopic individuals—those with a genetic predisposition to allergies. Eczema is a common allergic reaction in children, often beginning in infancy and believed to be due to allergies to milk, orange juice, or some other foods. Eczema in infants often disappears when the offending food is discontinued. Factors that can cause eczema include heredity, other diseases, allergies, and substances that irritate the skin.

■ **SYMPTOMS.** In adults, eczema often produces dry, leathery skin lesions characterized by itching, redness, vesicles, pustules, scales, and crust, appearing alone or in combination (Figure 18–12). Stress, humidity, and severe changes in temperature are a few of the identified factors causing an exacerbation or flare-up of the condition.

■ **DIAGNOSIS.** Diagnosis is made on the basis of clinical examination and history.

■ **TREATMENT.** Treatment is aimed at decreasing the occurrence and severity of the condition. Topical cortisone creams are often used along with antihistamines and sedatives to treat pruritus. Sunlight

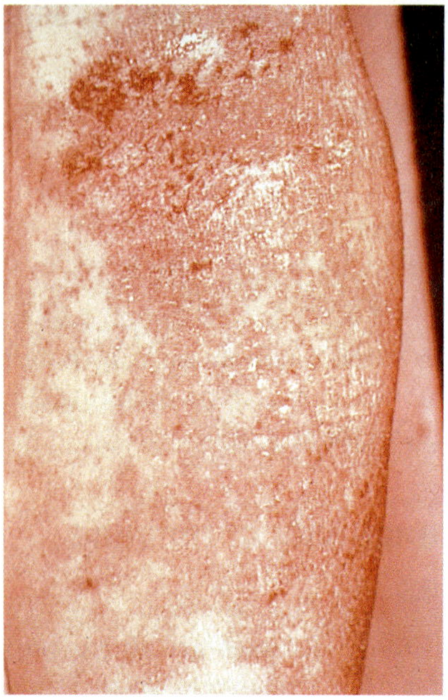

Courtesy of the Centers for Disease Control and Prevention

FIGURE 18–12 Eczema.

should be avoided, especially with light-sensitive eczema.

■ ***PREVENTION.*** Eczema is not preventable, but avoiding irritants reduces symptoms and exacerbation of the condition.

URTICARIA

■ ***DESCRIPTION.*** Commonly called hives or nettle rash, this is a vascular reaction of the skin.

■ ***ETIOLOGY.*** Urticaria is caused by contact with an external irritant such as insect bites, pollen, or plants. Urticaria also can be caused by internal irritants such as food, drugs, and contrast dye.

■ ***SYMPTOMS.*** Urticaria is characterized by slightly elevated lesions that are redder or paler than the surrounding skin and are associated with severe itching. The elevated areas are called **wheals** (WEELs) or hives. Scratching or rubbing the hypersensitive area can lead to formation of larger or additional wheals.

■ ***DIAGNOSIS.*** Diagnosis is made on the basis of physical examination of the characteristic wheal.

■ ***TREATMENT.*** Treatment includes antihistamines and avoidance of the allergen. (See Chapter 5, "Immune System Diseases and Disorders," for more information.)

■ ***PREVENTION.*** Avoiding exposure to the allergen and avoiding hot baths, showers, or exposure to the sun after a recent episode are preventive measures. Exposure to heat can cause the hives to return.

CONTACT DERMATITIS

■ ***DESCRIPTION.*** Contact dermatitis is an acute or chronic allergic reaction affecting the skin.

■ ***ETIOLOGY.*** Often, the allergen is some type of cosmetic, laundry product, plant, jewelry, paint, drug, plastic, or a variety of other agents. Frequently, it is difficult to determine the causative agent and, when found, sometimes impossible to avoid completely.

■ ***SYMPTOMS.*** Allergic lesions can range from small, red, localized lesions to vesicular lesions that cover the entire body. A common example of a contact dermatitis is poison ivy. (See Chapter 5 for more information.)

■ ***DIAGNOSIS.*** Diagnosis is not always easy. The location of the rash can help determine diagnosis if the rash appears under an item of clothing, jewelry, or an area exposed to sunlight. A use test is performed by placing a small spot of a suspected substance such as shampoo, laundry detergent, perfume, or cosmetic in another area away from the rash and watching for a reaction. Another helpful test is a patch test in which a patch containing common allergens are placed on the skin and observed for a reaction.

■ ***TEATMENT.*** Itching can be relieved with a number of over-the-counter topical medications containing camphor or menthol. Antihistamines such as diphenhydramine (Benadryl) also relieve itching but cause drowsiness. Cool tub baths can also help. Treatment will not be beneficial until there is no further contact with the allergen.

■ ***PREVENTION.*** Avoiding the allergen is the best preventive measure. If contact with a known allergen occurs, immediately washing with soap and water might prevent the rash from developing. Application of barrier creams and wearing protective clothing are also helpful.

SCLERODERMA

Scleroderma (SKLEHR-oh-DER-mah; sclero = hardening, derma = skin) is a chronic autoimmune disorder characterized by hardening, thickening, and shrinking of the connective tissues of the body, including the skin. It is thought that this autoimmune reaction begins with the skin and connective tissues, attracting lymph cells that stimulate the production of collagen, leading to the disorder. More information can be found in Chapter 5.

Idiopathic Diseases

Idiopathic diseases of the skin have no known cause but often tend to be familial. They can range from mild to severe and are generally treated symptomatically. They tend to be chronic with periods of remission and exacerbation of the disease process.

PSORIASIS

DESCRIPTION. Psoriasis (soh-RYE-uh-sis) is a very common, chronic skin disease that often affects individuals between the ages of 15 and 35. It can appear slowly or quite suddenly and usually has periods of remission (no symptoms) and exacerbation (flare up). Psoriasis is not contagious.

A classic characteristic of the condition is the rapid replacement of epidermal cells. Normally, in a square centimeter of skin, some 25,000 cells produce 1,250 new cells with a life of 300 hours. Epidermal cells in a square centimeter of skin affected by psoriasis will number around 52,000 (twice the normal) and will produce 35,000 new cells (28 times more) with a life of only 36 hours (approximately one-eighth as long as normal).

ETIOLOGY. The cause is unknown but some hereditary basis does exist. Stress, infection, skin trauma, and sunlight tend to cause an exacerbation of the condition.

SYMPTOMS. Psoriasis is characterized by red, raised lesions with distinct borders and silvery scales (Figure 18–13). These lesions generally occur on the elbows, knees, and scalp.

DIAGNOSIS. Diagnosis is usually made by physical examination of the skin condition. A skin biopsy might be performed to determine the exact type of psoriasis.

TREATMENT. Treatment includes medications to control itching, creams containing coal tar, creams to remove the scaling (salicylic acid), ultraviolet (UV) light treatments, steroids, and prescription medications for vitamin D or vitamin A. Oatmeal baths can also be helpful to loosen the scales.

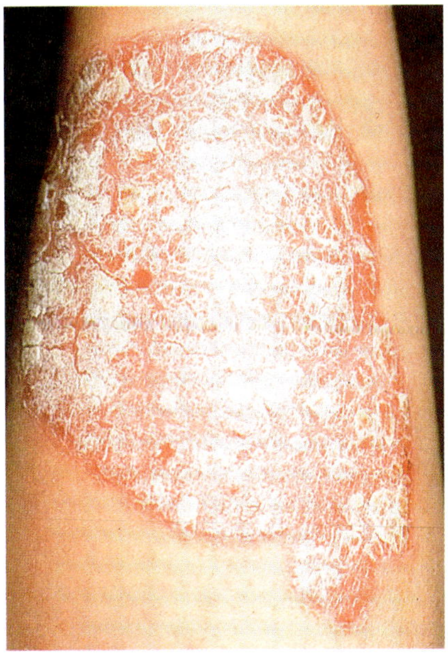

FIGURE 18–13 Psoriasis.

PREVENTION. There is no way to prevent psoriasis, but certain activities can reduce flare-up of symptoms. These activities include keeping the skin moist and avoiding cold climates, skin scratches, stress, infection, and smoking.

ROSACEA

DESCRIPTION. Rosacea is a chronic skin condition characterized by inflammation and redness of the forehead, nose, cheeks, and chin but is not dangerous or life-threatening. The individual's facial skin appearance can lead to psychological damage related to loss of self-esteem.

ETIOLOGY. The cause of rosacea is unknown, but individuals affected blush easily and tend to be fair-skinned, female, and between the ages of 30 and 50. Rosacea involves enlargement of the blood vessels just under the skin and might be associated with other skin conditions such as seborrhea and acne vulgaris.

SYMPTOMS. The facial skin appears red with swelling or skin eruptions similar to acne. Other symptoms include:

- A red, bulbous nose.
- Spider-like blood vessels called telangiectasia of the face.
- A burning or stinging sensation of the face.
- Bloodshot, irritated, watery eyes.

COMPLEMENTARY AND ALTERNATIVE THERAPY

Alternative Therapy for Psoriasis

Historically, traditional Chinese medicines (TCM) have been used for a variety of dermatological conditions. Several research studies have shown TCM to be beneficial for psoriasis and atopic dermatitis. Perhaps practitioners of Western medicine should investigate TCM for its benefits in relieving conditions such as psoriasis. The use of TCM along with conventional treatments may be the best practice in the future.

Source: Koo & Desai (2003).

■ ***DIAGNOSIS.*** Diagnosis is commonly made by physical examination of the skin condition.

■ ***TREATMENT.*** There is no known cure. Symptoms might be controlled by identifying triggers that cause the condition to become worse. Avoiding sun exposure, prolonged exertion in hot weather, stress, spicy foods, alcohol, and hot beverages might reduce symptoms.

Antibiotic ointments applied to the face might control skin eruptions, and laser surgery might reduce the redness. Surgical reduction of the enlargement of the nose might be preferred to improve appearance.

■ ***PREVENTION.*** There is no known prevention.

Benign Tumors

Benign tumors of the skin are relatively common. They tend to be familial and often are more common in older adults.

SEBORRHEIC KERATOSIS

■ ***DESCRIPTION.*** Seborrheic keratosis (SEB-oh-REE-ic KERR-ah-TOH-sis) is a benign overgrowth of epithelial cells. It is one of the most common types of benign skin growth in older adults. Most people as they age will have at least one of these lesions.

■ ***ETIOLOGY.*** The cause is unknown, although it does appear to be age related.

■ ***SYMPTOMS.*** The lesions usually appear as a tan, brown, or black growth with a well-defined border. The surface of the lesion is covered with a warty scale that is soft on the trunk but harsh, dry, and rough on the hands, arms, and face. These lesions are rather loose and appear to be tacked onto the skin.

■ ***DIAGNOSIS.*** This condition is easily diagnosed by physical examination of the lesion. Seborrheic keratosis does not become cancerous, but can appear that way at times. If this is the case, a skin biopsy might be ordered.

■ ***TREATMENT.*** They are often easily scraped off by curettage, the treatment of choice. These skin growths are normally painless and require no treatment. They are often removed for cosmetic reasons.

■ ***PREVENTION.*** There is no prevention for this condition.

KELOID

■ ***DESCRIPTION.*** A keloid (KEE-loid) is a raised, firm, irregularly shaped mass of scar tissue that develops following trauma or surgical incision. (See Chapter 4, "Inflammation and Infection," for photograph.)

■ ***ETIOLOGY.*** Keloids are an overgrowth of collagen during connective tissue repair; it is more common in the black population.

■ ***SYMPTOMS.*** Keloids can be unsightly but are generally considered harmless.

■ ***DIAGNOSIS.*** Diagnosis is easy and consists of a physical examination of the keloid.

■ ***TREATMENT.*** Surgical removal of keloids is usually not effective because it often results in the formation of another keloid. Radiation, injecting the lesion with steroids, and cryotherapy might be helpful in reducing the size of a keloid.

■ ***PREVENTION.*** There are no known preventive measures.

HEMANGIOMA

■ ***DESCRIPTION.*** Hemangioma (heh-MAN-jee-OH-mah; hem = blood, angio = vessel, oma = tumor) is the most common childhood tumor. In most cases, hemangiomas will disappear over time with as many as 50% disappearing by age 5 and the majority disappearing by puberty. Most hemangiomas appear on the face and neck and affect females more often than males. They are also more likely to appear in twin births. Hemangiomas are congenital and do not grow on adults.

■ ***ETIOLOGY.*** The cause of hemangioma is unknown.

■ ***SYMPTOMS.*** Hemagiomas are made up of small blood vessels forming a reddish or purplish birthmark. Sometimes they present as a flat red or pink area. Common types of hemangioma include port wine stain, strawberry, and cherry hemangioma (Figure 18–14).

- **Port wine stain** A dark red to purple birthmark usually appearing on the face
- **Strawberry hemangioma** A strawberry red, rough, protruding lesion commonly appearing on the face, neck, or trunk
- **Cherry hemangioma** A small, red, dome-shaped lesion

■ ***DIAGNOSIS.*** Diagnosis is easy and consists of a physical examination of the hemangioma.

■ ***TREATMENT.*** Treatment is usually not necessary because most hemangiomas will disappear with time. Surgical removal of lesions on the face is common for cosmetic reasons.

■ ***PREVENTION.*** There are no preventive measures.

Premalignant and Malignant Tumors

Skin cancer is the most common type of cancer in humans and, in most cases, is due to exposure to sun. Skin cancers generally occur in multiples and appear on the face, arms, and hands of middle-aged and older individuals. The most common skin cancer is basal cell carcinoma, but the most deadly is malignant melanoma. Diagnosis is made on the basis of clinical examination and positively confirmed by biopsy. Prevention for all forms of skin cancer consists of avoiding overexposure to the sun and lifelong use of sunscreen with a high sun protection factor (SPF).

ACTINIC KERATOSIS

■ ***DESCRIPTION.*** Actinic keratosis (ack-TIN-ick KERR-ah-TOH-sis; actinic = sun-related), is a premalignant skin condition more common in those with fair complexions, sun bathers, and individuals who have occupations in the sun such as fishermen, farmers, and construction workers.

■ ***ETIOLOGY.*** Actinic keratosis, also known as solar keratosis, is caused by excessive exposure to UV rays typically from the sun. These actinic lesions are slow growing, taking years to develop and often appear first in older adults.

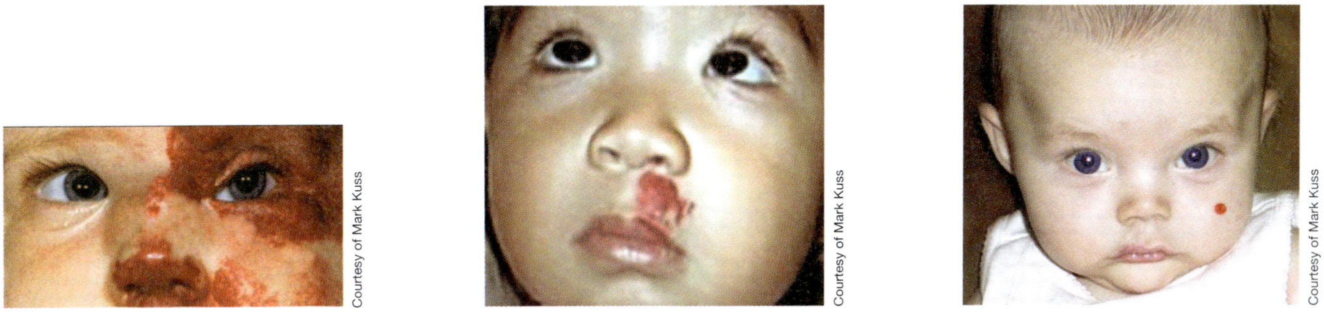

(A) (B) (C)

FIGURE 18–14 Hemangiomas. Port-wine hemangioma, Strawberry hemangioma, Cherry hemangioma.

■ ***SYMPTOMS.*** It is characterized by the growth of multiple wart-like lesions on sun-exposed areas of the body such as the face, backs of the hands, forearms, ears, and legs.

■ ***DIAGNOSIS.*** Diagnosis is made on the basis of clinical examination of the lesions.

■ ***TREATMENT.*** Left untreated, about 2% to 5% of actinic keratoses develop into a serious form of skin cancer called squamous cell carcinoma. Treatment is with topical medication such as Retin-A or removal by curettage or cryotherapy.

■ ***PREVENTION.*** Reducing sun exposure reduces or eliminates this condition.

BASAL CELL CARCINOMA

■ ***DESCRIPTION.*** Basal cell carcinoma is the most common type of skin cancer. It is most common in fair-skinned, blonde, and blue- or gray-eyed individuals. Basal cell carcinoma is a slow-growing, locally invading tumor that does not metastasize. This is not to say that left untreated it is not dangerous. Tumors near the eyes and mouth can invade these spaces and cause much concern. Tumors on the nose, lip, and ear can lead to the loss of these tissues.

■ ***ETIOLOGY.*** As with most cancers, the cause of basal cell carcinoma is unclear but does seem to be the result of a mixture of genetic and environmental factors. The most common identified environmental factor is excessive exposure to the sun.

■ ***SYMPTOMS.*** The appearance of this tumor varies, appearing as a raised nodule with a depressed or dented center; a smooth, shiny bump that is pink to pearly white in color; or a nonhealing lesion that bleeds easily (Figure 18–15).

■ ***DIAGNOSIS.*** Diagnosis is confirmed by biopsy.

■ ***TREATMENT.*** Treatment of basal cell carcinoma is surgical removal.

■ ***PREVENTION.*** Basal cell carcinomas that are related to sun exposure can be prevented by avoiding the strong midday sun, using sunscreen year round, and covering up with protective clothing if exposure is necessary.

SQUAMOUS CELL CARCINOMA

■ ***DESCRIPTION.*** Squamous cell carcinoma is less common than basal cell carcinoma, but it tends to grow more rapidly and become metastatic.

■ ***ETIOLOGY.*** This tumor, like basal cell, tends to occur on the sun-exposed skin of those with fair complexion. It most commonly appears on people over age 50. As a general rule, basal cell carcinoma occurs on the face above the lip line, and squamous cell occurs below the lip line. This tumor is often preceded by another skin lesion such as actinic keratosis, chronic ulcers, sinus tracts, or scars.

■ ***SYMPTOMS.*** Squamous cell carcinoma can appear as a firm, red nodule with crusts or a slightly elevated plaque (Figure 18–16). The nodule is usually located on the face, arm, neck, or hands but can appear in other areas. A sore that does not heal or bleeds easily might be a symptom of this cancer.

■ ***DIAGNOSIS.*** Diagnosis is confirmed by skin biopsy.

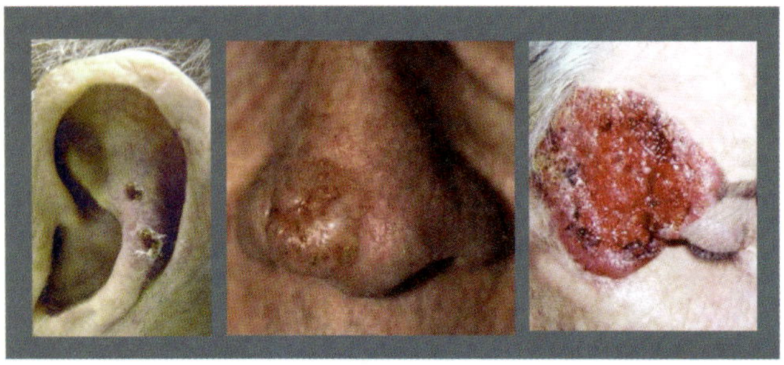

Ear (A) Nose (B) Near eye (C)

Courtesy of Mark L. Kuss

FIGURE 18–15 Basal cell carcinoma: (A) ear, (B) nose, (C) near eye.

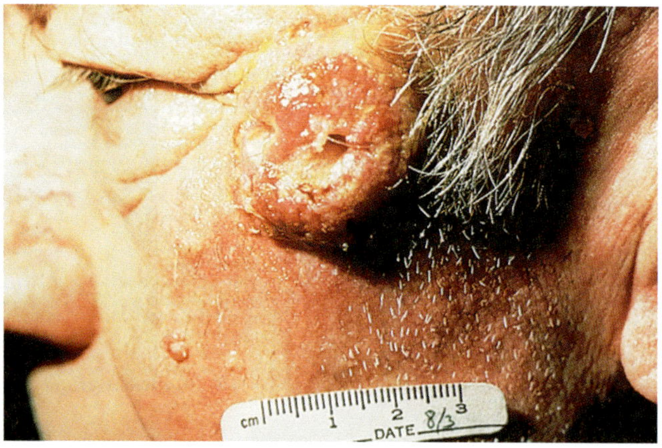

Courtesy of Robert A. Silverman, MD, Pediatric Dermatology, Georgetown University

FIGURE 18–16 Squamous cell carcinoma.

■ ***TREATMENT.*** Squamous cell skin cancer has a high rate of cure if caught early. Treatment depends on location and size of the tumor and if there is metastasis. Wide surgical excision with radiation treatments and follow-up for at least 5 years for signs of recurrence is often the recommended treatment.

■ ***PREVENTION.*** Reducing sun exposure, examining the skin frequently for suspicious growths or changes in existing skin lesions, and seeking immediate treatment for these are preventive measures.

MALIGNANT MELANOMA

■ ***DESCRIPTION.*** Malignant melanoma (melan = black, oma = tumor) is the most serious type of skin cancer. It occurs more commonly in men and is responsible for the majority of skin cancer deaths.

■ ***ETIOLOGY.*** Malignant melanoma is due to an uncontrolled growth of pigment, or skin coloring cells, called melanocytes. Growth of this tumor is caused by genetic and environmental factors, primarily sun exposure. Malignant melanoma rarely occurs before the age of 20 and can be related to a severe childhood sunburn.

■ ***SYMPTOMS.*** This tumor is usually tan, brown, or dark brown in color (Figure 18–17). Often, it arises in a mole and causes a change in size and color of the mole. Malignant melanoma metastasizes quickly and is highly malignant. It spreads into the lymph nodes and can metastasize to all organs of the body.

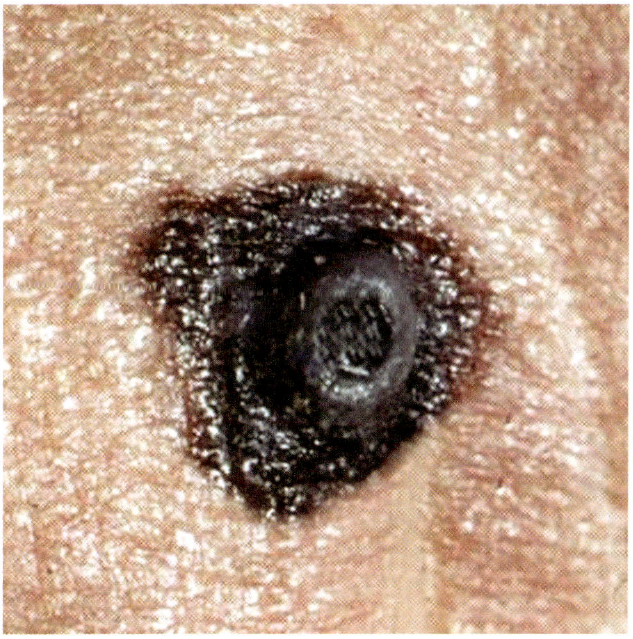

Courtesy of Mark L. Kuss

FIGURE 18–17 Malignant melanoma.

■ ***TREATMENT.*** Treatment depends on the degree of spread and might include wide surgical excision, radiation, and chemotherapy. Prognosis depends on the degree of spread when discovered, but approximately 20% of those diagnosed with this tumor die from effects of metastasis.

■ ***PREVENTION.*** Preventive measures include reducing sun exposure, examining the skin frequently for suspicious growths or changes in existing skin lesions, and seeking immediate treatment.

HEALTHY HIGHLIGHT

Sunburn Prevention

Fair-skinned persons and those working in the sun—sailors, farmers, ranchers, road crew workers, and construction personnel—are at the greatest risk for development of sunburn and, ultimately, skin cancer. Prevention of sunburn includes:

- Avoiding sun exposure between the hours of 10:00 A.M. and 3:00 P.M., when the sun's rays are the strongest.
- Using sunscreen with SPF of 30 or higher on all exposed skin.
- Wearing a large, brimmed hat to reduce sun exposure to the face, ears, and head.
- Avoiding tanning beds.

KAPOSI'S SARCOMA

■ ***DESCRIPTION.*** Prior to the discovery of AIDS, Kaposi's sarcoma (KAP-oh-seez sar-KOH-mah) was relatively rare, but with the recent epidemic of AIDS, the development of this neoplasm has increased drastically.

■ ***ETIOLOGY.*** The relationship between Kaposi's sarcoma and AIDS is not fully understood. Usually, this tumor is not highly malignant except in the case of AIDS, in which it tends to be widespread and is often the cause of death in these individuals.

■ ***SYMPTOMS.*** This sarcoma is a malignant vascular skin tumor characterized by bluish-red cutaneous patches that grow under the skin most often on the face and legs. About one third of the time, they show up in the lining of the nose, mouth, and throat and can lead to pain and difficulty with eating and swallowing. The patches are usually composed of blood and cancer cells and often cause no symptoms. Tumors developing on the toes, feet, and legs often increase in number and size and spread upward. If the cancer spreads to the digestive tract or lungs, bleeding can result.

■ ***DIAGNOSIS.*** Diagnosis is made on the basis of a physical examination of the skin revealing painless, flat, bluish-red lesions that do not itch or drain. A skin biopsy is definitive.

■ ***TREATMENT.*** The most important treatment is treating AIDS. Specific Kaposi's treatments include liquid nitrogen, chemotherapy, and radiation. As with AIDS, there is no cure for Kaposi's.

■ ***PREVENTION.*** Because most cases of Kaposi's are related to HIV infection, taking preventive measures to avoid HIV infection will usually prevent Kaposi's.

Abnormal Pigmented Lesions

The epidermis of normal skin contains melanocytes that produce melanin, the coloring pigment of skin. Skin color varies from light to dark, depending on the number of melanocytes present and protects the skin from burning. This explains why individuals with a fair or pale complexion burn more easily than individuals with a darker complexion. An individual's skin can contain several variations of abnormal lesions associated with pigment. These abnormal, pigmented lesions include ephelis, lentigo, nevus, albinism, vitiligo, and melasma. These conditions can be unsightly but are usually harmless and easily diagnosed by a physician. Moles can cause increased concern if they undergo a change in size and shape, possible indicators of cancer. Lesions can be biopsied if cancer is suspected. A brief description of abnormal pigmented lesions follows.

- **Ephelis** Commonly called a freckle and is indicative of skin damage due to sunburn. The melanocytes in a freckle area are hyperreactive to sunlight, causing the darkened lesion. Freckles commonly occur in children and tend to fade in adults.
- **Lentigo** A small brown spot occurring on the face, neck, and back of the hands of older adults. Commonly called liver spots, these lesions are not due to aging but to years of overexposure to the sun.
- **Nevus** Commonly called a mole. Nevi can be brown, black, or pink-colored and are often due to a collection of melanocytes, which can appear on any area of the body, vary in size and shape, and occur singly or in multiples. Suspicious or unsightly nevi are often removed surgically.
- **Albinism** A hereditary disorder characterized by a decrease or total absence of pigment in the skin, hair, and eyes. Individuals affected with albinism have pale skin, white hair, and pale blue or pink eyes. These individuals suffer from extreme sunburn if adequate protection is not provided.
- **Vitiligo** (VIT-ih-LYE-go) Characterized by destruction of melanocytes in small or large patches of skin (Figure 18–18). This condition can be due to an immune disorder.
- **Melasma** Characterized by dark patches of skin on the face, especially the cheeks (Figure 18–19) and common in pregnant females and those taking birth control pills. It is commonly called the mask of pregnancy. Melasma usually disappears after delivery or discontinuation of birth control pills.

Diseases of the Nails

Nails act as coverings for the toes and fingers and can be considered extensions of the skin. Diseases of the nail can cause abnormal shape, thickening, and color changes. Fungal and bacterial infections are the most common cause of nail disease.

Bacterial infection of the nails is **paronychia** (PAR-oh-NICK-ee-ah), an infection of the skin

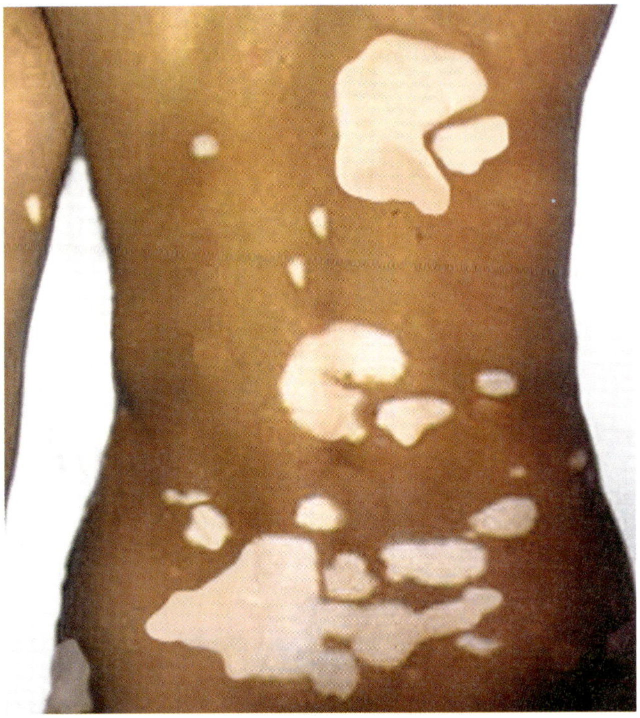

FIGURE 18–18 Vitiligo.

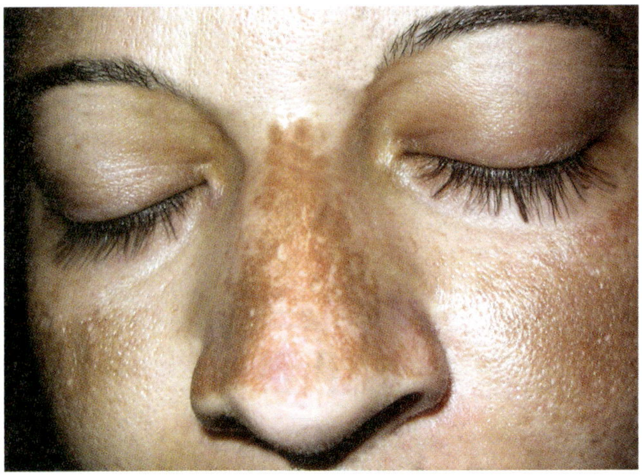

FIGURE 18–19 Melasma.

around the nail. This condition is commonly seen in individuals whose hands are in water for long periods of time, such as dishwashers, for example. This infection can cause the nail to lift away from the bed, causing acute pain. Antibiotics are usually an effective treatment.

Fungal infections frequently affect the feet, are often chronic in nature, and commonly cause permanent nail deformity. Tinea pedis (athlete's foot) is a common cause of fungal nail infections of the feet. Fungal infections, as discussed previously in the chapter, are difficult to treat, and recurrence is common.

Diseases of the Hair

Hair color, texture, and distribution are genetically determined and influenced by hormones.

HIRSUTISM

■ ***DESCRIPTION.*** **Hirsutism** (HER-soot-izm; Latin, meaning shaggy) is excessive growth of hair. Men typically have facial and chest hair due to stimulation by male sex hormones. Hair growth in these areas in females is quite distressing, however, and is usually caused by hormone abnormalities due to such disorders as adrenal tumors, ovarian tumors, and polycystic ovaries.

ALOPECIA

■ ***DESCRIPTION.*** **Alopecia** (AL-oh-PEE-shee-ah; Greek, meaning fox mange, which causes hair loss) is partial or complete hair loss, usually from the head.

■ ***ETIOLOGY.*** Alopecia can be caused by a number of factors, including aging, heredity, thyroid disease, iron deficiency, chemotherapy, radiation, and dermatitis. Alopecia can occur suddenly or over a period of time and can be temporary or permanent.

■ ***TREATMENT.*** Treatment of alopecia varies according to cause and usually restores hair growth. One of the most common causes of sudden, temporary alopecia is related to chemotherapy and radiation treatment. Hair growth normally returns when treatments are stopped.

MALE-PATTERNED BALDNESS

■ ***DESCRIPTION.*** Male-patterned baldness is a common cause of hair loss in men and is an inherited trait passed to males by their mothers. The mother does not have this type of hair loss because it is influenced by male sex hormones, but the pattern can easily be recognized in the mother's brothers or the affected individual's maternal uncles.

■ ***SYMPTOMS.*** Male-pattern baldness often begins around age 30 with a receding front hairline and loss of hair on the top and back portion of the head

(Figure 18–20). In some men, these areas of alopecia eventually meet, leaving hair on only the sides of the head. Alopecia in females is usually due to a hormonal or nutritional disorder.

■ ***TREATMENT.*** In the case of male-pattern baldness, hair growth can be restored to some degree by certain special medications. These medications are quite expensive, and loss of hair returns if treatment is discontinued. Other options include use of a wig, toupee, and hair transplantation.

TRAUMA

The skin is the outermost organ of the human body and the body's first line of defense. The position of the skin exposes it to high risk for receiving frequent trauma, which might be the result of mechanical, thermal, or electrical injury or radiation or pressure injury and insect or spider bites.

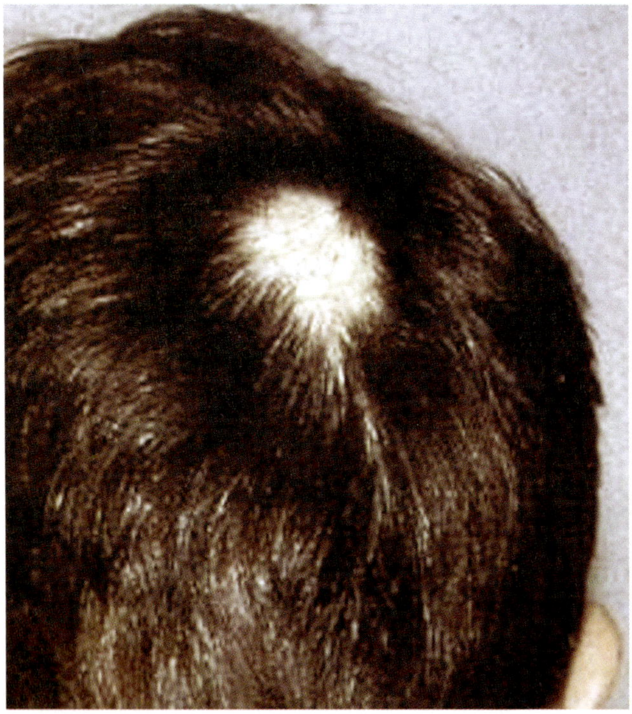

Courtesy of Mark L. Kuss

(A)

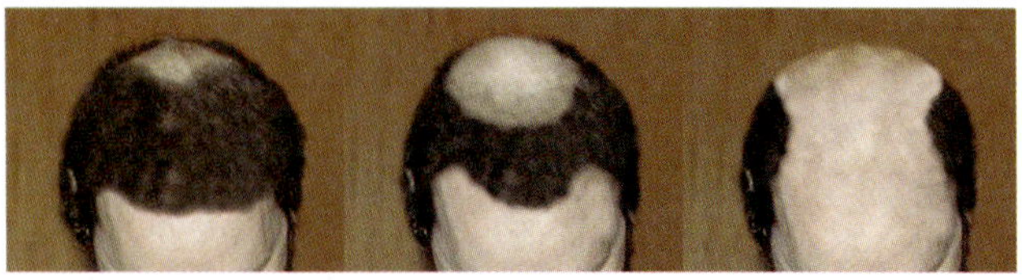

Courtesy of Mark L. K uss

(B)

FIGURE 18–20 (A) Alopecia. (B) Male pattern baldness.

Mechanical Skin Injury

Skin is exposed to mechanical trauma in a variety of ways. Mechanical trauma can be due to blunt or sharp objects and range from mild and insignificant to major and life-threatening. Types of mechanical skin injury include the following.

ABRASION

■ ***DESCRIPTION.*** A common mechanical trauma is caused by scraping away the skin surface. Abrasions are also called friction burns or rug burns.

■ ***SYMPTOMS.*** An **abrasion** is red, raw, and painful, but bleeding is usually minimal. A skinned knee is a typical example of an abrasion.

■ ***TREATMENT.*** Treatment generally consists of cleaning the area with soap and water, removing any embedded particles such as grass or rock, applying antibiotic ointment, and covering the area with a light sterile dressing.

BLUNT TRAUMA

■ ***DESCRIPTION.*** **Blunt trauma** can be caused when an individual is struck by items such as hammers and clubs or is thrown into objects such as steering wheels and walls. Falls also can cause blunt trauma.

■ ***SYMPTOMS.*** Blunt trauma often causes a large bruise called a **contusion** (kon-TOO-zhun), an accumulation of blood from injured or disrupted blood vessels in the tissue without breaking the skin (Figure 18–21).

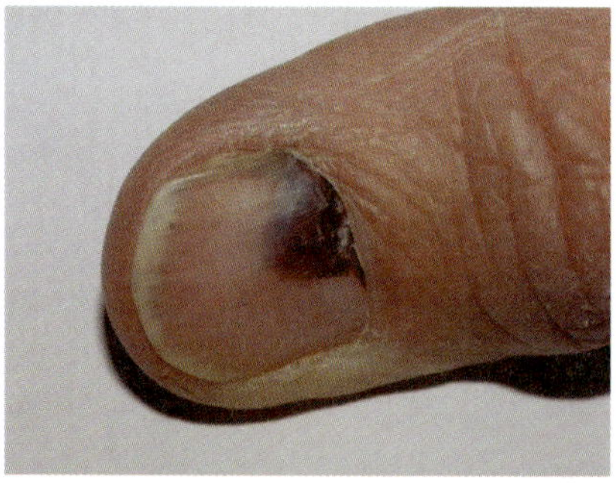

Courtesy of Larry J. Butler

FIGURE 18–21 Bruise of the finger due to blunt trauma.

AVULSION

■ **DESCRIPTION.** **Avulsion** occurs when a portion of skin or appendage is pulled or torn away. Avulsion injuries usually occur when tissue is caught up in some type of machinery. If an appendage is completely torn away, it is termed an amputation.

CRUSH TRAUMA

■ **DESCRIPTION.** Crush trauma occurs when tissue is caught between two hard surfaces. Crush injuries commonly involve fingers, hands, feet, and toes such as when hands and fingers are caught in doors or between objects or when heavy items are dropped on the fingers, hands, feet, and toes.

PUNCTURE INJURY

■ **DESCRIPTION.** Puncture injury occurs when a sharp object such as a knife, nail, or splinter of glass or metal is forced into the tissue. Bleeding is usually minimal. A feared complication of puncture injury is tetanus because puncture injuries set up an anaerobic condition favorable to tetanus bacteria.

LACERATION

■ **DESCRIPTION.** A **laceration** is a cut in the skin caused by a sharp object such as a knife, razor, glass, or metal. The edges of the laceration can be smooth, making repair easy, or the edges can be jagged, leading to a more difficult repair. A laceration with smooth, even edges is commonly called an **incision**.

Thermal Skin Injury

Thermal skin injury can be from excessive heat or cold or to short-term or long-term exposure to varying temperatures. Skin injury can range from mild to severe. Untreated severe skin injuries can become life-threatening.

HYPERTHERMIA

■ **DESCRIPTION.** Hyperthermia (hyper = excessive, thermia = temperature) occurs when the body is overheated from excessive exposure to the sun or a hot environment or to excessive exercise in a hot environment. There are two types of hyperthermia: heat exhaustion and heat stroke. The cause and treatment of these types of hyperthermia vary considerably.

HEAT EXHAUSTION

■ **DESCRIPTION.** Heat exhaustion is sometimes called heat prostration; it commonly occurs from excessive exercise or activity in a warm environment.

■ **SYMPTOMS.** The individual has profuse perspiration and loss of salt and water, leading to dehydration. The skin is cool and moist. The individual might feel weak and nauseated and might have muscle cramps. Body temperature is usually normal.

■ **TREATMENT.** The affected individual should lie quietly in a cool place. Fluid and salt replacement can include drinking tomato juice or other high-sodium drinks along with water. In extreme cases, the affected individual should be transported to the hospital.

HEAT STROKE

■ **DESCRIPTION.** Heat stroke is more serious than heat exhaustion. It occurs when the body's temperature-regulating mechanisms are no longer able to cope with the excessive exposure to heat.

■ **SYMPTOMS.** The body's core temperature rises above 105°F, and the skin is red and hot. The skin is dry with a noted absence of perspiration. The affected individual might feel nauseated and weak and can become mentally confused. In extreme cases, the confusion can progress to loss of consciousness with convulsions. Without rapid and effective treatment, brain damage and death can result.

■ **TREATMENT.** Treatment is aimed at immediate and aggressive cooling of the body by removing clothing and pouring cool water over the body or placing the body in a cool tub or pool. The affected individual should be immediately transported to a hospital.

BURNS

■ **DESCRIPTION.** Burns can be caused by fire, steam, exposure to hot liquids or items, chemicals, and electricity. The degree of tissue injury is related to the intensity of the heat and duration of exposure. Burns are classified by depth of skin injury and include first-, second- and third-degree burns.

■ **ETIOLOGY.** The main complications of burns are fluid loss and infection. Open tissue affected by second- and third-degree burns can leak pints to quarts of serous fluid per day, leading to dehydration and shock. *Pseudomonas*, the bacterium often causing infection, is noted for its ability to spread to the blood, leading to septicemia and death.

■ ***TREATMENT.*** Treatment of burns depends on the degree and type of burn. Generally, treatment will include cooling the tissue with cool water to prevent further burning. Pain is treated with analgesics ranging from over-the-counter products to narcotic analgesics, depending on the severity of pain. Antibiotics are given orally and intravenously to prevent or treat infection. Antibiotic ointments also can be applied directly to the burned area.

Surgical débridement might be needed to remove charred and necrotic tissue. In some cases, this can be accomplished by whirlpool treatments. Surgery is often necessary to graft skin, remove excessive scar tissue, and reshape deformities. Surgical treatment might be necessary multiple times over a period of months or years to obtain the desired results.

FIRST-DEGREE BURNS

■ ***DESCRIPTION.*** First-degree burns are fairly common and are characterized by pain, skin redness, and swelling. First-degree burns involve only the epidermis and are often the result of sunburn. Healing generally occurs within a week, followed by peeling of the damaged epidermis.

SECOND-DEGREE BURNS

■ ***DESCRIPTION.*** Second-degree burns are also called partial-thickness burns; they involve the epidermis and dermis and are characterized by extreme pain, redness, blisters, and open wounds. Second-degree burns usually heal in 2 to 3 weeks. If the burned area becomes infected, a second-degree burn can progress into a third-degree wound.

THIRD-DEGREE BURNS

■ ***DESCRIPTION.*** Third-degree burns are also called full-thickness burns; they involve the epidermis and entire dermis, exposing layers of fat, muscle, and bone. Tissue burned to the third degree is painless because the nerves in the dermis have been destroyed. This is not to say that individuals with third-degree burns do not have pain; there is extreme pain, but the pain is due to a layering of degrees of burn, with first- and second-degree areas surrounding the third-degree areas.

■ ***SYMPTOMS.*** This burn is characterized by charred and broken tissue layers. The affected individual can exhibit signs and symptoms of shock.

■ ***TREATMENT.*** Third-degree burns often need tissue grafting to heal. Scarring and deformity are common with third-degree tissue damage.

The amount of body surface burned generally correlates with the chance of survival for the affected individual. Body surface may be determined by applying the rule of nines (Figure 18–22). Burns exceeding 9% of the body are serious and should be treated in large medical centers with special burn units. Generally speaking, body burns of 25% to 30% of the body are extremely serious, and 60% body burns are usually fatal.

Other factors affecting the chance of survival include age, health, quality of care, and complications. Those who are older and the very young do not survive serious burns as well as other age groups.

COLD INJURIES

■ ***DESCRIPTION.*** Cold thermal injury is usually not as severe or life-threatening as heat or burn injuries. **Hypothermia** (hypo = low, therm = temperature) occurs when the body's core temperature falls below 95°F, which can occur when the body is cold for a long period of time or is exposed to extreme cold for even short periods of time. Exposure to wind and water increase the chilling effect and can lead to hypothermia in shorter amounts of time.

■ ***SYMPTOMS.*** Symptoms of hypothermia include extreme shivering, mental confusion, blue or cyanotic extremities, and weak pulse.

■ ***TREATMENT.*** Treatment includes removing wet clothing and warming the body with warm blankets, warm packs, or another person's body. Warm liquids can be given if the individual is conscious. The affected individual should be immediately transported to an emergency medical facility. Hypothermia can be fatal.

FROSTBITE

■ ***DESCRIPTION.*** **Frostbite** is the freezing of tissue, usually on the face, fingers, toes, and ears, and might or might not occur with hypothermia. Tissue affected by severe frostbite can become necrotic and need surgical débridement or amputation.

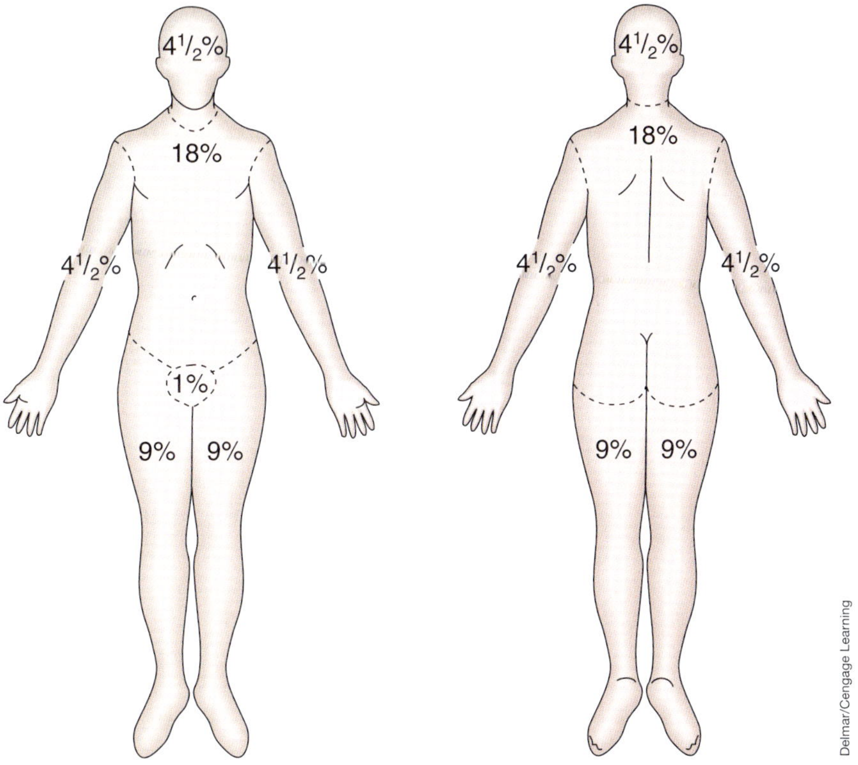

FIGURE 18–22 Rule of nines: used to calculate percentage of body surface burned.

■ ***SYMPTOMS.*** The tissue affected by frostbite usually is painless and white in color. With warming, the skin becomes painful and turns red.

■ ***TREATMENT.*** Treatment includes rapid warming in warm (not hot) water baths, not rubbing the affected tissue, and emergency treatment at a medical facility.

Electrical Injury

Electrical tissue injury is the result of contacting unprotected or inadequately insulated electrical wiring or coming in contact with lightning. Whatever the cause of injury, electrical tissue damage has a point of entry and an exit point. The point of entry is the area coming in contact with the electrical source and the exit point is the grounded area. Electricity travels through the body from point of entry to point of exit, causing burns and often causing deep tissue injury.

A common cause of death related to electrical injury is from respiratory and cardiac arrest. These conditions are caused by the physical jolt of electricity and the electrical current passing through the body interfere with the conduction system of the heart.

Radiation Injury

Radiation injury can be caused by ionizing radiation such as X-rays and by sunlight. Of the two, sunlight injury is the most common. Exposure to sunlight for short amounts of time leads to skin redness, but prolonged exposure can cause first- and second-degree burns to the skin. Fair-skinned persons are the most easily burned due to a lower number of pigment cells in the skin. Tanning of the skin occurs as a protective mechanism. Tanned skin returns to normal color when pigmented keratocytes in the epidermis are shed. Pigmented skin cells shed approximately every 30 days.

Radiation injury also can occur from exposure to tanning beds, which tan skin in the same manner as sun exposure. Tanning of the skin is a popular activity because of the cosmetically pleasant color produced, but the long-term effects of tanning are not so pleasant. Prolonged exposure to sun or tanning beds causes the skin to become prematurely dry, brittle, and wrinkled and to lose elasticity. These effects cause the skin to appear much older than its natural age. Another unpleasant effect of sun exposure is the development of skin cancers as discussed previously in this chapter.

Pressure Injury

Pressure injury is caused when placing pressure against tissue leads to a decrease in blood flow to this area. The most common type of pressure injury is a decubitus ulcer. Corns and calluses are also the result of pressure injury.

DECUBITUS ULCER

■ **DESCRIPTION.** Decubitus (dee-KYOU-bih-tus) ulcer is a pressure injury commonly called a bedsore or pressure sore. The term *decubitus* actually means the act of lying down or the position of lying down.

■ **ETIOLOGY.** Decubitus ulcers commonly affect the bony areas of the body such as the heels, sacrum, elbows, and head of individuals who spend prolonged amounts of time in bed. Increased pressure in these areas slows blood flow, thus leading to tissue ischemia and necrosis.

■ **PREVENTION.** Pressure sores can be avoided by frequent turning and repositioning to decrease tissue pressure and allow blood flow to the tissues. Massaging the affected area also can improve circulation.

CORNS AND CALLUSES

■ **DESCRIPTION.** Corns and calluses are protective hyperplasias of tissue as a result of pressure. The main difference between a corn and a callus is the location. Corns are commonly found on the feet and are due to ill-fitting shoes. Corns are usually painful, and the affected individual might seek to have them surgically removed.

Calluses are found in the palms of the hands and are related to pressure injury to the hands, generally due to working with hand tools or performing labor. Calluses are usually not painful and, in fact, protect the hands from repeated abrasions and blisters.

Insect and Spider Bites and Stings

There are thousands of varieties of insects and spiders. Most bites and stings are mild and cause only itching at the site, but in a few people, these can bring about serious reaction. Most bites and stings can be treated with home remedies.

INSECT BITES AND STINGS

■ **DESCRIPTION.** Insect bites and stings vary from bloodsucking mosquitoes, flies, and fleas, to the stings of bees, wasps, hornets, yellow jackets, and fire ants. Most of these bites and stings feel unpleasant and might cause swelling and itching at the site; however, insect bites also can transmit diseases such as malaria and yellow fever.

■ **SYMPTOMS.** Signs and symptoms of insect bites or stings often result from the injection of venom or poison into the skin. This venom incites an allergic reaction, the severity of which depends on the individual's sensitivity. Most symptoms are mild and disappear within a few days. An allergic reaction might cause intense itching, fever, and joint pain. A small percent of people develop a severe reaction called anaphylaxis, as discussed in Chapter 5.

■ **TREATMENT.** Treatment for mild reactions includes moving to an area to avoid more insects; if a stinger is involved, scraping or brushing it off with a knife or credit card; washing the affected area with soap and water; applying ice; applying hydrocortisone cream; and taking an antihistamine such as diphenhydramine (Benadryl). Pain can usually be controlled by a mild analgesic such as Tylenol.

If a severe reaction occurs with symptoms of difficulty breathing, swelling of the face or lips, hives, tachycardia, nausea, and vomiting, call 911 for immediate assistance.

Other emergency response includes laying the victim down on his or her back with feet higher than head, loosening tight clothing, covering with a blanket, and checking for special medications the individual might have for allergic reaction, such as an EpiPen. If vomiting occurs, turn the individual on his or her side to prevent aspiration. If breathing stops, begin cardiopulmonary resuscitation.

■ **PREVENTION.** To prevent bites and stings, use insect repellent, wear protective clothing, and watch for and avoid insect nests. If you have allergies to insects, always carry an emergency epinephrine kit.

SPIDER BITES

More than 20,000 species of spiders exist in the Americas, yet only 60 are capable of biting humans and, of these, only a few have a serious bite. Most spiders are not poisonous and are helpful to have around because they eat insects that can be annoying. However, two commonly poisonous spiders are the black widow and brown recluse.

BLACK WIDOW BITE

DESCRIPTION. The black widow is by far the most commonly known poisonous spider due to its famous red markings in the shape of an hourglass. The name comes from a mistaken belief that the female spider kills the male after mating. They are found mostly in the southern United States but appear in all states except Alaska. They try to avoid humans and tend to live in garages and attics. Only the female bites and this happens usually when she is disturbed or trying to protect her eggs.

ETIOLOGY. The venom of the black widow is a protein that affects the victim's nervous system. Even though this venom is one of the most potent produced by spiders, it causes severe response in only a few individuals.

SYMPTOMS. The first symptom is acute pain at the site. Other, more severe, symptoms include abdominal pain that mimics appendicitis, muscle cramps, nausea, fainting, dizziness, and chest pain.

The severity of the reaction to the bite depends on the age of the victim: the elderly and children are the most seriously affected. The bite is seldom fatal.

TREATMENT. Treatment includes cold compresses and pain relievers. Children, pregnant women, hypertensive individuals, and the elderly, if bitten, should be taken to the hospital for treatment.

PREVENTION. Prevention of bites includes taking care when reaching into dark areas where spiders might be living and eradication by professional pest services.

BROWN RECLUSE BITE

DESCRIPTION. The bite of the brown recluse spider can be very dangerous. Brown recluse spiders, also called fiddleback spider, violin spider, or brown fiddler, are native to the midwestern and southeastern United States. They live up to their name in that they have a distinctive violin shape on their backs and tend to hide in dark, warm, dry, areas such as attics, closets, porches, barns, and woodpiles and, in some instances, inside shoes. They are not aggressive and bite only when threatened and actually pressed against an individual's skin.

ETIOLOGY. The bite venom is a collection of enzymes that is extremely poisonous to a level that some say is more potent than a rattlesnake's. Even so, most bite sites become firm and heal within a few days with little scarring. On occasion, however, the reaction in the bite area will be more severe, with redness, blistering, and blue discoloration. The venom can cause destruction to tissues, often leading to necrosis of skin, fat, and blood vessels in areas immediately surrounding the bite site (Figure 18–23). Bites are rarely fatal, but deaths have been reported in children younger than 7 years of age.

SYMPTOMS. Symptoms of brown recluse spider bite include severe pain, severe itching, fever, nausea, and muscle pain.

TREATMENT. First aid consists of the application of an ice pack, administration of analgesic medications, and acquisition of prompt medical care. Further treatment includes pain medication, antihistamines, and antibiotics if infection occurs. No antivenin medication is available. A follow-up visit to the doctor might be necessary to monitor the wound, débride necrotic tissue if needed, and treat any secondary infection.

If possible, the spider should be caught in a clear, tightly closed container for future identification. It is important to seek medical treatment if a brown recluse bite is suspected because, in rare cases, necrosis can spread quickly, particularly when the venom reaches a blood vessel. When venom travels along a vein or artery, the resulting necrosis of tissue can be as large as several inches and might require extensive excising of tissue around the wound.

DIAGNOSIS. Diagnosis is based on a careful history and examination of the bite site, but no specific lab studies can confirm brown recluse bite. Diagnosis can be confirmed only if the spider is available for identification.

PREVENTION. Prevention of brown recluse spider bite includes activities to eliminate the spider by thorough house cleaning, installing tight-fitting windows and doors, and professional pest elimination services.

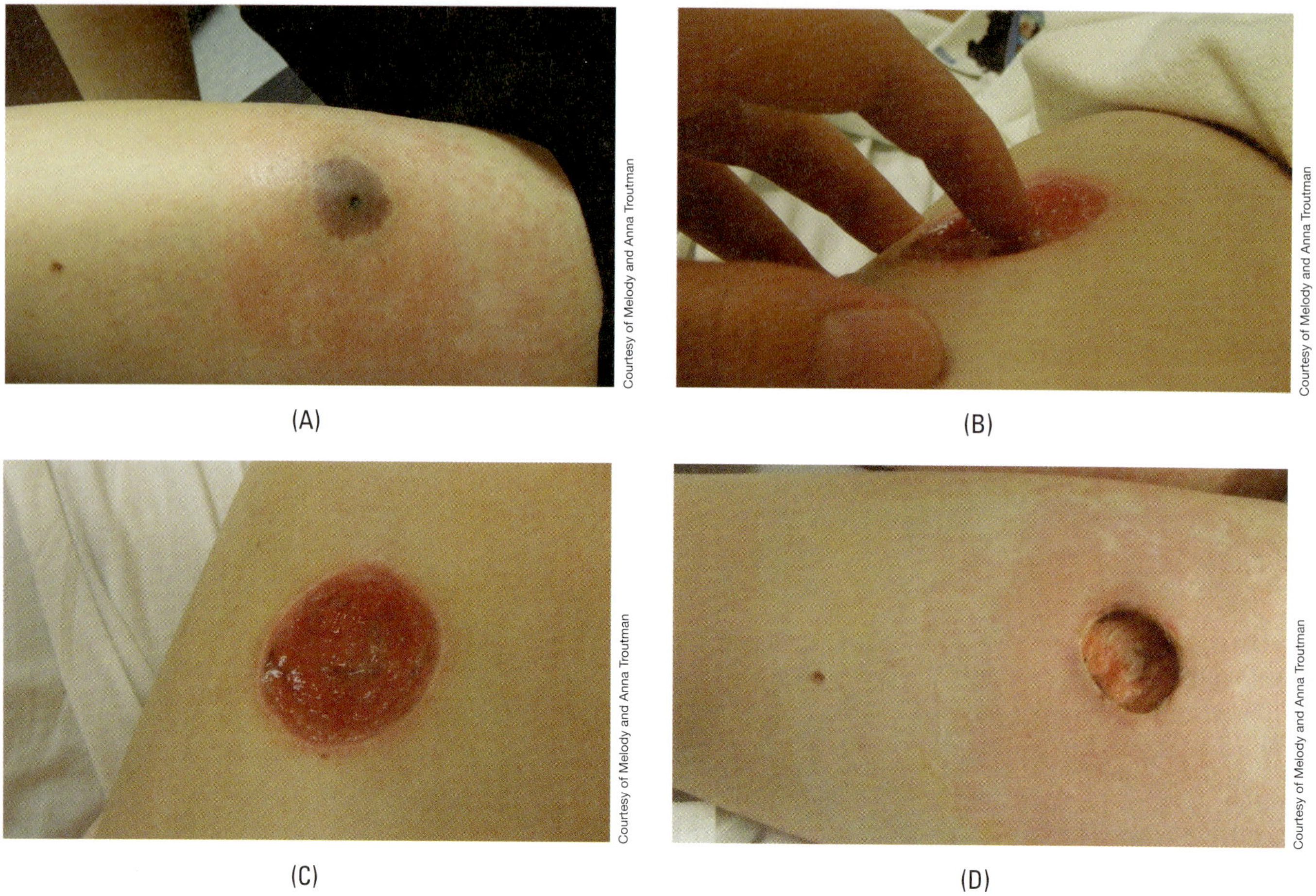

FIGURE 18–23 Stages of a recluse spider bite. (A) wound- a few hours after bite (B) wound- 1 day after bite (C) wound- 2 days after the bite (D) wound- after debridement of necrotic tissue.

RARE DISEASES

Elephantiasis

Elephantiasis is characterized by hypertrophy of the skin and subcutaneous tissue, giving it an elephant-like appearance. Inflammation of the lymphatic system also leads to fluid accumulation in the legs, causing them to become enlarged. Elephantiasis is caused by a parasitic worm that enters the lymphatic system and causes obstruction of drainage and accumulation of fluids. This disease is most commonly seen in tropical areas, such as central Africa, and is spread by mosquitoes and bloodsucking flies.

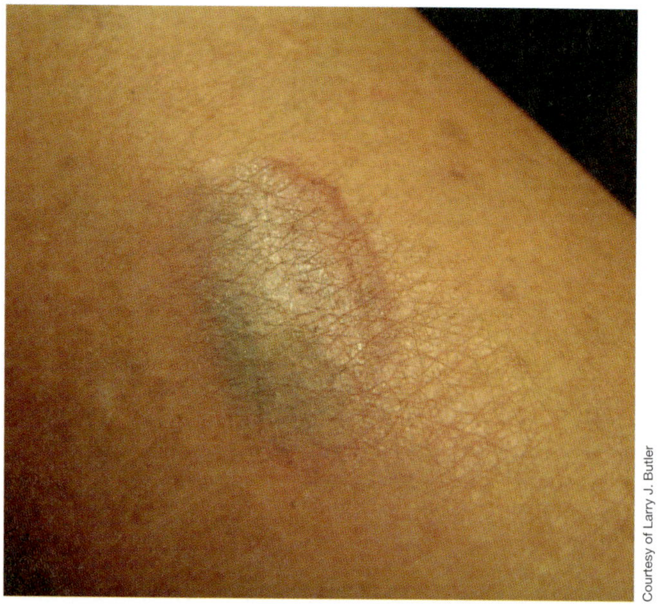

FIGURE 18–24 Senile keratosis.

EFFECTS OF AGING ON THE SYSTEM

Numerous changes develop in the integumentary system during the aging process. The epidermal layer becomes thinner and retains less water, which

GLIMPSE OF THE FUTURE

Improved Treatment for Vitiligo

Although topical or oral psoralen plus ultraviolet A (PUVA) has been one of the most commonly used treatments for vitiligo, in recent years research has shown that ultraviolet B (UVB) is also an effective therapy for the disorder. Using UVB treatment is simpler than PUVA and does not require using psoralen (a drug that reacts with UV light, causing darkening of the skin). It also may be safer in long-term therapy. More research needs to be completed to determine which treatment is the best for vitiligo, but since UVB does have advantages over PUVA, it may be the best alternative treatment for vitiligo in the future.

Source: Don, et al. (2006); MayoClinic.com (2008).

accounts for the easy tearing and dryness of the skin common in older adults. **Xerosis** (zee-ROE-sis; dry skin) is a major problem in older adults, who might have flaky, scaly skin and pruritis. The sweat and sebaceous glands do not function as well, further contributing to the dry skin problem. The youthful elasticity of the skin is lost, causing wrinkles and an aged appearance. If the individual has spent a great deal of time in the sun over the years, these problems will be exaggerated. The nails become thicker and might be difficult to trim. The hair becomes thinner and brittle. There might be extensive hair loss and graying.

Skin lesions are common in older people. Keratoses and skin cancers are the most common problems, especially in individuals who have been exposed to sunlight for many years without using protection (Figure 18–24). Seborrheic dermatitis, rosacea, and psoriasis are frequently seen disorders. Older adults with chronic disorders such as diabetes or peripheral vascular diseases are particularly prone to develop skin problems, especially pressure injuries. Older adults are also more likely to experience burn or cold injuries because they have decreased touch sensation.

SUMMARY

The skin is important in protecting the body from pathogens; in providing sensations of touch, heat, and cold; and in regulating body temperature. There are numerous skin conditions, some of which are manifestations of other body system diseases. Skin problems are very traumatic to the individual because they affect appearance and can cause extreme discomfort. Skin diseases range from mild to severe and from acute to chronic. Treatment for many of the skin conditions is symptomatic. Changes in the integumentary system in the older adult cause dry skin; thick, brittle nails; and gray, thinning hair. Older people are at increased risk for secondary skin disorders related to other system diseases.

REVIEW QUESTIONS

Short Answer

1. What is the main function of the integumentary system?

2. What are the most common symptoms of integumentary system disorders?

3. Which diagnostic tests are used to diagnose integumentary system disorders?

Matching

4. Match the skin condition in the left column with its description in the right column.

_____ Herpes	a. a form of cellulitis commonly involving the face
_____ Verruca	b. a chronic autoimmune disorder characterized by hardening and thickening of the skin and connective tissue
_____ Folliculitis	c. a condition caused by a tiny mite that burrows into the skin
_____ Erysipelas	d. an inflammation and infection of the hair follicle
_____ Tinea	e. a viral disease characterized by inflammation and fluid-filled blisters
_____ Scabies	f. a chronic skin condition characterized by red, raised lesions with distinct borders and silvery scales
_____ Eczema	g. a condition caused by papillomavirus that affects the keratin cells, causing hypertrophy
_____ Psoriasis	h. an inflammation of the skin also known as atopic dermatitis
_____ Scleroderma	i. a group of contagious fungal diseases of the skin

True or False

5. T F Genital warts are a sexually transmitted disease.

6. T F Carbuncles are most commonly caused by staphylococcus bacteria.

7. T F Pediculosis is an infestation of lice.

8. T F Tinea capitis is also known as jock itch because it is located in the groin area.

9. T F Comedones are plugged skin pores found in cases of acne.

10. T F A port wine stain is a type of erythema found on the neck or trunk of the body.

11. T F An avulsion is a traumatic crushing injury, often caused by heavy objects dropped on parts of the body such as the fingers.

12. T F Skin cancer is the most common type of cancer diagnosed in individuals.

13. T F Radiation injury can be caused by ionizing radiation such as X-rays and by sunlight.

14. T F In burn injuries, the amount of body surface burned generally correlates with the chance of survival of the affected individual.

15. T F Third-degree burns, also called partial thickness burns, involve the epidermis and dermis.

16. T F Cold thermal injury is usually more severe or life-threatening than heat or burn injuries.

17. T F In the aging process, the elasticity of the skin is lost, causing wrinkles and an aged appearance only if the individual has had constant exposure to sunlight over the years.

CASE STUDIES

■ Jenny Johnson is a 21-year-old college student who has vitiligo. She has some patchy areas on her legs and just a few on her arms. She visits the health clinic on campus where you work to talk about treatment for the disorder. What options are available for her? Is vitiligo detrimental to her overall health? What can you tell her about the progression of the problem? Where might she find out more information about her disorder?

■ Mrs. Moore is a 54-year-old school teacher who has been diagnosed with psoriasis. At the present time, she has a few patches on her arms and legs but not an extensive amount. She asks you to give her more information about the disorder. She wants to know whether it will get worse, if it will eventually heal, what she can do to relieve the symptoms, whether it is contagious, whether it is genetic, and what might cause it to get worse. How would you answer her questions? How much information should you give Mrs. Moore? Where might you refer her for more information? What is her long-term prognosis?

*Study*WARE™ Connection

To help you learn the content in this chapter, take a practice quiz or play an interactive game on your StudyWARE™ CD-ROM.

Workbook Practice

Go to your Workbook and complete the practice questions.

BIBLIOGRAPHY

American Social Health Association. (2008). Herpes Resource Center. American Social Health Association. *www.ashastd.org* (accessed March 28, 2008).

Bevins, C., & Fu-Tong, L. (2007). Rosacea: Skin innate immunity gone awry? *Nature Medicine 13*(8), 904–906.

Black widow spider. (2007). Survive Outdoors, Inc. *www.surviveoutdoors.com* (accessed July 2008).

Black widow spider bite. (2008). EMedicine Health. *www.emedicine.com* (accessed July 2008).

Brown recluse or fiddleback spider. (2008). Entomology and plant pathology. Oklahoma State University. *www.entoplp.okstate.edu* (accessed July 2008).

Buchannan, P., & Courtenay, M. (2007). Topical treatments for managing patients with eczema. *Nursing Standard 21*(41), 45–50.

Centers for Disease Control and Prevention. (2007). United States cancer statistics. *www.cdc.gov/uscs/* (accessed July 2008).

Clinical snippets. (2008). *Journal of Investigative Dermatology 128*(1), 1.

Dark side of ATP may hold clues to cause of rosacea. *Dermatology Nursing 19*(3), 306.

Don, P., Luga, A., Dacko, A., & Hardwick, K. (2006). Treatment of vitiligo with broadband ultraviolet B and vitamins. *International Journal of Dermatology 45*(1), 63–65.

Erbil, A., Sezer, E., Koc, E., Tunca, M., Tastan, H., & Demiriz, M. (2008). Acrokeratoelastiodosis treated with the erbium: YAG laser. *Clinical & Experimental Dermatology 33*(1), 30–31.

Grimsrud, T., & Andersen, A. (2008). Protective effect from solar exposure, risk of an ecological fallacy. *European Journal of Cancer 44*(1), 16–18.

Hemangioma. (2008). Mayo Clinic. *www.mayoclinic.com* (accessed July 2008).

Herpes simplex. (2008). Wipimedia Foundation, Inc. *www.wikipedia.org* (accessed July 2008).

Insect bites. (2007). E Medicine Health. *www.emedicinehealth.com* (accessed July 2008).

Issues in antifungal susceptibility testing. (2008). *Journal of Antimicrobial Chemotherapy 61*(0), 13.

Klevens, R., Morrison, M., Nadle, J., Petit, S., Gershman, K., Ray, S., et al. (2007). Invasive methicillin-resistant staphylococcus aureus infections in the United States. *JAMA 298*(15): 1763–1771.

Kockler, D., & McCarthy, M. (2007). Zoster vaccine live. *Pharmacology 27*(7), 1013–1019.

Koo, J. & Desai, R. (2003). Traditional Chinese medicine in dermatology. *Dermatologic Therapy, 16*(2), 98–105.

Luther, J., & Glesby, M. (2007). Dermatologic adverse effects of antiretroviral therapy: Recognition and management. *American Journal of Clinical Dermatology 8*(4), 221–233.

MayoClinic. (2008). Vitiligo. MayoClinic. *www.mayoclinic.com* (accessed March 28, 2008).

Meduri, N., Vandergriff, T., Rasmussen, H., & Jacobe, H. (2007). Phototherapy in the management of atopic dermatitis: A systematic review. *Photodermatology, Photoimmunology & Photomedicine 23*(4), 106–112.

MRSA Infections. (2008). Medicine Net, Inc. *www.medicinenet.com/mrsa* (accessed July 2008).

MRSA: Methicillin-resistant *Staphylococcus aureus* in healthcare settings. (2007). Centers for Disease Control and Prevention. *www.cdc.gov* (accessed July 2008).

Neil, S. (2006). You may not know about anogenital skin disorders. *Pulse 66*(46), 59–61.

Oliver, P. (2006). Topical photodynamic therapy: An introduction for nurses. *British Journal of Nursing 15*(15), 811–813.

Reid, F. (2007). Psoriasis treatment and management in primary care. *Primary Health Care 17*(9), 25–29.

Scabies. (2008). Mayo Foundaton for Medical Education and Research. *www.mayoclinic.com* (accessed July 2008).

Seborrheic dermatitis. (2007). Medline Plus. *www.nim.nih.gov/medline* (accessed July 2008).

Seghal, V., & Srivastava, G. (2006a). Lepra vaccine: Misinterpreted myth. *International Journal of Dermatology 45*(2), 164–167.

Seghal, V., & Srivastava, G. (2006b). Vitiligo: Autoimmunity and immune responses. *International Journal of Dermatology 45*(5), 583–590.

Sezer, E., & Etikan, I. (2007). Local narrowband UVB vs. local PUVA in the treatment of chronic hard eczema. *Photodermatology, Photoimmunology & Photomedicine 23*(1), 10–14.

Skin Drink. (2007). *Natural Health 37*(8), 30.

Spider bites. (2007). Bad Spider. *www.badspiderbites.com* (accessed July 2008).

Soeborg, T., Basse, L., & Halling-Sorensen, B. (2007). Risk assessment of topically applied products. *Toxicology 236*(1/2), 140–148.

Weatherhead, S., Robson, S., & Reynolds, N. (2007). Eczema in pregnancy. *British Medical Journal 335*(7611), 152–154.

UNIT III

Genetic and Developmental, Childhood, and Mental Health Diseases and Disorders

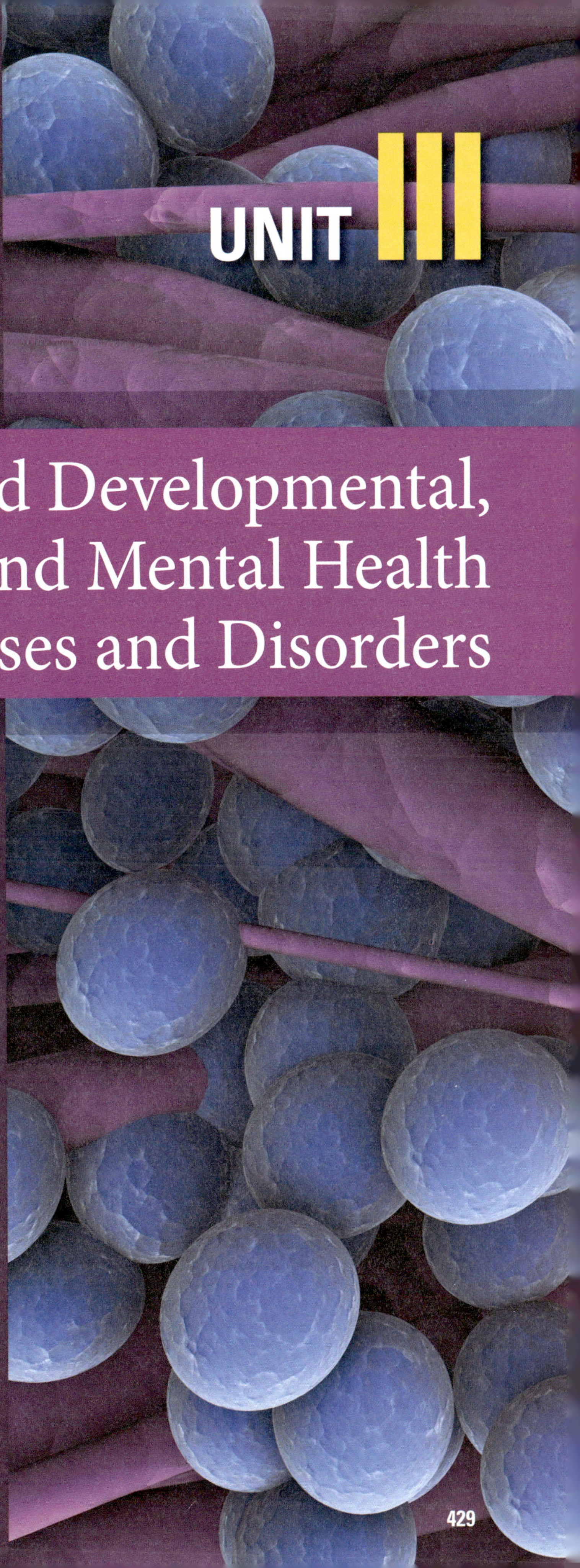

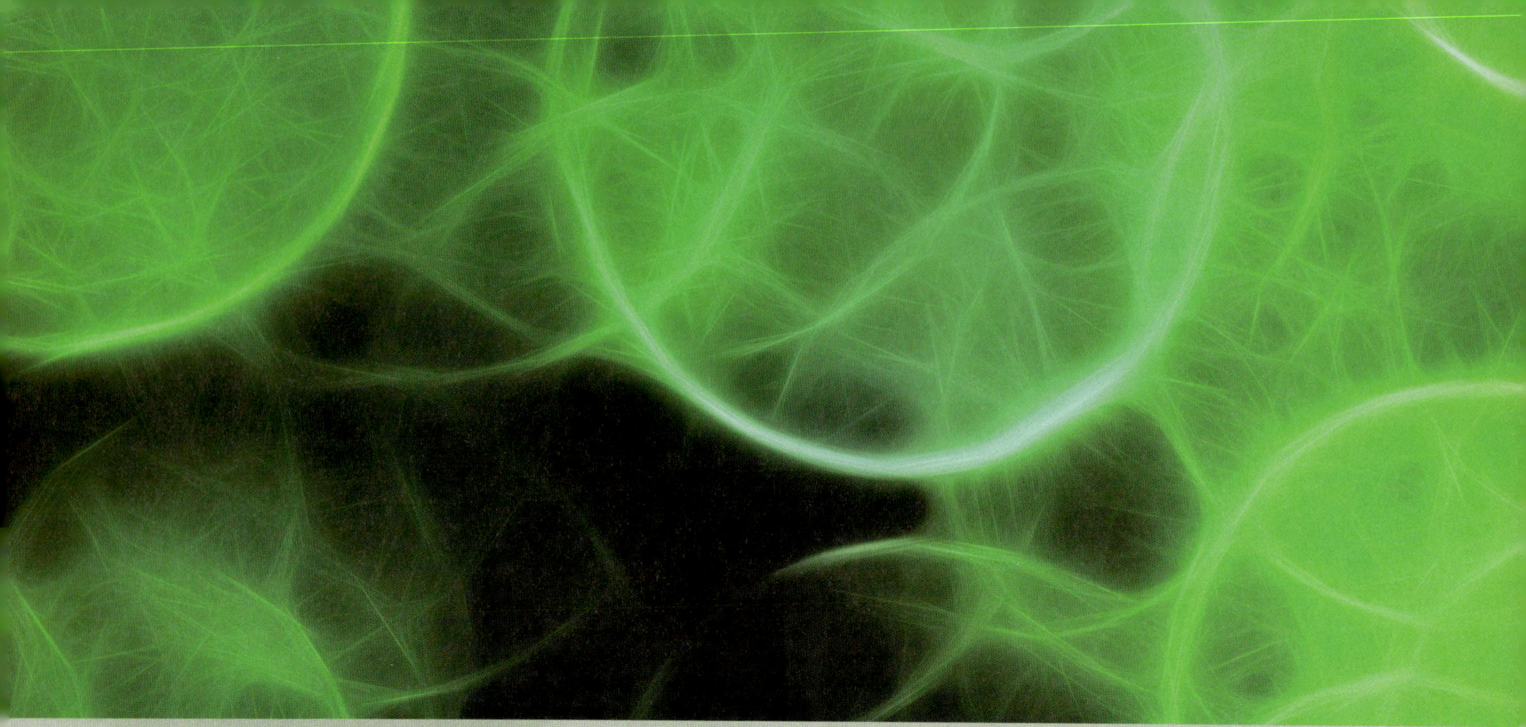

OUTLINE

- Anatomy and Physiology
- Common Signs and Symptoms
- Diagnostic Tests
- Common Genetic and Developmental Disorders
  Musculoskeletal
  Neurologic
  Cardiovascular
  Blood
  Digestive
  Urinary
  Reproductive
  Other Developmental Disorders
  Multisystem Diseases and Disorders
- Trauma
  Failure to Thrive
  Fetal Alcohol Syndrome
  Congenital Rubella Syndrome
- Rare Diseases
  Anencephaly
  Achondroplasia
  Tay–Sachs Disease
- Summary
- Review Questions
- Case Studies
- Bibliography

KEY TERMS

Alleles (p. 433)
Atresia (p. 443)
Auscultation (p. 441)
Autosomes (p. 432)
Buccal smear (p. 432)
Congenital anomaly (p. 436)
Delusions (p. 448)
Dominant (p. 433)
Epicanthus (p. 450)
Exocrine (p. 449)
Gene (p. 432)
Genotypes (p. 433)
Germ cells (p. 432)
Heterozygous (p. 433)
Homozygous (p. 433)
Karyotyping (p. 432)
Meiosis (p. 432)
Microcephaly (p. 451)
Mitosis (p. 432)
Murmurs (p. 441)
Phenotype (p. 433)
Pyloromyotomy (p. 445)
Recessive (p. 433)
Somatic (p. 432)
Stricture (p. 442)
Viscous (p. 449)

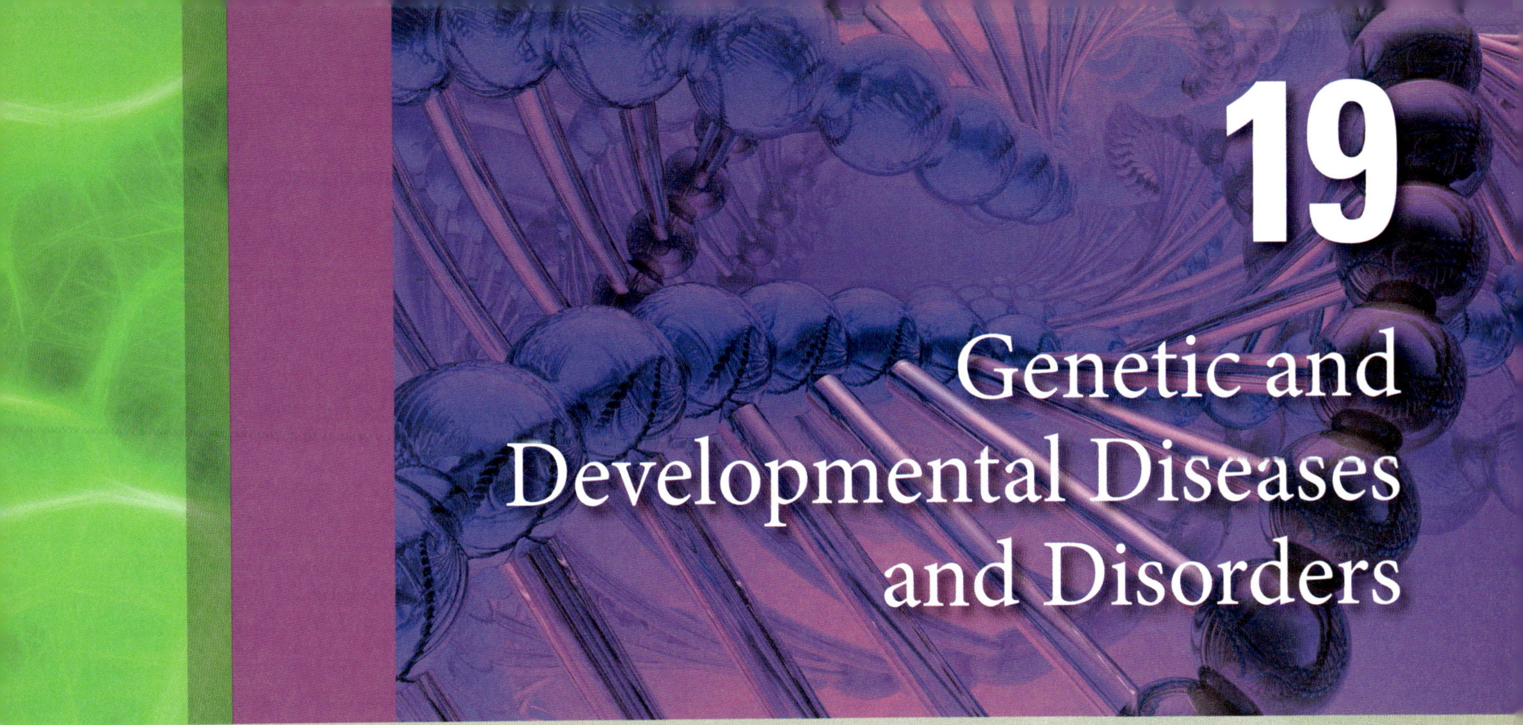

19

Genetic and Developmental Diseases and Disorders

LEARNING OBJECTIVES

Upon completion of the chapter, the learner should be able to:

1. Define the terminology common to genetic and developmental disorders.
2. Identify the important signs and symptoms associated with genetic and developmental disorders.
3. Describe the common diagnostics used to determine the type and cause of genetic or developmental disorders.
4. Identify the common genetic and developmental disorders.
5. Describe the typical course and management of the common genetic and developmental disorders.

OVERVIEW

Genetic and developmental disorders can first appear or be diagnosed at any age throughout the life span. Some are readily diagnosed at birth; others do not display symptoms until childhood, adolescence, or adulthood. Although some disorders have relatively few symptoms, others are profoundly disabling and can even result in early death. In disorders such as cystic fibrosis or Tay–Sachs disease, genetic testing can inform an individual of whether he or she is a carrier of the disease. There are many other disorders, however, for which testing is not yet available. ■

ANATOMY AND PHYSIOLOGY

The nucleus of each cell of the normal body has 46 chromosomes or 23 pairs of chromosomes. Most **somatic** (body) cells can reproduce in a process called **mitosis** (mi-TOE-sis), during which the 46 chromosomes duplicate and divide into two identical daughter cells, each containing 46 chromosomes (Figure 19–1).

Germ (sex) **cells**, specifically the ova and sperm, also have 46 chromosomes, but division in these cells is different—they do not duplicate before division. This process is called **meiosis** (my-OH-sis) and results in each cell carrying only half the number: 23 chromosomes (see Figure 19–1).

Meiosis is necessary to maintain the normal 46 chromosomes in a newly formed individual. When an ovum (carrying 23 chromosomes) is fertilized with a sperm (carrying 23 chromosomes), the newly formed individual will have a combined total of the normal 46 chromosomes. Half of these, or 23 chromosomes, will have come from each parent.

Of the 46 chromosomes each individual cell possesses, 44 chromosomes, or 22 pairs, determine somatic or body function and are called **autosomes** (auto = self, somes = body). One pair (or two chromosomes) are sex chromosomes and determine the sex of the individual.

Normal females have XX chromosomes as the sex chromosome, and males have XY chromosomes. A female germ cell, or ovum, undergoes meiosis and divides into two separate X chromosomes; thus, the only chromosome a female can give is an X, or female, chromosome. Male germ cells, or sperm, undergo meiosis and divide into two separate chromosomes, one X and one Y, so the male can give an X (female) or Y (male) chromosome. This explains why the male partner, or sperm, determines the sex of the fetus.

If an X sperm combines with the ova, the result is XX, and the fetus is female. If a Y sperm combines with the ova, the result is XY, and the fetus is male. Because each male germ cell division results in one X and one Y, there is a 50/50 chance of the fetus being male or female. These two chromosomes, the sex chromosomes, are in every cell of the body and are responsible for directing the activity of the cell specifically for a female or for a male.

Chromosomes can be visualized by a process known as **karyotyping** (CARE-ee-oh-TYPE-ing), which involves taking a picture of a cell during mitosis, arranging the chromosome pairs in order of largest to smallest, and numbering them 1 through 23.

Sex chromosomes can be evaluated by a simple **buccal smear**, performed by obtaining squamous epithelial cells from the buccal cavity of the mouth, staining the cell, and microscopically observing for X chromosomes called Barr bodies. Barr bodies can be visualized when two X chromosomes are present (female). If there is no Barr body, the individual is male.

X chromosomes are much larger than Y chromosomes and carry more genetic information. The X chromosome not only carries genes for female characteristics but also for other genes essential to life, such as those for blood formation, various activities of metabolism, and immunity. The Y chromosome carries only the genes related to maleness and masculinity.

Chromosomes are made of ultramicroscopic units of deoxyribonucleic acid (DNA) arranged in a specific order, each of which is called a **gene**. Each

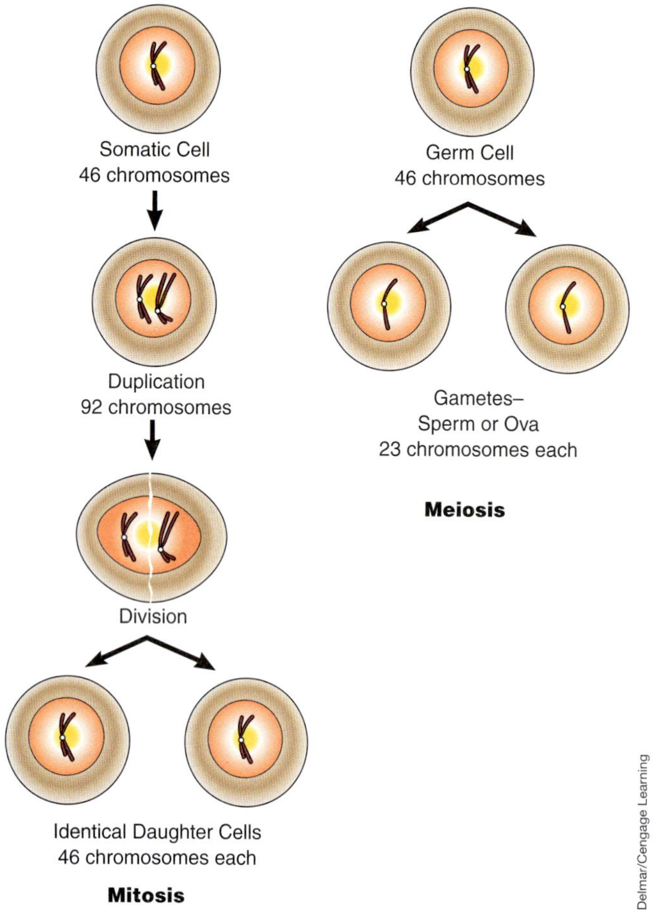

FIGURE 19–1 Cell division: mitosis and meiosis.

chromosome is composed of thousands of genes located at specific positions in the chromosome.

When the chromosomes (one from each parent) pair up during fertilization of the egg, the genes on the chromosomes align and are called **alleles** (ah-LEELS). This matched gene pair determines heredity or, in other words, expresses those characteristics inherited from parents. When one thinks of genes and heredity, we usually think of facial features such as hair and eye color, but genes also determine the entire physical makeup of the individual from the length of toes to the color and texture of skin.

As discussed in previous chapters, heredity is thought to play a part in many other processes such as the development of plaque in arteries and the occurrence of rheumatic fever, obesity, and alcoholism in families, to name only a few.

To understand basic heredity, one must look at individual **genotypes**—the genetic pattern of the individual. Each gene in an allele or matched pair of genes can be **dominant** (in control) or **recessive** (lacking control). Dominant genotypes are expressed with a capital letter (B, for example), whereas recessive genotypes are expressed with a small letter (b, for example).

If the alleles, or genes in a pair, match, such as BB or bb, they are said to be **homozygous** (homo = one, zygo = yoked or paired). If the alleles do not match, such as Bb, they are **heterozygous** (hetero = different, zygo = yoked or paired).

Expression of a trait such as brown hair or blue eyes is called **phenotype**. Generally speaking, homozygous alleles, whether dominant or recessive, will always express the trait. Heterozygous pairs will express the phenotype of the dominant gene only. Heterozygous pairs are often said to be carriers of recessive disorders because the recessive trait will not be expressed unless paired with another recessive gene (Figure 19–2).

Abnormalities can be due to chromosomal, genetic, or environmental factors or a combination of these. Chromosomal disorders are usually related to the number or placement of the chromosome. Chromosomes can fail to separate properly during cell division, causing one daughter cell to have an extra chromosome and the other daughter cell to have none.

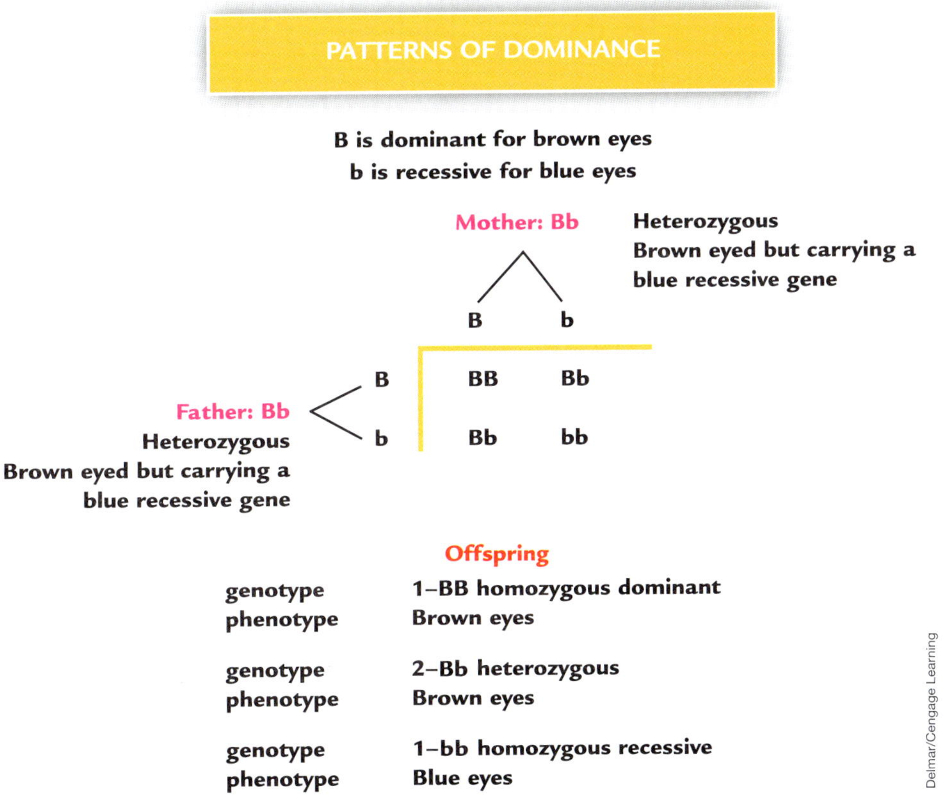

FIGURE 19–2 Patterns of dominance.

Abnormal number or structure of autosomal (or body) chromosomes is usually incompatible with life. These chromosomes carry a large number of essential genes, and such major chromosomal abnormalities usually lead to spontaneous abortion of the fetus. The most common autosomal chromosomal disorder is Down syndrome.

An abnormal number of chromosomes in the sex chromosomes is less serious but does lead to a number of abnormalities, disorders that are not usually apparent until puberty, when sexual characteristics are found to be abnormal.

An individual can acquire an abnormal gene in two ways: (1) by mutation of the gene during meiosis, affecting the newly formed fetus, or (2) by passage of the abnormal gene from the parents (heredity).

Genetic disorders are passed to offspring in four ways: autosomal dominant, autosomal recessive, sex-linked dominant, and sex-linked recessive.

1. **Autosomal dominant** Dominant disorders are easily recognized because presence of the disorder identifies those individuals with the dominant gene. The line of inheritance is easily followed from one generation to another.

   Dominant genes will always be expressed, whether homozygous (PP) or heterozygous (Pp). An example of an autosomal dominant disorder is polydactyly, evidenced by an excessive number of fingers or toes. Refer to Figure 19–3 to see how individuals carrying a dominant gene (P) would have polydactyly.

2. **Autosomal recessive** Recessive disorders are seen only when two recessive genes are paired (cc). Cystic fibrosis is an autosomal recessive disorder. Each parent might be phenotypically normal or without sign of the disorder but be a heterozygous carrier (Cc) of the disorder. If each parent is heterozygous, the chance of the offspring having the disorder is one in four (Figure 19–4a). If one parent has the disorder (cc), the chances increase to one in two (Figure 19–4b). If one parent is homozygous dominant (CC), none of the offspring will be affected (Figure 19–4c).

   The occurrence of recessive disorders is often quite surprising to a family because this disorder can skip generations and hundreds of years before it is paired with another recessive gene and expressed.

AUTOSOMAL DOMINANT PATTERN

Polydactyly is dominant (P)
Normal finger number is recessive (p)

Polydactyly father \ Normal mother	p	p
P	Pp	Pp
P	Pp	Pp

Offspring

genotype (all 4) **heterozygous**
phenotype **polydactyly**

FIGURE 19–3 Autosomal dominant pattern.

AUTOSOMAL RECESSIVE PATTERN

Genotype	Phenotype
cc (affected)	cystic fibrosis
CC	normal
Cc (carrier)	normal

Father Normal (carrier) \ Mother Normal (carrier)	C	c
C	CC	Cc
c	Cc	cc

Offspring

genotype	**1–CC homozygous dominant**
phenotype	**Normal**
genotype	**2–Cc heterozygous (carrier)**
phenotype	**Normal**
genotype	**1–cc homozygous recessive**
phenotype	**Cystic fibrosis**

If both parents are heterozygous, there is a 1 in 4 chance of having a child with cystic fibrosis.

(A)

FIGURE 19–4 Autosomal recessive pattern.

AUTOSOMAL RECESSIVE PATTERN

Genotype	Phenotype
cc (affected)	cystic fibrosis
CC	normal
Cc (carrier)	normal

Mother
Normal (carrier)

		C	c
Father Has cystic fibrosis	c	Cc	cc
	c	Cc	cc

Offspring

genotype 2–Cc heterozygous (carrier)
phenotype Normal

genotype 2–cc homozygous recessive
phenotype Cystic fibrosis

If one parent has the disorder, the chances of having a child with cystic fibrosis increase to 1 in 2.

(B)

AUTOSOMAL RECESSIVE PATTERN

Genotype	Phenotype
cc (affected)	cystic fibrosis
CC	normal
Cc (carrier)	normal

Mother
Normal (carrier)

		C	c
Father Normal (homozygous dominant)	C	CC	Cc
	C	CC	Cc

Offspring

genotype 2–CC homozygous dominant
phenotype Normal

genotype 2–Cc heterozygous (carrier)
phenotype Normal

If one parent is homozygous dominant, none of the offspring will be affected.

(C)

FIGURE 19–4 Autosomal recessive pattern (continued).

3. **Sex-linked dominant** Like autosomal dominant disorders, these are rarer than the recessive disorders and are easily recognized.
4. **Sex-linked recessive** These disorders are typically carried by females and passed to males. The reason for this is that recessive gene disorders on the X chromosome of the female are overridden by the dominance of the normal gene on the other X chromosome.

In males, the X disorder is expressed because there is no corresponding gene on the Y chromosome. X-linked disorders usually appear every other generation because they are passed from mother to son (Figure 19–5). The affected male (son) will pass this disorder to all of his daughters, who then become carriers.

The affected male is unable to pass this disorder to his sons because the male gives a Y chromosome to sons, not an X. All the carrier daughters can then pass the disorder to their sons. If the mother is a carrier

SEX-LINKED RECESSIVE PATTERN

Hemophilia is recessive X linked
X and Y are chromosomes
H and h are dominant and recessive genes
found only on the X chromosome

Mother
Normal (carrier)

		XH	Xh
Father Normal	Yo	**XHYo** boy normal	**XhYo** boy hemophiliac
	XH	**XHXH** girl normal	**XHXh** girl normal (carrier)

FIGURE 19–5 Sex-linked recessive pattern.

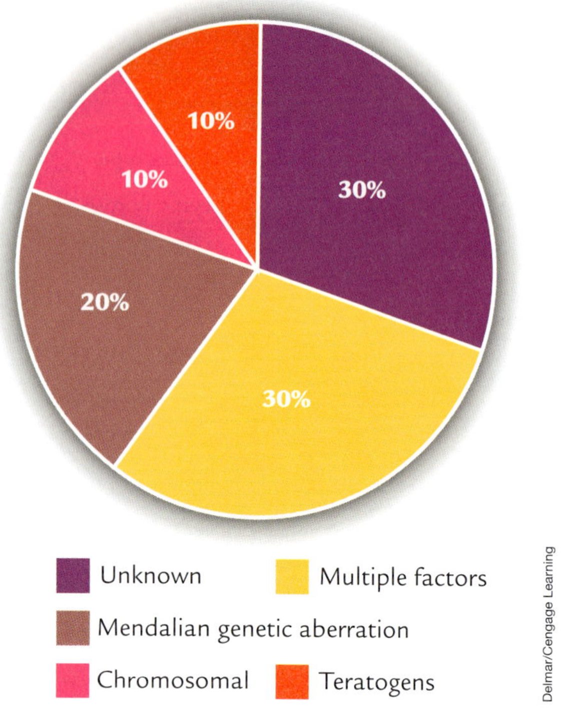

FIGURE 19–6 Causes of congenital anomalies.

(XX Hh), there is a possibility that some of her sons will not be affected. If the mother has the disorder (XX hh), which is very rare with X-linked disorders, all her sons will have the disorder. Hemophilia and muscular dystrophy are both sex-linked recessive disorders.

Approximately 2% of all newborns have a significant birth defect, or **congenital** (kon-JEN-ih-tahl; present at birth), **anomaly** (ah-NOM-ah-lee; abnormality). A high percentage of defects (60%) are due to an unknown cause.

Other causes are genetic (20%), chromosomal (10%), and teratogens (ter-AT-oh-gens) or environmental (10%) (Figure 19–6). Chromosomal and genetic causes have been discussed. Teratogens include any chemical, substance, or exposure that can cause a physical defect in a fetus during pregnancy. Teratogens are commonly thought of as environmental causes and include maternal radiation, infection, metabolic disorders, smoking, alcohol, drugs, and medications, to name only a few.

COMMON SIGNS AND SYMPTOMS

Signs and symptoms of the various genetic and developmental disorders vary, depending on the disorder, and are discussed individually with each disorder.

DIAGNOSTIC TESTS

Diagnosis of many of the genetic and developmental disorders begins with a physical examination of the affected individual. Diagnostic tests for these disorders vary, depending on the disorder, and are discussed individually with each disorder. Prenatal diagnosis of genetic and developmental disorders is beneficial for genetic and family counseling. Tests to diagnose prenatal disorders include:

- Ultrasonography of the fetus to detect malformations of the head, internal organs, and extremities.
- Amniotic fluid analysis to determine genetic and chromosomal disorders.
- Maternal blood analysis to observe for abnormal fetal substances.

COMMON GENETIC AND DEVELOPMENTAL DISORDERS

There are hundreds of genetic and developmental disorders among populations; however, most of them occur very rarely.

Genetic or developmental disorders might affect only one body system or involve several systems. Muscular dystrophy, for example, which affects the musculoskeletal system, can also be considered a neurological system disease because it affects the neurons, thereby affecting muscle movement.

Some of the more familiar genetic and developmental disorders are covered in this chapter.

Musculoskeletal

Genetic and developmental musculoskeletal disorders are some of the more familiar severe disorders. The severity of the disease varies with the particular disorder and other problems the individual has.

MUSCULAR DYSTROPHY

DESCRIPTION. Muscular dystrophy (MD) (dys = abnormal, trophic = nourishment, growth) is a group of genetically inherited diseases characterized by progressive degeneration, or weakening, of the muscles. The affected muscles are unable to store needed protein. Malnourished muscle fibers die and are replaced with fat and connective tissue. These fibers are unable

GLIMPSE OF THE FUTURE

A Potential New Muscular Dystrophy Drug

A new drug developed in the Netherlands may be a future treatment for Duchenne's muscular dystrophy. In this type of MD, the individual is unable to produce an essential muscle protein called dystrophin. This new drug allows the person to produce the necessary protein. The experimental drug is one of a group of drugs called antisense compounds. Some of these compounds are being studied for use in treating cancer, heart disease, and other disorders. Although the study was done on a small number of affected individuals, it has promise for others with the disease. However, the researchers say many more years of study are necessary to find the safe and therapeutic effects of antisense drugs.

Source: Grady (2007).

COMPLEMENTARY AND ALTERNATIVE THERAPY

Green Tea Extract for Muscular Dystrophy

A variety of herbal preparations and supplements, such as creatine, glutamine, and green tea extract, have been used to treat MD and related disorders. There has been some evidence that creatine (an amino acid found in muscle) and glutamine (a nonessential amino acid) have helped with some of the problems in MD. In one study, the effects of green tea extract were tested on dystrophic mice to see whether that did affect the muscles; the results showed improved muscle residual force and decreased necrosis of muscles. The results demonstrated that diet supplementation with green tea extract was beneficial in dystrophic mice. Whether the same findings would occur in humans is to be determined.

Source: Dorchies, et al. (2006).

to contract and function like muscle fibers. Over a period of time, the muscle digresses from weak to useless.

■ ***DESCRIPTION.*** The most common type of MD is Duchenne's MD, also called pseudohypertrophic (pseudo = false, hyper = excessive, trophic = nourishment, growth) MD. The affected muscles appear healthy and bulging when, in reality, it is bulking up in size from fat deposits. This bulking of muscle mass is especially noticeable in the calf muscle.

■ ***ETIOLOGY.*** Duchenne's MD is a sex-linked disorder generally passed from mother to son.

■ ***SYMPTOMS.*** Onset is usually between the ages of two to five years of age. The pelvic and leg muscles are usually affected first, leading to a characteristic waddling gait, toe walking, lordosis, and Gower's maneuver (a characteristic way of getting up from a squatting position that demonstrates the weakness of the pelvic muscles). (See Figure 19–7.)

Affected children are usually confined to a wheelchair by age 9. Life expectancy is usually in the late teens or early 20s, with death due to respiratory or cardiac complications.

■ ***DIAGNOSIS.*** Diagnosis is made on the basis of physical examination, muscle biopsy, and electromyography.

■ ***TREATMENT.*** Although there is no cure for MD, physical therapy, orthopedic appliances such as leg braces, and exercise are quite effective in maintaining mobility and quality of life.

■ ***PREVENTION.*** There are no preventive measures other than genetic counseling.

GLIMPSE OF THE FUTURE

New Treatment for Problems in Cerebral Palsy

Problems with hypertonicity (increased muscle tension or stiffness) associated with cerebral palsy may be reduced with botulinum toxin A (BTX-A). This is a poisonous toxin that is used medically in small doses. It is most commonly known as Botox and has been widely used in cosmetic treatments. In a recent study, high-dose BTX-A was found to be an effective treatment for the increased muscle stiffness problems in children with cerebral palsy. Although the study concluded that high-dose BTX-A is safe and can be tolerated by children with cerebral palsy, more research needs to be done to ensure the benefits and safety of this treatment.

Source: Willis, et al. (2007).

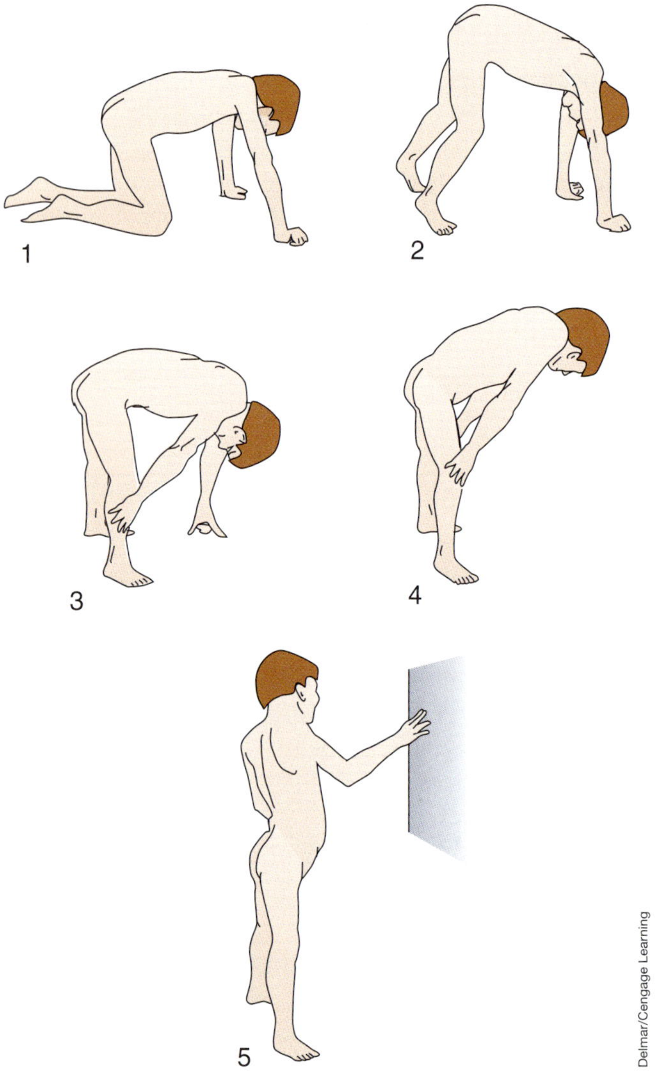

FIGURE 19–7 Gower's maneuver.

CONGENITAL HIP DISLOCATION (CHD)

■ ***DESCRIPTION.*** CHD is an abnormality of the hip joint, or acetabulum, resulting in the femoral head, or ball, slipping out of the normal position. CHD is more common in girls and is usually obvious during the first few months of life.

■ ***ETIOLOGY.*** It is thought that this disorder occurs as a result of (1) improper positioning of the fetus in the uterus prior to or during birth or (2) the maternal hormones, which relax the mother's pelvic ligaments during labor, also relaxing the joint ligaments in the infant.

■ ***SYMPTOMS.*** The affected infant might exhibit asymmetrical folds of the affected thigh, a difference in leg length, and limited abduction, called a positive Ortolani's sign (Figure 19–8).

■ ***DIAGNOSIS.*** Diagnosis is confirmed by physical examination and hip joint X-ray studies.

■ ***TREATMENT.*** Treatment involves closed reduction (placing the femoral head in proper position) and maintaining the normal position with a splint or cast for approximately 2 to 3 months. Treatment might require surgery in older children. The earlier the treatment is begun, the better the prognosis.

■ ***PREVENTION.*** Prevention is aimed at prenatal care to determine the position of the baby in the womb to assess and treat for possible CHD. The practice of swaddling, or wrapping the baby's body tightly in a blanket with legs forced into a closed, straight-together

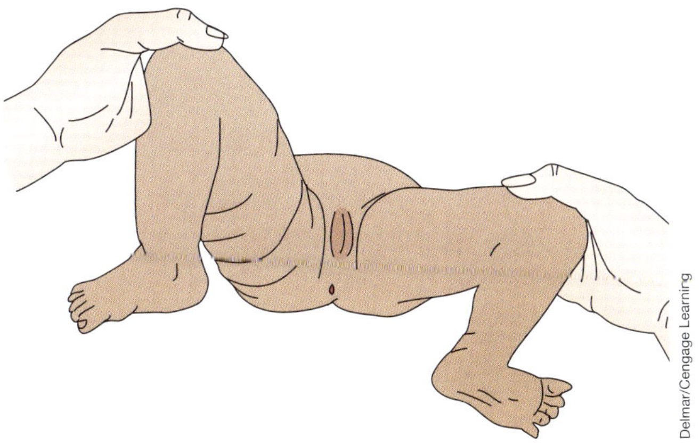

FIGURE 19–8 Asymmetrical thigh folds and Ortolani's sign in congenital hip dislocation.

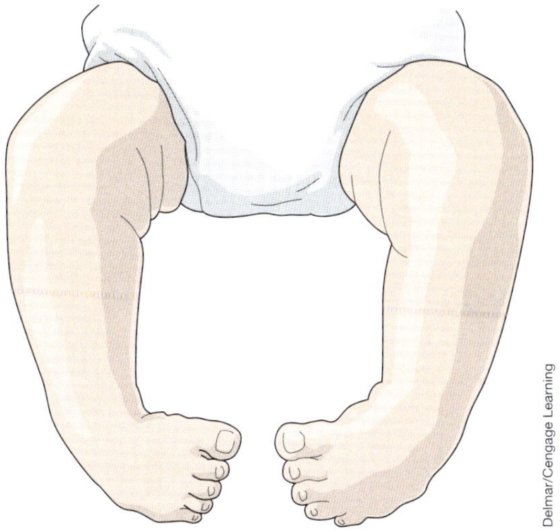

FIGURE 19–9 Talipes equinovarus (clubfoot).

position can lead to CHD. This position places undue stress on the hip joints.

CLUBFOOT (TALIPES EQUINOVARUS)

DESCRIPTION. Clubfoot, or talipes (talus = ankle, pes = foot) equinovarus (TAL-eh-peas ee-KWI-no-VAY-rus; equine = horse or toe walking, similar to a horse, varus = bent inward), is a frequently occurring congenital deformity of the foot.

ETIOLOGY. The cause of clubfoot is unknown, but it is thought to be due to genetic factors or fetal position in the uterus. Some positional deformities can be straightened with manipulation, but a true clubfoot deformity will not straighten with manipulation.

SYMPTOMS. The affected foot or feet turn inward with the toes pointed downward and the heel drawn upward (Figure 19–9).

DIAGNOSIS. Clubfoot is easily diagnosed with physical examination. X-rays help determine the severity of the disorder.

TREATMENT. Treatment, quite successful if begun during infancy, can involve application of a cast or splints to straighten the foot gradually. The cast or splints are changed frequently until the desired position is achieved. If casting and splinting do not achieve the desired results, surgery might be indicated. Attention must be given to the position of the child's feet throughout childhood to ensure that normal position is maintained.

PREVENTION. There are no known preventive measures.

OSTEOGENESIS IMPERFECTA

DESCRIPTION. Osteogenesis (osteo = bone, genesis = beginning) imperfecta (not perfect or normal) is characterized by abnormally brittle bones, often leading to frequent fractures.

ETIOLOGY. Osteogenesis imperfecta is an inherited condition caused by gene mutation.

SYMPTOMS. Undiagnosed children affected with osteogenesis imperfecta might be suspected as victims of child abuse due to the frequency of bone fractures. Other significant signs are an abnormally blue coloration of the sclera of the eyes, otosclerotic deafness, translucent skin, and thin dental enamel of the teeth.

DIAGNOSIS. Diagnosis is made primarily with history and physical examination. X-rays of the bones can be helpful.

TREATMENT. There is no cure for osteogenesis imperfecta, but the tendency of bones to fracture decreases with age and often disappears by adulthood.

PREVENTION. There are no preventive measures for osteogenesis imperfecta.

Neurologic

Genetic and developmental neurologic disorders are some of the most severe because of their long-term debilitating effects. Two of the most common severe disorders in this category are hydrocephalus and cerebral palsy.

HYDROCEPHALUS

■ ***DESCRIPTION.*** Hydrocephalus (high-droh-SEF-ah-lus; hydro = water, cephal = brain) is an abnormal accumulation of cerebrospinal fluid in the brain.

■ ***ETIOLOGY.*** Hydrocephalus is generally caused by obstruction of the flow of cerebrospinal fluid out of the brain, which can be from a congenital defect, an infection, or a tumor.

■ ***SYMPTOMS.*** The head of the affected child might be normal at birth but will rapidly enlarge over the first few months of life as the fluid accumulates. The brain tissue becomes compressed, and the skull begins to bulge. Other signs include bulging eyes, a tight scalp, prominent head veins, and a shrill, high-pitched cry. The infant is unable to lift its head, fails to develop normally, and is mentally challenged.

■ ***DIAGNOSIS.*** Diagnosis is confirmed with skull X-rays and angiography.

■ ***TREATMENT.*** Treatment of choice is surgical correction by placing a shunt from the brain to the peritoneal cavity or right atrium of the heart to drain the excess fluid (Figure 19–10). Even with early surgical intervention, the prognosis is guarded. Mortality rate is high without surgical correction.

■ ***PREVENTION.*** There are no preventive measures.

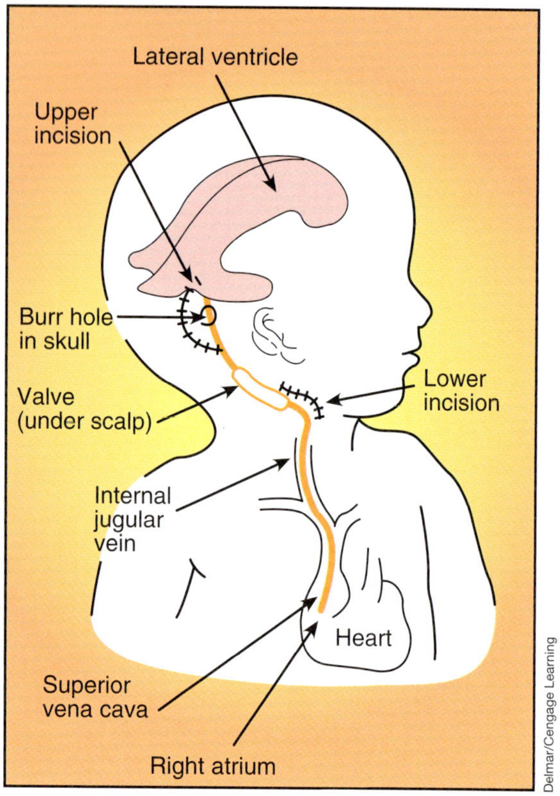

FIGURE 19–10 A ventricle shunt drains spinal fluid in an infant with hydrocephalus.

CEREBRAL PALSY

■ ***DESCRIPTION.*** Cerebral palsy (CP) (SER-eh-bral PAWL-zee) is a congenital bilateral paralysis that results from inadequate blood or oxygen supply to the brain during fetal development, the birthing process, or in infancy. CP is the most common crippler of children and more often affects premature infants and males.

■ ***ETIOLOGY.*** Causes of CP include maternal rubella, toxemia, birthing difficulties such as prolonged labor, anoxia, hypoxemia, asphyxia from the umbilical cord being wrapped around the infant's neck, head trauma, and meningitis. Often, the cause of CP is unknown.

■ ***SYMPTOMS.*** This disorder usually affects motor or muscle performance and can be noticed if the infant has difficulty sucking or swallowing. Other complications include visual and hearing deficits, seizure activity, and mental challenges. CP is characterized by hyperactive reflexes, rapid muscle contraction, and muscle weakness. The affected child commonly has a scissors gait, exhibited by toe-walking and crossing one foot over the other with each step.

■ ***DIAGNOSIS.*** Diagnosis is based on clinical symptoms including posture, oral motor patterns, strabismus, muscle tone, postural reaction, and tendon reflexes.

■ ***TREATMENT.*** There is no cure for CP. Treatment involves physical therapy, speech therapy, orthopedic casting, braces, and, often, surgery to help the child reach full potential. Anticonvulsant and muscle relaxant medications also can be beneficial.

■ ***PREVENTION.*** There are no preventive measures.

SPINA BIFIDA

■ ***DESCRIPTION.*** Spina bifida (SPY-nah BIF-ih-dah), a neural tube defect (NTD) is a congenital disorder in which one or more of the vertebrae of the bony spinal column fails to close over the spinal cord, leaving an opening in the column. *Bifid* means split in two parts, which describes the vertebra in this condition. Development of the spinal cord and column occurs during the first trimester of pregnancy.

■ ***ETIOLOGY.*** The cause of this malformation is unknown, but risk factors include maternal radiation, virus, and genetic factors. Children born with spina bifida are more often born to mothers who have other children with this defect. There are several other conditions that tend to accompany spina bifida, including hydrocephalus, cleft palate, and clubfoot. The several forms of spina bifida are illustrated in Figure 19–11 and described as follows:

- **Spina bifida occulta** The most common form of spina bifida. A spina bifida is present, but it is asymptomatic and hidden (occulta). Signs of the malformation often include a dimpling of the skin and a tuft of hair or port wine nevus on the skin surface above the defect.
- **Meningocele** Occurs when the meninges of the spinal cord protrude through the opening in the vertebral column, forming a fluid-filled sac on the skin surface. Because nerve tissue is not involved, the infant usually does not have neurologic problems.
- **Myelomeningocele** The most serious spina bifida because the meninges and a portion of the spinal cord protrude through the opening in the vertebral column, causing neurologic symptoms.

■ ***SYMPTOMS.*** Depending on the type and cause, common symptoms include skeletal malformation, deformed joints, paralysis of the legs, and bowel and bladder incontinence.

■ ***DIAGNOSIS.*** The condition is suspected in the presence of a skin defect over the spinal area along with muscular abnormalities in the legs and deformities of the feet. The diagnosis is confirmed by X-ray examination or myelography.

■ ***TREATMENT.*** Surgical intervention to correct the condition is usually performed in the first 24 hours of life. Additional procedures might be needed as the child grows. Some of these children are unable to walk and might die before the age of 2 or 3 years.

■ ***PREVENTION.*** There are no preventive methods, although there is a link between folic acid (a B vitamin) levels in pregnant women and major birth defects in the baby's brain and spine from NTDs. For this reason, women need to take folic acid every day, starting before they become pregnant, to help prevent NTDs.

Cardiovascular

The heart and its related great vessels are the most common sites of congenital defects. The defects can be small or quite large, and consequences of these deformities can range from asymptomatic to life-threatening. Collectively, these malformations of heart structure are called congenital heart defects.

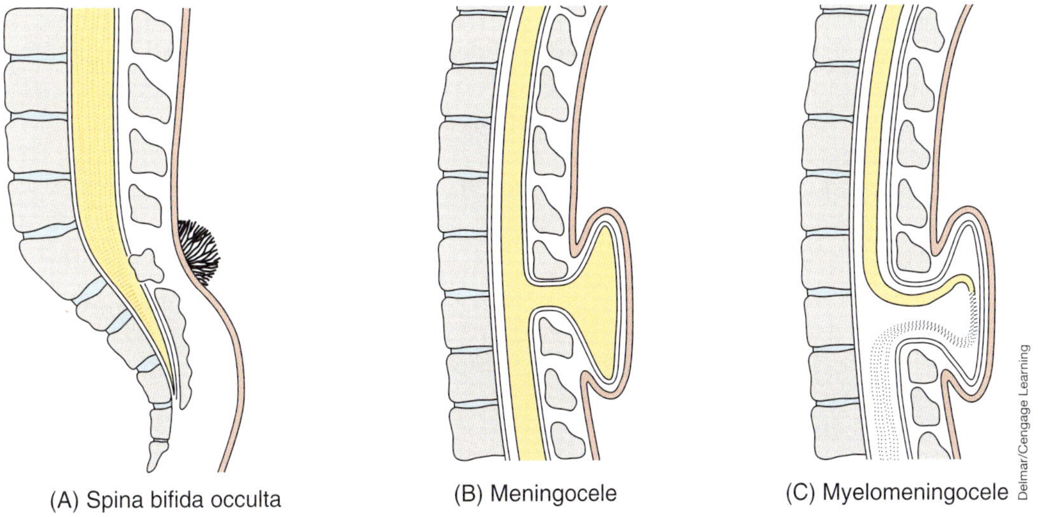

FIGURE 19–11 Types of spina bifida.

CONGENTIAL HEART DEFECTS

ETIOLOGY. The cause of these defects is unknown, but a genetic tendency is strongly suspected. Certain risk factors include maternal rubella, poor maternal nutrition, smoking, and alcoholism.

SYMPTOMS. Symptoms of congenital heart defects can vary from mild cases that are asymptomatic to extreme conditions with symptoms of extreme cyanosis, breathing difficulties, and very audible heart murmurs.

DIAGNOSIS. Diagnosis is made by electrocardiogram and physical examination, including **auscultation** (listening to the chest with a stethoscope), which usually reveals heart **murmurs** (abnormal heart sounds) if present.

TREATMENT. Early diagnosis and surgical correction of these defects have improved drastically in recent years and have significantly reduced the mortality rate of infants born with heart defects.

PREVENTION. Controlling risk factors is the only preventive measure.

ATRIAL SEPTAL DEFECT

DESCRIPTION. Atrial septal defect is an opening between the right and left atria (Figure 19–12a), commonly due to the foramen ovale not closing at birth. The foramen ovale is a natural opening between the atria that allows blood to bypass the nonfunctional lungs during fetal life. After the infant is born, the act of breathing causes a change in chest cavity pressure that normally closes the foramen ovale. Atrial septal defects allow oxygenated blood to be pumped from the left atria to the right atria, which is again pumped to the right ventricle and to the lungs without ever circulating through the body. This repumping causes an increased workload on the right side of the heart. This defect occurs more commonly in girls than in boys.

VENTRICULAR SEPTAL DEFECT

DESCRIPTION. Ventricular septal defects are the most common heart defects, accounting for approximately 25% of all heart defects. As the name suggests, this defect is a hole between the right and left ventricle (Figure 19–12b) that allows blood from the left ventricle to flow into the right ventricle. Like the atrial septal defect, this oxygenated blood has to be repumped, causing an increased workload on the right side of the heart.

PATENT DUCTUS ARTERIOSUS

DESCRIPTION. A ductus arteriosus is a connection between the pulmonary artery and the aorta of the normal fetal heart (Figure 19–12c) that allows blood to flow from the pulmonary artery to the aorta, thus bypassing the nonfunctional lungs. The ductus arteriosus, like the foramen ovale, normally closes off shortly after birth. If the structure does not close, or remains patent, the condition is called patent ductus arteriosus. With this condition, oxygenated blood shunts abnormally from the higher-pressured aorta back to the pulmonary artery. Once in the pulmonary artery, the blood is recirculated to the lungs. This condition causes an increased workload on the heart and pulmonary system and occurs twice as frequently in girls as in boys.

COARCTATION OF THE AORTA

DESCRIPTION. Coarctation is a **stricture** or narrowing. A coarctation of the aorta is a narrowing of the descending or thoracic aorta (Figure 19–12d), a condition that causes a high blood pressure proximal to the stricture and lower blood pressure distal to the stricture. Infants or children affected with coarctation of the aorta can have a high blood pressure in the arms but a lower blood pressure in the legs. Coarctation increases the workload on the heart because the heart attempts to pump blood through the narrowed vessels.

TETRALOGY OF FALLOT

DESCRIPTION. Tetralogy of Fallot (TET-traw-law-gee of fall-OH) is a combination of four (tetra) defects (Figure 19–12e) and is one of the most serious of congenital heart defects. The four defects are as follows.

1. **Pulmonary valve stenosis** The opening into the pulmonary artery is too small, restricting the amount of blood flow to the lungs.
2. **Right ventricle hypertrophy** This is due to the increased workload on the right ventricle as it attempts to pump blood through the stenotic valve.
3. **Ventricle septal defect** Allowing oxygenated blood to flow from the left ventricle to the right.
4. **Abnormal placement of the aorta** The aorta opens over the ventricle septal defect, allowing blood from both ventricles to be pumped into the aorta. The unoxygenated blood from

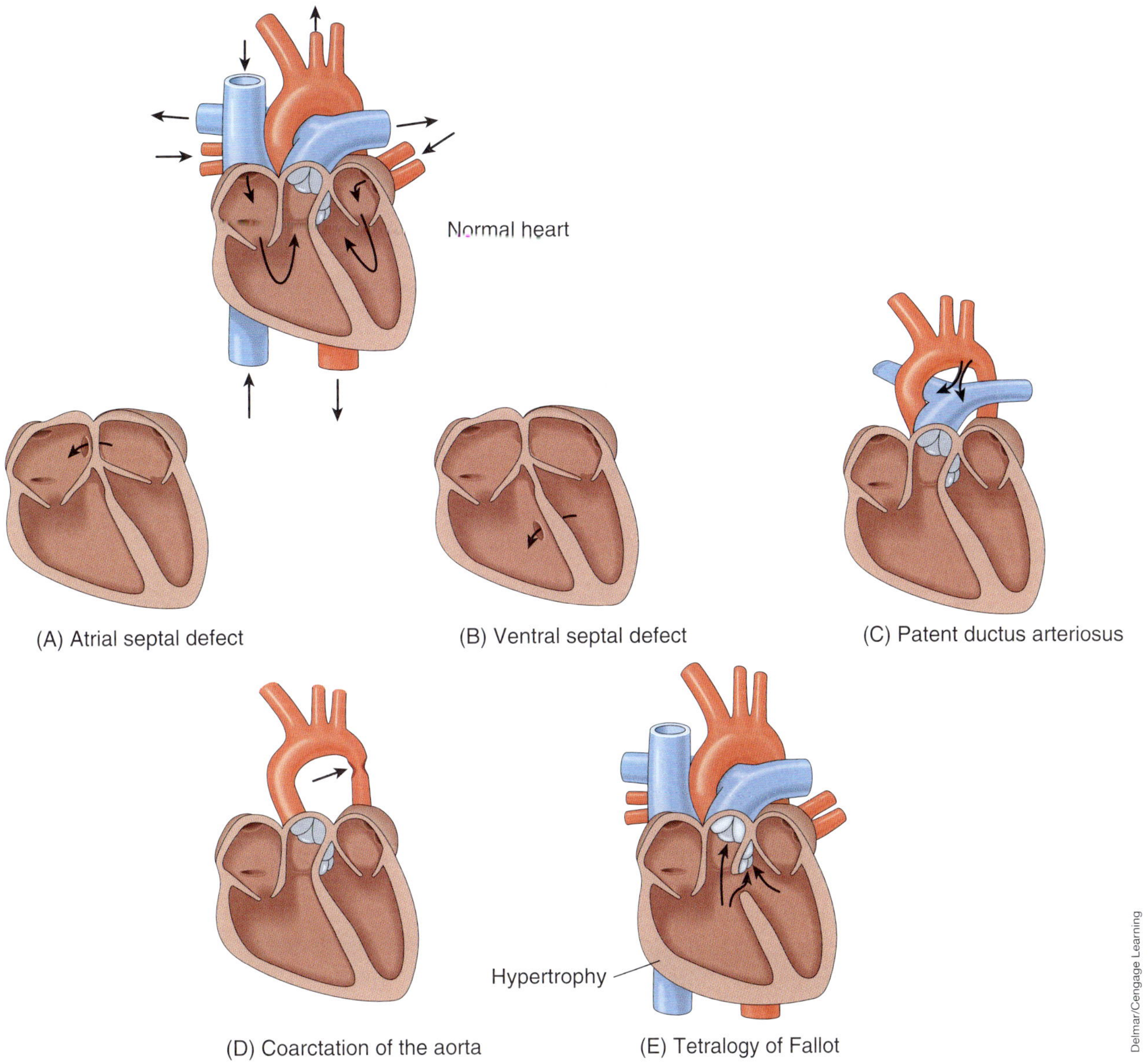

FIGURE 19–12 A normal heart and congenital heart defects (A-E).

the right ventricle enters the general circulation without passing through the lungs to become oxygenated. This unoxygenated blood from the right ventricle causes the tissues to become cyanotic (blue).

■ ***SYMPTOMS.*** Infants and children with tetralogy of Fallot are truly blue babies. Cyanosis increases with age, and clubbing of fingers and toes becomes evident. Older children will rest in a squatting position to breathe easier. This position also increases venous return. Other symptoms are growth retardation, severe dyspnea with exercise, and frequent respiratory infections.

Blood

Genetic and developmental disorders of the blood are more common in certain population groups. For example, some anemias are most commonly found in black populations, whereas other anemias are more common in European populations. Sickle cell anemia and hemophilia are both discussed in more detail in Chapter 7, "Blood and Blood-Forming Organs Diseases and Disorders."

SICKLE CELL ANEMIA

Sickle cell anemia is a chronic hereditary form of anemia found predominately in African American individuals.

HEMOPHILIA

Hemophilia is an X-linked hereditary bleeding disorder passed from a carrier mother to a son.

Digestive

Digestive system disorders, both genetic and developmental, range from mild to severe. Many are diagnosed at birth, especially if the disorder interferes with ingestion, digestion, or elimination. Some of them are incompatible with life and must be corrected immediately, or the infant will not survive.

DEVELOPMENTAL MALFORMATIONS

■ ***DESCRIPTION.*** Several developmental malformations occur in the digestive system.

■ ***ETIOLOGY.*** The cause of these disorders is unknown but might be related to genetic tendencies or to maternal risk factors, including maternal rubella, poor maternal nutrition, smoking, and alcoholism.

A few of the more common malformations are briefly discussed here.

MECKEL'S DIVERTICULUM

■ ***DESCRIPTION.*** This is an outpouching, or diverticulum, of the ileum (Figure 19–13a). During fetal life, the intestine is connected to the yolk sac by a duct. Failure of the duct to disappear leads to formation of this diverticulum. Meckel's diverticulum is the most common malformation of the gastrointestinal (GI) system, occurring in approximately 2% of the population. The diverticulum might be asymptomatic the entire life of the individual and found only on autopsy.

■ ***SYMPTOMS.*** If symptoms do occur, it is usually during infancy. The most common symptom is painless, bloody stools.

ESOPHAGEAL ATRESIA

■ ***DESCRIPTION.*** This is the absence of part of, or abnormal closure of, the esophagus. An **atresia** (ah-TREE-ze-ah) is the congenital absence or closure of a normal opening or lumen in the body and can occur in a variety of areas. Esophageal atresia is often accompanied by a fistula, called a trachealesophageal fistula, connecting the trachea to the esophagus (Figure 19–13b). This is an emergency condition that allows food to pass directly into the lung.

■ ***SYMPTOMS.*** Reflux regurgitation of food occurs with both atresias. If a fistula is present, extreme coughing, cyanosis, and respiratory difficulties will appear.

CONGENITAL DIAPHRAGMATIC HERNIA

■ ***DESCRIPTION.*** This is a congenital hole in the diaphragm. Abdominal organs might herniate through this opening and into the chest cavity (Figure 19–13c).

■ ***SYMPTOMS.*** Difficulty breathing and chest pain are common symptoms.

IMPERFORATE ANUS

■ ***DESCRIPTION.*** This is a failure of the anus to connect to the rectum (Figure 19–13d). Infants with imperforate anus commonly have other developmental anomalies such as those affecting the heart, kidneys, esophagus, and spine.

■ ***SYMPTOMS.*** The primary symptom is not passing stool. Other symptoms are abdominal cramping and vomiting.

■ ***DIAGNOSIS.*** Diagnosis is commonly made on the basis of X-ray examination and ultrasound.

■ ***TREATMENT.*** Surgical correction is the treatment of choice for these malformations.

■ ***PREVENTION.*** There are no preventive measures other than controlling maternal risk factors.

CLEFT LIP AND PALATE

■ ***DESCRIPTION.*** Cleft (a split) lip consists of one or more abnormal splits in the upper lip (Figure 19–14a). This is a common anomaly, occurring in approximately 1 in 1,000 births. The defect occurs more frequently in boys and can vary from slight to severe.

A cleft palate involves the palate or roof of the mouth (Figure 19–14b)and is more serious than a cleft lip because it forms an opening between the nasopharynx and the nose. Cleft palate is more common in girls.

Both conditions can occur separately or in combination and can range from mild to severe.

■ ***ETIOLOGY.*** The cause of clefts appears to be related to a hereditary factor coupled with an alteration in intrauterine environment.

■ ***SYMPTOMS.*** Symptoms of cleft lip are related to difficulty feeding, speaking, and, if not corrected

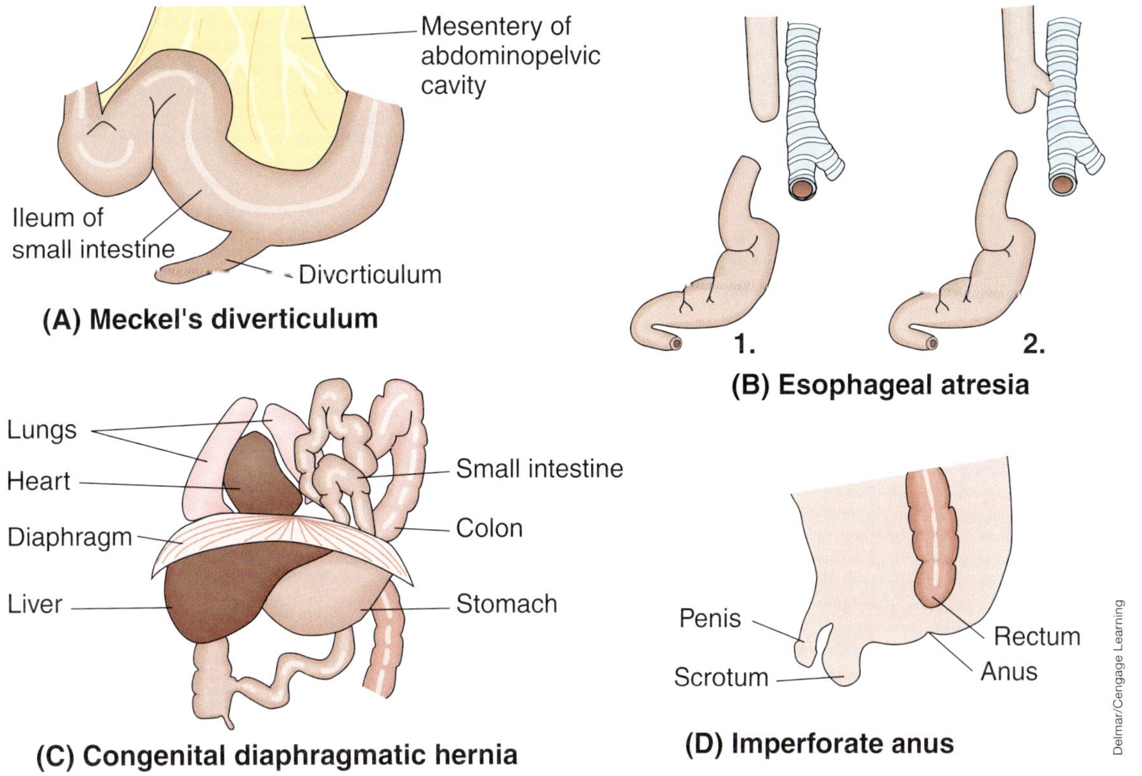

FIGURE 19–13 Digestive developmental malformations.

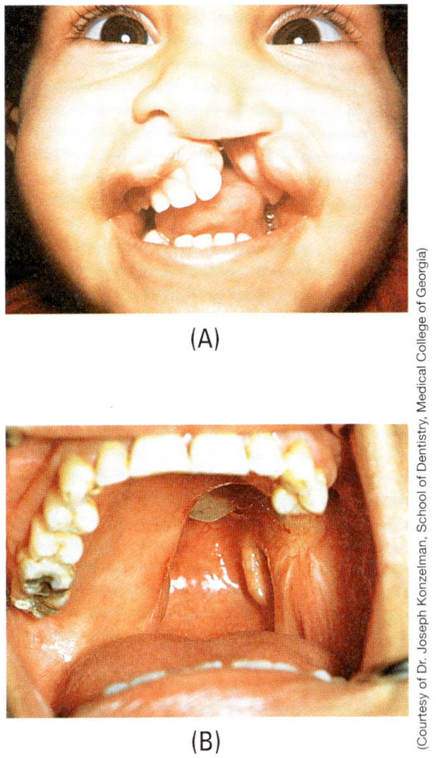

FIGURE 19–14 (A) Cleft lip, (B) cleft palate.

during infancy, a struggle with positive self-image. Cleft palate includes these symptoms plus an increased risk of respiratory and middle ear infections.

■ ***DIAGNOSIS.*** Physical examine easily reveals this disorder. X-ray and computerized tomography (CT) may be utilized to determine the extent of the malformation.

■ ***TREATMENT.*** Surgical repair for cleft deformities is usually performed as soon as possible after birth. Several surgeries might be neecessary to achieve the desired results. Special feeding devices and speech therapy are common needs.

■ ***PREVENTION.*** The only prevention is contolling maternal risk factors.

PYLORIC STENOSIS

■ ***DESCRIPTION.*** Pyloric stenosis is a narrowing (stenosis) of the outlet of the lower end of the stomach, the pylorus (Figure 19–15). This condition is one of the most common developmental abnormalities of the digestive tract.

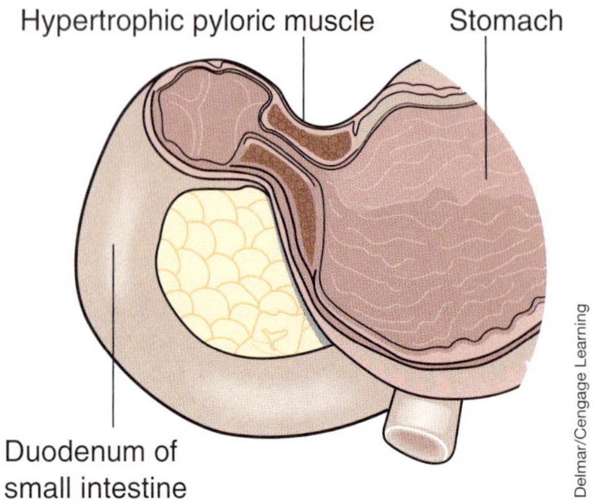

FIGURE 19–15 Pyloric stenosis.

■ ***ETIOLOGY.*** Pyloric stenosis is caused by a hypertrophy, or thickening, of the pyloric sphincter, which controls the flow of contents out of the stomach or pyloric area. The hypertrophy of the pyloric sphincter slows the flow of stomach contents, resulting in a backup.

■ ***SYMPTOMS.*** The most common symptom of pyloric stenosis is projectile, or forceful, vomiting. Symptoms of pyloric stenosis usually begin at 2 to 4 weeks of age. This condition occurs almost exclusively in boys.

■ ***DIAGNOSIS.*** Diagnosis is made from history and X-ray examination (upper GI).

■ ***TREATMENT.*** A simple operation called a **pyloromyotomy** (pyloro = pyloric, myo = muscle, otomy = cut into), which involves incising and suturing the pyloric sphincter muscle, can be performed to correct the problem. This surgery is the standard treatment and is usually very effective.

■ ***PREVENTION.*** There are no known preventive measures.

HIRSCHSPRUNG'S DISEASE

■ ***DESCRIPTION.*** Hirschsprung's disease is due to an absence of nerves (ganglion) in a segment of the colon, usually the sigmoid colon. Without normal ganglion, the affected segment of colon lacks peristalsis, causing massive distention of the colon with feces (Figure 19–16).

■ ***ETIOLOGY.*** Hirschsprung's disease is seen more often in boys and those affected with Down syndrome. It has a familial tendency and occurs in approximately 1 in 5,000 births.

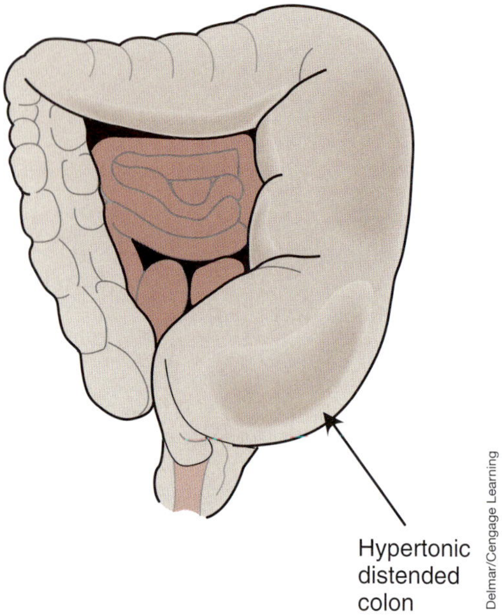

FIGURE 19–16 Hirschsprung's disease.

■ ***SYMPTOMS.*** Common symptoms include chronic constipation and abdominal distention.

■ ***DIAGNOSIS.*** Diagnosis is made on the basis of a biopsy to determine the absence of ganglion cells.

■ ***TREATMENT.*** Treatment is surgical removal of the affected segment. A temporary colostomy might be necessary to allow adequate healing of the colon.

■ ***PREVENTION.*** There is no known prevention. Genetic counseling can be offered to discuss risk and treatment options with a couple with a previous child with the condition and with those with the condition who are considering pregnancy.

PHENYLKETONURIA (PKU)

■ ***DESCRIPTION.*** PKU is an abnormal or faulty metabolism of the phenylalanine protein.

■ ***ETIOLOGY.*** PKU is a recessive genetic disorder.

■ ***SYMPTOMS.*** Affected individuals do not produce the enzyme necessary to break down the phenylalanine protein, which then builds up in the blood and becomes present in the urine. Phenylalanine is toxic to brain cells and causes mental disability if the condition is not corrected.

■ ***DIAGNOSIS.*** Diagnosis is made by PKU blood testing 72 hours after birth or after the infant has ingested proteins. This testing is mandatory in the United States.

■ ***TREATMENT.*** Affected infants are placed on a protein-restrictive diet. If the disease is discovered and treated early, prognosis for normal intelligence is good. If the condition is not discovered until after age 2 or 3 years, mental challenges are inevitable and irreversible.

■ ***PREVENTION.*** There are no preventive measures. Genetic counseling can be offered to discuss risk and treatment options with a couple with a previous child with the condition and to those with the condition who are considering pregnancy.

Urinary

Some genetic and developmental disorders of the urinary system, such as hypospadias or epispadias, can be obvious at birth. Other disorders, such as Wilms' tumor, might not present symptoms for many years. If the condition interferes with elimination of urine, it is incompatible with life.

HYPOSPADIAS AND EPISPADIAS

■ ***DESCRIPTION.*** Hypospadias is an abnormal congenital opening of the male urinary meatus on the undersurface of the penis (Figure 19–17a). This abnormality can be mild, with the opening located just under the tip of the penis, or it can be more severe, with locations midshaft or near the scrotum. Hypospadias is fairly common, occurring in 1 in 250 boys.

Hypospadias can be accompanied by an abnormally downward curvature of the penis called chordee (COR-dee) (Figure 19–17b). The cause of chordee is an abnormal fibrous band of tissue.

Another, similar but less common, condition is epispadias, characterized by the urinary meatus located on the upper surface of the penis (Figure 19–17c).

■ ***ETIOLOGY.*** The cause of these conditions is unknown.

■ ***SYMPTOMS.*** Abnormal position of urethra is the only symptom. Chordee becomes worse with erection and can lead to difficulty with sexual intercourse.

■ ***DIAGNOSIS.*** Diagnosis is easily made with physical examination.

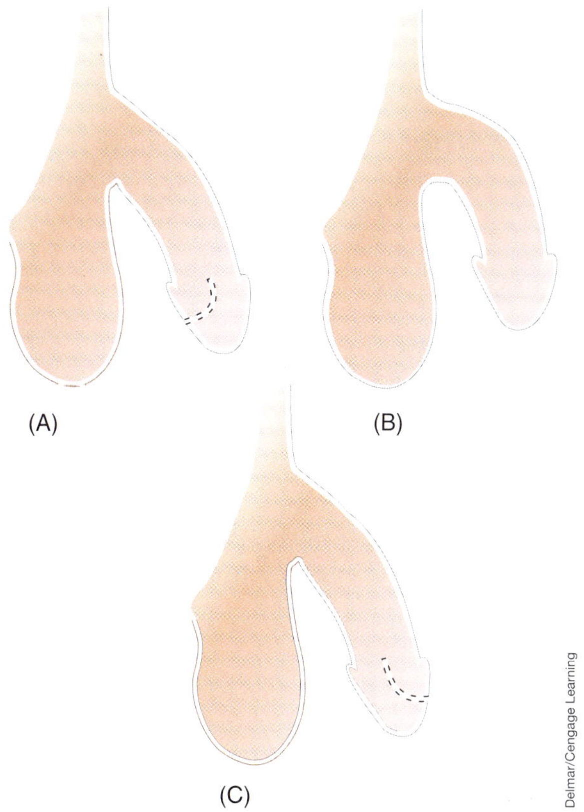

FIGURE 19–17 (A) Hypospadias, (B) chordee, (C) epispadias.

■ ***TREATMENT.*** Mild cases of all these conditions can be left untreated. Surgical repair is the treatment of choice for severe cases.

■ ***PREVENTION.*** There are no known preventive measures.

WILMS' TUMOR

■ ***DESCRIPTION.*** Wilms' tumor is the most common solid tumor affecting children and infants. Most tumors are thought to be present at birth, usually appearing between the ages of 2 to 4 years.

■ ***ETIOLOGY.*** The cause is thought to be genetic. It is highly malignant and usually replaces one entire normal kidney but rarely affects both kidneys.

■ ***SYMPTOMS.*** The tumor is usually asymptomatic until it becomes large enough to feel in the child's abdomen.

■ ***DIAGNOSIS.*** Most tumors are discovered by palpation of the abdomen during a routine examination by a pediatrician or by a parent.

■ ***TREATMENT.*** Current treatment involving chemotherapy and surgery has improved a previously dismal prognosis to a survival rate of approximately 85%.

■ ***PREVENTION.*** There are no preventive measures. Genetic counseling might be helpful for those who have a history of a family member affected with this condition.

Reproductive

Genetic and developmental disorders of the reproductive system are very rare disorders. Although they are not usually incompatible with life, they can have serious psychological effects on the individual because of the changes they can cause in the appearance of the person and the gender differences expected in our population.

CRYPTORCHIDISM

This developmental condition of undescended testes (crypt = hidden) is discussed in detail in Chapter 17, "Reproductive System Diseases and Disorders."

TURNER'S SYNDROME

■ ***DESRIPTION.*** Turner's syndrome is a condition affecting females. At birth, the ovaries are abnormal or absent. Turner's syndrome is less common than Klinefelter's syndrome, a similar condition that affects males.

■ ***ETIOLOGY.*** Turner's Syndrome is caused by a chromosomal disorder and affects approximately 1 in 3,000 females. Affected females have only one X chromosome rather than the normal XX.

■ ***SYMPTOMS.*** This individual fails to develop normal female secondary sex characteristics at puberty. General physical features of affected females include a short stature, broad neck, wide chest, amenorrhea, sterility, dwarfism, and impaired intelligence.

■ ***DIAGNOSIS.*** Physical examination and blood hormone testing aid in diagnosis.

■ ***TREATMENT.*** Symptoms can be reduced with growth hormone and estrogen therapy. Counseling and emotional support are often needed for the affected individual and family members to help cope with altered body image and self-esteem issues.

■ ***PREVENTION.*** There is no prevention for Turner's syndrome.

KLINEFELTER'S SYNDROME

■ ***DESCRIPTION.*** Klinefelter's syndrome affects approximately 1 in 1,000 males.

■ ***ETIOLOGY.*** Klinefelter's syndrome is caused by a chromosomal disorder. Affected males have an extra X chromosome (XXY) in addition to the normal XY.

■ ***SYMPTOMS.*** This disorder is usually not diagnosed until puberty, when the affected individual fails to exhibit normal male sexual development. General physical features of affected males include sterility, abnormally small penis and testes, enlarged breasts, absent or scant body hair, decreased muscle development, and impaired intelligence. The affected individual has a general appearance of a eunuch with a tall, slender body and long legs.

■ ***DIAGNOSIS.*** Physical examination and blood hormone testing aid in diagnosis.

■ ***TREATMENT.*** Symptoms can be improved with testosterone therapy. Emotional and psychological counseling are often needed for the affected individual and family members to help cope with altered body image and self-esteem issues.

■ ***PREVENTION.*** There is no known prevention for this condition.

Other Developmental Disorders

Developmental disorders that do not fit into the previous categories of musculoskeletal, neurologic, cardiovascular, blood, digestive, urinary, or reproductive disorders are autism and stuttering.

AUTISM

■ ***DESCRIPTION.*** Autism, also called autistic disorder, is a severe type of developmental disorder characterized by a preoccupation with inner thoughts, daydreams, fantasies, and **delusions** (a false belief that is firmly adhered to although it is not shared by others).

■ ***ETIOLOGY.*** The cause of autism is unknown, although there might be a physical cause.

■ ***SYMPTOMS.*** Symptoms of autism are usually apparent in infancy when the infant exhibits an eye-to-eye gaze and blank facial expression. Affected children are so involved with themselves that they become inaccessible to others, including parents. These children might play alone happily for hours and become angry if interrupted. Approximately 10% of autistic children possess an outstanding skill such as rote memory or musical ability. An example is a child who can play a very difficult piano piece after hearing it only one time. Such children are often called autistic savants.

■ **DIAGNOSIS.** Diagnosis is confirmed on the basis of observation of behavior.

■ **TREATMENT.** Behavioral therapy to teach the child how to adapt to situations is beneficial. Prognosis is still relatively poor, and affected children rarely recover.

■ **PREVENTION.** There is no recognized prevention, although some cases can be linked to chemical exposure during pregnancy. Not taking drugs or drinking alcohol and checking with the physician before taking any medications during pregnancy might aid in prevention.

STUTTERING

■ **DESCRIPTION.** Stuttering, also called stammering, is a developmental speech disorder, a common condition in young children that most of them will outgrow. If the problem persists, speech therapy might be necessary.

■ **ETIOLOGY.** Stuttering often occurs when children address an impatient or angry parent or someone who is in authority. The child's anxiety often leads to stuttering. The listener's reaction often enforces the child's anxiety, leading to more difficulties.

■ **SYMPTOMS.** Stuttering is characterized by hesitancy of starting and finishing a sound or word and prolonged pauses between words or sounds.

■ **DIAGNOSIS.** Diagnosis is usually confirmed upon physical examination, which includes talking with the child.

■ **TREATMENT.** Treatment is often based on some type of behavior modification and positive reinforcement of proper speech.

■ **PREVENTION.** There are no preventive methods, although speech therapy might help overcome the condition.

Multisystem Diseases and Disorders

Multisystem disorders are complex diseases that affect several body systems. Because of this effect, treatment is complicated and usually long term.

CYSTIC FIBROSIS

■ **DEFINITION.** Cystic fibrosis is a life-threatening disorder that requires constant management of symptoms. It commonly causes nutritional deficiencies and severe lung damage.

■ **ETIOLOGY.** Cystic fibrosis is a hereditary recessive disorder affecting young children. It is passed to the child by a recessive gene from each parent.

■ **SYMPTOMS.** Cystic fibrosis affects all the **exocrine** glands (glands that excrete through a duct) of the body, causing **viscous** (thick) secretions. These viscous secretions cause obstruction in body passageways. The most serious complication of cystic fibrosis is in the lungs. The thick secretions block bronchi, causing difficulty with breathing. These thick secretions also trap bacteria and increase the risk of respiratory infections, including pneumonia. The most common cause of death from this disease is respiratory failure.

The pancreas is also affected because blockage of these ducts decreases the amount of pancreatic enzymes delivered to the intestine, resulting in poor digestion and weight loss.

The sweat glands are also affected. Affected children perspire excessively and lose large amounts of salt (sodium). This loss of sodium causes an increase in the risk for heat exhaustion and electrolyte imbalances. This abnormal excretion of salt is usually the first sign that parents recognize as abnormal. Parents might take the child to the physician and complain that the child, when kissed, tastes salty or has sweaty baby kisses.

■ **DIAGNOSIS.** This excessive salt excretion is the basis for the sweat test that confirms the diagnosis of cystic fibrosis.

■ **TREATMENT.** Major improvements in treatment of cystic fibrosis have been made in the past few decades, but it is still considered a fatal disease. Life expectancy can reach into the late 20s or early 30s. Treatment is directed toward reducing complications and improving quality of life. Aggressive respiratory treatments include postural drainage, chest-clapping, antibiotics, bronchodilators, expectorants, and oxygen therapy. A high-calorie, high-sodium diet is provided with pancreatic enzyme supplementation. Emotional support and extensive education are needed for the affected individual and family members.

PREVENTION. There are no preventive measures. Genetic counseling can be offered to a couple with a previous child with the condition.

DOWN SYNDROME

DESCRIPTION. Down syndrome is also called Trisomy 21 because it is a condition resulting in three (tri) chromosomes instead of the normal two in the 21st position of the chromosome chain. Down syndrome occurs in approximately 1 of every 700 births. It is the most common cause of genetic mental disability.

ETIOLOGY. The cause of Down syndrome is not known, but it is known that during germ cell division (usually affecting the ovum), the twenty-first chromosome pair fails to separate. This results in a pair of chromosomes in position 21; if fertilized, this ovum—carrying two chromosomes—combines with the sperm—carrying one chromosome—resulting in three chromosomes in position 21. This condition is more common in children born to women 35 years or older, suggesting that chromosomal division is affected by maternal age.

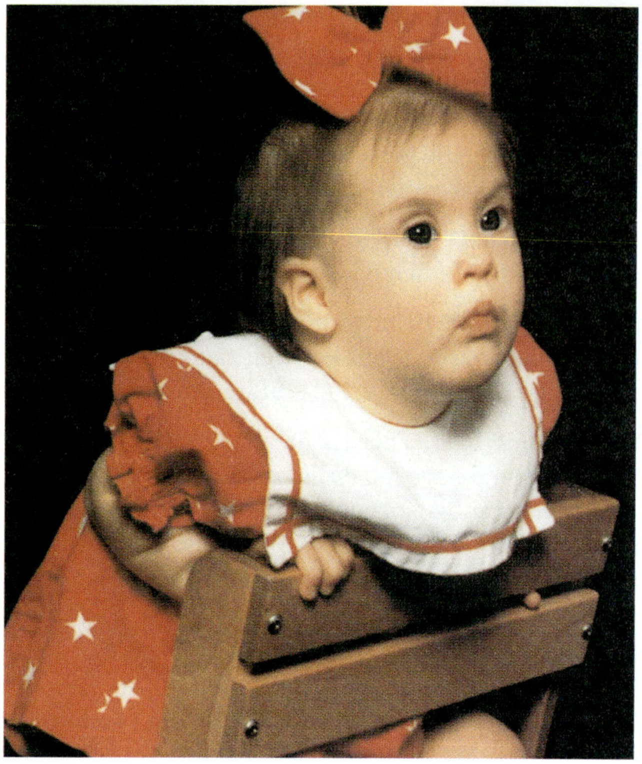
Marijane Scott, Marijane's Designer Portraits, Down Right Beautiful 1996 Calendar

FIGURE 19–18 Down syndrome.

SYMPTOMS. Signs of Down syndrome include:

- Mild to severe mental disability.
- Facial features that include a flat nasal bridge, low-set ears, slanted eyes with **epicanthus** (a vertical fold of skin across the medial canthus of the eyes, giving them an Oriental appearance), and a thick, protruding tongue (Figure 19–18).
- Abnormal extremities, including short arms and legs. The hands are short and wide with a crease across the entire width of the palm called a simian crease. The little finger is short and often crooked. There is an abnormally wide gap between the first (big) and second toes.
- Organ defects, especially congenital heart defects. Infertility is common in males but might not affect females.
- Other diseases are common, including anemia, leukemia, immune deficiencies, and respiratory infections.

DIAGNOSIS. Prenatal tests used to diagnosis Down syndrome include ultrasound, amniocentesis, and maternal blood testing showing abnormal levels of pregnancy hormones, including human chorionic gonadotropin (HCG), are indicative of the condition.

Diagnosis of newborns includes physical examination for symptoms along with a chromosomal karyotype that looks for the extra chromosome 21.

TREATMENT. There is no cure, but amniocentesis is an effective tool for discovery. The treatment plan is highly individual and is directed toward maximizing mental and physical abilities. Improved surgical techniques and antibiotic therapies have increased the life expectancy of affected individuals to an average of 55 years. Individuals affected with Down syndrome are known for their loving, affectionate personalities.

PREVENTION. There are no preventive measures. Genetic counseling might be beneficial.

TRAUMA

Failure to Thrive

Failure to thrive is a lack of physical growth and development in an infant or child. The condition of failure to thrive is usually reserved for infants and children who are not growing and developing due to emotional or psychological causes.

This condition was first noticed by a European psychiatrist who studied the development of infants institutionalized during their early years and who were deprived of emotional warmth and security.

The cause of failure to thrive appears to be a disturbance in the mother–child relationship or a failure to bond. This condition tends to be associated with alcohol and drug abuse, economic stress, parental immaturity, and single parenthood. Involved mothers are often found to be victims of maternal deprivation themselves.

Symptoms of failure to thrive include weight loss or failure to gain weight and grow, irritability, anorexia or lack of appetite, vomiting, and diarrhea. Affected infants often are weak and exhibit rag-doll limpness. They can be unresponsive to affection or wary of parents or caregivers and might avoid eye contact and stiffen when cuddled.

Treatment includes teaching nurturing and mothering behaviors for the mother, promoting her self-esteem, and providing for the physical and emotional needs of the child. The prognosis for infants and children with this condition is often unknown. Decreased intelligence and social and language disabilities have been noted in children with failure to thrive. A significant number of these children die early in life.

Fetal Alcohol Syndrome

Fetal alcohol syndrome (FAS) is a group of symptoms and birth defects in an infant born to a mother who consumed alcohol during pregnancy. Infants born to mothers who chronically abuse alcohol can go through physical alcohol withdrawal shortly after birth.

Signs and symptoms of FAS include varying degrees of mental challenges, decreased physical development, irritability in infants and hyperactivity in children, **microcephaly** (micro = small, cephal = brain), and an increased occurrence of ventricular septal heart defects.

The exact amount of alcohol consumption needed to cause defects is unknown, so alcohol consumption during pregnancy should be avoided. The greatest risks for defects occur when alcohol is consumed during and after the third month of pregnancy.

Congenital Rubella Syndrome

Transmission of the rubella virus across the placenta to the unborn fetus can result in spontaneous abortion or birth of an infant with major birth defects. The most common defects are microcephaly, learning disorders, deafness, growth retardation, heart defects, and ocular lesions such as cataracts, glaucoma, nystagmus, and strabismus.

Prevention includes immunization of all children and women of childbearing age. Women should avoid becoming pregnant for 3 months after immunization and should not be immunized during pregnancy.

RARE DISEASES

Anencephaly

Anencephaly is a severe congenital malformation resulting in the absence of the brain or cranial vault. This condition is not compatible with life. Infants born with anencephaly are stillborn or die shortly after birth if they are not kept alive by artificial means.

Achondroplasia

Achondroplasia is a rare genetic disorder characterized by abnormal development of the epiphyseal cartilage, resulting in decreased long bone growth and a type of dwarfism. Interestingly, a similar condition affects basset hounds. Affected individuals might die at birth or shortly thereafter or live to a normal life expectancy.

Tay–Sachs Disease

Tay–Sachs disease is an autosomal recessive disorder primarily affecting families of Eastern Jewish origin. This condition is due to a genetic error in lipid metabolism and results in an accumulation of toxins in the brain. As a result, the brain tissue degenerates, causing mental and physical disabilities.

Symptoms usually occur by 6 months of age and include lack of developmental skills, convulsions, and blindness. A cherry-red spot on the retina of the eye is one indicative diagnostic test. Affected children usually die before age 4 years. There is no cure and no specific treatment other than symptomatic treatment.

SUMMARY

Although there are literally hundreds of genetic and developmental disorders, overall, most are relatively rare. Some are obvious at birth and can be incompatible with life; others might not be diagnosed until later in the individual's life. Because some disorders have no distinct diagnostic tests, a variety of testing might be necessary to obtain a definitive diagnosis. Other disorders can be diagnosed by genetic testing.

Many of the genetic and developmental disorders have lifelong effects on the individual and can be progressively disabling. Because of new research and extended health care services, most individuals with these disorders have longer life expectancy than in past years.

REVIEW QUESTIONS

Short Answer

1. How many chromosomes are in the nucleus of each body cell?
2. Which body cells can reproduce in a process called mitosis?
3. What is a germ cell?
4. Describe the process called meiosis.
5. What is karyotyping?
6. Why is DNA considered to be so important?
7. Name an autosomal dominant disorder.
8. Name an autosomal recessive disorder.
9. Define genotype.
10. Define phenotype.

Multiple Choice

11. Which of the following statements is the best description of MD?
    - **a.** MD is a degenerative disorder of the nervous system.
    - **b.** MD is a group of genetically inherited diseases characterized by degeneration or weakening of the muscles.
    - **c.** MD is a genetic disorder most common in male children.
    - **d.** MD is a neuromuscular disorder affecting children.

12. Which of the following statements is the best description of CP?
    a. CP is a congenital bilateral paralysis that results from inadequate blood or oxygen supply to the brain during fetal development.
    b. CP is a crippling disease caused by a genetic inherited disorder.
    c. CP is an abnormal accumulation of cerebrospinal fluid in the brain.
    d. CP is a condition of spastic movements and inability to walk caused by a genetic anomaly.

13. Coarctation of the aorta is ___________.
    a. a combination of four tetra defects of the heart.
    b. a constriction or stricture of the major artery of the heart.
    c. an abnormal connection of the pulmonary artery and the aorta.
    d. a small hole in the artery at birth.

14. Some of the problems for the infant with a cleft lip and palate might include ___________.
    a. a fistula connecting the trachea to the esophagus.
    b. increased risk for elimination problems.
    c. increased risk for difficulty with feedings, respiratory distress, and middle ear infections.
    d. projectile or forceful vomiting.

15. PKU is best described as ___________.
    a. an absence of nerves in a particular segment of the colon, causing constipation and distention of the colon.
    b. a recessive genetic disorder of metabolism of protein.
    c. an autosomal-dominant genetic disorder of digestion and absorption.
    d. a constriction of the valve in the stomach, causing a backup of food and fluid.

16. Which of the following is the most common solid tumor affecting children and infants?
    a. Osteoma
    b. Sarcoma
    c. Ewing's tumor
    d. Wilms' tumor

17. Which of the following factors are usually present in Down syndrome?
    a. Dwarf-like body, mental disability, spastic movements
    b. Organ defects, small stature, epicanthal folds, and epispadias
    c. Mental disability, immune deficiencies, and abnormal brain size
    d. Epicanthal folds, small stature, mild to severe mental disability

18. When is FAS most likely to occur?
    a. If the mother drinks alcohol during and after the third month of pregnancy.
    b. If the mother drinks more than one glass of alcohol per day during the last trimester.
    c. If the mother drinks alcohol during the first 2 months of pregnancy.
    d. Only if the mother drinks more than two glasses of alcohol per day during the pregnancy.

19. Tay–Sachs disease is an ___________.

a. autosomal-dominant disease affecting the brain.

b. autosomal-dominant disease affecting metabolism, causing mental disability.

c. autosomal-recessive disease affecting metabolism, causing mental disability.

d. autosomal-recessive disease affecting the brain.

20. Failure to thrive is defined as which of the following?

a. It is a lack of growth and development due to a genetic disease.

b. It is a lack of physical growth and development in an infant or child.

c. It is an inborn error of metabolism, causing delayed growth and development.

d. It is an inherited disease affecting growth in the infant.

CASE STUDIES

■ Heather Lee is an 8-month-old infant who is brought to the clinic because of chronic respiratory infections. Heather is weak, inactive, and underweight; she has poor skin turgor and seems very quiet except for spells of coughing. She is subsequently diagnosed with CF. Heather's mother is very upset with this diagnosis, thinking it is her fault the baby is not doing well. Is she correct in thinking this? What can you tell her about this disorder? What is the cause of CF? What is the usual treatment prescribed? What is the prognosis for Heather?

■ Abnormalities in children might be due to genetic factors. Because individuals have dominant and recessive genes, some predictions can be made about such things as color of eyes or genetic disease probabilities. If the mother has brown eyes but has a recessive gene for blue eyes and the father has blue eyes (homozygous recessive), what is the likelihood of them having a blue-eyed child? What is the likelihood of them having a brown-eyed child?

*Study*WARE™ Connection

To help you learn the content in this chapter, take a practice quiz or play an interactive game on your StudyWARE™ CD-ROM.

Workbook Practice

Go to your Workbook and complete the practice questions.

BIBLIOGRAPHY

Abdel-Aziz, M. (2007). Treatment of submucous cleft palate by pharyngeal flap as a primary procedure. *International Journal of Pediatric Otorhinolaryngology 71*(7), 1093–1097.

Abbeduto, L., Warren, S., & Conners, F. (2007). Language development in Down syndrome: From the prelinguistic period to the acquisition of literacy. *Mental Retardation & Developmental Disabilities Research Reviews 13*(3), 247–261.

Abelson, R. (February 20, 2008). Lacking cure, a new tack on a muscle disease. *New York Times 157*(54266), A1–A16.

Birth Defect Research for Children, Inc. (2008). *www.birthdefect.org* (accessed July 2008).

Chen, Y., Kang, L., Chuang, T., Doong, T., Lee, S., Tsai, M., Jeng, S., & Sung, W. (2007). Use of virtual reality to improve upper-extremity control in children with cerebral palsy: A single-subject design. *Physical Therapy 87*(11), 1441–1457.

Christiansen, A., & Lange, C. (2008). Intermittent versus continuous physiotherapy in children with cerebral palsy. *Developmental Medicine & Child Neurology 50*(4), 290–293.

Cleft Palate Foundation. (2008). *www.cleftline.org* (accessed July 2008).

Delefave, L., & McNally, E. (2007). Cardiomyopathy in neuromuscular disorders. *Progress in Pediatric Cardiology 24*(1), 35–46.

Dorchies, O., Wagner, S., Vuadens, O., Waldhauser, K., Buetler, T., Kucera, P., & Ruegg, U. (2006). Green tea extract and its major polyphenol (-)-epigallocatechin gallate improve muscle function in a mouse model for Duchenne muscular dystrophy. *American Journal of Physiology: Cell Physiology 290*(2), C616–2C65.

Down syndrome. (2007). Mayo Foundation for Medical Education and Research. *www.mayoclinic.com* (accessed July 2008).

Down Syndrome Foundation (2008). *www.downsyndromefoundation.org* (accessed July 2008).

Dykens, E. (2007). Psychiatric and behavioral disorders in persons with Down syndrome. *Mental Retardation & Developmental Disabilities Research Reviews 13*(3) 272–278.

Gardner, J. (2007). What you need to know about cystic fibrosis. *Nursing 37*(7), 52–55.

Genetic Disease Foundation. (2008). *www.geneticdiseasefoundation.org* (accessed July 2008).

Grady, D. (December 12, 2007). Promising drug clears early test. *New York Times* Section A, late edition, 16.

Herper, M. (2007). Stopping the nonsense. *Forbes 180*(5), 72–73.

Hsiao, K., & Nixon, G. (2008). The effect of treatment of obstructive sleep apnea on quality of life in children with cerebral palsy. *Research in Developmental Disabilities 29*(2), 133–140.

Law, M., Dreyer, Z., Heinle, J., & Dickerson, H. (2007). Staged single-ventricle palliation in infant with hemoglobin SC disease. *Texas Heart Institute Journal 34*(4), 439–441.

Lott, I., Patterson, D., & Seltzer, M. (2007). Toward a research agenda for Down syndrome. *Mental Retardation & Developmental Disabilities Research Reviews 13*(3), 288–289.

Muscular Dystrophy Foundation. (2008). *www.mda.org* (accessed July 2008).

Operation Smile. (2008). *www.OperationSmile.org* (accessed July 2008).

Pediatrics electronic pages. (2007). *Pediatrics 119*(2), 383–394.

Price, F., Kuroda, K., & Rudnicki, M. (2007) Stem cell based therapies to treat muscular dystrophy. *BBA-Molecular Basis of Disease 1772*(2), 272–283.

Rahoma, A. (2007). Complete cleft palate: A new scheme of treatment. *Internet Journal of Plastic Surgery 4*(1), 3. *www.ispub.com/journal/the_internet_journal_of_plastic_surgery.html*

Rando, T. (2007). Non-viral gene therapy for Duchenne muscular dystrophy: Progress and challenges. *BBA-Molecular Basis of Disease 1772*(2), 263–271.

Sandrio G. (2006). Surgical treatment of neck, hyperextension in Duchenne muscular dystrophy by posterior interspinous fusion. *Spine 31*(16), 1805–1809.

Senechal, C., Serge, R., & Englebert, M. (2007). Hyperbaric oxygenation therapy in the treatment of cerebral palsy: A review and comparison of accepted therapies. *Journal of American Physicians & Surgeons 12*(4), 109–113.

Turner's syndrome. (2007). National Institutes of Health. *www.nim.nih.gov* (accessed July 2008).

United Cerebral Palsy. (2008). *www.ucp.org* (accessed July 2008).

Wagner, K., Lechtzin, N., & Judge, D. (2007.) Current treatment of adult Duchenne muscular dystrophy. *BBA-Molecular Basis of Disease 1772*(2), 229–237.

Ward, K., Adams, J., Freemont, T. & Mughai, M. (2007). Can biphosphonate treatment be stopped in a growing child with skeletal fragility? *Osteoporosis International 18*(8), 1137–1140.

Willis, A., Crowner, B., Brunstrom, J., Kissel, A., & Recette, B. (2007.) High dose botulinum toxin A for the treatment of lower extremity hypertonicity in children with cerebral palsy. *Developmental Medicine & Child Neurology 49*(11), 818–822.

Wilms' tumor. (2007). Mayo Foundation for Medical Education and Research. *www.mayoclinic.com* (accessed July 2008).

Appendix A

Common Laboratory Values

Test	Explanation/Normal Values
Complete blood count (CBC)	Indicates oxygen-carrying capacity of blood and presence of infection.
White blood cells (WBCs)	5,000–10,000 mm^3
Red blood cells (RBCs)	4.2–5.4/mm^3
Hemoglobin (Hg)	
males	13.5–17.5 g/dl
females	12–16 g/dl
Hematocrit (Hct)	
males	40–54%
females	37–47%
Electrolytes	Test determines blood electrolyte levels.
Sodium (Na)	136–145 mEq/L
Potassium (K)	3.5–5 mEq/L
Chloride (Cl)	98–106 mEq/L
Carbon dioxide (CO_2)	22–30 mEq/L
Magnesium (Mg)	1.5–2.5 mEq/L
Arterial blood gases (ABGs)	Indicates respiratory and metabolic functioning. pH = 7.35–7.45 PCO_2 = 35–45 mm Hg HCO_3 = 21–28 mEq/L PO_2 = 80–100 mm Hg O_2 saturation = 95–100%
Culture and sensitivity (C&S)	Culture determines presence of microorganism. Sensitivity determines antibiotic that will kill or inhibit growth of microorganism. Normal value is negative for microorganism growth.
Urinalysis	Diagnoses problems in the urinary system
Color	Clear to amber
Odor	Pleasantly aromatic
Albumin (protein)	Negative
Acetone	Negative

(Continued)

Test	Explanation/Normal Values
Red blood cells	2–3/HPF
White blood cells	4–5/HPF
Bilirubin	Negative
Glucose	Negative
Specific gravity	1.005–1.030
Bacteria	Negative
Casts	Rare
pH	4.6–8.0

Appendix B

Metric Conversion Tables

LENGTH	Centimeters	Inches	Feet
1 centimeter	1.00	0.394	0.0328
1 inch	2.54	1.00	0.0833
1 foot	30.48	12.00	1.00
1 yard	91.4	36.00	3.00
1 meter	100.00	39.40	3.28

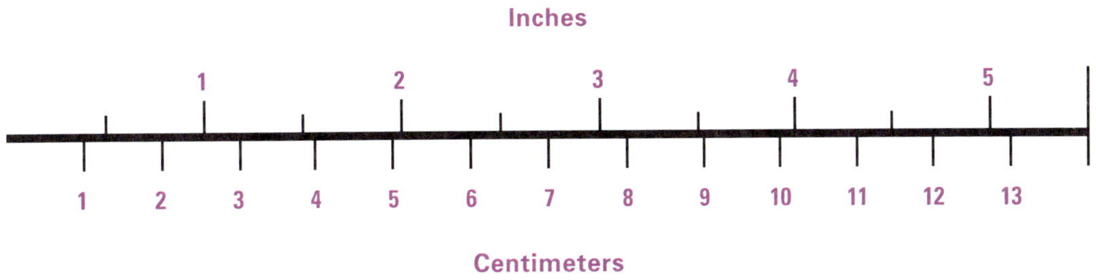

Comparison of Centimeters and Inches

VOLUMES	Cubic Centimeters	Fluid Drams	Fluid Ounces	Quarts	Liters
1 cubic centimeter	1.00	0.270	0.033	0.0010	0.0010
1 fluid dram	3.70	1.00	0.125	0.0039	0.0037
1 cubic inch	16.39	4.43	0.554	0.0173	0.0163
1 fluid ounce	29.6	8.00	1.00	0.0312	0.0296
1 quart	946.00	255.00	32.00	1.00	0.946
1 liter	1000.00	270.00	33.80	1.056	1.00

WEIGHTS	Grains	Grams	Apothecary Ounces	Pounds
1 grain (gr)	1.00	0.064	0.002	0.0001
1 gram (gm)	15.43	1.00	0.032	0.0022
1 apothecary ounce	480.00	31.1	1.00	0.0685
1 pound	7000.00	454.00	14.58	1.00
1 kilogram	15432.00	1000.00	32.15	2.205

Rules for Converting One System to Another

Volumes

Grains to grams	divide by 15
Drams to cubic centimeters	multiply by 4
Ounces to cubic centimeters	multiply by 30
Minims to cubic millimeters	multiply by 63
Minims to cubic centimeters	multiply by 0.06
Cubic millimeters to minims	divide by 63
Cubic centimeters to minims	multiply by 16
Cubic centimeters to fluid ounces	divide by 30
Liters to pints	divide by 2.1

Weights

Milligrams to grains	multiply by 0.0154
Grams to grains	multiply by 15
Grams to drams	multiply by 0.257
Grams to ounces	multiply by 0.0311

Temperature

Multiply centigrade (Celsius) degrees by $\frac{9}{5}$ and add 32 to convert Fahrenheit to Celsius

Subtract 32 from the Fahrenheit degrees and multiply by $\frac{5}{9}$ to convert Celsius to Fahrenheit

Common Household Measures and Weights

1 teaspoon	= 4–5 cc or 1 dram	1 cup	= 8 fluid ounces or $\frac{1}{2}$ pint
3 teaspoons	= 1 tablespoon	1 tumbler or glass	= 8 fluid ounces or 240 cc
1 dessert spoon	= 8 cc or 2 drams	1 wine glass	= 2 fluid ounces or 60 cc
1 tablespoon	= 15 cc or 3 drams	16 fluid ounces	= 1 pound
4 tablespoons	= 1 wine glass or $\frac{1}{2}$ gill	4 gills	= 1 pound
16 tablespoons (liquid)	= 1 cup	1 pint	= 1 pound
12 tablespoons (dry)	= 1 cup		

Appendix C

Glossary

A

abdominocentesis (ab-DOM-ih-no-sén-**TEE**-sis) pacentesis of the abdomen; a procedure in which a puncture is made into the abdominal cavity to withdraw fluid.

abrasion a scraping away of skin surface.

abscess a localized collection of pus.

achlorhydria (a-klor-HIGH-dree-ah) absence of hydrochloric acid.

acromegaly (ACK-roh-**MEG**-ah-lee; acro = extremity, megaly = enlargement) a condition of extremity enlargement as a result of excessive growth hormone in the adult.

acute (a-CUTE) a disease that is short term.

addiction a physical and/or psychological dependence on a substance.

Addison's disease hypoadrenalism; an uncommon under-secretion of hormones by the adrenal cortex.

adenoidectomy (AD-eh-noy-**DECK**-toh-me; ectomy = removal) surgical removal of the adenoids.

adenoma (AD-eh-**NO**-ma; adeno = gland, oma = tumor) a tumor of glandular tissue.

adhesions (ad-HE-zhun) parts of tissue that cling to the surface of adjoining organs as normal fibrous scar tissue develops in an operative site, resulting in a fibrous band.

affect outward expression of emotions.

AIDS acquired immunodeficiency syndrome.

albumin (al-BYOU-men) a blood protein distributed throughout the body; responsible for osmotic pressure of the blood.

albuminuria (al-BYOU-mih-**NEW**-ree-ah; albumin = a blood protein, uria = urine) albumin in the urine; usually albumin but may also be globulin; usually indicative of a disease process.

aldosterone (al-doh-STER-ohn) a mineralocorticoid; acts on the kidney to assist in maintaining electrolyte balance.

alleles matched pairs of genes; the term used to refer to the product when the chromosomes (one from each parent) pair up during fertilization of the egg; the genes on the chromosomes align.

allergen the environmental substance that causes a reaction.

allergy the state when the immune response is too intense or hypersensitive to an environmental substance.

alopecia (AL-oh-**PEE**-shee-ah; in Greek, meaning fox mange, which caused hair loss) a partial or complete hair loss, usually from the head.

amblyopia (AM-blee-**OH**-pee-ah) a decrease in the vision of the affected eye due to a lack of visual stimuli.

amenorrhea (ah-MEN-oh-**REE**-ah; a = without, menorrhea = menses) the absence or cessation of menses.

amnesia (am-NEE-zee-ah) loss of memory.

amylase an enzyme; often elevated in pancreatic disorders.

anaerobic (an = without, aerobic = air) living without oxygen.

analgesic (AN-al-**GEE**-sick) a medication that relieves pain.

anaphylaxis (AN-ah-fih-**LACK**-sis) an immediate allergic reaction characterized by contraction of smooth muscle and dilation of capillaries, leading to severe respiratory distress or failure.

anaplastic (AN-ah-**PLAST**-ic) abnormal tissue, the more undifferentiated tissue.

androgens hormone's secreted by the adrenal cortex and responsible for male characteristics.

anemia (ah-NEE-me-ah; an = without, emia = blood) any decrease in oxygen carrying ability of the red blood cell.

angiogenesis (AN-jee-oh-**JEN**-eh-sis; angio = vessel, genesis = formation) new growth of blood vessels.

angiography (AN-jee-**OG**-rah-fee; angio = vessel, graphy = procedure to record) a radiographic study of blood vessels after injection of fluorescein dye.

angioplasty (AN-jee-oh-**PLAS**-tee; angio = vessel, plasty = surgical repair) a procedure that involves passing a catheter into the artery and inflating a balloon on the catheter to push the plaque against the vessel wall, thus widening the lumen of the vessel.

Ankle-brachial index (ABI) a comparison of the blood pressure in the lower legs to the blood pressure in the arms.

anomaly (ah-NOM-ah-lee) any abnormality.

anorexia nervosa (AN-oh-**RECK**-see-ah; an = without, orexia = appetite) a disorder of self-imposed starvation, resulting from a distorted body image.

anoxia (ah-NOCK-see-ah) no oxygen.

antibody(ies) immunoglobulins that develop in response to an antigen; also called immune bodies; proteins that the body produces to react to and render the antigen harmless.

antigen(s) (AN-tih-jens) a cell marker that induces a state of sensitivity after coming in contact with an antibody; any substance that causes the body some type of harm, thus setting off this specific reaction.

antipyretics (anti = against, pyretic = fever) a class of medications given to reduce an elevated temperature.

anuria (ah-NEW-ree-ah; an = without, uria = urine) no urine output.

apnea (ap-NEE-ah; a = without, pnea = breathing) the condition of not breathing; a term used to describe the absence of respirations for a period of time.

arterial blood gases (ABGs) the laboratory test that measures the amounts of oxygen and carbon dioxide in blood.

articular relating to a joint surface.

articular fracture one that involves a joint surface.

ascites (ah-SIGH-teez) fluid in the abdomen (peritoneal cavity).

asymptomatic (a = without, symptomatic = symptoms) not displaying symptoms.

atresia the congenital absence or closure of a normal opening or lumen in the body; it may occur in a variety of areas.

atrophy (AT-tro-fee) a decrease in cell size, which leads to a decrease in the size of the tissue and organ.

audiometry (AW-dee-**OM**-eh-tree; audio = sound, metry = measure) the basic test used to measure hearing.

aura symptoms occurring at the onset of a partial epileptic seizure or migraine headache; it may include tingling of the fingers, ringing in the ears, and visual disturbances.

auscultation (AWS-kul-**TAY**-shun) using a stethoscope to listen to body cavities and organs.

autodigestion autolysis or digestion of self or one's own cells.

autoimmunity or autoimmune the state when the immune response attacks itself.

autosomes (auto = self, somes = body) a chromosome other than a sex chromosome; they determine body function.

avulsion skin pulled or torn away.

avulsion fracture one where there is a separation of a small bone fragment from the bone where a tendon or ligament is attached.

B

bacteria a one-celled microorganism that may be aerobic or anaerobic and free-living, saprophytic, parasitic, or pathogenic.

Bence Jones protein a special protein found in the blood and urine, indicative of multiple myeloma.

benign (beh-NINE) having limited growth, noncancerous.

bimanual examination (bi = two, manual = handed) an examination in which the physician places one hand on the abdomen and inserts fingers of the other hand into the vagina to feel the female organs between the two hands.

biopsy (BYE-op-see) removing a small piece of tissue for microscopic examination.

bleeding time a test to determine the length of bleeding time or time it takes the blood to clot.

blood urea nitrogen (BUN) a test to determine the level of urea nitrogen or waste in the blood.

blunt trauma a wound or injury (trauma) caused by an object with a flat, dull, or not sharp area (blunt).

bone mass density (BMD) a measure of bone density or weight. A thinning bone results in a lower bone density.

bronchiectasis (BRONG-key-**ECK**-ta-sis) a chronic or long-term dilatation of a bronchus or bronchi along with an infection.

bronchoscopy (brong-KOS-koh-pee; broncho = bronchus or lung passageways, oscopy = procedure to look into) a diagnostic or surgical procedure in which a scope is passed through the mouth into the bronchus.

bronchospasm (BRONG-ko-**SPA**-zm) muscular constriction of the bronchi of the respiratory tract.

buccal smear a test for evaluating chromosomes; this test is performed by obtaining squamous epithelial cells from the buccal cavity, staining the cell, and microscopically observing for X chromosomes called Barr bodies.

bulimia (boo-LIM-ee-ah) an eating disorder characterized by episodes of binge eating (an intake of approximately 5,000 calories in 1 to 2 hours) followed by activities to negate the calorie intake by purging.

C

cachexia (ca-KACK-see-ah) a term used to describe any individual who has an ill, thin, wasted appearance.

calcaneal the heel area of the foot.

cancer a malignant tumor.

caput medusae tortuous, unsightly varicosities spreading from the umbilicus outward across the front of the abdomen.

carcinogen (kar-SIN-oh-jen) cancer-causing agent or substance.

carcinogenesis (KAR-sin-oh-**JEN**-eh-sis) cancer development.

carcinoma (KAR-sih-**NO**-mah) the most common type of malignant neoplasm arising from epithelial tissue.

carcinoma in situ atypical cells residing in the epithelial layer of tissue, not having broken through the basement membrane and invading other local tissues.

cardiac catheterization (KATH-eh-ter-eye-**ZAY**-shun) an invasive procedure used to sample the blood in the chambers of the heart to determine the amount of oxygen content and blood pressure in the chambers.

cardiac palpitations an unusually strong, rapid, or irregular heart rate that is so abnormal the individual can feel it.

carotid endarterectomy (END-ar-ter-**ECK**-toh-me; endo = inside, arter = artery, ectomy = excision of) surgical intervention to remove plaque in the carotid arteries to improve blood flow and reduce the risk of a thrombus.

catarrhal (ka-TAR-all) inflammation of mucous membranes of the head and mouth with increased mucus flow.

catheterization (KATH-er-ter-eye-**ZAY**-shun) a sterile procedure consisting of passing a soft catheter through the urethra and into the bladder for the purpose of (1) instilling or pouring fluids or medication into the bladder or (2) removing urine.

cauterization (KAW-ter-eye-**ZAY**-shun) the electrical burning of tissue to stop bleeding; used most frequently during surgery to stop bleeding from vessels.

cerebrovascular accident (CVA) poor blood flow to the brain, commonly called a stroke.

cellulitis (SELL-you-**LYE**-tis) inflammation of connective tissue.

cephalalgia (SEF-ah-**LAL**-jee-ah; cephal = head, algia = pain) headache.

cerumen (se-ROO-men) ear wax.

cervicitis (SER-vih-**SIGH**-tis) inflammation of the cervix.

chancre (SHANG-ker) a painless, highly contagious lesion occurring in the primary stage of syphilis.

chemotaxis the movement of cells or organisms in response to chemicals.

chemotherapy using pharmacologic therapy in the treatment of cancer.

cholecystectomy (KOH-lee-sis-**TECK**-toh-me; chole = gall or bile, cyst = bladder, ectomy = removal) surgical removal of the gallbladder.

chorea (ko-REE-ah) a constant, jerky, uncontrollable movement.

chronic a disease that persists for a long time.

circadian rhythm a normal 24-hour cycle of biological rhythms including sleep, metabolism, and glandular secretions.

clean catch a term used to describe a clean urine collection method involving cleansing the urethal area prior to urinating and catching the voided urine specimen.

closed or simple fracture a fracture that does not break through the skin.

clubbing a condition affecting the distal portion of the finger; characterized by soft tissue enlargement and an abnormal curvature of the nail.

Colle's fracture a fracture of the lower end of the radius with displacement of the fragment.

colorectal pertaining to both the colon and rectum.

comedones (KOM-eh-dohns) plugged skin pores; the open form is a blackhead; the closed form is a whitehead.

comminuted fracture one in which there are more than two ends or fragments.

complete blood count (CBC) a laboratory test that identifies the number of red blood cells (RBCs), white blood cells (WBCs), and platelets per cubic millimeter.

complete fracture the fracture is completely through the bone.

complication the onset of a second disease or disorder in an individual who is already affected with a disease.

compound (open) fracture a fracture involving the bone puncturing through the skin, or an object puncturing the skin, making an opening through the skin to the fracture site.

compression fracture one in which the bone appears to be mashed down.

compulsion a repetitive act the affected individual is unable to resist performing.

computerized axial tomography (CAT or CT) imaging by a cross-sectional plane of the body; also called computed tomography.

congenital (kon-JEN-ih-tahl) present at birth; usually concerning a congenital anomaly or an abnormality present at birth.

congenital anomaly (kon-JEN-ih-tahl ah-NOM-ah-lee; congenital = present at birth, anomaly = abnormality) a birth defect.

contusion (kon-TOO-zhun) a large bruise.

convulsion an abnormal muscle contraction; a violent spasm or jerking of the face, trunk, or extremities.

corticosteroids (KORT-ti-ko-**STEHR**-oyds) powerful anti-inflammatory hormones.

cortisol hydrocortisone; a steroid hormone secreted by the adrenal cortex.

cortisone a glucocorticoid; it affects carbohydrate metabolism, and influences the nutrition and growth of connective tissues.

creatinine (kree-**AT**-in-in) one of the two most common nitrogenous waste products that are normally filtered from the blood, the final product of creatine catabolism.

creatinine clearance test a diagnostic test for kidney function that measures the rate the kidneys excrete creatinine, a waste product from muscle contraction that is carried in small amounts in the blood, filtered by the kidney, and excreted in urine. An increased blood or urine level indicates a disturbance in kidney function.

cretinism congenital hypothyroidism.

cryptorchidism (krip-TOR-kih-dizm; crypt = hidden, orchid = testicle, ism = condition) undescended testicle(s).

culture and sensitivity a test to identify a pathogen and the type of treatment needed.

curative something that corrects or cures the disease or condition.

cyanosis (SIGH-ah-**NO**-sis; cyano = blue, osis = condition) a bluish condition of the skin due to lack of oxygen in the blood.

cystogram (cysto = bladder, gram = picture) an X-ray picture of the bladder that helps determine the shape and function of the bladder.

cystoscopy (sis-TOS-koh-pee; cysto = bladder, scopy = procedure to look) an invasive procedure to look into the urethra and bladder by using a lighted scope.

cytologic (SIGH-toe-**LAW**-gic) pertaining to cytology.

cytology (SIGH-**TOL**-oh-jee; cyto = cell, logy = study) the examination or study of cells.

cytotoxic (cyto = cell, toxic = killing) something that kills cells.

D

débridement (day-breed-MENT) a process of washing or cutting away necrotic tissue and foreign material.

decompress a release of pressure.

defecate to have a bowel movement.

degenerative diseases related to aging, or destruction of tissue, functions, and use.

dehiscence (dee-HISS-ens) separation of tissue margins.

delirium tremens (DTs) (dee-LIR-ee-urn **TREE**-mens) a serious form of delirium due to alcoholic withdrawal after a period of sustained intoxication.

delusions false beliefs that are firmly adhered to although they are not shared by others.

dementia (dee-MEN-she-ah) a loss of mental ability due to the loss of neurons or brain cells.

densitometry measurement of bone thickness.

dental plaque tough, sticky material that adheres to the tooth enamel; caused by bacteria.

dependency a psychological craving for a substance that may or may not be accompanied by a physical need.

diabetic retinopathy (DYE-ah-**BET**-ick RET-ih-**NOP**-ah-thee, retino = retina, opathy = disease) disease of the retina of the eye, often resulting in blindness; caused by, degeneration due to diabetes mellitus.

diagnosis (DIE-ag-**KNOW**-sis) the identification or naming of a disease.

diapedesis (DYE-ah-pe-**DEE**-sis) passage of blood, or its formed elements, through the intact walls of blood vessels.

diastolic (dye-as-TOL-ick) relating to cardiac diastole; the process of the heart resting as the chambers refill with blood.

differential a detailed white blood cell count identifying the number of each type of leukocyte.

differentiation the process of individual specialization of cells.

digital rectal examination a manual examination in which the physician feels the prostate for abnormal enlargement (hypertrophy or hyperplasia) and tumors.

dilitation and curettage (**KYOU**-reh-TAHZH) or D&C, a procedure that involves a dilation of the cervix (dilatation) and scraping (curettage) of the uterine endometrial tissue; a D&C is commonly performed for abnormal uterine bleeding and following a spontaneous abortion.

diplopia (dih-PLOH-pee-ah) double vision.

disease a change in structure or function within the body that is considered to be abnormal; any change from normal.

diskectomy surgery to remove a vertebral disk.

disorder a derangement or abnormality of function.

displaced fracture one in which fragments are out of position.

dominant in control.

Doppler a device that may be placed over arteries to magnify the sound of blood flow.

dormant state of being inactive.

dowager's hump abnormal curvature in the upper thoracic spine.

dual-energy X-ray absorptiometry (DEXA) the most widely used technology to measure bone density. Two X-ray beams are aimed at the patient's bones and the density of the bone is determined by the absorption of each X-ray beam.

dwarfism a decrease in growth hormone (GH) that leads to impaired growth of all body tissues.

dysentery an acute inflammation of the colon; colitis.

dysmenorrhea (DIS-men-oh-**REE**-ah; dys = painful, menorrhea = menses) pain with menstrual periods.

dyspareunia (DIS-pa-**ROO**-nee-ah) painful sexual intercourse.

dysphagia (dis-FAY-jee-ah; dys = difficulty, phagia = swallowing) difficulty swallowing.

dysphasia (dis-FAY-zee-ah; dys = difficulty, phasia = speaking) difficulty speaking.

dysplasia (dis-PLAY-zee-ah) an alteration in size, shape, and organization of cells.

dyspnea (disp-NEE-ah; dys = difficult, pnea = breathing) difficulty breathing.

dysuria (dis-YOU-ree-ah; dys = difficult or painful, uria = urine) difficulty or pain with urination.

E

ecchymoses (ECH-ih-**MOH**-ses) large areas of bruising or hemorrhage.

eclampsia (eh-KLAMP-see-ah) a condition of pregnancy characterized by all the symptoms of toxemia or preeclampsia, plus the symptoms of convulsions.

ectopic (eck-TOP-ick) out of normal place.

electrocardiogram (ECG or EKG; ee-LECK-troh-**KAR**-dee-oh-GRAM; electro = electrical, cardio = heart, gram = picture) the graphic drawing produced by an electrocardiograph, a machine that receives electrical information and draws heart action.

electromyography (EMG; ee-LEK-troh-my-**OG**-ra-fee) a diagnostic test in which a small needle is inserted into muscle tissue and the electrical activity is recorded.

embolus (EM-boh-lus) material floating in the blood that may stick in a vessel and occlude or stop blood flow, leading to ischemia or death of the organs supplied by that vessel.

empyema (EM-pye-**EE**-mah) an accumulation of pus in a body cavity.

encapsulated enclosed in a capsule.

encephalopathy (en-SEF-ah-**LOP**-ah-thee; encephalo = brain, opathy = disease) any disease or disorder of the brain.

endarterectomy (END-ar-ter-**ECK**-toh-me; endo = inside, arter = artery, ectomy = excision) a surgical procedure involving opening an artery and cleaning out the plaque.

endometritis (EN-doh-me-**TRY**-tis) inflammation of the uterus lining.

enteral relating to the small intestine.

enterotoxin intestinal poison.

enucleation removal of the eyeball.

epicanthus a vertical fold of skin across the medial canthus of the eye, giving the eyes an Oriental appearance.

epidural (hematoma) (EP-ih-**DOO**-ral; epi = above, dural = dura, outer meninges) blood collecting between the skull and the dura mater.

epistaxis (EP-i-**STACK**-sis) hemorrhage or bleeding from the nose; nosebleed.

erythema (ER-ih-**THEE**-mah) skin redness.

erythrocytopenia (erythrocyte = red cell, penia = decrease) a deficiency of red blood cells.

erythrocytosis (erythrocyte = red cell, osis = condition) a condition of increased red blood cells.

esophageal varices (eh-**SOF**-ah-JEE-al **VAYR**-ih-seez) varicosities (varicose veins) of the esophagus.

estrogen a term used to describe the hormones responsible for female characteristics.

etiology (ET-tee-**OL**-oh-jee) the study of cause or the cause of a disease.

euphoric a sense of well-being.

exacerbation (x-AS-er-**BAY**-shun) a time when symptoms flare up or become worse.

exocrine (glands) glands that excrete through a duct.

exophthalmos (ECK-sof-**THAL**-mos) abnormal protrusion of the eyeballs.

exsanguination loss of circulating blood volume.

extracapsular fracture a fracture outside or not involving the joint capsule.

exudate (ECKS-you-dayt) fluid that has seeped out of tissue or capillaries because of injury or inflammation.

F

familial runs in or common to a family; for example, a disease that tends to occur in several members of the same family.

fascia (FASH-ee-ah) a thick fibrous connective tissue.

fatal inevitable or causing death.

feces evacuated bowel contents; commonly called bowel movement or BM.

femoral neck fracture a fracture involving the neck of the femur.

fibrillation (FIH-brih-**LAY**-shun) a heart rhythm that is wild and uncoordinated; a cardiac arrhythmia.

fissure a crack, split, or ulcer-like sore; a groove or slit.

fistula (FIS-tyou-lah) a tract that connects two organs or cavities to each other or to the surface of the skin.

flatulence excessive gas in the stomach or intestine.

frequency how often the individual urinates.

frostbite the freezing of tissue, usually on the face, fingers, toes, and ears.

frozen section a technique that enables a pathologist to make a rapid determination of a tumor condition, either malignant or benign.

fulminant (FULL-ma-nant) occurring suddenly, rapidly, and intensely.

fungi forms of yeast and molds; microscopic plant-like organisms.

G

gangrene (GANG-green) a condition occurring when saprophytic (dead tissue–loving) bacteria become involved in necrotic tissue.

gene the unit on the chromosome that carries DNA information.

genotypes the genetic pattern of the individual.

germ cells sex cells.

giantism a condition of overgrowth due to hyperpituitarism occurring before puberty and during the growing years.

gingivitis inflammation of the gums.

glucagon a hormone secreted by the alpha cells in the islets of Langerhans in the pancreas; responsible for elevating blood glucose concentration.

glucocorticoids a group of steroids of the adrenal cortex that affects metabolism such as causing glycogen storage and causing an anti-inflammatory effect.

glycogen (GLYE-ko-jen) the form that extra sugar is stored in, primarily in the liver.

glycosuria (GLYE-koh-**SOO**-ree-ah; glyco = glycogen or sugar, uria = urine) the spilling of sugar into the urine; a common symptom of diabetes mellitus.

goiter (GOI-ter) noticeable protrusion of the thyroid gland.

goitrogenic goiter producing, as in foods or drugs such as turnips, cabbage, and lithium.

gonad a sex organ; a testis or an ovary.

grading determining the degree of differentiation of cells through microscopic examination.

grand mal a term applied to seizures that are the type most often thought of as epilepsy; these seizures are characterized by convulsions, loss of consciousness, urinary and fecal incontinence, and tongue biting.

greenstick fracture A common incomplete fracture that occurs in children; it appears to have broken partially like a sap-filled green stick.

gumma (GUM-mah) a characteristic soft, gummy lesion caused by bacteria that invade organs throughout the body; found in the tertiary stage of syphilis.

gynecomastia (GUY-ne-koh-**MAS**-tee-ah) abnormal breast enlargement.

H

hallucinations (hah-LOO-sih-**NAY**-shun) false sensations of sight, touch, sound, smell or taste.

hallucinogenic (hah-LOO-sih-no-**JEN**-ick) producing psychedelic or bizarre alterations in mental functioning.

heat exhaustion a reaction to heat, marked by prostration, weakness, and collapse; caused by severe dehydration.

heat stroke a serious and possibly fatal illness caused by exposure to excessively high temperatures.

helminths intestinal parasites; also called worms; nematodes, cestodes, and trematodes.

hemarthrosis (hem = blood, arthro = joint, osis = condition) bleeding into joints.

hematemesis (HEM-ah-**TEM**-eh-sis; hema = blood, emesis = vomiting) vomiting blood.

hematochezia (HEM-at-toe-**KEE**-zee-ah) bright red blood in the feces.

hematocrit (he-MAT-oh-krit) a measurement of the amount of red cell mass as a proportion of whole blood.

hematoma (HEM-ah-**TOH**-mah) a large tumor or swelling filled with blood; also called a bruise or contusion.

hematuria (HEM-ah-**TOO**-ree-ah; hema = blood, uria = urine) blood in the urine.

hemiparesis (HEM-ee-**PAR**-ee-sis; hemi = one half, paresis = paralysis) weakness or paralysis affecting one side of the body.

hemoglobin (Hgb) a measurement of the amount of hemoglobin, or oxygen-carrying potential, available in the blood.

hemolytic (HE-moh-**LIT**-ick) destruction of red blood cells.

hemolyzed broken-down cells.

hemoptysis (he-MOP-tih-sis; hemo = blood, ptysis = saliva) coughing up blood.

hemothorax (hemo = blood, thorax = chest) blood in the chest cavity.

hepatomegaly (HEP-ah-toh-**MEG**-ah-lee) enlarged liver.

heterozygous (hetero = different, zygo = yoked or paired) having different paired genes.

hirsutism (HER-soot-izm) abnormal hair on the face and body of the female.

histamine a substance that causes local arterioles, venules, and capillaries to dilate, resulting in an increase in blood flow to the area; released in response to injury or irritation.

holistic medicine the concept of considering the whole person rather than just the physical being.

homeostasis (HOME-ee-oh-**STAY**-sis) the state of sameness or normalcy that the body strives to maintain.

homozygous (homo = one, zygo = yoked or paired) having identical genes.

hydrocortisone a steroid hormone secreted by the adrenal cortex.

hydrophobia (hydro = water, phobia = fear) fear of the water.

hyperemia (HIGH-per-**EE**-me-ah; hyper = increased, emia = blood) can increased blood flow in response to a release of histamine.

hyperglycemia (HIGH-per-glye-**SEE**-me-ah; hyper = excessive, glyc = glycogen or glucose, emia = blood) high blood sugar level.

hyperplasia (HIGH-per-**PLAY**-zee-ah) an increase in cell number; overgrowth in response to some type of stimulus.

hypersensitivity a condition in which there is an excessive response by the body to the stimulus of a foreign body.

hypertrophy (HIGH-**PER**-tro-fee) an increase in the size of the cell, leading to an increase in tissue and organ size.

hypoglycemia (HIGH-poh-gly-**SEE**-me-ah; hypo = decreased, glyc = glucose, emia = blood) a low blood sugar level.

hypothermia (hypo = low, thermia = heat or temperature) a significantly low body temperature.

hypovolemia (HIGH-poh-voh-**LEE**-me-ah) low or decreased blood volume.

hypoxemia (high-**POX**-SEE-me-ah; hypo = not enough, ox = oxygen, emia = blood) not enough oxygen in the circulating blood.

hypoxia (HIGH-**POX**-see-ah) not enough oxygen in tissues.

hysterosalpingogram (hystero = uterus, salpingo = fallopian tubes, gram = picture) an X-ray picture of the uterus and fallopian tubes.

I

iatrogenic (eye-AT-roh-**JEN**-ick; iatro = medicine, physician, genic = rising from) a problem arising due to or related to a prescribed treatment.

idiopathic (ID-ee-oh-**PATH**-ick) an unknown cause of disease.

ileus (ILL-ee-us) absence of peristalsis.

immunodeficiency the state when the immune response is unable to defend the body due to a decrease or absence of leukocytes, primarily lymphocytes.

impacted fracture one that has a bone end forced over the other end.

impotent (IM-poh-tent) inability in the male to achieve or maintain a penile erection.

in and out catheterization a catheterization procedure in which the catheter is removed as soon as the urine is drained; the catheterization is temporary.

incision a laceration or cut with smooth, even edges.

incomplete fracture the bone is fractured but not in two.

incubation period the time between exposure to the disease and the presence of symptoms, which might last several days.

induration (IN-dur-**RAY**-shun) hardened tissue.

indwelling catheter a catheter that is placed for a longer period of time than an in and out catheter as commonly occurs for urinary incontinence; a balloon on the end of the catheter is inflated to hold the catheter in the bladder.

infarct (in-FARKT) necrosis of cells or tissues due to ischemia.

infection (in-FECT-shun) invasion of microorganisms into the tissue, causing cell or tissue injury, thus leading to the inflammatory response.

inflammation (IN-flah-**MAY**-shun) a basic pathologic process of cytologic and chemical reactions that occur in the blood vessels and tissues in response to an injury or irritation; a protective immune response that is triggered by any type of injury or irritant.

inspiratory stridor (STRYE-dor) high-pitched sound during inspiration due to blocked airways.

insulin a hormone secreted by the beta cells in the islets of Langerhans in the pancreas; responsible for glucose usage.

intermittent claudication (KLAW-dih-**KAY**-shun) the condition of developing muscle cramps that are relieved with rest and increased with activity.

interphalangeal (inter = between, phalangeal = finger bones) usually referring to joints between the finger bones.

intertrochanteric fracture one that is in the trochanteric area of the femur.

intoxicated when the blood alcohol level reaches 0.10% or more.

intracapsular fractures a fracture inside the joint capsule.

intractable difficult to stop or control.

intrathecal (IN-trah-**THEE**-kal; intra = within, thecal = spinal cord) injected into the spinal fluid.

intravenous pyelogram (IVP) (IN-trah-**VEE**-nus **PYE**-eh-loh-GRAM) an X-ray picture taken after injecting dye into the individual's bloodstream; the dye accumulates in the urinary tract and improves the ability to identify obstructions, tumors, and deformities.

intrinsic factor a substance secreted by the stomach lining necessary for absorption of vitamin B_{12}.

intussusception (IN-tus-sus-**SEP**-shun) the telescoping of one part of the intestine over the adjoining section.

invasion spreading into surrounding or local tissue.

ischemia (iss-**KEE**-me-ah) hypoxia of cells or tissues caused by decreased blood flow.

islets of Langerhans specialized cells in the pancreas that act as an endocrine gland secreting hormones, primarily insulin.

isoimmune a high level of a specific antibody as a result of antigen stimulation from the red blood cells of another individual; isoimmunization may occur when an Rh-negative person is treated with a transfusion of Rh-positive blood.

J

jaundice (JAWN-dis) a yellowish color in the skin and sclera due to increased bile pigments in the blood.

K

Kaposi's sarcoma (KAP-oh-seez sar-KOH-ma) blood vessel cancer that causes reddish-purple skin lesions.

karyotyping a method of identifying chromosomes; this process involves taking a picture of a cell during mitosis, arranging the chromosome pairs in order from largest to smallest, and numbering them 1 to 23.

keloid (KEE-loid) excessive collagen formation, often resulting in a hard, raised scar.

keratin a tough protein substance in nails, hair, and body tissues.

ketoacidosis acidosis seen in diabetes mellitus caused by overproduction of ketone bodies.

ketones waste products produced when tissue cells burn fats and proteins.

kidneys-ureter-bladder (KUB) a common X-ray of the structures of the urinary tract to determine abnormalities.

Koplik's spots spots seen in the mouth in the early stage of measles; these spots are rather unique to measles and are often the definitive symptom that confirms the diagnosis.

L

laceration a cut in the skin.

laminectomy surgery to cut away part of the vertebra to open the area around the spinal nerve.

laparoscopy (LAP-ah-**ROS**-ko-pee; laparo = abdomen, scopy = scope procedure) looking inside the abdominal cavity with a lighted scope; commonly used to view the female organs for abnormalities, diagnose endometriosis, and to perform a tubal ligation.

lesion (LEE-zhun) any discontinuity of tissue.

lethal something that kills.

leukemia (loo-KEE-me-ah; leuk = white, emia = blood) a progressive overgrowth of abnormal leukocytes; a malignant disease of the bone marrow.

leukocytopenia (leukocyte = white cell, penia = decrease) a decrease in white cell count.

leukocytosis (leuko = white, cyto = cell, osis = condition) an increase in white cell count.

leukorrhea (LOO-koh-**REE**-ah; leuk = white, orrhea = flow or discharge) a white, usually foul-smelling, vaginal discharge.

lipids fats or fat-like substances.

lithotripsy (litho = stone, tripsy = breaking) a procedure for breaking kidney or gallbladder stones.

longitudinal fracture one that runs the length of the bone.

lumen (LOO-men) the inner open space or width of a tubular structure or anatomical part.

lymph a clear liquid similar to plasma containing many white cells.

lymphadenopathy (lim-FAD-eh-**NOP**-ah-thee; lymph = lymph, adeno = gland, opathy = disease) any disease of the lymph glands.

lymphangiography (lim-FAN-jee-**OG**-rah-fee; lymph = lymph, angio = vessel, ography = procedure) a radiographic procedure consisting of injecting a contrast dye and taking X-rays of lymphatic vessels.

lymphangiopathy (lim-FAN-jee-**OP**-ah-thee; lymph = lymph, angio = vessel, opathy = disease) a general term to describe any disease of the lymph vessels.

lymphedema (lymph = lymph, edema = swelling) an abnormal collection of lymph fluid, usually observed in the extremities.

lymphocytes white blood cells formed in lymphatic tissue.

lymphocytopenia or lymphopenia a decrease in lymphocytes.

lymphocytosis increase in number of lymphocytes.

lymphoma (lim-FOH-ma) malignant neoplasms of blood-forming organs.

M

macrophage (macro = large, phage = eat) a monocyte that leaves the bloodstream and moves into the tissue and becomes phagocytic.

magnetic resonance imaging (MRI) a diagnostic radiological test using nuclear magnetic resonance technology.

malaise general ill feeling.

malignant (mah-LIG-nant) deadly or progressing to death; cancerous.

mammography (mam-OG-rah-fee; mammo = breast, ography = procedure to take a picture) a procedure of taking an X-ray picture of breast tissue.

mammoplasty (**MAM**-oh-PLAS-tee; mammo = breast, plasty = surgical repair or restructuring) a surgical procedure that involves reconstruction of the breast with plastic surgery and prosthetic breast implants.

mania extreme elation or agitation.

mast cells also called tissue histocytes; found in all tissues of the body; play a major role in the inflammatory process.

mastectomy (mas-TECK-toh-me; mast = breast, ectomy = excision) surgical removal of the breast.

mastoidectomy (MAS-toy-**DECK**-toh-me; ectomy = removal or excision) a procedure used to prevent complications and preserve hearing by removing the bony partitions forming the mastoid cells.

medical ethics values and decisions in medical practice including relationships to patient, patient family, peer physicians, and society.

meiosis the process of reproduction of germ cells in which they divide before duplication.

melena (meh-LEE-nah) dark tarry stool due to blood in feces.

meniscus semilunar articular cartilage found inside the knee joint.

metacarpophalangeal (meta = beyond, carpo = wrist, phalangeal = finger bones) referring to the metacarpus and the phalanges; specifically, the articulations between them.

metaplasia (MET-ah-**PLAY**-zee-ah) a cellular adaptation in which the cell changes to another type of cell.

metastasis (meh-TAS-tah-sis) spreading to distant sites.

metastasize (meh-TAS-tah-sighz) move or spread.

metastatic (MET-ah-**STAT**-ic) moves from a site of origin to a secondary site in the body.

metatarsophalangeal (meta = between, tarso = foot, phalangeal = toe bones) referring to the metatarsus and the phalanges; specifically, the articulations between them.

microcephaly (micro = small, cephal = brain) having an abnormally small head; usually associated with mental retardation.

mineralization a process that causes the characteristic hardness of bones.

mineralocorticoids one group of steroids of the adrenal cortex that influences sodium and potassium metabolism.

mitosis the process of reproduction of cells in which the 46 chromosomes duplicate and divide into two identical daughter cells, each containing 46 chromosomes.

mood emotion.

morbidity the state of being diseased.

mortality the quality of being mortal or destined to die.

motility ability to move.

multiparity (mul-TIP-ah-rah-tee) multiple births.

murmur an abnormal sound in the heart or vascular system.

MVAs motor vehicle accidents.

myelogram an X-ray picture taken after injecting dye into the spinal canal to reveal compression on the spinal cord or spinal nerves.

myringotomy (MIR-in-**GOT**-oh-me; myringo = eardrum, tomy = incision into) incision into the eardrum to remove fluid.

myxedema (MECK-seh-**DEE**-mah) advanced hypothyroidism in an adult.

N

necrosis (nee-CROW-sis) cellular death.

neoplasia (nee-oh-PLAY-zee-ah) the development of a new type of cell with an uncontrolled growth pattern.

neoplasms (new growths) an increase in cell number, leading to an increase in tissue size; commonly called tumors.

nephrectomy (neh-FREC-toh-me; nephr = kidney, ectomy = excision or removal) the surgical removal of the kidney.

neutropenia a decrease in neutrophils.

nits lice eggs.

nocturia (nock-TOO-ree-ah; noc = night, uria = urine) excessive voiding at night.

nondisplaced fracture one in which the fragments are still in correct position.

nosocomial (NOS-oh-**KOH**-me-al) a disease acquired from the hospital environment.

nuchal rigidity a stiffness in the neck that resists bending the neck forward or sideways.

O

oblique fracture a fracture that runs in a transverse pattern.

obsession repetition of a thought or emotion.

occult blood hidden blood; invisible except under microscopic examination.

oliguria (OL-ih-**GOO**-ree-ah; olig = scanty or few, uria = urine) a decrease in urine output.

oncology (ong-KOL-oh-jee) the study of tumors.

oophoritis (OH-of-oh-**RYE**-tis) inflammation of the ovary.

open (compound) fracture a fracture involving the bone puncturing through the skin, or an object puncturing the skin, making an opening through the skin to the fracture site.

ophthalmoscope (aft-THAL-moh-skope; ophthalm = eye, scope = instrument used to look) the instrument used for a basic examination of the eye.

opportunistic normal flora bacteria that take the "opportunity" to cause infection in the host.

orchiectomy (OR-kee-**ECK**-toh-me; orchi = testicle, ectomy = removal) removal of the testicle(s).

orchitis (or-KYE-tis) inflammation of a testis.

organ rejection when the body recognizes an organ (after a transplant) as foreign and attacks it, leading to organ death.

organic related to an organ or physical component.

ORIF (open-reduction internal fixation) surgical opening over a fracture site and internally fixing the fracture with plates, screws, or pins.

orthopnea (or-THOP-nee-ah; ortho = straight, pnea = breathing) the condition in which an individual has difficulty breathing in a lying position, or is able to breathe with less difficulty when standing or sitting straight up.

osteomyelitis inflammation or infection of the marrow of the bone.

otalgia (oh-TAL-gee-ah; oto = ear, algia = pain) ear pain.

otoscope (OH-toh-skope; oto = ear, scope = instrument to look) the instrument used to examine the ear.

ova and parasite (O&P) an examination of a stool specimen for the presence of adult parasites or their eggs (ova).

P

palliative (PAL-ee-ay-tiv) something that is directed toward relief of symptoms but does not cure.

pallor (PAL-or) lack of color; paleness.

palmar erythema (ER-ih-**THEE**-mah) unusual redness of the palms of the hands.

palpation feeling lightly or by pressing firmly on internal organs or structures.

pancytopenia (pan = all, cyto = cell, penia = decrease) severe decrease or total absence of erythrocytes, leukocytes, and thrombocytes.

panhypopituitarism (pan = all, hypo = decreased) the condition in which the secretion of all anterior pituitary hormones is inadequate or absent; caused by a variety of disorders.

panhysterectomy (pan = all, hyster = uterus, ectomy = excision) the surgical removal of the ovaries, fallopian tubes, and uterus.

Pap test also called Papanicolaou test; a screening for cancer using and examining the cells scraped from the cervical area.

paralytic obstruction a decrease or absence of peristalsis that causes intestinal blockage.

paraplegia (PAR-ah-**PLEE**-jee-ah; para = beyond or two like parts, plegia = paralysis) a loss of movement and feeling in the trunk and both legs.

parenteral (pah-REN-ter-al) a delivery route for fluid or medications that includes subcutaneous, intramuscular, or intravenous administration.

paresthesia (PAR-es-**THEE**-see-ah) abnormal sensation, burning, tingling, or numbness.

paronychia (PAR-oh-**NICK**-ee-ah) an infection of the skin around the nail.

parotid glands the salivary glands located just in front of the ears.

paroxysmal (PAR-ock-**SIZ**-mal) spasm or convulsion.

patency openness.

patent open.

pathogenesis (PATH-oh-**JEN**-ah-sis; patho = disease, genesis = arising) a description of how a particular disease progresses.

pathogens (PATH-oh-jens) microorganisms or agents that cause disease.

pathologic (path-oh-LODGE-ick) caused by a pathogen or a disease.

pathologic fracture (path-oh-LODGE-ick) a fracture caused by weakness from another disease.

pathologist (pah-THOL-oh-jist; patho = disease, logist = one who studies) one who studies disease.

pathology (pah-THOL-oh-jee; patho = disease, ology = study) the study of disease.

percussion (per-KUSH-un) tapping over various body areas to produce a vibrating sound.

perforation an abnormal opening in an organ or tissue.

perfusion (per-FYOU-zuhn) to pour through or supply with blood.

peristalsis the contraction of muscles along the gastrointestinal tract to move food and fluid.

peritonitis (PER-ih-toe-**NIGH**-tis) an inflammation of the peritoneum.

petechiae (pee-TEE-kee-ee) small hemorrhages in the skin.

petit mal a term applied to a type of seizure; these seizures consist of a brief change in the level of consciousness without convulsions; the involved individual may show symptoms of blank staring, blinking, and/or twitching of the eyes or mouth.

phenotype the physical expression of a genetic trait such as eye, hair, and skin color.

phimosis (figh-MOH-sis) abnormally tight foreskin of the penis.

photophobia (photo = light, phobia = fear) an abnormal fear of light.

pilonidal cyst (PYE-loh-**NIGH**-dal) a particular type of sebaceous cyst found in the midline of the sacral area.

plaque (PLACK) a patch; dental plaque is a sticky mass of microorganisms growing on teeth.

pneumocystis carinii (NEW-moh-**SIS**-tis kah-RYE-nee-eye) **pneumonia** a protozoan infection of the lungs, commonly occurring in immunodeficient individuals.

polydipsia (POL-ee-**DIP**-see-ah; poly = many, dipsia = thirst or drinking) excessive thirst.

polyp (POL-ip) an inward projection of the mucosal lining of the colon.

polyuria (POL-ee-**YOU**-ree-ah; poly = many, uria = urine) excessive urination.

portal hypertension increased pressure in the portal system frequently seen in cirrhosis.

Pott's fracture fracture of the lower part of the fibula and tibia, with outward displacement of the foot.

precocious (puberty) premature (early) sexual development.

predisposing factors also known as risk factors; make a person more susceptible to disease.

preeclampsia (PREE-ee-**KLAMP**-see-ah) the development of hypertension with proteinuria and/or edema due to pregnancy; also called toxemia.

prevalent occurring more often.

preventive something that reduces risk.

primary union also called healing by first intention; involves approximating the edges of the wound.

primigravid (PRE-mih-**GRAV**-id; primi = first, gravid = pregnancy) the term used to describe a female who is pregnant with her first child.

productive cough coughing up sputum or excessive mucus.

progesterone (pro-**JESS**-ter-ohn) a female sex hormone produced by the ovary.

prognosis (prawg-KNOW-sis) the predicted or expected outcome of the disease.

prone positioned face down on the stomach.

prophylactic (pro-fil-LACK-tic) something that works to prevent.

prosthesis (pros-THEE-sis) an artificial part.

proteinuria protein in the urine; specific protein or albumin, may be identified, resulting in albuminuria.

protozoa a parasite of the phylum Protozoa; a single-celled microscopic member of the animal kingdom.

pruritus (proo-RYE-tus) itching.

puerperal (pyou-ER-pier-al) relating to childbirth.

purpura (PER-pew-rah) a bleeding disorder characterized by bleeding into the skin and mucus membranes initially turning the affected areas purplish in color.

purulent (PURR-you-lent) loaded with dead and dying neutrophils, tissue debris, and pyogenic (pus-forming) bacteria.

pus white or yellow exudate due to death of numerous neutrophils mixed with exudate or blood fluid.

pustules (PUS-tyoul) small, pus-filled lesions.

pyloromyotomy (pyloro = pyloric, myo = muscle, otomy = cut into) a surgical procedure that involves incising and suturing the pyloric sphincter muscle.

pyoderma (PYE-oh-**DER**-mah) inflammatory, purulent dermatitis.

pyogenic (PIE-oh-**JEN**-ick; pyo = pus, genic = arising) pus forming.

pyuria (pye-YOU-ree-ah; py = pus, uria = urine) pus in the urine.

Q

quadriplegia (KWAD-rih-**PLEE**-jee-ah; quadri = four, plegia = paralysis) the loss of movement and feeling in the trunk and all four extremities with the accompanying loss of bowel, bladder, and sexual function.

R

radial keratotomy (KER-ah-**TOT**-oh-me; kerato = cornea, otomy = incision) a surgical procedure to correct myopia; incisions are made in a radial fashion in the cornea to flatten the cornea, thus shortening the length of the eyeball and correcting the refractive error.

radiation the process of using light, short-waves, ultraviolet or X-rays, or any other rays.

radical cystectomy (radical = a treatment that seeks to cure, aggressive, not paliative or conservative, sis-TECT-toh-me, cyst = bladder, ectomy = excision or removal) the removal of the entire bladder, usually done as treatment for cancer of the bladder.

radiologic relating to medical imaging using X-rays, ionizing radiation, nuclear magnetic resonance, or ultrasound.

rales (RALZ) an abnormal discontinuous breath sound caused by narrowed bronchi and heard primarily on inspiration during auscultation of the chest.

recessive lacking control; weak.

Reed–Sternberg cell a large connective tissue cell found in lymphatic tissue indicative of Hodgkin's disease.

remission a time when symptoms are diminished or temporarily resolved.

rhinitis (RYE-**NIGH**-tis) inflammation of the nasal mucous membrane.

rhinorrhea (rhino = nose, orrhea = run through) a runny nose.

rhonchi (RONG-kigh) abnormal wheezing breath sounds caused by partial airway blockage and heard during inspiration, expiration, or both during auscultation of the chest.

RICE acronym for Rest, Ice, Compression, and Elevation, the activities to manage soft tissue trauma like those often associated with sports injuries.

rickettsiae (ric-KET-see-ah) microscopic organisms that are intermediate between bacteria and viruses. They live in the host and are spread by lice, fleas, ticks, and mites.

RPR (rapid plasma reagin) a blood test for syphilis.

S

salmonella (SAL-moh-**NEL**-ah) a group of gram-negative bacteria often responsible for intestinal infections.

salpingitis (SAL-pin-**JIGH**-tis; salping = fallopian tube, itis = inflammation) inflammation of the fallopian tube.

sarcoma (sar-KO-mah) a malignant neoplasm arising from connective tissue.

scar skin lesion resulting from fibrous connective tissue repair.

sciatica pain along the sciatic nerve, often radiating down the leg and caused by pressure on the spinal nerve.

sebum oil produced by the sebaceous glands.

secondary union also called healing by secondary intention; the same process as primary union, but involving a larger degree of tissue damage and more inflammation to resolve.

seizure a sudden onset or attack, but the term is commonly used to indicate a convulsive seizure as occurs in epilespy.

self-antigen the body's own antigen.

septicemia (SEP-tih-**SEE**-me-ah; septic = dirty, contaminated, emia = blood) a systemic disease caused by the spread of microorganisms in the blood; also called blood poisoning.

signs observable or measurable factors used to determine a diagnosis.

simple (closed) fracture a fracture that does not break through the skin.

sinus a tract or opening to the surface of the body formed by a large ruptured abscess.

somatic related to the body.

spasms uncontrolled muscle contractions.

spider angiomas telangiectasis or small dilated vessels in the skin; commonly seen on the face and chest of individuals with cirrhosis of the liver.

spinal stenosis (stenosis = narrowing) the condition of narrowing of nerve root openings in the spinal column.

spiral fracture a fracture that twists around the bone.

splenomegaly (SPLEE-no-**MEG**-ah-lee) enlargement of the spleen.

sputum (SPYOU-tum) fluid or secretions coughed up from the lungs.

staging determining the degree of spread of a malignant tumor.

stapedectomy (STAY-peh-**DECK**-toh-me; stape = stapes, ectomy = removal or excision) a procedure that removes the stapes bone in the middle ear and replaces it with a prosthesis.

status asthmaticus (AZTH-**MAH**-ti-kus) a severe asthma attack that lasts for several days.

status epilepticus a life-threatening event; a state of continued convulsive seizure with no recovery of consciousness; it is a medical emergency.

stellate fracture a fracture that forms a star-like pattern.

sterility inability to conceive. In the female, an inability to become pregnant. In the male, an inability to impregnate a female, often related to sperm quality or quantity.

stool fecal matter; feces; bowel movement (BM).

strep throat an acute form of pharyngitis caused by *Streptococcus*.

streptococcal (**STREHP**-toh-KAHK-al) relating to the organism *Streptococcus*; an anaerobic, gram-positive bacteria.

stress fracture related to too much weight or pressure.

striae stretch marks on the skin.

stricture a narrowing.

subcapital fracture a fracture below (sub) the head (caput) of the femur.

subdural (hematoma) (SUB-**DOO**-ral) blood collecting between the outer (dura mater) layer and the middle (arachnoid) layer of the meninges.

supine (SUE-pine) positioned on the back.

suppurative (SUP-you-**RAY**-tive) formation of pus.

suprapubic catheter a catheter that is inserted surgically through the pelvic wall as is often done after urinary tract surgeries.

symptoms what patients report as their problem or problems.

syncope (SIN-koh-pee) fainting.

syndrome (SIN-drome) a group of symptoms that may be caused by a specific disease but also may be caused by several interrelated problems.

systemic refers to the entire or whole body rather than to a part or region.

systolic (sis-TALL-ick) relating to cardiac systole; the process of cardiac contraction (heartbeat) when blood is ejected into the systemic circulation.

T

tachycardia (TACH-ee-**KAR**-dee-ah; tachy = rapid, cardia = heart rate) a rapid heart rate; usually a rate over 100 beats per minute.

tachypnea (TACK-ihp-**NEE**-ah; tachy = rapid, pnea = breathing) a severely increased respiratory rate.

tetany (TET-ah-nee) hyperirritability of muscles causing a spasm-like condition; usually the result of a lack of calcium.

thoracentesis (THOR-rah-sen-**TEE**-sis; thora = chest, centesis = puncture) a procedure in which a puncture is made into the chest cavity to withdraw air (or fluid); a chest tube also may be inserted to help the lung reexpand.

thrombocytopenia (THROM-boh-SIGH-toh-**PEE**-nee-ah; thrombocyte = platelet, penia = decrease) a decrease in platelets, leading to a coagulation problem.

thrombocytosis (THROM-boh-sigh-**TOH**-sis; thrombocyte = platelet, osis = condition of) an increase in platelets.

thrombus (THROM-bus) a blood clot attached to a vein or artery.

thyroid storm a sudden life-threatening exacerbation of all symptoms of hyperthyroidism.

tinnitus (tin-EYE-tus) ringing in the ears.

tolerance the ability to endure a larger amount of a substance without an adverse effect, or the need for a larger amount or dose of the drug to have the same effect.

tonometry (toh-NOM-eh-tree; tono = tone or pressure, metry = measurement) a procedure to measure the pressure inside the eye.

tonsillectomy (TON-sih-**LECT**-toh-me; ectomy = removal) the surgical removal of the tonsils.

tophi small, whitish nodules of uric acid.

topical placed on the skin.

TPN total parenteral nutrition; intravenously giving a special solution that meets, the total nutritional needs of the individual.

transurethral resection (TUR) (trans = through, urethral = uretha; resection = partial excision) a surgical procedure that may be performed to remove a tumor, visualize a structure, or take a piece of tissue for biopsy; a cystoscope is passed through the urinary meatus and the urethra for this procedure.

transverse fracture one that runs across or at a 90-degree angle.

trauma (TRAW-mah) a physical or mental injury.

triage (tree-AUZH) the prioritizing of care.

trichomonas (TRICK-oh-**MOH**-nas) a parasitic protozoan that commonly infects the vagina and causes trichomoniasis.

tumor "swelling" or growth, originally used in the description of the swelling related to inflammation.

tympanoplasty (TIM-pah-no-**PLAS**-tee; tympano = eardrum, plasty = surgical correction) surgery to repair the tympanic membrane.

tympanostomy (TIM-pan-**OSS**-toh-me; tympano = eardrum, ostomy = new opening) a procedure in which tubes, commonly called PE tubes or pediatric ear tubes, are placed through the tympanic membrane to prevent the accumulation of fluid.

U

ulcer a crater-like lesion in the skin or mucous membranes.

undifferentiated change in a cell that is more general or appears more malignant; not clearly or easily identified.

urea a common nitrogenous waste product that is normally filtered from the blood.

uremia (you-REE-me-ah; ur = urine, emia = blood) a toxic condition of the blood due to high levels of waste products.

urgency the severe need to urinate.

urinalysis (YOU-rih-**NAL**-ih-sis; urine analysis) a laboratory urine test for pH, specific gravity, protein, glucose or sugar, and blood; it also includes a microscopic examination to determine the presence of bacteria, crystals, and casts.

urine culture and sensitivity (C&S) a laboratory analysis that determines the type of bacteria present and the most effective antibiotic to prescribe for treatment.

urticaria (UR-tih-**KAR**-ree-ah) an allergic reaction resulting in a skin eruption of wheals that causes intense itching.

V

vasopressin antidiuretic hormone (ADH) secreted by the posterior portion of the pituitary gland.

venereal disease research laboratory (VDRL) a blood test to screen for syphilis.

vermiform (VER-my-form) worm-like.

vertigo (VER-tih-go) dizziness.

vesicles (VES-ih-kuls) blister-like eruptions on the skin.

virilism (VIR-ill-izm) masculinization; used to describe the occurrence or presence of male characteristics in a female or prepubescent male.

virulent (VIR-u-lent; infectious) difficult to kill; able to produce disease.

viruses a large group of infectious agents; they are much smaller than bacteria and must be viewed with an electron microscope. They can pass through fine filters that would retain most bacteria.

viscous (VIS-cuss) thick.

volvulus (VOL-view-lus) the bowel twisted on itself.

W

wheal(s) round, slightly reddened, spot(s) on the skin, usually accompanied by intense itching; also called urticarial lesion(s) or hives; caused by an allergic reaction to something such as food or medication.

wheezing a whistling, musical, or raspy sound during breathing, usually indicative of partially blocked respiratory passages.

withdrawal the unpleasant physical and psychological effects resulting from stopping the use of a substance after an individual is addicted.

X

xerosis (zee-ROE-sis) dry skin.